Operative Gynecologic Endoscopy

Springer
New York
Berlin
Heidelberg
Barcelona
Budapest
Hong Kong
London
Milan
Paris
Santa Clara
Singapore
Tokyo

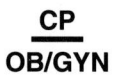 Clinical Perspectives in Obstetrics and Gynecology

Series Editor: Isaac Schiff, M.D.

Published Volumes:

Shoupe and Haseltine (eds.): *Contraception (1993)*
Lorrain (ed.): *Comprehensive Management of Menopause (1993)*
Gonik (ed.): *Viral Diseases in Pregnancy (1994)*
Flamm and Quilligan (eds.): *Cesarean Section: Guidelines for Appropriate Utilization (1995)*

Forthcoming Volumes:

Reindollar and Gray (eds.): *Molecular Biology for the Obstetrician-Gynecologist*
Stovall and Guido (eds.): *Acute Care Gynecology*

Published Volumes (*Series Editor:* The Late Herbert J. Buchsbaum, M.D.):

Buchsbaum (ed.): *The Menopause (1983)*
Aiman (ed.): *Infertility (1984)*
Futterweit: *Polycystic Ovarian Disease (1984)*
Lavery and Sanfilippo (eds.): *Pediatric and Adolescent Obstetrics and Gynecology (1985)*
Galask and Larson (eds.): *Infectious Diseases in the Female Patient (1986)*
Buchsbaum and Walton (eds.): *Strategies in Gynecologic Surgery (1986)*
Szulman and Buchsbaum (eds.): *Gestational Trophoblastic Disease (1987)*
Cibils (ed.): *Surgical Diseases in Pregnancy (1990)*
Collins (ed.): *Ovulation Induction (1990)*
Sanfilippo and Levine (eds.): *Operative Gynecologic Endoscopy (1990)*
Altchek and Deligdisch (eds.): *The Uterus (1991)*

Joseph S. Sanfilippo, M.D. ❖ Ronald L. Levine, M.D.
Department of Obstetrics and Gynecology
University of Louisville School of Medicine
Editors

Operative Gynecologic Endoscopy

Second Edition

With 321 black and white illustrations and 55 color plates

Foreword by Byron J. Masterson, M.D.

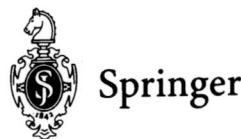

Editors:
Joseph S. Sanfilippo, M.D. ❖ **Ronald L. Levine, M.D.**
Department of Obstetrics and Gynecology, University of Louisville School of Medicine, Louisville, KY 40292, USA

Library of Congress Cataloging-in-Publication Data
Operative gynecologic endoscopy / Joseph S. Sanfilippo, Ronald L. Levine, editors. — 2nd ed.
    p. cm. — (Clinical perspectives in obstetrics and gynecology)
  Includes bibliographical references and index.
  ISBN 0-387-94467-2 (hardcover : alk. paper)
  1. Generative organs, Female—Endoscopic surgery. I. Sanfilippo, J. S. (Joseph S.) II. Levine, R. L. (Ronald L.) III. Series.
  [DNLM: 1. Genitalia, Female—surgery. 2. Laser Surgery. 3. Endoscopy. WP 660 061 1996]
RG104.7.0635 1996
618.1′059—dc20
DNLM/DLC
for Library of Congress   95-25735

Printed on acid-free paper.

© 1996, 1989 Springer-Verlag New York, Inc.
All rights reserved. This work may not be translated or copied in whole or in part without the written permission of the publisher (Springer-Verlag New York, Inc., 175 Fifth Avenue, New York, NY 10010, USA), except for brief excerpts in connection with reviews or scholarly analysis. Use in connection with any form of information storage and retrieval, electronic adaptation, computer software, or by similar or dissimilar methodology now known or hereafter developed is forbidden.
The use of general descriptive names, trade names, trademarks, etc., in this publication, even if the former are not especially identified, is not to be taken as a sign that such names, as understood by the Trade Marks and Merchandise Marks Act, may accordingly be used freely by anyone.
While the advice and information in this book are believed to be true and accurate at the date of going to press, neither the authors nor the editors nor the publisher can accept any legal responsibility for any errors or omissions that may be made. The publisher makes no warranty, express or implied, with respect to the material contained herein.

Production managed by Robert Wexler; manufacturing supervised by Jacqui Ashri.
Typeset by Princeton Editorial Associates, Inc., Princeton, NJ.
Printed and bound by Maple-Vail Book Manufacturing Group, York, PA.
Printed in the United States of America.

9 8 7 6 5 4 3 2 1

ISBN 0-387-94467-2 Springer-Verlag New York Berlin Heidelberg SPIN 10491538

We dedicate this book to our families for their patience and to our patients, whom we care for as family.

Foreword

While the technical development of pelvic endoscopy began in the late 1800s and early 1900s, its wider application in the United States occurred during the 1960s. The principal procedures were diagnostic or tubal interruption. Where the instrument maker and instrument user were closely aligned, creative solutions to surgical problems began to appear. Dr. Kurt Semm and other members of his family business were most innovative, and physicians from around the world began to visit him at the Christian Albrechts University in Kiel, Germany. They returned home with a new appreciation of what could be accomplished in the abdominal cavity via the endoscope. Many of the early procedures in gynecology that did not necessarily merit a laparotomy were worth the minimally invasive approach, and studies assessing cost of a laparoscopic procedure and additional information in the areas of pelvic pain management, endometriosis, and infertility were reported.

In 1986, the University of Louisville hosted the first university course in operative laparoscopy given in the United States. The faculty members were prominent in the conference that facilitated the aggressive adoption of the expanded view of pelvic endoscopy. Standards of technical excellence for endoscopic surgery soon developed. Just as the first bilateral ovarian tumor removal in Kentucky spawned a whole era of abdominal gynecologic surgery, many new operative procedures, techniques, and instruments sprang from an expanding array of creative and energetic minds. The first studies of appropriate suture materials (endoloops), knot strengths, and other technical advances in endoscopic surgery were conducted in the Wound Laboratory at the University of Louisville Department of Obstetrics and Gynecology. The investment necessary for the development, purchase, and maintenance of the very highly successful technical innovations in a commercially acceptable environment was due to the long term vision of the administration of the University of Louisville affiliated hospitals Alliant Health System and Jewish Hospital. Making these innovations commercially acceptable was and is a significant advance. One of the earliest studies on cost accounting of these procedures was published by Dr. Ronald Levine. The very careful and critical future analysis of miniaturization, virtual reality, multimodal imaging and molecular manipulation of the disease processes found endoscopic surgery to hold great promise for the future. I look forward most enthusiastically to the leadership of Drs. Sanfilippo and Levine, as well as the physicians they have trained in this new and exciting era in gynecologic surgery.

Byron J. Masterson, M.D.
J. Wayne Reitz Professor of Gynecologic Surgery
Co-Director, Wound Institute
University of Florida

Preface

Our first edition of *Operative Gynecologic Endoscopy*, published in 1989, included what seemed at that time to be revolutionary ideas of laparoscopic and hysteroscopic gynecologic surgery. The preface to that edition contained the well-known quote from Dr. Alan DeCherney (*Fertil Steril* 1985;44:299): "The obituary of pelvic reconstructive surgery has been written: it is only its publication that remains." His view of the future was remarkably clear, as operative endoscopic surgery has indeed supplanted laparotomy in a great proportion of gynecologic operations.

We were convinced then, and our belief has been reaffirmed, that operative endoscopy would contribute significantly to the enhancement of health care for women. Our prediction of decreased costs of this modality has been altered only by widespread and often injudicious use of disposable instruments and by inappropriately high charges by some health care providers. Even so, the impact of this technique on the total health care economics of the United States is startling in its potential. The return of women to the workplace 10 days to 3 weeks earlier than if they had a laparotomy must impress most observers and has particular importance to industry.

In 1988 the American Association of Gynecologic Laparoscopists (AAGL) survey of more than 800 physicians demonstrated that operative endoscopic procedures fell mainly in the area of laser vaporization of endometrial implants, lysis of adhesions, ovarian cystectomy, surgical treatment of ectopic pregnancy, tuboplasty, myomectomy, and management of pelvic abscesses. Multiple operative laparoscopic procedures were performed by the respondents with a "serious complication rate" of 15.4 per 1000 procedures. In a 1993 survey the complication rate appeared to be similar to that in a previous report (1991) but with a clear increase in the number of unintended laparotomies, hemorrhage, and gastrointestinal and urinary tract injuries (*J Am Assoc Gyn Laparosc* 1995; 2:134).

Similarly, operative hysteroscopic procedures have taken on a new dimension. In 1988 a hysteroscopic complication rate (most frequently uterine perforation not requiring transfusion) of 13 per 1000 procedures was reported. In 1993 a complication rate of 14.2 per 1000 was reported, including uterine perforations, hyponatremia in association with water intoxication, pulmonary edema, and a number of other complications: hospital readmission, transfusion requirement, laparotomy, neurologic injury, and gastrointestinal and genitourinary tract injuries.

This wealth of experience enables clinicians to determine the risk/benefit ratio preoperatively, identify and manage intraoperative complications, and perhaps most importantly offer patients technologic advances in the field of endoscopic surgery. Thus we have embarked on the second edition of our textbook. It provides clinicians with an update regarding instrumentation, current knowledge of electrosurgical principles, new laser technology, and procedures to avoid bowel and ureteral injury and postoperative problems.

The contributors to this edition include many of the original chapter authors, most of whom were among the pioneers of operative endoscopy. They obviously have the depth and breadth of knowledge and the clinical experience to enhance the usefulness of this text. Several of the contributors were on the faculty of the first American university-sponsored course on operative laparoscopy that was held in Louisville, Kentucky in April 1986. All of the present contributors have great experience in teaching both laparoscopic and endoscopic surgery.

Clinicians must realize that technologic advances afford us the opportunity to offer patients a number of alternatives to open surgery, including endoscopic vaginal reconstruction, new approaches to management of acute pelvic inflammatory disease, laparoscopic-assisted hysterectomy, the Classic Assisted SEMM Hysterectomy (CASH) procedure, the laparoscopic Burch procedure and vaginal suspension. These techniques are of increasing importance in pediatric adolescent gynecology. Increasingly gynecologists are called upon to assist their surgical colleagues when dealing with such entities as laparoscopic lymphadenectomy and laparoscopic intervention in the pregnant patient as well as in pediatric laparoscopy.

The Council on Resident Education in Obstetrics and Gynecology (CREOG) has embarked on an intensive effort to provide clinicians with defined goals and objectives when teaching endoscopic surgery to residents. Included are cognitive and technical objectives to ensure the competence of these residents in specific areas.

Rapid advances in the arena of operative hysteroscopy continues to enhance our clinical acumen. Management of abnormal uterine bleeding with endometrial ablation, current techniques with respect to hysteroscopic myomectomy, and ultrasonographic Doppler flow studies also provide us with new vistas regarding preoperative and intraoperative management of specific endoscopic surgical procedures. As we come full circle, fetal endoscopic surgery takes on a new dimension. Clinical perspectives beyond the year 2000 must be kept in mind. Innovations in instrumentation and technology have set the stage for the second edition of our textbook *Operative Gynecologic Endoscopy*.

Joseph S. Sanfilippo, M.D.
Ronald L. Levine, M.D.

Acknowledgments

We are indebted to Alliant Health System and Jewish Hospital, for their generous support in making this book possible. We owe special thanks to our former colleague, now retired, Douglas M. Haynes, M.D., for his translation of Professor Kurt Semm's chapter on history and for his many years of scholarly guidance. We are greatly appreciative to the University of Louisville School of Medicine for continuing its tradition of excellence in teaching and research and for providing us the environment and encouragement to see our ideas and goals become reality. Thanks also must go to our secretarial staff and our editorial assistant Ms. Leta Weedman for their help and unending enthusiasm to see this text through to completion. Most importantly, we acknowledge the support and guidance of our wives, Patricia and Sonia, and our families. Once again, we thank them not only for their help and forbearance but most importantly for understanding the demands of our "mistress medicine."

Contents

Foreword vii
  Byron J. Masterson
Preface ix
  Joseph S. Sanfilippo and Ronald L. Levine
Acknowledgments xi
Contributors xvii

Section I History

1. History 3
   Kurt Semm, translated by Douglas M. Haynes

Section II Instrumentation

2. Instrumentation 21
   Ronald L. Levine
3. Lasers 43
   Anthony A. Luciano
4. Electrosurgery 58
   Roger C. O'Dell
5. Documentation 72
   John M. Leventhal

Section III Laparoscopic Techniques

6. Laparoscopic Myomectomy 89
   Harrith M. Hasson
7. Ovarian Surgery 104
   Ronald L. Levine
8. Laparoscopic-Assisted Hysterectomy: American Perspective 116
   C. Y. Liu and D. Alan Johns

9. Pelviscopic Intrafascial Hysterectomy Without Colpotomy   128
   PAUL F. VIETZ
10. Vaginal Prolapse and Bladder Suspension: Role of Endoscopic Surgery   142
    C. Y. LIU
11. Ectopic Pregnancy   153
    DWIGHT PRIDHAM and HARRY REICH
12. Distal Tubal Reconstructive Surgery   182
    LISA PEACOCK and JOHN A. ROCK
13. Laparoscopic Tubal Reanastomosis   192
    D. ALAN JOHNS
14. Endometriosis   199
    DAVID B. REDWINE
15. Laparoscopic Treatment of Tuboovarian and Pelvic Abscess   215
    HARRY REICH and F. MICHAEL SHAW
16. Laparoscopic Pelvic Lymph Node Dissection for Urologic Malignancies   228
    J. MATTHEW GLASCOCK and HOWARD WINFIELD
17. Endoscopic Surgical Procedures During Pregnancy   241
    MARCELLO PIETRANTONI and JOSEPH S. SANFILIPPO
18. Principles of Pediatric Laparoscopy   257
    JOSEPH S. SANFILIPPO and THOM E. LOBE
19. Laparoscopic Suturing Techniques   270
    HOWARD C. TOPEL
20. Assisted Reproductive Technology Versus Tubal Surgery   278
    CLAUDIO A. BENADIVA, ISAAC KLIGMAN, and ZEV ROSENWAKS
21. Current Perspectives   306
    LOTHAR W. POPP

Section IV   Hysteroscopic Techniques

22. Operative Hysteroscopy and Resectoscopy   315
    RAFAEL F. VALLE
23. Abnormal Uterine Bleeding and Endometrial Ablation   348
    RICHARD J. GIMPELSON

Section V   Supportive Techniques and Procedures

24. Anesthesia   361
    LINDA F. LUCAS and BENJAMIN M. RIGOR
25. Complications   380
    BARBARA S. LEVY
26. Adhesion Prevention and Lysis: Indications for Laparotomy and Laparoscopy   391
    MICHAEL P. DIAMOND and ESAT ORHON
27. Role of Pelvic Ultrasonography and Color Doppler in Laparoscopy   404
    RESAD PASIC
28. Operating Room Personnel   412
    WENDY K. WINER
29. Teaching Operative Endoscopy   423
    MICHAEL J. SAMMARCO

30. Learning, Certification, and Credentialing for Endoscopic Surgery ... 435
    CARL J. LEVINSON and RAYMOND H. KAUFMAN
31. Legal Issues Regarding Operative Gynecologic Endoscopy ... 442
    STEVEN R. SMITH

Section VI General Surgery and New Horizons

32. Laparoscopic Overview: General Surgery Perspective ... 463
    GARY C. VITALE
33. Fetus as an Endoscopic Surgical Patient ... 476
    RUBÉN A. QUINTERO
34. Clinical Perspectives: The Year 2000 ... 499
    PATRICK J. TAYLOR

Index ... 507

Contributors

CLAUDIO BENADIVA, M.D., Center for Fertility and Reproductive Endocrinology, New Britain General Hospital, New Britain, CT 06050, USA

MICHAEL P. DIAMOND, M.D., Division of Reproductive Endocrinology and Infertility, Departments of Obstetrics and Gynecology, and Physiology, Wayne State University, Detroit, MI 48201, USA

RICHARD J. GIMPELSON, M.D., Department of Obstetrics and Gynecology, St. Louis University School of Medicine, St. Louis, MO 63110, USA

J. MATTHEW GLASCOCK, M.D., Department of Urology, The University of Iowa College of Medicine, Iowa City, IA 52242-1101, USA

HARRITH M. HASSON, M.D., University of Chicago Hospitals, Gynecologic Endoscopy Center at Weiss Memorial Hospital, Chicago IL 60640, USA

D. ALAN JOHNS, M.D., Richland Medical Center, Fort Worth, TX 76180, USA

RAYMOND H. KAUFMAN, M.D., Department of Obstetrics and Gynecology, Texas Medical Center, Baylor College of Medicine, Houston, TX 77030-3498, USA

ISAAC KLIGMAN, M.D., Center for Fertility and Reproductive Endocrinology, New Britain General Hospital, New Britain CT 06050, USA

JOHN M. LEVENTHAL, M.D., Department of Obstetrics and Gynecology, Harvard Medical School, Boston, MA 02120, USA

RONALD L. LEVINE, M.D., Department of Obstetrics and Gynecology, University of Louisville School of Medicine, Louisville KY 40292, USA

CARL J. LEVINSON, M.D., Department of Obstetrics and Gynecology, Stanford University School of Medicine, Stanford CA 94305-5317, USA

BARBARA S. LEVY, M.D., Department of Obstetrics and Gynecology, University of Washington School of Medicine, Seattle WA 98195, USA

C.Y. LIU, M.D., Chattanooga Women's Laser Center, Chattanooga, TN 37421, USA

THOM E. LOBE, M.D., Section of Pediatric Surgery, University of Tennessee, Memphis, Memphis, TN 38163, USA

LINDA F. LUCAS, M.D., Department of Anesthesiology, University of Louisville School of Medicine, Louisville, KY 40292, USA

ANTHONY A. LUCIANO, M.D., Department of Obstetrics and Gynecology, University of Connecticut School of Medicine, Farmington, CT 06030, and Center for Fertility and Reproductive Endocrinology, New Britain General Hospital, New Britain, CT 06050, USA

ROGER C. ODELL, Electroscope, Inc, Boulder, CO 80301, USA

ESAT ORHON, M.D., Department of Obstetrics and Gynecology, Division of Reproductive Endocrinology and Infertility, Gulhane Military Medical Academy, School of Medicine, Ankara, TURKEY

RESAD PASIC, M.D., Department of Obstetrics and Gynecology, University of Louisville School of Medicine, Louisville KY 40292, USA

MARCELLO PIETRANTONI, M.D., Division of Maternal-Fetal Medicine, Department of Obstetrics and Gynecology, University of Louisville School of Medicine, Louisville, KY 40292, USA

LISA M. PEACOCK, M.D., Department of Gynecology and Obstetrics, Emory University School of Medicine, Atlanta, GA 30329, USA

LOTHAR W. POPP, M.D., Clinic Dr. Guth, Arzt für Gynäkologie und Geburtshilfe, 22609 Hamburg, GERMANY

DWIGHT PRIDHAM, M.D., Department of Obstetrics and Gynecology, University of Louisville School of Medicine, Louisville, KY 40292 USA

RUBÉN A. QUINTERO, M.D., Center for Fetal Diagnosis and Therapy, Fetal Endoscopy Program, Wayne State University, Detroit, MI 48201, USA

DAVID B. REDWINE, M.D., Endometriosis Institute of Oregon, Department of Gynecologic Surgery, St. Charles Medical Center, Bend, OR 97701, USA

HARRY REICH, M.D., Wyoming Valley GYN/OB Associates, Kingston, PA 18704, and Department of Obstetrics and Gynecology, Advanced Laparoscopic Surgery,

Columbia University College of Physicians and Surgeons, New York, NY 10032, USA

BENJAMIN M. RIGOR, M.D., Department of Anesthesiology, University of Louisville School of Medicine, Louisville KY 40292, USA

JOHN A. ROCK, M.D., Department of Gynecology and Obstetrics, Emory University School of Medicine, Atlanta, GA 30329, USA

ZEV ROSENWAKS, M.D., The Center for Reproductive Medicine and Infertility, The New York Hospital-Cornell Medical Center, Department of Obstetrics and Gynecology, New York, NY 10021, USA

MICHAEL J. SAMMARCO, M.D., Department of Obstetrics and Gynecology, Northwestern University Medical School, Chicago, IL 60611, USA

JOSEPH S. SANFILIPPO, M.D., Division of Reproductive Endocrinology, Department of Obstetrics and Gynecology, University of Louisville School of Medicine, Louisville, KY 40292, USA

KURT SEMM, M.D., Klinik für Gynäkologie und Geburtshilfe, Im Klinikum der Christian-Albrechts-Univeristät und Michaelis-Hebammenschule, D-24105 Kiel, GERMANY

F. MICHAEL SHAW, M.D., Division of Gynecology, Westchester County Medical Center, New York Medical College, Valhalla, NY 10595, USA

STEVEN R. SMITH, Cleveland-Marshall College of Law, Cleveland, OH 44115, USA

PATRICK JAMES TAYLOR, M.D., Department of Obstetrics and Gynecology, University of British Columbia, Vancouver, B.C. V6Z 1Y6, CANADA

HOWARD C. TOPEL, M.D., Parkside Medical Center, Park Ridge, IL 60068, USA

RAFAEL F. VALLE, M.D., Department of Obstetrics and Gynecology, Northwestern University Medical School, Chicago, IL 60611, USA

PAUL F. VIETZ, M.D., Carroll County General Hospital, Westminster, MD 21157, USA

GARY C. VITALE, M.D., Department of Surgery, University of Louisville School of Medicine, Louisville, KY 40292, USA

WENDY K. WINER, R.N., B.S.N., Center for Women's Care and Reproductive Surgery, Atlanta, GA 30327, USA

HOWARD N. WINFIELD, M.D., Department of Urology, The University of Iowa College of Medicine, Iowa City, IA 52242-1101, USA

Section I
History

1
History of Operative Gynecologic Endoscopy

Kurt Semm, translated by Douglas M. Haynes

The development of general surgery began with the introduction of chloroform narcosis by the obstetrician Sir James Y. Simpson of Edinburgh, Scotland in 1847. This technique later received the historical designation *l'anesthésie à la reine* because Simpson had used it for the painless delivery of Queen Victoria. The next leap forward took place 100 years later, in 1947, when Sir Alexander Fleming was honored with the Nobel Prize for the discovery of penicillin. With the introduction of intensive care and medical transfusion technology, the groundwork was laid for surgical transplantation procedures. In 1965 there began the transformation of "classic" surgery to "minimally invasive" surgery as a result of new technical advances.

The first endoscopic inspection of the abdomen was performed in a dog in 1901 in Germany by Kelling[1]; He called his technique coelioscopy and performed it two times in humans. Less than a decade later in Sweden Jacobaeus[2] extended the technique to human subjects and spoke about laparoscopy. The method was hazardous, as adequate illumination required introduction of a hot incandescent light source into the abdominal cavity. The hazards of burns and embolism were eliminated after 1963 with the advent of "cold" illumination using fiberoptic glass cables and the introduction of the CO_2-pneu technique by Semm[3] in 1967, which allowed safe pneumoperitoneum. Tubal sterilization via laparotomy (and its operative risks) was replaced by a laparoscopic procedure that could be performed in a matter of minutes.

The feasibility of performing tubal sterilization endoscopically resulted in an exponential worldwide dissemination of pelviscopy[4,5]/laparoscopy utilization from 1968 to 1972. Simultaneously, experience with pelviscopy was extended to other operations on the fallopian tubes, notably to tubal reconstruction to relieve sterility and to ovarian and uterine procedures. The breakthrough into general surgery followed on September 12, 1980 in Kiel, when gynecologist Semm[6,7] performed the first successful endoscopic appendectomy in a patient with endometriosis—an advance roundly condemned by the abdominal surgery establishment.

In 1985 the surgeon Mühe[8] removed a gallbladder using an instrument called a cholecystoscope, which he designed for that purpose. After having performed 54 successful laparoscopic cholecystectomies, he was the target of a lawsuit alleging "improper surgical action," which resulted in a court sentence officially prohibiting his laparoscopic surgical activity. In Bordeaux two years later Mouret[9] was more fortunate: Using standard gynecologic instrumentation, he performed his first laparoscopic cholecystectomy. Mühe was not officially exonerated by the German Surgical Society until 1992.

As early as the middle of the nineteenth century, more than a century earlier, gynecologists Aubinais[10] and Pantaleon[11] had been experimenting with hysteroscopy although gynecologists were unwilling to abandon standard abdominal surgical approaches for operative gynecology. In contrast, within 2 years after the first reports of successful laparoscopic cholecystectomy general surgeons all over the world had become proficient in the new field of laparoscopic surgery (i.e., performing cholecystectomy, appendectomy, selective sympathectomy, resection of the rectum, and operations on the sigmoid colon, small intestine, and stomach ulcers). These developments, during the last decade of the twentieth century, have ushered in an end to the era of classic surgery, best characterized by the equation "big incision = big surgeon." This new discipline of minimally invasive surgery, sometimes facetiously called "keyhole surgery," or "small incision = small brain," has been adopted not only by general surgeons but by specialists in thoracic surgery (thoracoscopy), orthopedics (arthroscopy), and most recently neurosurgery.

In gynecology a long road led via laparoscopic-assisted vaginal hysterectomy or classic intrafascial Semm hysterectomy (CISH) from the siphopherot (see next section) to vaginoscopy and pelviscopic hysterectomy. Since the late 1980s the surgical establishment has come to grips with a comprehensive concept, namely, that gynecologists have been the pioneers of operative pelviscopy. The 1980 appendectomy and the cholecystectomy five years later were in effect the wake-up call for general surgery.

How Did It Happen?

The first description of an endeavor to reflect light into the human body in order to become conversant with its innermost structure is found in the Babylonian Talmud (about 200 CE; Niddah, V. 65b). In that tract there is a description of a lead pipe (*siphopherot*) with an inwardly tilted mouthpiece furnished with a *mechul* (wooden drain). Both of these devices were introduced into the vagina to determine if bleeding originated in the uterus or the vagina.

The concept of "mirroring" (i.e., visualization of internal organs) was attributed by Avicenna (980–1047 CE) to the Arab physician Abulkasim (912–1013 CE), who had placed a mirror in front of the spread vulva and used its reflected light for purposes of illumination, notably of internal body parts. We are indebted to Tulio Cesare Aranzi for the first endoscopic light source. In the treatise *Tumores Praeter Naturam* (Venice, 1587, Chap. 21, p. 171) he described use of the *camera obscura* for medical purposes. The *camera obscura*, discovered by the Benedictine monk Don Panuce, was mentioned by Leonardo da Vinci (1519) and was first described as such by Porta (1589) in his *Medica Naturalis*. In his work, the rays of the sun shining through the aperture of a shutter were focused through a spherical glass vessel and projected into the nasal cavities. Even then, artificial light sources were recommended in the event of overcast skies.

Development of the vaginal speculum over the centuries received a new impetus in the *Memoires Gynécologiques* of gynecologist Arnaud (1768). He first made a practical medical application of the functionally effective small "thief's lantern," widely used at the time as a light source for endoscopic visualization. Modern endoscopy was born at the beginning of the nineteenth century with the work of Bozzini,[12] who devised the first light reflector. It consisted of an apparatus that directed light rays into the innermost cavity of the live animal body, reflecting them in turn to the eye of the observer (Fig. 1.1). The historical development of endoscopy resulted in the first portable endoscope, described by Desormeaux[13] (Fig. 1.2). His endoscope, presented to the Royal Academy of Medicine in Paris on November 29, 1843 and recommended by him for the inspection of both vagina and uterus, shared the Argenteuil Prize.

Photography and television have come to the fore in connection with the further development of endoscopic abdominal surgery. This phase was inaugurated in Frankfurt, Germany a century ago by Stein, who as early as 1874 demon-

1. History of Operative Gynecologic Endoscopy

Although gynecologists were the pioneers in the systematic evolution of endoscopy, its further technical elaboration was principally achieved by the field of cystoscopy. The first fully functional and clinically applicable endoscope was devised by Nitze[15] in 1878. An incandescent lamp installed on the tip of the endoscope posed no burn hazard, as the requisite cooling was provided by circulating water inside the urinary bladder (Fig. 1.4).

In 1902, the German, Kelling[1] (Munich, 1901) was the first to inspect the viscera of the dog using air insufflation of the abdomen, an advance he called "celioscopy," and he used it two times in humans. The Swedish investigator Jacobaeus[2] repeated this procedure in the human, designating the technique "laparoscopy" (in German *Lendenschau,* in English "flank inspection"). This methodology was supposedly reinvented on two occasions, first by Steiner[16] (American, 1924), who called it "abdominoscopy" and by Redi[17] (Italy, 1935), who gave his technique the designation "splanchnoscopy." Two years later in Munich Korbsch[18] published the first textbook of laparothoracoscopy (1927).

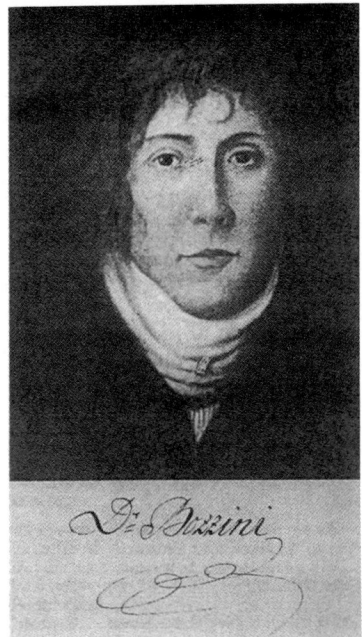
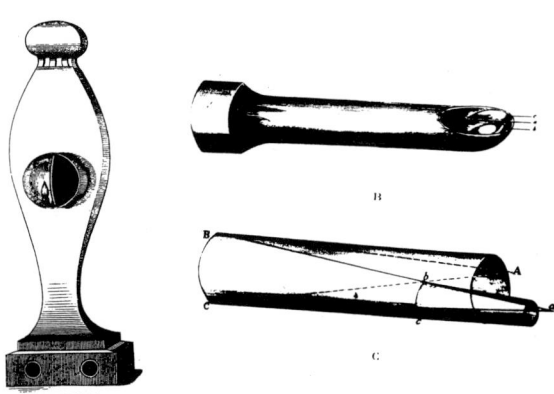

Figure 1.1. Dr. Bozzini was the inventor of the first endoscope and his illuminating device for reflecting light rays from the body cavity to the naked eye: Dr. Bozzini (1805)—self portrait.

strated his "photoendoscope" and "endocamera" (Fig. 1.3).

The earliest steps in the development of endoscopy were initiated by gynecologists. Désormeaux,[13] Aubinais,[10] and Pantaleoni[11] carried out the first attempts to inspect the uterine cavity, calling it "hysteroscopy." Unfortunately, further developments in gynecologic endoscopy during the nineteenth century came to an end with the efforts of these physicians.

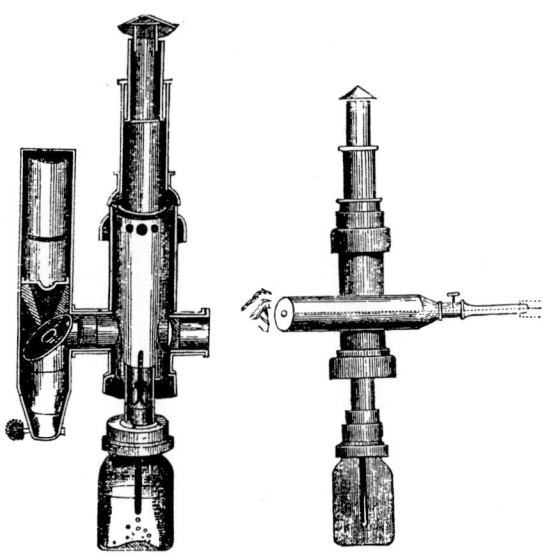

Figure 1.2. Original illustration of Desormeaux's portable endoscope, awarded the Argenteuil Prize (Paris, Nov. 29, 1843).

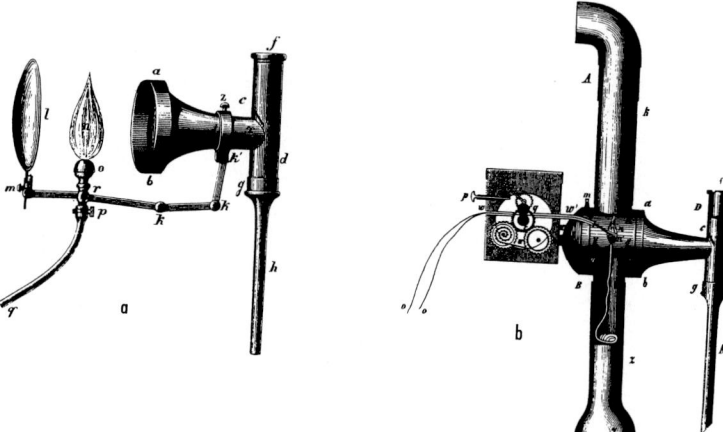

Figure 1.3. Original illustration of Stein's photoendoscope (left) and endo-camera (right), introduced in Frankfurt in 1874.

The first laparoscopic surgeon was a gynecologist. The endoscopic technique was applied directly in 1933 during a surgical procedure by Fervers.[19] He cut intraabdominal adhesions using the coagulating tip of a cystoscope.

In 1936, Bösch[20] (Aarau, Switzerland), in a paper on laparoscopy, reported "a wonderful overview of freely mobile internal female genitalia, and the ability to achieve lysis of adhesions of fixed organs such as the ovaries using a grasping instrument." He went on: "At last the

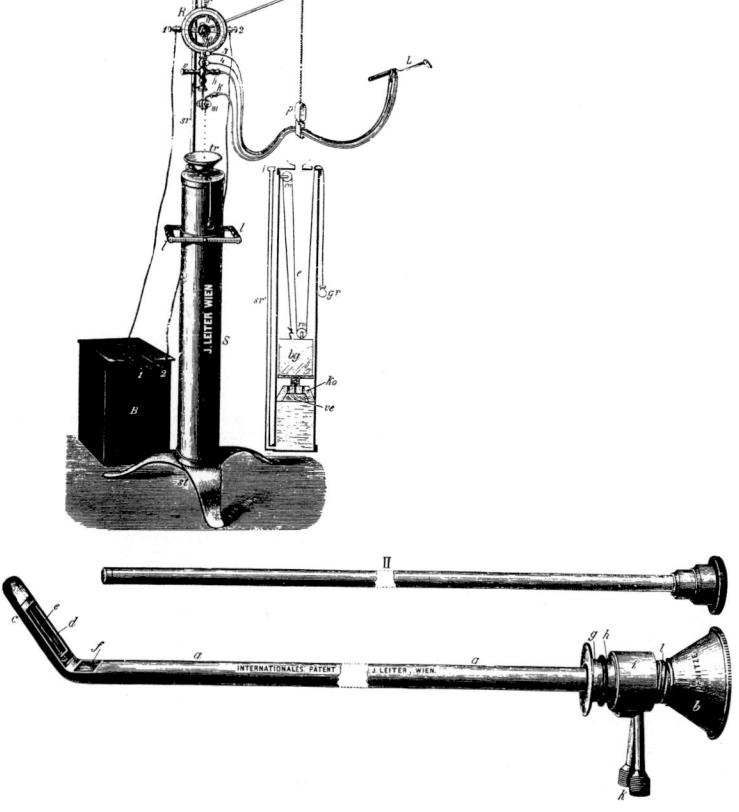

Figure 1.4. Original illustration (1878) of Nitze's cytoscope, the first to be furnished with electricity. (Manufactured by J.. Leiter, Vienna).

laparoscope provides us with a way to perform indicated tubal sterilization without a laparotomy. By means of a suitably grounded cautery terminal it is possible to perform endoscopic coagulation of several tubal areas under direct visual contact." The identical technique was redescribed in 1941 by Power and Barnes[21] in Ann Arbor, Michigan. They used a peritoneoscope for a tubal sterilization procedure.

As early as 1918 Goetze[22] had used a mechanically engineered needle for the safe puncture and insufflation of the abdominal wall and chest and had recommended filling the abdominal cavity with oxygen.

In the field of internal medicine, the work of Kalk[23] contributed to making laparoscopy a recognized method during the 1930s by performing diagnostic biopsy procedures on the liver and spleen under local anesthesia. It was a pioneering achievement when Raoul Palmer[24] in Paris in 1946 redirected the laparoscope from the upper to the lower abdomen. This maneuver was a high risk procedure because of the hot, incandescent tip of the laparoscope and the still unperfected creation of a pneumoperitoneum. Palmer originally used local anesthesia, then customary in internal medicine, for the gynecologic application of laparoscopy. A few years later he reported to me personally that after the first two years he carried out his celioscopies exclusively under general anesthesia because he did not encounter a single woman who was willing to submit herself to this modality a second time.

The abdominal route, and its inherent difficulties led Decker[25] in the United States in 1946 to suggest the vaginal approach as being a more suitable one for gynecologic purposes. He dubbed his technique "culdoscopy," derived from the cul-de-sac of Douglas. Although there was immediate wide acceptance of this technique in the United States, it was less than trailblazing, as culdoscopy was not only ineffective for diagnostic purposes, it forestalled the development of surgical advances using this approach. Furthermore, the practical application of culdoscopy was fraught with the difficulty of requiring either an exaggerated Trendelenburg position or the knee-chest position, both of which posed problems for the anesthesiologist. In Germany Frangenheim[26] in 1958 and Schwalm[27] in 1964 promulgated the trend toward laparoscopy.

Laparoscopy of the epigastrium under local anesthesia is more or less nonproblematic and entails no significant hazard. Laparoscopy of the hypogastrium is a riskier matter because of the bowel and great vessels. During the early 1960s the latter was proscribed on principle for gynecologic purposes as constituting a prohibitively hazardous procedure. During the foundational era of gynecologic laparoscopy in Europe a high complication rate was not unusual.[28] In fact, complications were the basis for the total ban on laparoscopy in Germany, where it was listed in the index of proscribed procedures. Not until the change of name to pelviscopy was it possible to focus the attention of gynecologists on endoscopy of the hypogastric region.

In 1955 Fikentscher and Semm developed a new tubal insufflation apparatus first described by Rubin[29] in 1920. These elaborate physical devices were pertinent to insufflation of a fallopian tube using carbon dioxide gas. This technique resulted in the creation of a multipurpose insufflation apparatus.[30] It was oscillographically highly sophisticated considering what was mechanically possible at that time. It realized a myriad of diagnostic possibilities involving tubal insufflation.

Stimulated by this concept of carbon dioxide insufflation of a body cavity, the definitive physical data pertinent to insufflation of the abdominal cavity were worked out in 1963, resulting in a reliable insufflation apparatus, the CO_2-Pneu,[3] which eventually took over the field of laparoscopy. Adaptation of the apparatus to the pressure conditions applying within the abdomen in connection with the vena cava and diaphragm led Semm[3] to elaborate the first CO_2-Pneu for laparoscopic application in internal medicine.[31] It eventuated in further devices: CO_2-Pneu-Automatic in 1967[3,32] and a decade later the CO_2-OP-Pneu-Electronic.[33,34]

The routine adoption of the insufflation procedure for pneumoperitoneum in 1964 by the First Medical Clinic of the University of Munich led the Munich Gynecological Clinic in 1964 to introduce laparoscopy, initially for diagnostic purposes only. This restriction theoretically averted the principal hazards attendant on the introduction of laparoscopy into gynecology: burns induced by the incandescent light source of the laparoscope and the possibility of gas embolism from carbon dioxide, even though monitored with respect to pressure and volume under physiologic conditions.

Under these ground rules, laparoscopy and pelviscopy[4,5] were introduced into the German surgical milieu with dissemination beginning in 1966. Whereas before 1960 only nine clinics were performing laparoscopy, by 1969 there were 95 additional, and by 1974 another 221 clinical departments had been added.

In America the development of laparoscopy followed a dissimilar course. Early on, laparoscopy was not, as in Europe, an outright taboo; it was simply an unknown entity. In 1967 Melvin R. Cohen was the sole demonstrator of his laparoscopic technique at the American Fertility Society convention. For production of a pneumoperitoneum he made use of a large glass cylinder furnished with a piston with which he forced gas into the abdomen. His demonstration did not attract favorable attention. Laparoscopy was similarly ignored in the United States. Cohen[35] seized on my personal recommendation to utilize the CO_2-Pneu for the induction of pneumoperitoneum, and in 1970 he published a small book on the significance of laparoscopy in gynecology.[35] In this work, he reproduced a visual representation of the CO_2-Pneu; two such devices placed at his disposal had convinced him of their mechanical dependability. Cohen's book proved to be the cornerstone of American gynecologic laparoscopy. Because of it, Cohen is today highly esteemed as the "father of laparoscopy" in the United States. In contradistinction to the situation in Europe where the method was used almost exclusively for diagnostic studies in patients with infertility problems, laparoscopy became the method of choice in the United States for 95 percent of tubal sterilization procedures, using the very technique that Bösch[20] had recommended and demonstrated in practice 35 years earlier.

Unfortunately, the term "laparoscopy" led to conceptual confusion when it came to designing the specific instrumentation for gynecologic pelviscopy. Lack of knowledge of the physical principles governing the use of high frequency current in closed body cavities (the "Faraday's cage") was the cause of accidents with severe sequelae. These two circumstances impeded introduction of the method into use in the United States during the 1970s, as it had in Europe during the 1960s.

The triumphant advance of pelviscopy/laparoscopy that had started in Europe and had evolved into a routine methodology began in the United States in 1971, in particular following the founding by Jordan Phillips of the American Association of Gynecologic Laparoscopists (AAGL). This point marks the birth of the history of advanced pelviscopic surgery. The history can be categorized into three subdivisions.

1. Development of surgical instruments and apparatus for operative pelviscopy
2. Accumulation of pelviscopic surgical experience
3. Simultaneous transmission of diagnostic and operative pelviscopy to the video screen

With respect to item one above, laparoscopic abdominal surgery is widely recognized today. It is no longer necessary to make a defensive presentation of the development of individual instruments, as I had to do in the preceding edition of this book. A less technical recounting of the pertinent historical information should now suffice.

The high-frequency current,[20] introduced into laparoscopy in 1935 for purposes of tubal cauterization, was superceded in 1965 by the endocoagulator[36] for the treatment of benign leukoplakia of the cervical portioepithelium and in 1972 introduced in laparoscopy. Also in 1965 the introduction of "cold" illumination and the CO_2-Pneu reduced the surgical hazard of hypogastric laparoscopy to a minimum. The CO_2-Pneu-Automatic system drastically simplified the performance of operations under general anesthesia.

There followed a period[33,37,38] of instrumentation development (1968: pelviscope, hook scis-

1. History of Operative Gynecologic Endoscopy

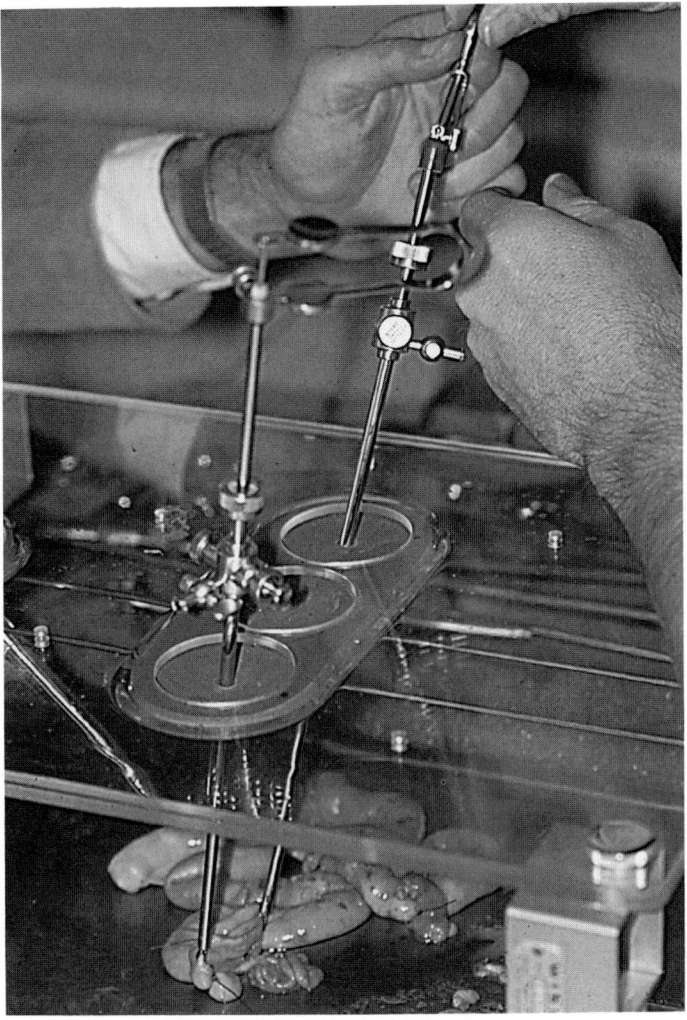

Figure 1.5. Pelvi-trainer for instruction in intraabdominal pelviscopy/laparoscopy for grasping, cutting and suturing following the 4-step principle.

sors, uterine mobilizer; 1971: bipolar high-frequency coagulation; 1972: endocoagulation with crocodile forceps). Significant advances were ligature of bleeding vessels by means of loop ligation (1976),[39] endoligation (1979), and especially the endosuture (1980). Parallel developments were the CO_2-Pneu (1982), the tissue morcellator (1976), and the Aquapurator by Semm (1977). This technology made possible the constant evolution of new surgical approaches. The hot-knife myoma enucleator (1982) ushered in the era of conservative uterine surgery.[33,37]

Despite these advances, pelviscopic surgery (Semm, 1978[32]) was still considered unacceptable. The breakthrough to general acceptance took place with the invention of the Pelvi-Trainer[38] in 1985 (Fig. 1.5 A and B). Since 1986 the latter has shown gynecologists how simple it is to use the appropriate instruments for grasping, cutting, and suturing inside the unopened abdomen.

From 1986 on, endoscopists have had available a complete operating kit with an emergency needle. In 1991 the serrated edged macro-morcellator (SEMM) became available, making it possible to morcellate myomas as large as a fist.[39] It obviated the need to open the abdomen via laparotomy or posterior colpotomy. Further suturing and knot-tying techniques and ultimately (1991) the calibrated uterine resection tool (CURT) made possible the

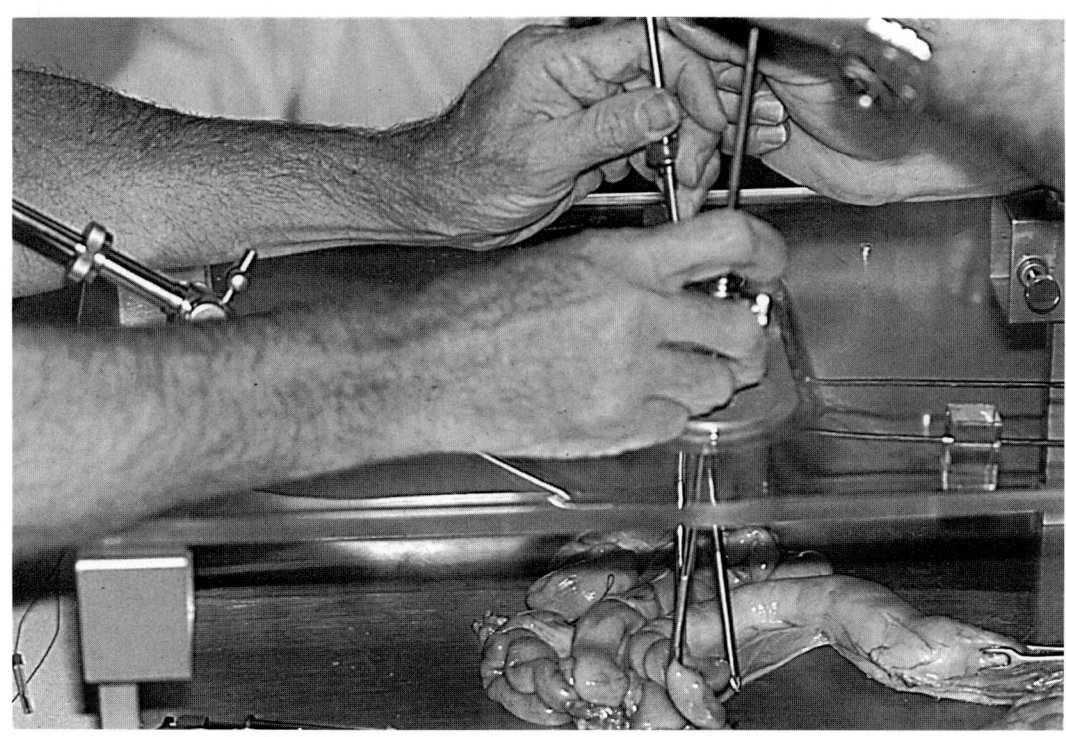

Figure 1.5. (*Continued*)

performance of subtotal hysterectomy[40] by the CISH method without colpotomy (Fig. 1.6).

In 1989 Reich et al.[41] suggested a new approach in operative gynecology, with the laparoscopic assisted vaginal hysterectomy (LAVH). This technique was present in its primitive stage in 1984[33,37] for endoscopic abdominal surgery as pelviscopy-assisted vaginal hysterectomy (Fig. 1.7). The emphasis then was on "vaginal hysterectomy,"[41] not, as Reich was to write in 1989, on "laparoscopic hysterectomy." In 1984, however, the thought of an endoscopic hysterectomy was enough to cause gynecologists everywhere to burst into gales of laughter. In 1992 motorization of the morcellizing instruments was introduced by the Wisap²-Auto-Moto-Drive (Sauerlach, Germany).[42–47] In 1995 these advancements led to the development of the

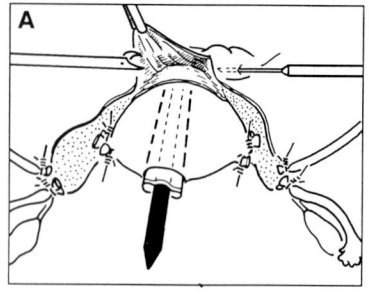 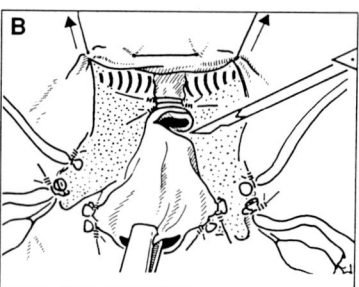

Figure 1.6. The first intrafascial (CISH) hysterectomy without colpotomy, performed in Kiel Germany on Sept. 7, 1991: (A) transvaginal excoriation of a cylinder incorporating the cervix, uterine cavity and fundus with dissection of bladder peritoneum under aqueous irrigation; (B) subtotal extirpation of the uterus with preservation of the cardinal and uterosacral ligaments, uterine arteries, etc.

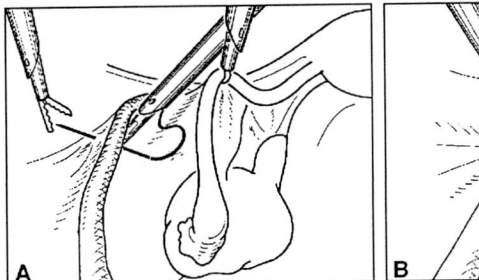
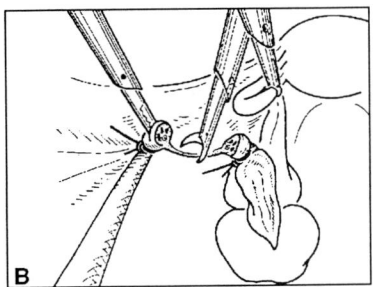

Figure 1.7. Original illustration for the surgical manual on endoscopic abdominal surgery (1984): pelviscopic separation of the left infundibulopelvic ligament (A) preliminary to the pelviscopically assisted vaginal hysterectomy (B).

motorized macromorcellator, available in diameters of 15 or 20 mm. The new technique of "horizontal" morcellation[48] (Fig. 1.8) allows for tumors (e.g. uterus, myomas, kidney) up to 15 cm in diameter to be morcellated intracorporeally without bloodloss in minimal time.

The manufacturers of pelviscopic operating instruments and devices had difficulty selling their products also in the United States before 1990. However, between 1991 and 1993 a manufacturing industry for minimal invasive surgical instrumentation emerged in the United States, making its first appearance at the 1993 AAGL convention in San Francisco. It was presented as a potential industry, offering a broad spectrum of technologic possibilities not only for gynecology but for general surgery as well.

With respect to item two above, the accumulation of pelviscopic operative experience began with tubal sterilization using high frequency current (1936)[20] and continuing with endocoagulation in 1972.[42] Salpingoplasty and salpingostomy followed in 1974.[33,37] As early as 1975 myomas were enucleated to the extent permitted by hemostasis via endocoagulation. In 1976, with the introduction of the triple-loop ligation technique, the radical treatment of ectopic pregnancy came into being.[38] In 1977 extensive adnexal resections were undertaken, and for the first time conservative management of tubal pregnancy was initiated. It involved suturing a longitudinal incision or a "rupture site."[37] The operative technique of the three-loop ligature for removal of the adnexa[37] was in place by 1978 and salpingostomy by endoscopic suture to produce fimbrial eversion was successfully performed in 1978.

The first laparoscopic repair of the small intestine was performed on April 20, 1983 in Kiel. After hysterectomy and postoperative radiotherapy for endometrial carcinoma in this patient, extensive lysis of adhesions succeeded in producing normal diameter of the bowel lumen. Microsuture was performed via laparoscopy, and the patient was discharged from the hospital within 4 days.[33,37]

September 12, 1980 saw the first successful appendectomy in a patient with endometrio-

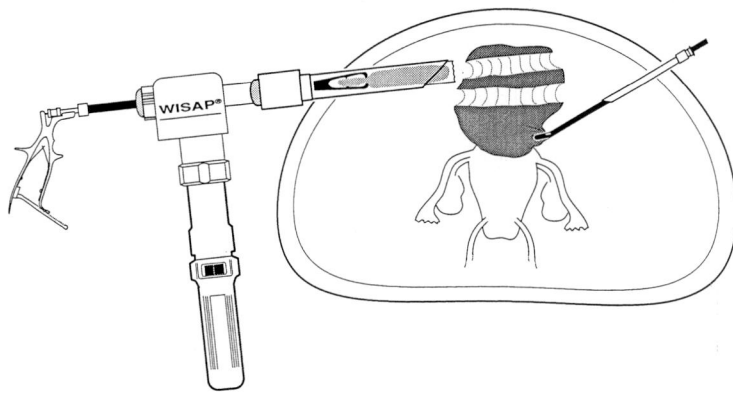

Figure 1.8. Horizontal macromorcellation with a new power driven morcellator for effectively and quickly reducing intra-abdominally the size of tissue specimens.

sis.[6,7] An article on the subject submitted to a German publisher in October 1981 was returned 11 months later with the editorial comment: "The publisher would become a laughing-stock if such an absurdity were published." Hence laparoscopic appendectomy continued to be an unknown entity in the German literature during 1982. However, at a meeting of the American Fertility Society in Puerto Rico in February 1982 this report was accorded the Chairman's Award of the United States International Foundation for Studies in Reproduction. In June 1982 the article in question, "Advances in Pelviscopic Surgery (Appendectomy)," was published in the United States.[6] Pelviscopic operative procedures were further refined in Kiel during subsequent years, but international acceptance was not forthcoming until American gynecologists drew attention to the reports from Kiel.

In September 1983, Dr. Ronald Levine from Louisville, Kentucky, visited Kiel to observe pelviscopic surgery. He subsequently published a paper entitled "The Economic Impact of Pelviscopic Surgery" in September 1985.[49] This paper gave impetus to the spread of operative laparoscopy in the United States with the description of a laparoscopic bilateral oophorectomy. In October 1985 Jordan Phillips, the founder of the AAGL, came to Kiel along with 16 colleagues. They were convinced that not only the chief of the department, nicknamed "Member of the Magic Club," but all his assistants were able to carry out endoscopic procedures in equally talented fashion.

As early as January 1986 the first teaching course on operative pelviscopy was offered at the Fontainebleau Hotel in Miami under the direction of Jordan Phillips. The 189 participating physicians were not unanimously won over to the technique demonstrated by four members of the Kiel faculty. Jordan Phillips then invited the Kiel team to present three subsequent courses in operative pelviscopy in New York, Chicago, and Los Angeles. In connection with each course the Kiel team caused a memorial medallion to be bestowed in honor of Raoul Palmer and Kiel.

Even though the "eccentric" method was not covered by the insurance companies, a few U.S. gynecologists began to perform pelviscopic and laparoscopic procedures. After some 26 courses in 18 states had been organized by the Kiel group between 1980 and 1991, this new technique was gradually introduced into the United States, as attested to by the large number of presentations at the annual conventions of the AAGL since 1992.

As early as 1982 a syllabus of pelviscopic operations appeared and was arranged according to organ systems. As of today, this endoscopic technique has disclosed a broad spectrum of possibilities for the expansion of intraabdominal operative gynecology and general surgery, even extending to cancer surgery. Figure 1.9 serves as a minisurvey of current routine endoscopic surgical techniques, a method that only a decade ago evoked smirks, yet today constitutes the subject of the present volume.

The first manual, *Pelviscopy and Hysteroscopy*,[38] a 12,000-copy edition comprising 329 pages and 471 color illustrations printed in German, English, French, Spanish, and Portuguese, brought about no greater acceptance of diagnostic and operative pelviscopy than did the "*Operative Manual for Endoscopic Abdominal Surgery,*"[33,37] a 1200-copy edition in German, English, Greek, Italian, and Japanese, with 485 pages and 387 illustrations in full color. These publications received worldwide attention but were virtually ignored by gynecologists.

For historic reasons, mention should be made of the fact that the surgical technique was described in individual illustrated leaflet collections and distributed at no charge to the reader[44–47,50] (edition of more than 40,000 copies in several languages: German, Serbo-Croatian, French, English, Spanish, Russian, Chinese). In addition, 10,000 videocassettes (a 60-minute presentation demonstrating 20 pelviscopic operations including appendectomy) were disseminated, reaching even the most out-of-the-way teaching venues.

In Semm's operative pelviscopy manual[33,34,43] several illustrations show how vaginal hysterectomy, in the presence of sizable ovarian enlargements, can be facilitated by pelviscopically freeing the adnexa from the infundibulopelvic ligament and other points of attachment. This

1. History of Operative Gynecologic Endoscopy

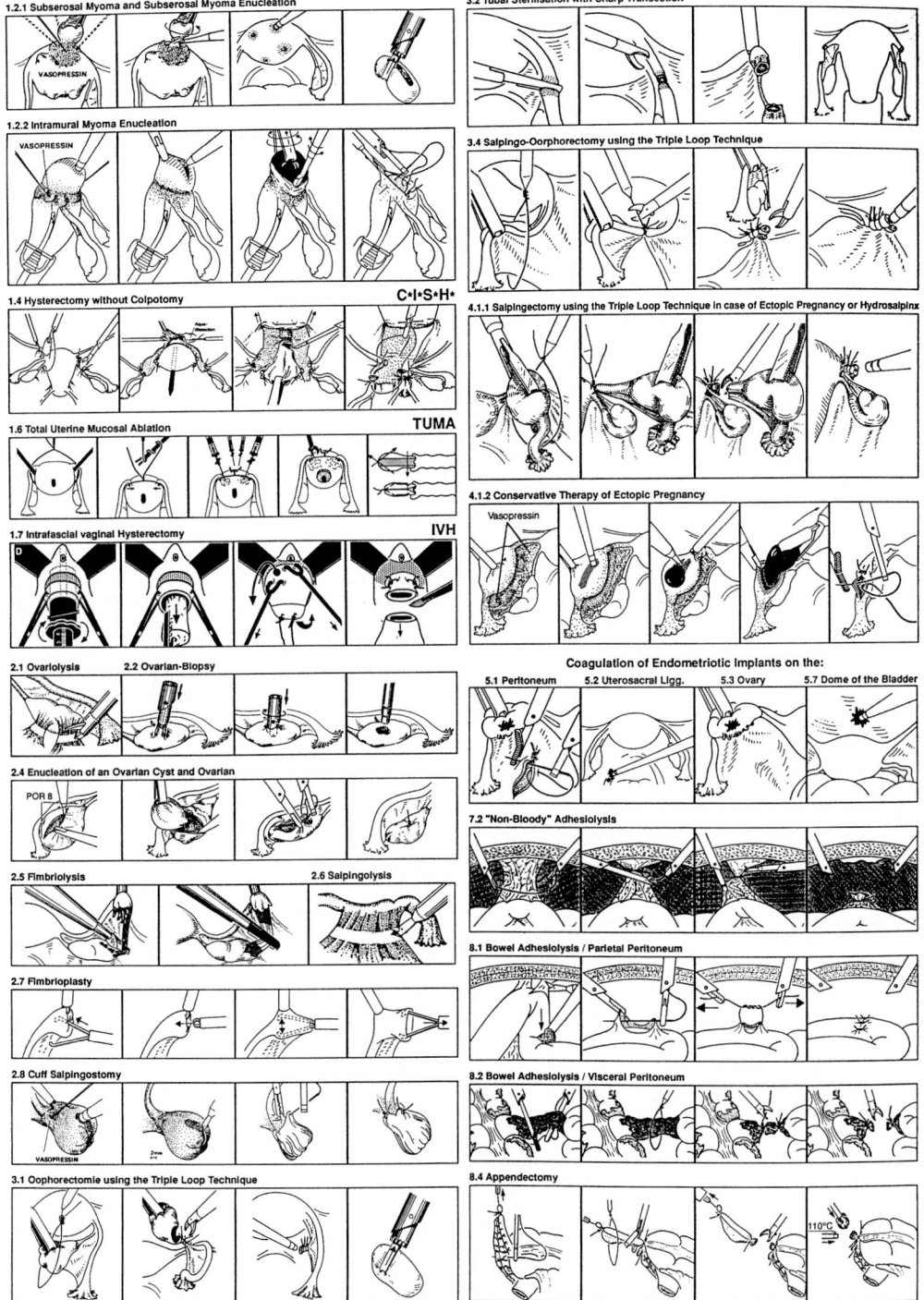

Figure 1.9. Schematic synopsis of the pelviscopic surgical procedures developed in Kiel, Germany for their 80 percent substitution for laparotomy in gynecologic surgery.

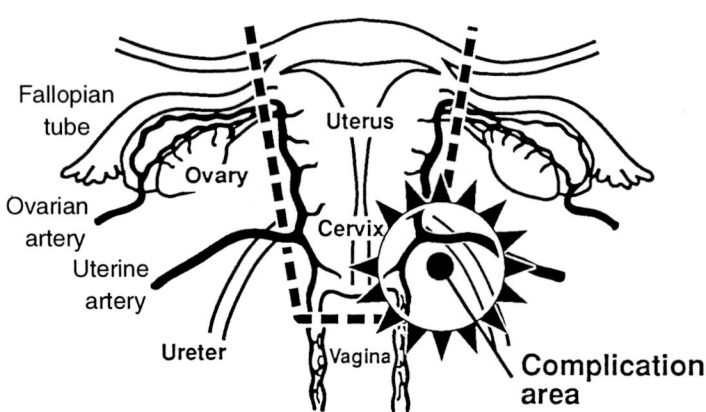

Figure 1.10. Schematic drawing of the step-by-step evolution of LAVH (Laparoscopic Assisted Vaginal Hysterectomy) from 1989–1993.

technique marked the beginning of pelviscopically assisted vaginal hysterectomy, even though in 1984 it was the subject of ridicule. In the United States Reich et al.[41] began to perfect laparoscopic hysterectomy one step at a time, setting aside all bias. This operation, the LAVH, has come of age all over the world as a routinely applicable technique for total pelviscopic hysterectomy (Fig. 1.10). This extrafascial vaginal hysterectomy cannot of course be regarded as a form of minimally invasive endoscopic surgery. Total hysterectomy can represent overtreatment. When benign indications for hysterectomy exist, there is no rationale for transection of the cardinal and uterosacral ligaments, amputation of the vagina, and ligation of the uterine arteries. So it was that in September 17, 1991 the first intrafascial hysterectomy[40] in conjunction with removal of a paracervical myoma *without colpotomy* (CISH) was successfully demonstrated in Kiel. The CISH (Classic Intrafascial SEMM Hysterectomy) technique preserved the anatomy of the pelvic floor via a subtotal hysterectomy, eliminating the need for a colpotomy incision (Fig. 1.11). Vietz introduced this procedure in 1994[51] in the U.S.

Hysteroscopic "endometrial ablation" may be significantly improved in the future by total uterine mucosa ablation (TUMA). This procedure produces a significant diminution of uterine volume by means of total ablation of the mucosal lining,[52] due to lysis of the myometrium by endocoagulation (Fig. 1.12).

It must be pointed out that the development of pelviscopic/laparoscopic hysterectomy has also led to changes in the vaginal hysterectomy technique. The latter operation may also be carried out using the CISH technique, the so-called intrafascial vaginal hysterectomy (IVH). By means of this supravaginal[53] operation (Fig. 1.13) the important structural elements of the female pelvic floor alluded to above are preserved. Sexual function is likewise unaffected. These considerations point the way to fundamental changes in the hitherto classic operative technique for pelvic floor reconstruction in

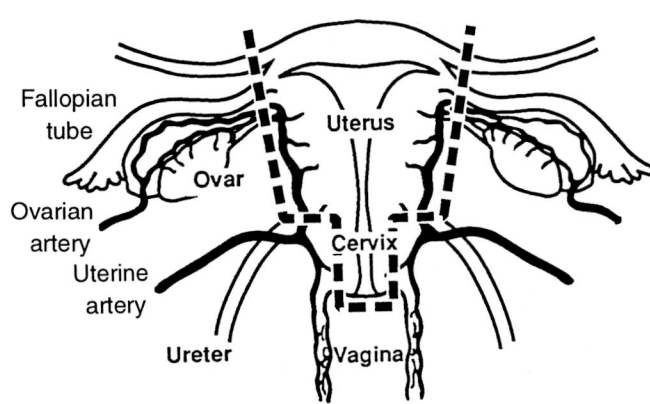

Figure 1.11. Schematic drawing of the CISH technique (Subtotal Pelviscopic Hysterectomy minus colpotomy) first performed by Semm in Kiel, Germany on September 7, 1991.

Figure 1.12. Schematic drawing of TUMA (Total Uterine Mucosal Ablation) with temporary fundus ligature and excoriation of a cylinder of mucosa (A), and total endometrial ablation using myometrolysis via a 120°F cautery (B).

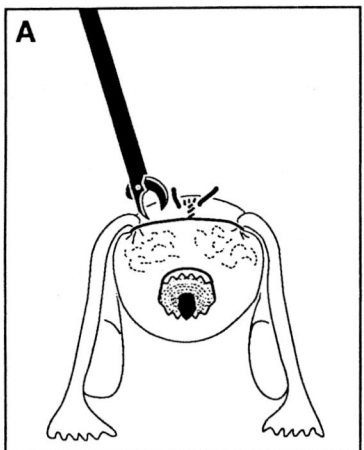 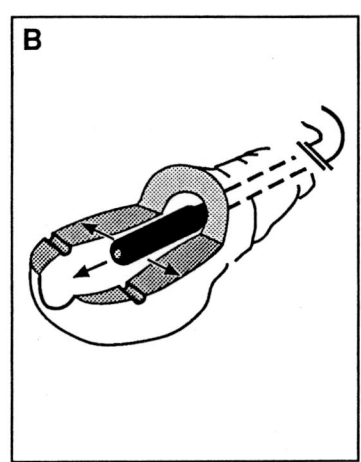

cases of genital prolapse. New endoscopic methods thus lead to fresh approaches to uterine suspension.

With respect to item 3, above, the earliest technology for simultaneous image transmission during diagnostic and operative pelviscopy was demonstrated at the First European Congress for Endoscopy, organized in Munich in October 1970. On that occasion, the procedure was used for the first time to project the female genitalia in full detail on a 12 × 16 meter screen and to demonstrate peristalsis of the right ureter. Subsequent attempts to transfer the endoscopic picture to 16 mm film encountered difficulties because of illumination problems. At first it was possible to secure only brief records on 16 mm film at the cost of severe physical hardship. The surgeon had to operate behind the camera with auxiliary lighting arrangements. Yet in Munich during 1967–1970 and in Kiel beginning in 1970, several hours of 16 mm celluloid film were recorded, depicting the broad spectrum of pelviscopic diagnostic procedures as well as the beginning stages of operative pelviscopy, from tubal procedures to enucleation of myomas. These efforts were recognized worldwide and were awarded gold medals and other prizes. However, even worldwide recognition failed to awaken appreciable interest.

In 1982 the Wittmoser transmission system permitted the general transition to video. The camera weighed more than 30 kg; and to produce videofilms of excellent color and resolution, the operator required a robust physical constitution.

The definitive video breakthrough did not occur until 1988 when tiny microchip cameras became available. They made it possible to perform large segments of laparoscopic operations while looking at a monitor rather than bent over looking through the laparoscope. Nezhat et al.[54] were among the first operators in the United States to attain prominence in this area.

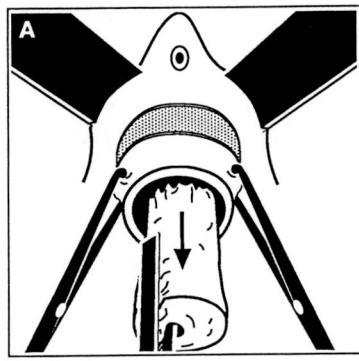 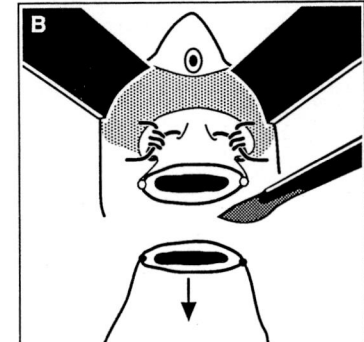

Figure 1.13. Schematic drawing of IVH (Intrafascial Vaginal Hysterectomy) with (A) excoriation of the cervix, and (B) pelviscopically assisted adnexectomy.

Since 1967 the production of 16 mm long-playing pelviscopy celluloid films, and videofilms since 1982, have been vital for promoting what is now an exponential acceptance of operative pelviscopy. These media materials depict 20 pelviscopic operations in minute detail and with outstanding technical quality, still produced using the Wittmoser transmitting system.

Ignorance might have prevented this pioneering gynecologic discipline from seeing the light of day in the surgical world at the end of the twentieth century if the field of general surgery had not adopted the principle of minimally invasive surgery in 1988.

References

1. KELLING G: Über oesophagoskopie, Gastroskopie und Cölioskopie. Münch. Med. Wochenschr. 1902;49:21–24.
2. JACOBAEUS HC: Über die Möglichkeit die Zystoskopie bei Untersuchungen seröser Höhlungen anzuwenden. Münch. Med. Wochenschr. 1910; 57:2090–2092.
3. SEMM K: Das Pneumoperitoneum mit CO_2, Visum 1967;6:144–146.
4. SEMM K: Gynecological Pelviscopy and Instrumentation. Acta Europ. Fert. 1 (1969) 81–97.
5. SEMM K: Weitere Entwicklung in der gynäkologischen Laparoskopie; Gynäkologische Pelviskopie, Klin. d. Frauenheilk. 1971; Bd. I, 326;1–39.
6. SEMM K: Advances in pelviscopic surgery (appendectomy) in: Current Problems in Obstetrics and Gynecology, Chicago, Year Book Medical Publishers, 1982, vol. 5, No. 10.
7. SEMM K: Endoscopic Appendectomy, Endoscopy 1983; 15:59–64.
8. MÜHE E: Die erste Cholezystektomie durch das Laparoskop. Langenbecks Arch. Klin. Chir 369: 804.
9. MOURET P: From the first Laparoscopic Cholecystectomy to the frontiers of Laparoscopic surgery: The future prospectives. Dig. Surg. 1991; Vol. 8, 124.
10. AUBINAIS: Id. Provence (C Marseille) Un Med. 1864, 24:591.
11. PANTALEONI D: On endoscopic examination of the cavity of the womb. Med Press and Circ. 14. July Canst. Jahres b. 1860);III:582.
12. BOZZINI P: Der Lichtleiter oder Beschreibung einer einfachen Vorrichtung und Anwendung zur Erleuchtung innerer Höhlen und Zwischenräumen des lebenden animalischen Körpers. Weimar Landes-Industrie-Comptoir 1807.
13. DÉSORMEAUX AJ: Proceedings of the Société de Chirurgie, Paris. Gazette des Hôp. 1865.
14. STEIN S: Das Photo-Endoskop. Berl. Klin. Wochenschr. Part 3, 1874.
15. NITZE H: Über eine neue Behandlungsmethode der Höhlen des menschlichen Körpers, Wien Med. Wochenschr. 1879;24:851–858.
16. STEINER OP: Abdominoskopie. Schweiz. Med. Wochenschr. 1924;54:84–87.
17. REDI R: Über ein neues endoskopisches chirurgisches Instrument, das Splanchnoskop, Zentralbl. Chir. 1935;558.
18. KORBSCH R: Lehrbuch und Atlas der Laparoskopie und Thorakoskopie. Munich, Lehmann 1927.
19. FERVERS C: Die Laparoskopie mit dem Cystoskop. Ein Beitrag zur Vereinfachung der Technik und zur endoskopischen Strangdurchtrennung in der Bauchhöhle. Med. Klin. Chir. 1933;178:288.
20. BOESCH PF: Laparoskopie. Schweiz Krankenhaus Anstaltsw. 1936;6:62.
21. POWER FH, BARNES AC: Sterilization by means of peritoneoscopic tubal fulguration: a preliminary report. Am. J. Obstet. Gynecol. 1941;41:1038.
22. GOETZE O: Die Röntgendiagnostik bei gasgefüllter Bauchhöhle; eine neue Methode Münch. Med. Wochenschr. 1918;65:1275–1280.
23. KALK H: Erfahrung mit der Laparoskopie (zugleich mit Beschreibung eines neuen Instrumentes). Z. Klin. Med. 1929;111:303–348.
24. PALMER R: Gynecologic celioscopy: Rapport of Prof. Mocquot. Acad. de Chir. 1946;72:363–368.
25. DECKER A: Pelvic culdoscopy. In Meigs JV, Sturgis, SH (eds): Progress in Gynecology New York, Grune & Stratton, 1946.
26. FRANGENHEIM H: Die Bedeutung der Laparoskopie für die gynäkologische Diagnostik. Fortschr. Med. 1958;76:451.
27. SCHWALM H: Die Laparoskopie in der gynäkolgishcen Diagnostik. In: Schwalm, H. G. Döderlein: Klinik der Frauenheilkunde und Geburtshilfe, Bd.I. S. 315. Uran & Schwarenberg, München 1964.
28. SEMM K: Statistical survey of Gynecologic Laparoscopy/Pelviscopy in Germany till 1977 Endoscopy 1979;11:101–106.
29. RUBIN IC: A. Amer. med. Ass. 75:661 (1920).
30. FIKENTSCHER R, SEMM K: Beitrag zur Methodik der utero-tubaren Perturbation. Geburtsh. u. Frauenheilk. 1955;15:313.

31. EISENBURG J: Über eine Apparatur zur schonenden und kontrollierbaren Gasfüllung der Bauchhöhle für die Laparoskopie. Klin. Wochenschr. 1966;44:593.
32. SEMM K: Die Laparoskopie in der Gynäkologie. Geburtsh. u. Frauenheilk. 1967;27:1029.
33. SEMM K: Operationslehre für endoskopische Abdominalchirurgie—operative Pelviskopie, Schattauer, Stuttgart 1984.
34. SEMM K: Operative Manual for Endoscopic Abdominal Surgery, Friedrich, ER (Trans. ed) Chicago, Year Book Medical Publishers, 1987 (German: Stuttgart, Schattauer, 1984; Japanese: Tokyo Central Foreign Books, 1986; Chinese: Shanghai, Shanghai Scientific & Technical Publishers, 1988; Italian: Naples, Martinucci, 1988.
35. COHEN MR: Laparoscopy, Culdoscopy and Gynecography, Technique and Atlas. Philadelphia, Saunders 1970.
36. SEMM K: Die kontrollierte und dosierbare Wärmekoagulation der gutartigen Portio-Veränderung. Geburtsh. u. Frauenheilk. 1965; 25: 795–802.
37. SEMM K: Tissue-puncher and loop ligation—new aids for for surgical therapeutic pelviscopy/laparoscopy = endoscopic intraabdominal surgery Endoscopy 1978;10:119–124.
38. SEMM K: Pelvi-Trainer, ein Übungsgerät für die operative Pelviskopie zum Erlernen endoskopischer Ligatur und Nahttechnik. Geburtsh. u. Frauenheilk. 1986;46:60–62.
39. SEMM K: Morzellieren und Nähen per pelviskopiam—kein Problem mehr. Geburtsh. u. Frauenheilk. 1991;51:843–846.
40. SEMM K: Hysterektomie per laparotomiam oder per pelviskopiam. Ein neuer Weg ohne Kolpotomie durch CASH. Geburtsh. u. Frauenheilk. 1991;51:773–777.
41. REICH H, DECAPRIO J and MCGLYNN F: Laparoscopic Hysterectomy. J. Gyecol. Surg. 1989; 5:213.
42. SEMM K: Tubal sterilization finally with cauterization or temporary with ligation via pelviscopy, in: Phillips JM and Keith L (eds): Gynecological Laparoscopy—Principles and Techniques. New York, Grune & Stratton 1974, pp 337–359.
43. SEMM K: Pelviskopie und Hysteroskopie—Farbatlas und Lehrbuch F.K. Schattauer, Stuttgart - New York 1976. (Translations: English: Saunders, Philadelphia 1977, French: Masson, Paris 1977; Spanish: Masson S.A., Barcelona 1977; Portuguese: Editoria Manole Sao Paulo 1977).
44. SEMM K: Endoscopic intraabdominal surgery Kiel, ISBN 3-922 500-16-1, 68 Seiten
45. SEMM K: Pelviskopie ein operativer Leitfaden 1991 Nach einer Organ-orientierten, Klassifizierung für "Minimal Invasive Chirurgie" Kiel, ISBN 3-922500-41-2, 05 Seiten.
46. SEMM K: Pelviscopy—operative guideline 1992 For "Minimally Invasive Surgery" following an Organ-orientated Classification Kiel, ISBN 3-922500-46-3, 92 Seiten.
47. SEMM K: Intrafasziale Hysterektomie per laparotomiam/per pelviskopiam durch CISH (Classical Intrafascial S(errated) E(dged) M(acro) M(orcellated) Hysterectomy und TUMA (Total Uterine Mucosa Ablation) 1993 Kiel, ISBN 3-922500-47-1, 123 Seiten.
48. SEMM K: Morcellation at Endoscopy. The Journal for European Private Hospitals Winter Edition 1995, page 69–72.
49. LEVINE RL: Economic impact of pelviscopic surgery. J Reprod Med 1985;30:655.
50. SEMM K: Intrafascial Hysterectomy per laparotomiam/per pelviscopiam/per vaginam using the CISH (Classic Intrafascial S(errated) E(dged) M(acro) M(orcellated) Hysterectomy— technique, TUMA (Total Uterine Mucosa Ablation) and IVH (Intrafascial Vaginal Hysterectomy) 1993 Kiel, ISBN 3-922500-52-8, 131 Seiten.
51. VIETZ PF, TS AHN: A new approach to hysterectomy without colpotomy: Pelviscopic intrafascial hysterectomy. Mosby Year Book, Inc., 1994, p. 609–613.
52. SEMM K: Totale Uterus Mucosa Ablatio (TUMA)-CURT anstelle Endometrium-Ablation. Geburtsh. u. Frauenheilk. 1992;52:773–777.
53. SEMM K: Intrafasziale vaginale Hysterektomie (IVH) mit oder ohne pelviskopischer Assistenz. Geburtsh. u. Frauenheilk. 1993;53:873–878.
54. NETZHAT, C, CROWGEY S, GARRISON C, HOOD J, WINER W, NETZHAT F: Videolaseroscopy and laser laparoscopy in gynecology Br. J. Hosp. Med. 1987;38:219–224.

Section II
Instrumentation

2
Instrumentation

Ronald L. Levine

The ever increasing number of instruments available to the surgeon with advanced gynecologic endoscopic skills continues to expand the horizon of operative laparoscopy. The terms operative laparoscopy and pelviscopic surgery are all encompassing designations for this approach to endoscopic surgery. In recent years the medical community in the United States has generally accepted operative laparoscopy as the preferred designation. The term "pelviscopy," as noted in Chapter 1, was originally coined by Professor Kurt Semm in Kiel, Germany for describing his laparoscopic surgical procedures. However, the terms operative laparoscopy and pelviscopic surgery are both used in a broad context to apply to all advanced gynecologic laparoscopic surgical procedures, utilizing all energy modalities, such as laser and electrosurgery.

There are numerous advantages to operative laparoscopy, among which are less postoperative pain and morbidity and in many cases decreased cost. This reduction of cost has been reported to be almost 50 percent.[1] Moreover, the patient's rapid return to the workplace and to normal activity has a marked economic impact when she may return to work one to three weeks earlier.[2]

Many gynecologic surgical procedures presented in subsequent chapters are amenable to the operative laparoscopic approach. The instruments required for operative laparoscopy should be viewed in much the same manner as the surgical instruments used for open laparotomy. All laparotomy sets have basic instruments that are found in almost any operating room. Just as some of the instruments that are used for one operative procedure differ from those used in another open case, so it is for operative laparoscopy. The basic instruments are discussed, and some special surgical requirements are outlined.

Regardless of the equipment used, the cardinal rule governing the use of all instruments is that the operator should be as familiar with them as a soldier is with his or her rifle. The surgeon should be able to take most instruments apart and reassemble them and should be familiar with how they work and how they are cleaned and maintained. Unfortunately, many surgeons depend solely on operating room personnel with their knowledge and training to assemble and maintain these complex, delicate instruments. Perhaps the best trademark of the laparoscopic surgeon, aside from dexterity, is the ability to be a gadgeteer who feels competent to trouble-shoot instrumentation problems. It is unavoidable, indeed inevitable, that occasional problems occur when using complex instruments. Trouble-shooting is a learned skill

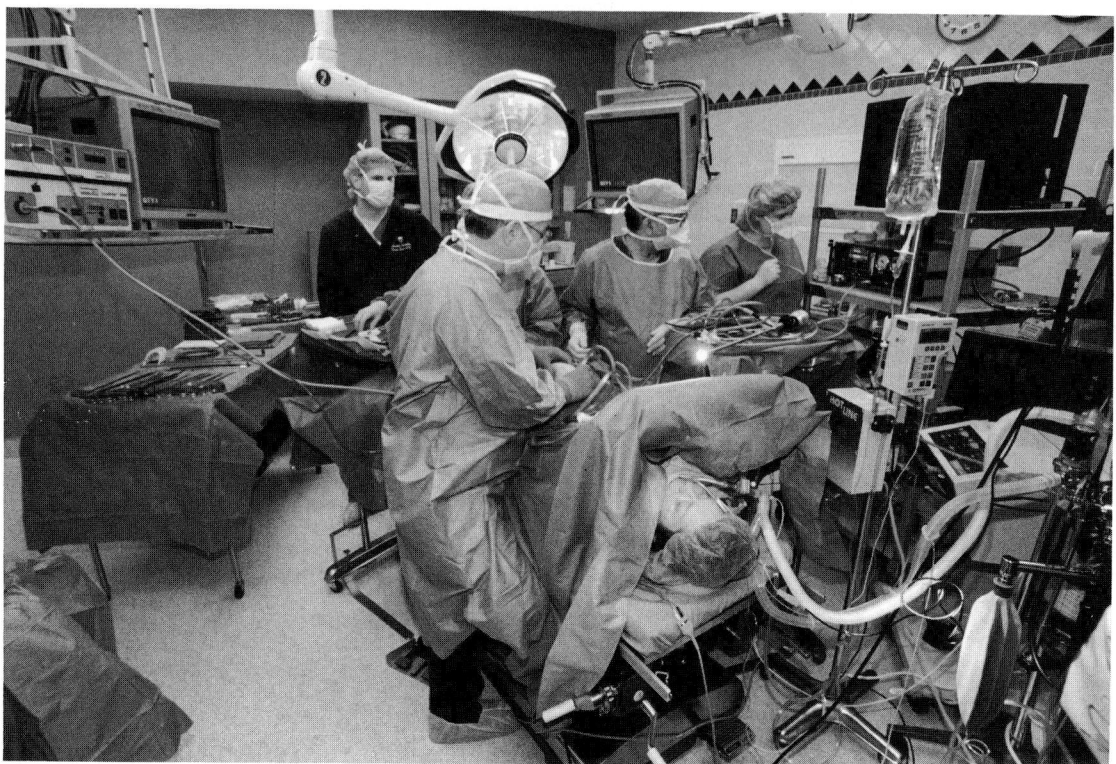

Figure 2.1. The modern operating room is brimming with equipment. Note the use of a video system that is suspended from the ceiling. The main instrument cart, opposite the surgeon, contains the insufflator and other electronic equipment. Two back tables are used to hold instruments. Two Mayo stands, one above the chest and one between the patient's legs, hold frequently used instruments. A biotechnician is present in the room to address any video or instrument problems. (Courtesy Jewish Hospital, Louisville, KY; and Christina M. Freitag, Photojournalist, Louisville, Ky)

and is possible only by throughly understanding the mechanics of the problem. One must start with the basics of the instrument, be able to work through the functions, and review the operation of the individual components. Many surgeons have witnessed the frustration and embarrassment that occurs when a large, complex gadget fails to work and it is finally discovered that the machine was not plugged in. The best answer to the failure of many instruments is to have backup for key pieces, although this situation is often financially prohibitive.

The modern laparoscopic operating room is laden with an array of electronic equipment, video equipment, and tables with operating instruments (Fig. 2.1). From the time the patient is brought into the operating room until the time she leaves, many instruments and varied equipment are used to perform the operative laparoscopy. This chapter presents an overview of basic equipment and introduces some innovative instruments that may be used for laparoscopic surgery. It is obvious that all instruments cannot be illustrated, but many of them from various manufacturers are presented.

Patient Positioning

Most standard operating tables can be used for operative laparoscopy if they allow placement in both steep Trendelenberg and Fowler positions. The table should accommodate stirrups and shoulder braces and have a support bridge for the surgeon's arm. The bridge allows the arm to remain steady while holding the camera.

2. Instrumentation

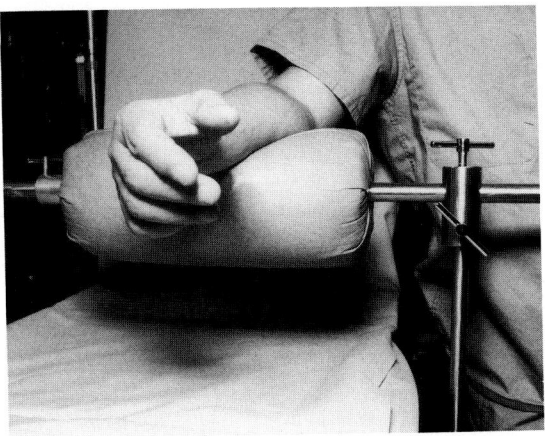

Figure 2.2. Hasson-Levine arm rest (Resnick Instrument, Skokie, IL) is attached to the side of the table and may be adjusted to any position over the patient's chest or neck to prevent the surgeon from leaning on her. The surgeon may rest an elbow when holding the laparoscope.

Such bridges are available commercially and can be adjusted to any position using sliding bars (Fig. 2.2). A homemade bridge can easily be constructed from a common ether screen using a padded board fitted to the crossbar of the screen, thus serving the purpose of support. It is important that the bar or bridge be securely fastened to the table to prevent the surgeon from accidentally falling onto the patient.

The patient's lower extremities must be properly placed in stirrups that provide adequate support but allow a proper amount of flexion of the thigh in relation to the trunk. If the flexion angle is too acute it becomes impossible to manipulate the lower instruments properly from both sides. An angle of about 145° allows adequate room for moving the instruments. The stirrups should be well padded to avoid compression of the popliteal nerve. The buttocks should extend slightly beyond the end of the table to allow full depression of a uterine manipulator to antevert the uterus. The stirrups should be able to be repositioned so the lower extremities may be placed in the traditional lithotomy position for procedures such as a laparoscopic-assisted vaginal hysterectomy (LAVH) (Fig. 2.3).

One of the first instruments used at the initiation of operative laparoscopy is a uterine manipulator. This device should be able not only to antevert the uterus but to position the uterus as needed depending on the procedures. There are many types of uterine manipulators, including the Semm vacuum cannula, Hulka uterine elevator, Cohen-Eder cannula, Valtchev uterine mobilizer, or perhaps something as simple as a small dilator taped to a tenaculum. A good manipulator not only should be able to mobilize the uterus well but should allow chromopertubation. The Valtchev mobilizer is popular as it permits manipulation of the fundus in all directions and is a totally reusable instrument. The Endopath Uterine Manipulator encompasses all of the above attributes but is available

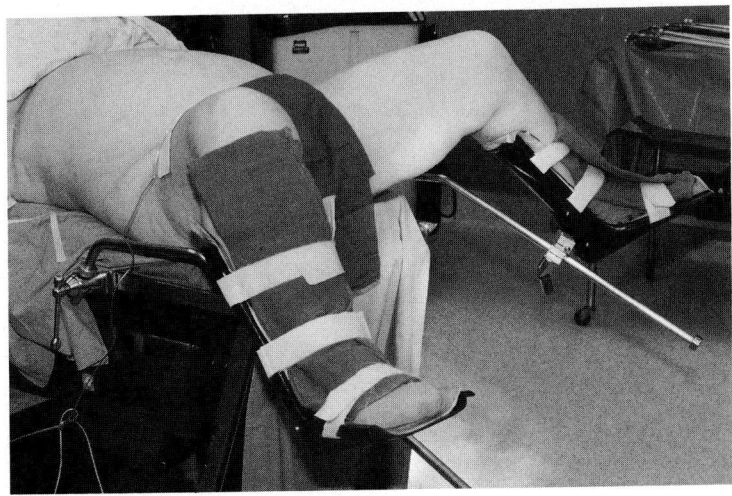

Figure 2.3. Allen Stirrups (Allen Medical Systems, Bedford Heights, OH) are ideal for supporting the lower extremities. Even in the case of an obese patient, positioning the legs can be accomplished with relative ease and safety. Note the padding and the position with little or no pressure on the popliteal nerve. (Courtesy Christina M. Freitag, Photojournalist, Louisville, Ky)

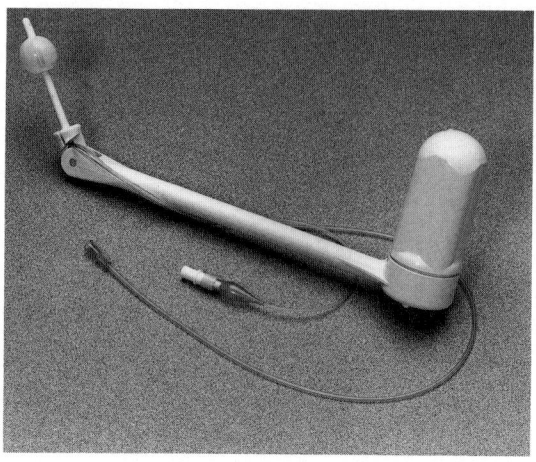

Figure 2.4. Endopath™ Clear View Uterine Manipulator (Ethicon Endosurgery, Cincinnati, OH) may be used as a uterine manipulator and permits excellent hydrotubation as well. When the balloon is inflated it provides a good seal and secures the device inside the uterine cavity. By turning the handle the fundus may be positioned in full anteversion or retroversion and easily held there.

at this time only as a disposable device (Fig. 2.4). Shoulder braces are imperative during operative laparoscopic surgery, as frequently it is necessary for patients to be placed in steep Trendelenburg position (more than 15°–20°) for a prolonged period. Without proper support the patient may rapidly slide toward the anesthesiologist. The padded shoulder braces must be placed with care over the acromion, keeping them as far lateral as possible to avoid compromising the neck (Fig. 2.5). It is recommended that a space the width of a finger be left between the shoulder and the brace to avoid undue pressure on the skin over the acromion. Casual use of the shoulder brace may lead to nerve injury in the neck or shoulder.

Insufflation

The standard procedures used to produce a pneumoperitoneum have been noted by many authors, with an excellent chapter describing the techniques written by Kleppinger in the *Manual of Endoscopy*, published by the American Association of Gynecologic Laparoscopists.[3] Because operative laparoscopic cases may be of relatively long duration and may involve cauterization, carbon dioxide is recommended over nitrous oxide as the insufflating agent. Carbon dioxide is also safer should a blood vessel inadvertently be punctured.[4] In a series of the author's patients, when monitoring end-tidal PCO_2, blood pH, and CO_2 partial pressures during prolonged laparoscopic cases, there have been no significant changes noted during normal general anesthetic ventilation.

In all but the most obese patient we use a standard 80 mm Veress needle to produce the pneumoperitoneum (these needles may also be

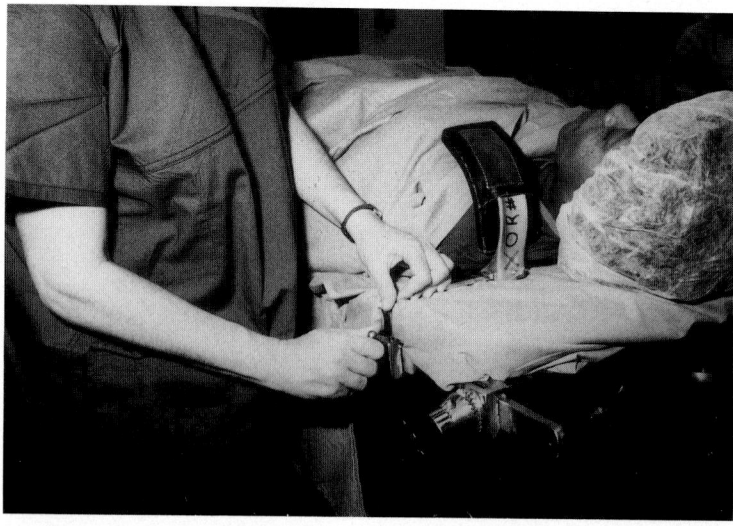

Figure 2.5. Shoulder braces are important for preventing the patient from sliding down the table when she is placed in a steep Trendelenburg position. The brace must be well padded and placed over the acromion, well away from the neck.

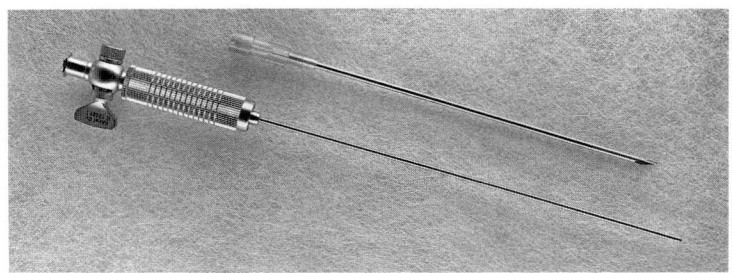

Figure 2.6. Semidisposable Veress-type needle. The outer metal sleeve is reusable, but the inner needle part is disposable and consequently is always sharp. (Courtesy of Advanced Surgical, Princeton, NJ)

purchased in longer lengths). Several types of Veress needle may be used. The standard reusable Veress needle has the disadvantage of becoming dull even after a few uses. If the reusable metal Veress needle is sharpened frequently, however, it is as functional and certainly less expensive than the disposable type. The disposable Veress needle has an advantage in always being sharp, which enhances its use, but the cost of disposable equipment must be considered. Some companies have developed a partially disposable product such as the eXcel-DR pneumoneedle (Fig. 2.6). This instrument consists of a reusable needle holder with a spring-loaded safety tip and a disposable needle, which combines economy and sharpness. Passage of the Veress needle is a blind procedure that sometimes creates difficulty by causing preperitoneal insufflation or omental or mesenteric emphysema. An instrument that has been designed to decrease injury secondary to insertion of the Veress needle is described as a pressure sensor-equipped Veress needle (Janicki Needle) (Fig. 2.7). It is a disposable instrument that contains a calibrated vacuum sensor and small light-emitting diodes that signal the moment the needle enters the negative pressure of the elevated peritoneal cavity. The surgeon can then immediately stop advancing the needle, should be relatively confident of the placement, and may begin insufflating.[5]

It is of utmost importance to use a high flow insufflator. If the insufflator cannot supply on demand a gas flow of approximately 4 L/min or more, adequate visualization cannot be maintained. Ideal insufflators can deliver rapid, accurate flow rates up to 15 L/min. However, it is obvious that the gas flow supplied at the outlet of the machine is not that delivered intraabdominally owing to the diameter and the distance of the connecting tubes. In actual measurements the true delivered amount at the end of the tubing may be only 60–70% of the capable flow rate of the insufflator.[6] Multiple punctures and frequent instrument changes result in a large loss of gas pressure unless high flow rates are available. For safety precautions it is mandatory that the operator be able to preset the insufflator to limit the insufflation pressure. Overpressurization of the peritoneal cavity has actual and theoretic dangers, not the least of which is possible occlusion of the inferior vena cava with subsequent loss of venous return to the heart. The instruments best suited for high flow insufflation are the electronic insufflators (Fig. 2.8). This equipment continually monitors the pressure and should be able to

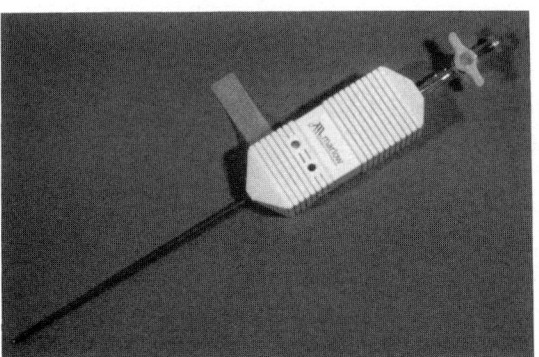

Figure 2.7. Janicki needle is used for insufflation. It has green and red light-emitting diodes and a pressure sensor. As soon as the negative pressure of the abdominal cavity is entered the light changes from red to green. (Courtesy of Marlow Surgical Technologies, Willoughby, OH)

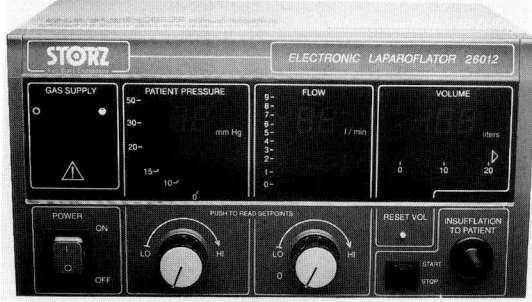

Figure 2.8. Electronic insufflators are a required necessity for modern operative laparoscopy. The basic insufflator must be able to provide a gas flow of at least 4L/ min. It must have dials to indicate the patient's intraabdominal pressure and flow rate. The volume dial is not needed, as the total volume used is unnecessary information. The insufflator should have adjustable pressure settings and should have a warning signal if intraabdominal pressure exceeds the surgeon's preset limits. (Courtesy Karl Storz Endoscopy-America, Culver City, CA)

reflect the true static intraabdominal pressure.[7] Regardless of the insufflator used, it is important that CO_2 be supplied from an external tank as well as an internal tank. Insufflators that use only internal tanks of CO_2 limit the quantity of gas available and may require frequent pauses to refill the internal supply. Some insufflators have the ability to warm the gas, thus decreasing the intraabdominal hypothermic effect of cold CO_2 gas and decreasing fogging of the distal lens of the laparoscope.

Gasless Insufflation

Several gasless insufflation techniques have been described, and theoretically there are advantages to these systems. They *may* avoid injury to bowel or large vessels by avoiding blind insertion of the Veress needle and the initial trocar. With this technique there is less danger of complications of pneumoperitoneum, such as hypercarbia or CO_2 embolism, as mentioned in the previous section. It is not necessary to check pressures or to depend on keeping the abdomen airtight, and the surgeon does not have to worry about gas leaks or suctioning out too much gas when evacuating smoke or suctioning out fluids. The Lift Retractor System (LRS) (Origin Medsystems, Menlo Park, CA) uses a fan-shaped retractor that is inserted inside the peritoneal cavity through a periumbilical incision; it is then opened, and the abdominal wall is lifted via an electrically powered lifting arm. Room air then enters the peritoneal cavity and allows enough room for visualization. Although the safety benefits have been stated, the disadvantages include decreased visibility and mechanical bruising of the abdominal wall. The cost of the initial equipment is high, and the use of elevators in the presence of severe adhesions is questionable.[8]

Optics

Numerous reports have been published on laparoscopy, laparoscopes, and video equipment; and the subject of video documentation and equipment is addressed in Chapter 5. It is important to address here the specific requirements of operative laparoscopic surgery as they relate to the laparoscope. It is important that a true perspective be obtained with as panoramic a view as possible, allowing the operator to coordinate the instruments properly, particularly for fine suturing or dissection. To obtain maximum resolution and imaging, we prefer a large scope: either 10 or 11 mm with a visual angle of 0° (180°). The 0° scope allows the more natural head on approach, permitting the surgeon to use normal perspective. The large scope is best suited for the video display. It is advantageous, however, to have the availability of a 5 mm laparoscope to be used through a secondary puncture site in a variety of operative situations, such as for lysis of adhesions. An operating laparoscope is almost mandatory during many procedures. If the surgeon uses a CO_2 laser, the instrument channel of the operating laparoscope may be utilized for conducting the laser beam into the abdomen to the target site (see Chapter 3). It is also advantageous to be able to use the operating channel for other instruments, such as dissecting scissors or grasp-

2. Instrumentation

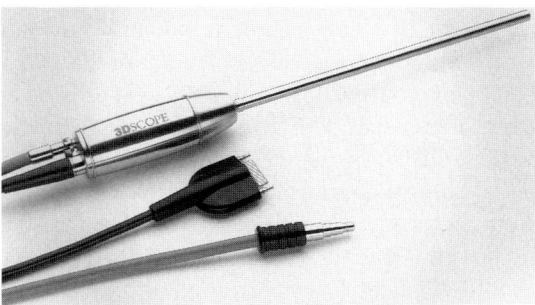

Figure 2.9. 3DScope system permits a three-dimensional view of laparoscopic surgery using a SteroLaparoscope, illustrated here. The scope produces two images that are merged by a digital processing system. The operating team wears special polarized glasses to view the procedure on a stereo video monitor. (Courtesy of American Surgical Technologies, Chelmsford, MA)

ers. Several three-dimensional laparoscopes have been developed allowing a three-dimensional video system to be used for laparoscopic surgery. The 3DScope produces two images that are then merged by a digital image processing technique. The surgeon and others in the operating room wear special polarized glasses and view the procedure on a stereo video monitor producing a three dimensional image. This system may be helpful when training surgeons and may facilitate suturing techniques (Fig. 2.9).

The bottom line with the use of any endoscope is the surgeon's ability to see well; therefore it is vital that fogging be prevented. Antifogging solutions are available; and it is recommended that they be applied prior to commencing surgery and be available for reapplication if needed during the procedure. Some laparoscopes (Hydro laparoscope, Circon ACMI, Stamford, CT) now have built in washers to clean the lens with water while operating. All experienced laparoscopists, however, are familiar with the technique of touching the fogged end of the scope to a piece of omentum or the uterus for rapid defogging. Fogging between the camera and the scope, which occurs at times, can be an annoying problem. The newer cameras have incorporated a number of methods to obviate this difficulty.

Support Cart

A large, movable cart is positioned on the side of the table opposite the surgeon. It can hold most of the electrical devices necessary for the operative laparoscopic surgery. By placing the cart on the opposite side, the surgeon is able to view all the dials. Basic equipment includes the insufflator, the light source, possibly the electric generator for bipolar and unipolar instruments, and an irrigator pump of some type, such as the Nezhat-Dorsey (American Hydro-Surgical Instruments, Delray Beach, FL). An endocoagulating device may be on the cart as well as the generator for the Harmonic scalpel (UltraCision, Smithfield, RI).

Instruments

Instruments may be divided into several groups and subgroups according to size, function, and ability to be reused or disposed. The debate regarding disposable instruments has been waged for some time and has fierce proponents on each side. Any discussion involving disposable instruments must address economics, safety, sterility, function, and environmental impact. Such a discussion would involve a chapter of and by itself. There are obvious benefits to some of the disposable instruments, and some are so beneficial as to outweigh the marked disadvantages of cost and disposal.[9]

The argument of disposable versus reusable equipment may be focused on *trocars and sheaths*. There has also been a continuing area of contention regarding the style of the tip used on the trocar. Some surgeons favor the pyramidal tip, whereas others extol the virtues of the conical tip. Each has its advantages, but the most important issue is sharpness. If the trocar is sharp, punctures are safer and easier regardless of the tip employed.[10] If reusable metal trocars are used, it is the responsibility of the surgeon to check the sharpness of the trocar and ensure that it is on a scheduled sharpening program. Many types of disposable and reusable trocars and sheaths are obtainable. One of the advantages of disposable trocars (other than sharpness) is the availability of stabilizing de-

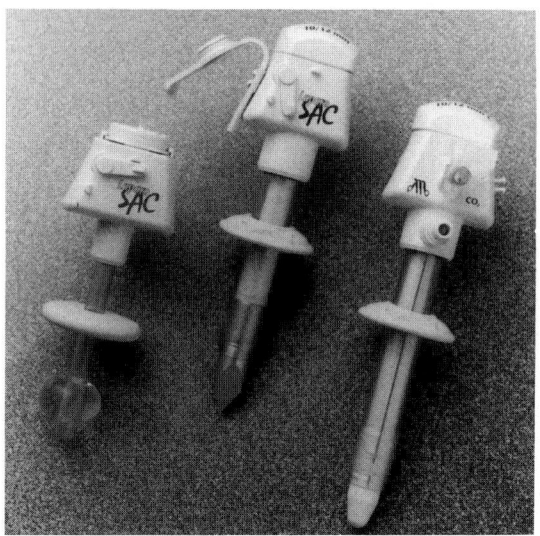

Figure 2.10. Trocar sleeves frequently are pulled out because of the numerous instrument changes necessary during operative laparoscopy. There are several ways to prevent sleeve removal. The stable access cannula (SAC) shown here, has a balloon on the end that is inflated with water and pulled up tight against the abdominal wall; the upper sleeve is then pushed down against the skin, stabilizing the cannula and preventing its accidental removal. (Courtesy Marlow Surgical Technologies, Willoughby, OH)

vices such as the Stable Access Cannula (SAC) (Fig. 2.10); it uses a balloon that is inflated after insertion to prevent accidental withdrawal. Other disposables, such as the Surgiport (US Surgical Corp., Norwalk, CT) and the Endopath, use a screw type apparatus to hold the cannula in place (Fig. 2.11). Another advantage of the disposable cannula is the ability to use various attachments to permit changing the diameter of the entry with step up and step down additions to the top of the cannula. Some reusable trocars also have reducers that permit a change in diameter (Karl Storz Endoscopy-America, Culver City, CA).

The retractable covering over the tips of many disposable trocars are said to help protect against injury to major vessels, but injury is still possible to the bowel and even to the vessels. One must have proper training on insertion techniques and not depend on the so-called safety shields. The argument may also be made for the open laparoscopy technique of Hasson.[11] The open laparoscopy cannula is best utilized as a reusable instrument, although equivalent disposable instruments are available. A technique called blunt trocar laparoscopy[12] utilizes a blunt, conical tip in an operative sleeve that has an integral thread to produce an airtight seal (Apple Medical Corporation, Bolton, MA). A unique approach to possibly safer entry with a trocar has been introduced by the ConMed Aspen Surgical Systems (Utica, NY). They describe an electronic trocar system in which the trocar uses a pure cut electrical current delivered from a special electrosurgical unit that stops the current as soon as the body wall is penetrated. Theoretically, this device is less likely to cause damage to underlying tissue, as the tip is dull and the cutting is performed strictly by the cutting current, which instantly stops as soon as the pneumoperitonealized cavity is breached. If bowel is stuck to the anterior abdominal wall, however, injury is unavoidable. In an attempt to preclude any damage to either bowel or blood vessels, the US Surgical Company has introduced a disposable 10.5 m trocar with a port through which a laparoscope is placed; the trocar is advanced through the tissue under direct vision while a small blade makes progressive tiny cuts (Fig. 2.12). This style instrument may have some use in patients with

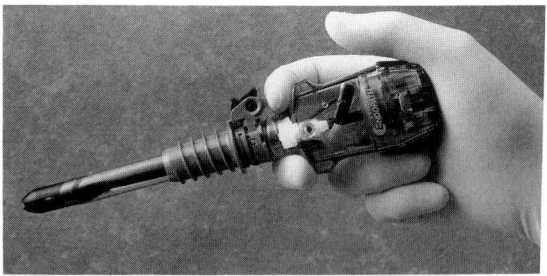

Figure 2.11. Technique for holding a trocar sleeve in place. An Endopath TriStar trocar has a screw type stabilizer in place. When the sleeve is twisted into the incisional site, the threads hold the cannula in the abdominal wall, helping to avert accidental withdrawal of the cannula. (Courtesy of Ethicon Endo-Surgery, Cincinnati, OH)

2. Instrumentation

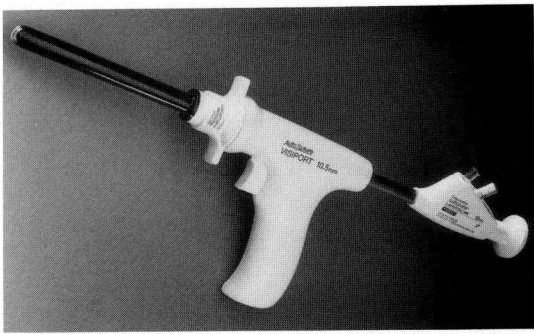

Figure 2.12. Visiport uses a laparoscope in the sleeve. The tip is translucent, allowing a view through it and permitting the tip to be held tight against the tissue. Each time the trigger is pulled a tiny knife makes progressive, small cuts; the surgeon can then visualize the tissues layer by layer, thus attempting to prevent inadvertent entry into bowel when entering the abdominal cavity. (Courtesy US Surgical, Norwalk, CT)

suspected multiple adhesions, although no system is completely protective against injury to bowel. Another innovative system has been described, the Step system (InnerDyne Medical, Sunnyvale, CA), but at this time the technique has had only limited trials. With this system a special Veress needle is inserted through an expandable sheath. The needle is then withdrawn, and the sheath may be subsequently dilated to a 5, 10, or 12 mm diameter, depending on the surgeon's needs, without the danger of a sharp entry. Original entry ports are most often 10 or 11 mm, and secondary ports may range from 3 to 12 mm. Some surgeons prefer ports that have no valves and that have the self-retaining screw as part of the instrument (Reich self-retaining sleeve; Richard Wolf Medical Instruments, Vernon Hills, IL).

Operating Instruments

Instruments may be divided into several categories: grasping, cutting, hemostatic, suturing, irrigation, and specialty. Within these categories are several subcategories such as disposable and nondisposable and various sizes (i.e., 5 mm or 10–12 mm).

Grasping Instruments

Graspers come in a multitude of shapes and sizes with a variety of handles and tips. Generally this type of instrument has two forms of tip: traumatic and atraumatic. Atraumatic instruments are used to hold and move tissue that is to remain in the abdomen, such as the fallopian tube or the bowel, with minimal trauma. The tips should appear dull (Fig. 2.13). When purchasing equipment, it is best to test how atraumatic a grasper is by gripping the web space of the hand between the thumb and forefinger with the grasper; there should be no discomfort, and it should feel gentle. Traumatic graspers have sharper tips and are used to immobilize tissue that either does not bleed or presents no concern to the surgeon if it is damaged. There are several tip configurations, including multipronged graspers such as the bulldog type as described by Hasson (Fig. 2.14). Large 10 or 11 mm graspers also have different shapes and usage. The large alligator tips may be used to extract segments of tissue from the abdomen (Fig. 2.15) and spoon forceps (Fig. 2.16) may be used to remove soft tissue and clots; the latter are useful for ectopic pregnancy surgery.

Several handles are available, some with traditional surgical grips with or without a box-lock, and others with spring operated mechanisms designed to be self-retaining. Other handles may appear strange to the surgeon but may have some utility, such as round-handled instruments (Fig. 2.17). These instruments can be eas-

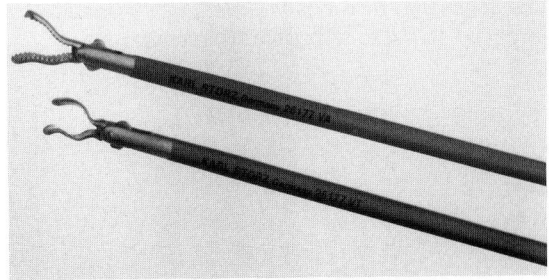

Figure 2.13. Two types of atraumatic grasper tip. Vancaille ovarian and mesoovarian forceps. (Courtesy of Karl Storz Endoscopy-America, Culver City, CA)

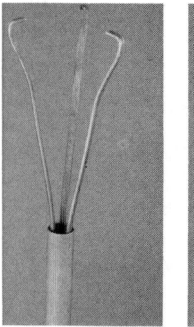 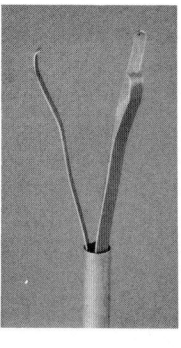 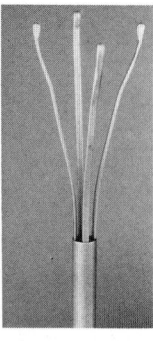

Figure 2.14. Multiprong forceps designed by Hasson. The sharp tip style on the left is called the bulldog because of the firm but traumatic grasp it provides.

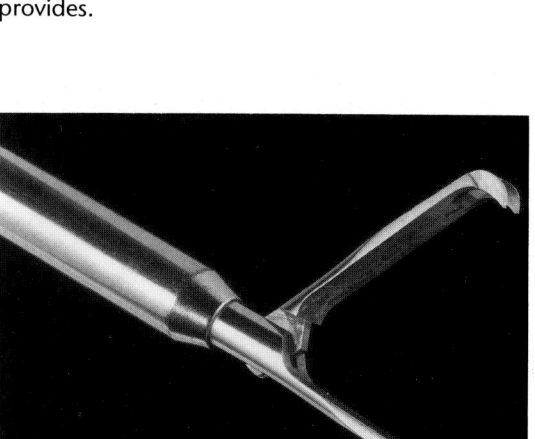

Figure 2.15. Large alligator jaw forceps are used through a 10 mm port and provide a firm grasp on tissue to be extirpated. The jaws may be opened wide and the teeth are sharp, so care must be taken to grip only tissue that does not bleed. Using this instrument through a large port with a twisting technique to compress tissue affords the ability to remove a sizable amount of material.

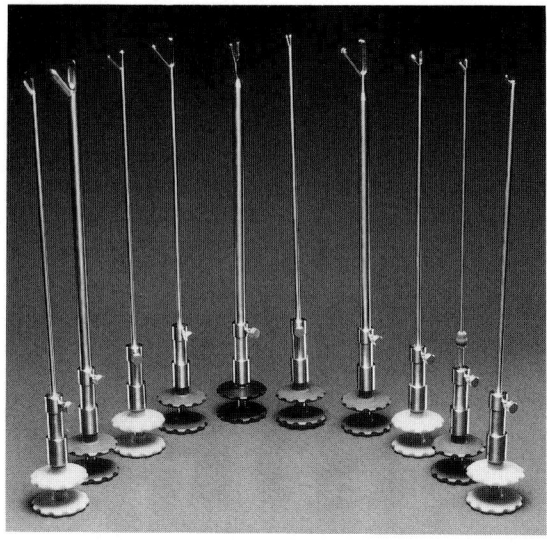

Figure 2.17. Round handles on a variety of instruments are also color coded. These handles are particularly good for graspers and needle holders, as they can easily be turned in any direction and still provide a firm grasp. (Courtesy of Wisap USA, Lenexa, KS)

ily oriented in any plane within the body and they provide a firm grasp.

When acquiring new instruments it is important that the surgeon test the various types of handle. A handle that is appropriate for a 220 pound man may be unmanageable for a 90 pound, 5 foot tall woman. Many instruments are now available in disposable form, but I do not believe it is cost-effective or necessary to use disposable graspers. The one justification for the purchase of disposable graspers is to keep one on a backup cart as a reserve in case a reusable instrument is broken and unrepairable during a case.

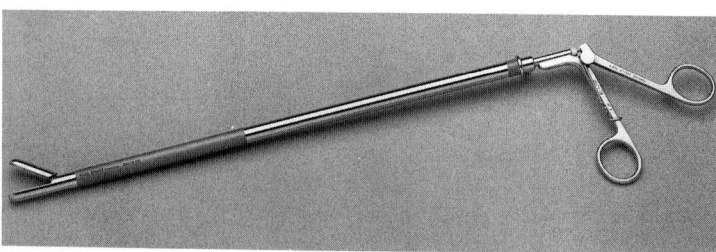

Figure 2.16. Semm spoon forceps is a 10 mm instrument with large trough-shaped jaws that permit removal of large amounts of tissue or clots. (Courtesy Karl Storz Endoscopy-America, Culver City, CA)

2. Instrumentation

Cutting Instruments

Scissors are an important cutting tool of laparoscopy. The hooked type is the most common variety and is usually strong with wide-ranging utility. Unfortunately, they frequently become dull rapidly. Hence disposable scissors have gained popularity, although the problem of cost-effectiveness remains a hotly debated issue. The most practical answer to the problem of cost versus utility was answered by the semi-disposable instruments, which have replaceable tips and reusable handles. This type of instrument cuts the cost by more than one-third and allows use of different styles of scissors, such as straight or curved, and the advantage of always having sharp blades on the scissor tips. Most scissors are 5 mm instruments; 10 mm scissors are available but are rarely if ever needed. Microscissor tips are available on the end of some 3 or 5mm instruments. The fine tips are excellent for dissecting the fimbria, but maintaining the sharpness of this instrument continues to be a problem.

Laparoscopic cutting may also be performed with electrosurgical needles, knife or hook electrodes, lasers, and the Harmonic scalpel. These modalities are discussed later in special areas.

Hemostatic Instruments

Without the ability to maintain adequate hemostasis, surgery is not possible, as the ultimate consequence of incising living tissue is bleeding. The surgeon must be able to control mild bleeding, not only from small capillaries or veins but also from some moderately large vessels, such as the uterine and ovarian arteries.

Electrocoagulation

High frequency electrical energy has been used during surgery for nearly a century, but only recently has the theory regarding its use during operative laparoscopy been reported. The use of unipolar and bipolar energy is presented in Chapter 4. It is important that the laparoscopic surgeon know that both unipolar and bipolar instrumentation should be available for both dissection and coagulation purposes to facilitate hemostasis. Without this modality operative laparoscopy would be virtually impossible. The electrosurgical generator must be able to supply both modes of energy (bipolar and unipolar). Most generators have two controls to regulate the power output: one to produce the coagulation waveform and the other for cutting. It is important to understand that the number setting on one machine has no relation to another company's model. Some units show the wattage output directly with a digital readout dial, whereas others have only a chart that indicates the power for a particular setting. It is most important to have a unit that has a built in ammeter to assist the surgeon using bipolar forceps in determining an endpoint of coagulation/desiccation. The ammeter, which displays the current flow, indicates no current when the tissue is completely desiccated and hence coagulated, signaling hemostasis.

The most popular bipolar instrument is the Kleppinger-type forceps. These forceps are also available with a microtip, allowing small vessels (such as are found when dissecting the fimbria) to be coagulated. Unipolar electrode tips may be obtained in numerous styles, from hook ends, spatula tips, needle tips, ball tips, to a host of other forms. They may be reusable or disposable. The bipolar and unipolar electrodes are most often controlled by a foot pedal switch, although some unipolar electrodes have hand-switching capability (Valleylab, Boulder, CO).

Cabot Medical (Langhorn, PA) has introduced the Seitzinger Tripolar cutting forceps. This instrument is a bipolar grasping forceps with a built-in blade. Tissue may be grasped and then bipolar-coagulated; then, while still grasping the tissue a guillotine-type blade may be activated to transect the tissue between the jaws of the forceps. This instrument theoretically can save time and cost by decreasing the number of instrument changes and eliminating the need for a stapler.

Endocoagulation

The endocoagulator is a Semm innovation that uses direct heat in the range of 90°–120°C for hemostasis. The basic instrument is switched on and off with a foot pedal, and the temperature of the tip and the coagulation time are preset.

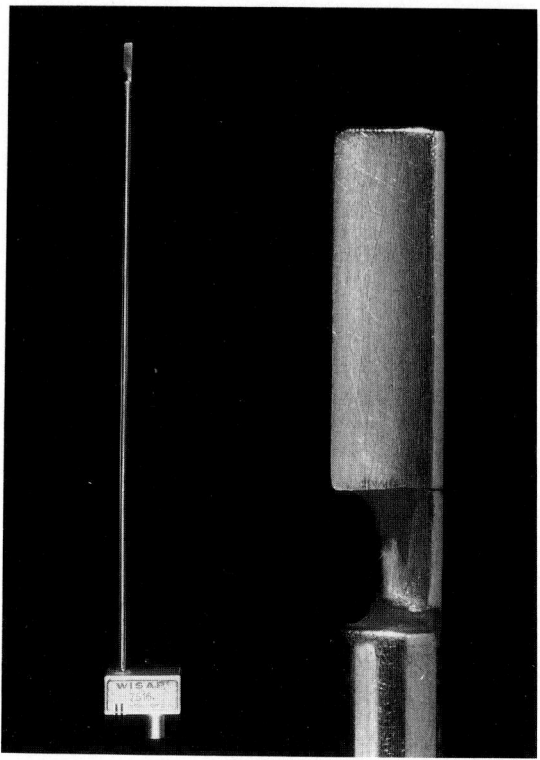

Figure 2.18. Myoma enucleator may be passed through a 5 mm port. The knife-type tip shown here uses direct heat to facilitate cutting while it coagulates. It is a safe, simple method for enucleating a myoma or for cutting across the base of a pedunculated tumor.

including a blunt tip for point coagulation, an alligator-type grasper for coagulating pedicles, and a knife-type instrument called a myoma enucleator (Fig. 2.18). The enucleator may be used with maximum safety for a myomectomy. With the advent of newer hemostatic modalities, however, endocoagulation has assumed a decreased role in laparoscopic surgery.

Lasers

The subject of laser energy is discussed in Chapter 3. Lasers can be used not only for cutting but for hemostasis by coagulating protein. The necessity of having lasers available is a controversial subject. The proponents of fiber lasers (KTP, argon, Nd:YAG) and supporters of the CO_2 laser have cogent arguments to support their particular prejudice toward each energy source. Each wavelength has different characteristics in regard to tissue effects, absorption, smoke production, and other parameters (Table 2.1). Many surgeons now use lasers only in a limited way because of the cost, although certain applications for this energy source are desirable.

Harmonic Energy

The Harmonic Scalpel (UltraCision, Smithfield, RI) system uses mechanical energy to both cut and coagulate. The Harmonic generator (Fig. 2.19) sends an electrical signal through a shielded coaxial cable to a transducer in the instrument. The transducer then converts the electrical energy to mechanical motion, resulting in a vibration of 55,500 cycles per second (cps) at either the blade tip or the anvil tip of the laparoscopic

There is an acoustic musical tone that increases and decreases according to the temperature. The surgeon can determine when the intraabdominal instruments are hot or cool by listening to the tone. There are varied tip styles,

Table 2.1. Comparison of various lasers

Parameter	CO_2	Nd:YAG	KTP	Argon
Wavelength (nm)	10,600	1064	532	488–514
Penetration (mm)	0.2	5.0	2.0	1.0
Beam delivery	Articulated arm	Fiber	Fiber	Fiber
Smoke production	High	High	Low	Moderate
Cutting	Good	Fair	Good	Poor
Coagulation	Poor	Good	Good	Fair

Note: The characteristics are different, permitting diverse application of each wavelength laser.

2. Instrumentation

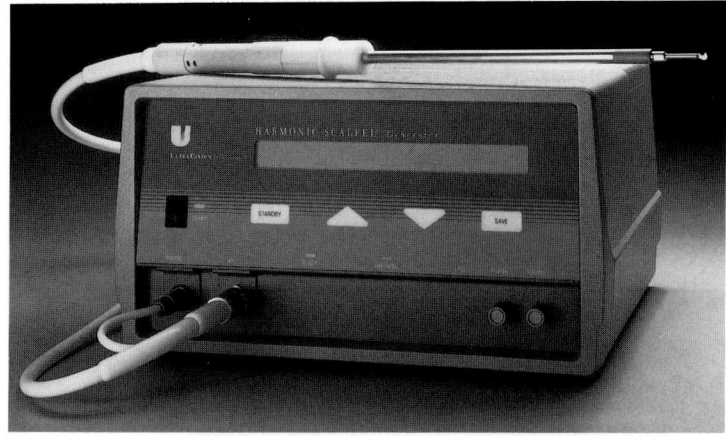

Figure 2.19. Harmonic Scalpel generator is self contained. It provides a range of power and has controls to supply either variable or full power and an acoustic signal. No cooling or special electrical connection is necessary. (Courtesy of UltraCision, Smithfield, RI)

coagulating shears (LCS). The Harmonic Scalpel vibrates over a distance of 80 μm, and protein in the tissue is denatured mechanically, forming a coagulum. The protein coagulum "welds" tissues around bleeding vessels, and larger vessels are sealed as they are coapted and then "welded." The advantage of this system seems to be the fact that the tip remains cool; consequently little heat is generated, and the thermal injury zone is claimed to only be 50–150 μm. There is no charring, and little smoke is produced. The tip of the 5 mm probes may be a dissecting hook used to cut and coagulate (Fig. 2.20) or a ball tip used only for coagulation (Fig. 2.21). The grasper-like instrument with jaws that may be used for cutting or coagulation is called the LCS (Fig. 2.22). The disadvantages of the Harmonic system include the fact that the LCS instrument requires a 12 mm port, and at this time the tips are disposable, which adversely affects the cost.

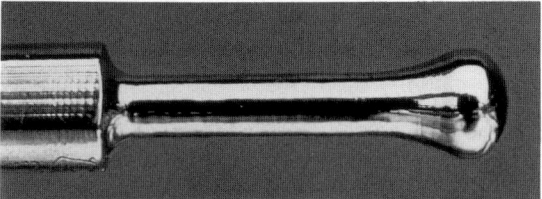

Figure 2.21. Ball coagulator tip for the Harmonic blade system. This tip is useful for coagulating large surfaces, such as the defect created during myomectomy. (Courtesy of UltraCision, Smithfield, RI)

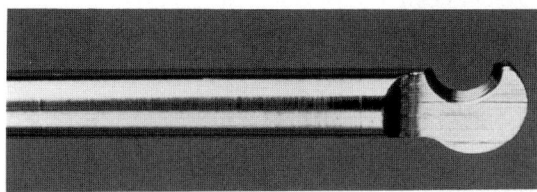

Figure 2.20. A 5 mm laparoscopic blade called a dissecting hook. This instrument is 32 cm in length with a sharp hook end that can be used for cutting. The flat side may be used for coagulation. The sharp tip may be used for incising a uterine tube to remove an ectopic pregnancy. (Courtesy of UltraCision, Smithfield, RI)

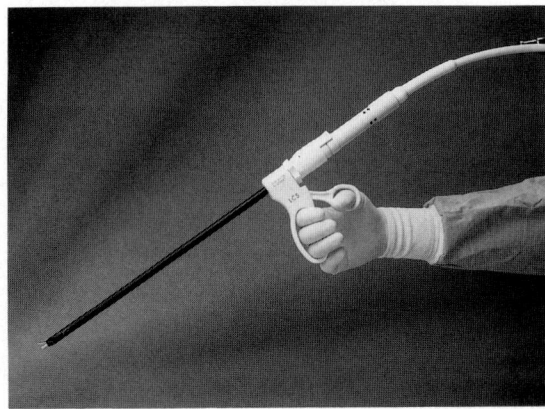

Figure 2.22. Laparoscopic coagulating shears (LCS) must be used through a 12 mm port. The tip has one jaw that is an anvil, which receives the energy; the other jaw does not. The nonactivated jaw may be rotated to expose a blunt edge (used for coagulation) or a sharp edge (used for cutting). (Courtesy of UltraCision, Smithfield, RI)

Argon Beam Coagulator

The argon beam coagulator (ABC) produces a jet of argon gas at 4L or more per minute and a high voltage current to create an electrical arc that fulgurates and does not penetrate tissue deeply. The effect is similar to that of the unipolar electrosurgery used for fulguration. The ABC creates a "blast effect" on the tissue before impact and has been found by some authors to be an excellent coagulator.[13] The ABC produces powerful fulguration and so is useful for coagulating a large area such as is found during myomectomy. A major difficulty that may be encountered because of the high flow rate of the argon gas is a marked increase in intraperitoneal pressure. The surgeon must be aware of this possibility and use some type of suction evacuation to maintain the pressure at the usual 16–20 mm Hg. The probe may be a 5 or 10 mm instrument and may be used to paint over the tissue thereby forming an eschar and controlling the bleeding. When the ABC was used as the primary technique to control hemostasis in a study involving 200 women the results were favorable, and the speed of tissue coagulation was reported to be faster than that of conventional bipolar and unipolar techniques.[14]

Suturing and Ligating Instruments

Laparoscopic suturing is often not necessary for most operative laparoscopic procedures. Laparoscopic ligation has been infrequently required since the advent of stapling and clip application. There are some techniques, however, that still require suturing and knot tying skills. The main instrument for suturing, as for open laparotomy, is the needle holder. Most needle holders or drivers are 5 mm, although 3 mm instruments are also available. Laparoscopic needle holders must maintain a strong hold on the needle and ideally be able to prevent a curved needle from rotating. The Cook endoscopic curved needle driver has a spring-loaded handle and a tip with a hook that pulls into a sleeve, thus anchoring the needle rather securely (Fig. 2.23). The force holding the needle is dependent on the spring tension. This instrument is available in right- and left-handed versions that hold the needle at a 45° angle rather then the traditional 90°. A different type of needle

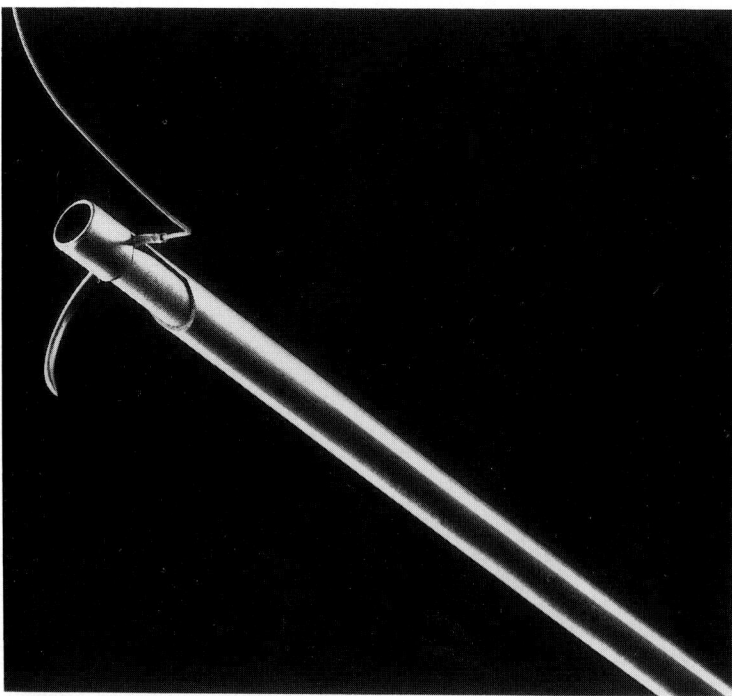

Figure 2.23. Cook needle driver has a tip that holds the needle securely in the correct position in relation to the axis of the shaft of the instrument. The tip may also be obtained in a 45° angle that is available as a left handed or right-handed instrument. (Courtesy of Cook Ob/Gyn, Spencer, IN)

2. Instrumentation

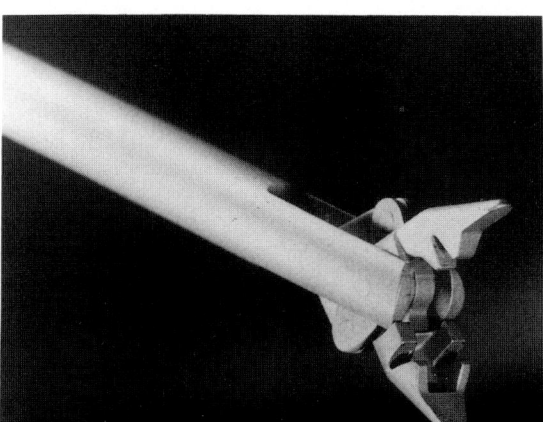

Figure 2.24. The Levine needle holder has notched jaws to hold the needle tight in the correct position. It also has a flat platform tip that enables the surgeon to grasp the suture without cutting it. (Courtesy of Marlow Surgical Technologies, Willoughby, OH)

driver is the Levine needle holder, which grips the needle in notched jaws and uses a traditional-type handle; thus the harder the surgeon grips the handle, the firmer is the grasp of the needle. The notch holds a curved needle in place, preventing the needle from twisting as might occur with traditional jaws (Fig. 2.24). The same principle applies to the round handles of the Wisap needle holders (Wisap USA;

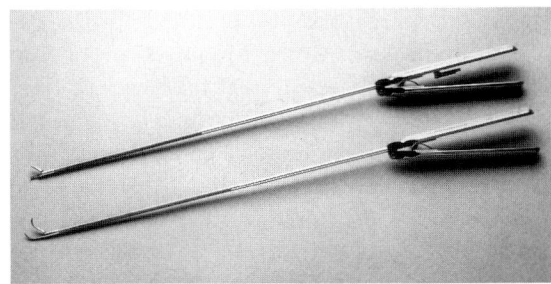

Figure 2.25. Szabo-Berci needle driver set has a needle holder and an instrument to assist in driving the needle through the tissue and grasping the suture. The handles on these instruments allow a firm grasp on the needle and are ergonomically advantageous. (Courtesy of Karl Storz Endoscopy-America, Culver City, CA)

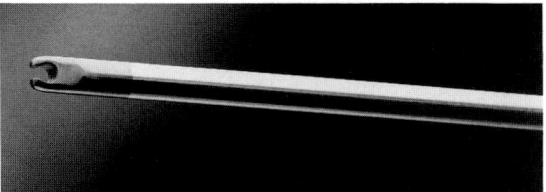

Figure 2.26. The Clarke-Reich knot ligator is available as a 5 mm or 3 mm instrument. A single throw of a knot, usually a square knot, can be pushed with the notched end of this instrument into the abdomen and tightly set. (Courtesy of Marlow Surgical Technologies, Willoughby, OH)

Leneka, KS), which have hooked ends: the tighter the grip the tighter the grasp of the needle. Other needle drivers have tips similar to those of the classic needle holder used for open laparotomy, with tungsten carbide inserts to encourage a tighter grasp on the needle. Some of these instruments are designed with tips that are right-handed, left-handed, or universal; others have a different style handle, such as the Szabo-Berci needle driver set. This instrument has a unique coaxial handle design that allows complete instrument rotation (Fig. 2.25).

Suturing, as originally described by Semm, may use 3 and 5 mm needle holders with classic type jaws and usually involves the use of the loop ligature for extracorporeal ties.[15] Extracorporeal knot-tying is performed using the Clarke-Reich ligator (Fig. 2.26), which is available in 3 and 5 mm sizes. It is used to push a knot, formed outside the abdomen, down through a trocar port.[16] Suturing and knot-tying techniques are described in Chapter 19.

Irrigation Instruments

Irrigation and aspiration are necessary for operative laparoscopy because without a clear surgical field the surgeon is literally blinded. Irrigation is used to clear away debris, blood clots, and the char that may be produced by electrosurgery or laser treatment. The ideal irrigator must be able to produce enough hydraulic pressure to disrupt clots and allow "aquadissection," but it also should have an easily controlled hand valve for suction aspiration.

Aspiration may be used not only for fluid but to remove smoke and plume that can limit visibility. It is also important to have as large a flow channel as possible so large clots may be evacuated rapidly without clogging the instrument. If the probe tip is to be used for suctioning near bowel, it is imperative that it have several small holes near its end to avoid pulling bowel into the probe, resulting in possible damage to the viscera. In contrast, if aquadissection is required, the tip should be solid. Many instruments are available, but I mainly use the Nezhat-Dorsey system because the probes can be changed to a variety of configurations and are reusable. The pump system supplies adequate pressure and may use a variety of irrigating solutions (Fig. 2.27). Other companies have similar instruments with different cannulas, some of which have a flexible tip that can be used without damaging the bowel (Gleeson FloVac, ConMed, Aspen Surgical Systems, Utica, NY). Other systems are simple and utilize only a syringe apparatus to supply the fluid pressure and suction (Pump Vac Plus; Marlow Surgical Technologies, Willoughby, OH). A number of systems have a pulsatile fluid jet that produces high-pressure liquid pulsations by using compressed nitrogen (Gyne-Flo Pump; Bard Instruments, Franklin Lakes, NJ). This type of system is excellent for breaking up large clots.

Specialty Instruments

Staples and Clips

Staples and clips play an important role in operative laparoscopy. Disposable stapling instruments can place six staggered rows of titanium staples and then sever the tissue between the rows, with three rows on each side of the cut. The stapling instrument requires a 12 mm sleeve. The usual instrument takes a 3 cm bite; newer instruments take even more tissue (6 cm) but require a larger trocar sleeve. If one bite is not adequate, another cartridge of staples may be placed in the instrument (Fig. 2.28). Although these instruments allow rapid hemostasis with minimal production of necrotic tissue, there have been numerous detractors of this technique. The argument against this type of instrumentation is based mainly on its cost. Johns stated that when four to eight cartridges are used during an LAVH any economic advantage of the procedure over abdominal hysterectomy is quickly lost.[17] The two most popular

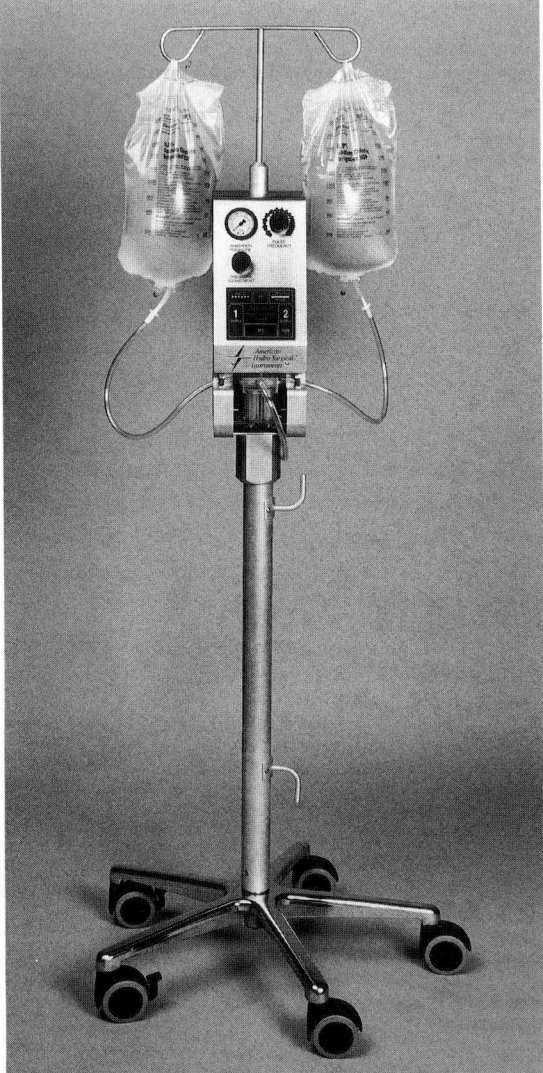

Figure 2.27. Nezhat-Dorsey system II pump is pneumatically powered and uses compressed gas to supply the power for irrigation. It can operate in either a continuous flow or a pulsed irrigation mode with irrigation pressures controllable from 0 to 2500 mm Hg. This type system uses irrigation bags in lieu of bottled irrigation fluid, which is cost-effective. (Courtesy of American Hydro-Surgical Instruments, Delray Beach, FL)

2. Instrumentation

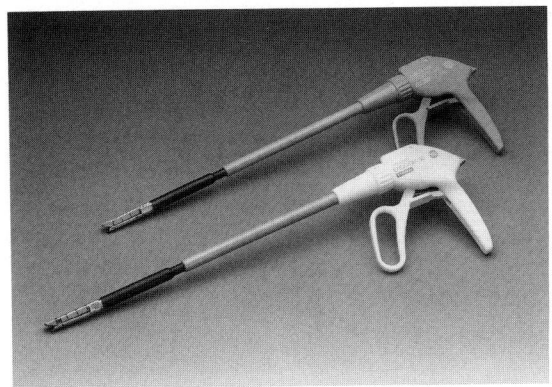

Figure 2.28. Endo GIA is introduced through a 12 mm trocar sheath. The jaws permit a 3 cm bite; and when fired, a double row of titanium staples are placed. The instrument simultaneously incises the tissue between the rows. (Courtesy US Surgical, Norwalk, CT)

among general surgeons. The individual clips are made of titanium. The most popular use has been for cholecystectomy, special clip applicators have now been used for hernia repair and fixing a nonabsorbable mesh over a defect. Stapling instruments use a 10 mm port and usually are supplied with about 20 staples per cartridge.

Mini-Instruments

Several instruments with small diameters have been described. They range from small laparoscopes to mini-trocars and grasping instruments. The Cook mini-retractor set has an introducing shaft of only 8F (2.7 mm) and 14 cm length. The grasping instruments are 5F (1.7 mm) and 30 cm in length, and they are controlled by a spring tension handle. The grasping tip may be a rat-tooth forceps or an alligator forceps. The introducing sheath is held in place with a silicon retention disk (Fig. 2.29). This type of instrument may be useful with delicate tissues, such as fimbria.

instruments are produced by the US Surgical Corporation (Norwalk, CT) and Ethicon Endo-Surgery (Cincinnati, OH).

Stapling instruments are valuable for hemostasis of large vessels and have become popular

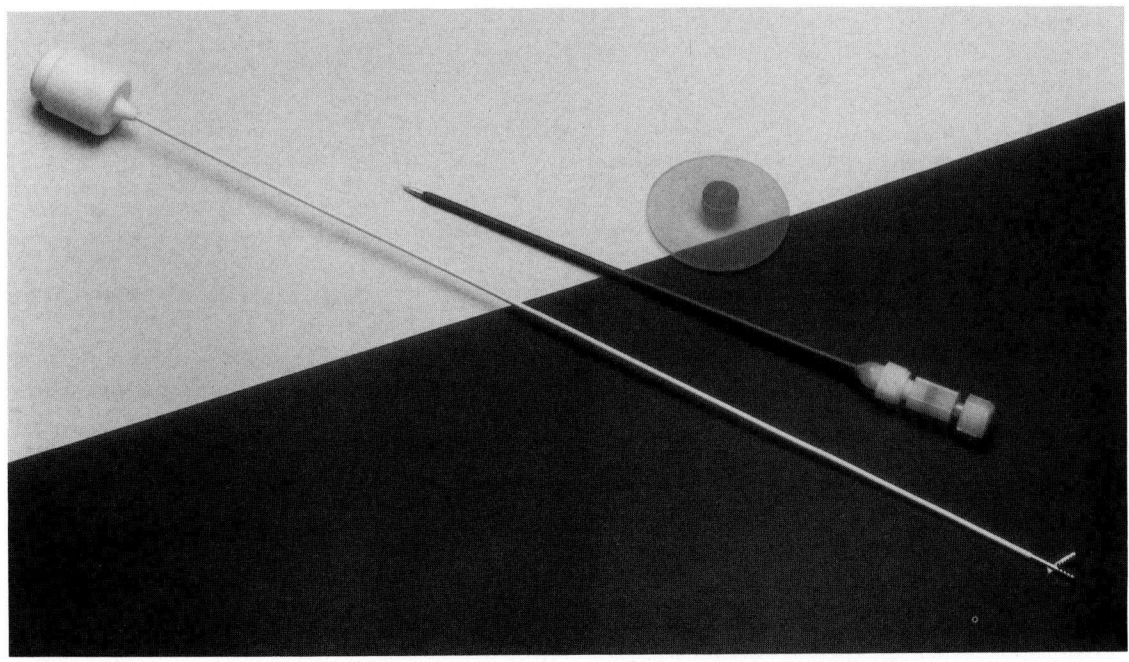

Figure 2.29. Laparoscopic mini-retractor set (Cook Ob/Gyn, Spencer, IN). The instrument is a 5F nylon grasper with the jaws operated by a push button. The disposable instument is used through a percutaneous access port that is secured onto the abdomen with the retention disk.

Myoma Screw

The myoma screw is a corkscrew-type instrument that is available in 5 or 10 mm size. The myoma screw is used to fix or stabilize the leiomyoma during the performance of a myomectomy. The instrument, twisted into the leiomyoma, is the most efficient way to hold larger tumors (Fig. 2.30).

Morcellating Instruments

An effective method for extirpating tissue from the body is perhaps the "Holy Grail" of laparoscopy. The ideal method would be safe and efficient, and prevent spillage of material within the abdominal cavity. As of this writing, the perfect method has yet to be described. If tissue is relatively small, if its structure is not critical for pathologic diagnosis, and if there is no fear of spillage, some type of morcellator may be considered. The original Semm tissue extractor (Wisap) still has significant use for morcellation, but it is cumbersome and if used on a large amount of tissue its use becomes arduous. If a large fibroid must be morcellated, a cork-boring type of instrument, described by Semm,[18] is available. This instrument (Wisap) cores out cylinders of tissue while the leiomyoma is still in the uterus: It is passed over a corkscrew device

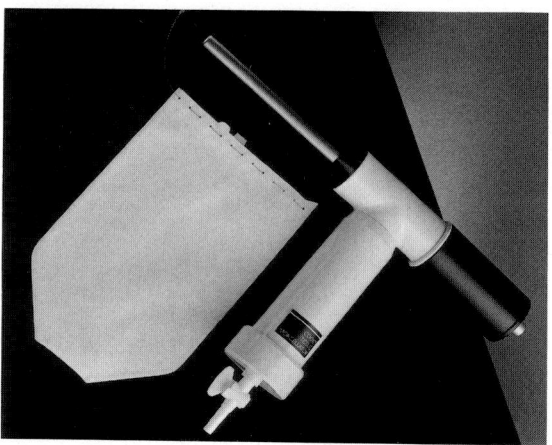

Figure 2.31. Cook morcellator is used in conjunction with the LapSac. The tissue to be extirpated is placed in the sack, which is impermeable. The tissue is pulled into the instrument with suction and is then morcellated into small pieces by the mechanically driven blades and suctioned away into a specimen container. This instrument is not useful for debulking thick tissue such as a leiomyoma. (Courtesy of Cook Ob/Gyn, Spencer, IN)

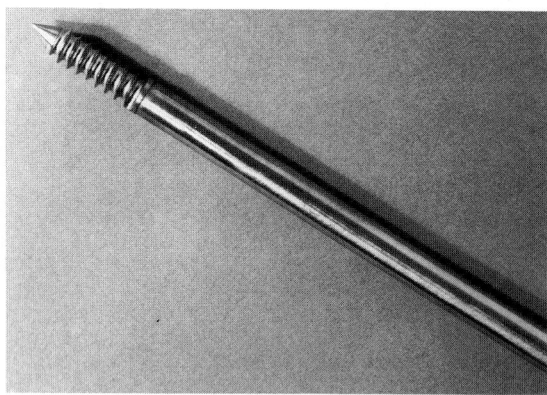

Figure 2.30. Myoma screw is a threaded rod that may be obtained in a variety of sizes. Some myoma screws have tips that are more similar to a corkscrew than the simple threads shown here The myoma screw is turned into a leiomyoma and can fix the tumor in place and provide excellent traction.

that is screwed into the leiomyoma, and the device is then twisted into the tissue and a cylindrical portion of tissue is removed. This process is repeated until the largest amount of tissue possible is removed. Steiner et al[19] described a similar instrument that was electrically powered, but it is not yet available in the United States and indeed may not be a completely safe approach.

Cook Ob/Gyn has developed a motorized morcellator and suction device. The tissue to be removed is placed in a bag (Lapsac) that is reinforced nylon with a polyurethane inner coating, rendering it impermeable. The suction pulls the tissue into a circular saw that morcellates the tissue into small pieces. Although this device seems to work well on soft tissue (it has been used to remove a kidney), it has not been useful for morcellating leiomyomas (Fig. 2.31).

Specimen Bags

Organ containment and retrieval bags play a vital role in laparoscopic surgery. They have been found to be necessary during general surgery for extirpating the gallbladder, removing stones and isolating an inflamed organ. Most importantly, specimen bags may be used to remove ovarian tissue in a manner that obviates dissemination of possibly malignant cells and prevents spillage during removal of a benign teratoma thereby precluding chemical peritonitis.[20] Several bags have been described. Companies such as Ethicon, Marlow, and US Surgical, among others, have produced disposable bags made from polyethylene or other clear plastic materials. Each is introduced through a plastic sleeve placed through a 10 or 11 mm trocar site. The bags are closed with a drawstring. These bags are relatively fragile and can tear when exposed to a moderate amount of tension. They are useful, however, if used appropriately. There are stronger bags that are more resistant to tearing, such as the Lapsac, a large (5 × 8 inch) nylon bag with a nylon drawstring (Fig. 2.31). The eXtract specimen bag (Fig. 2.32) has a unique design: It has an inflatable channel that allows easy deployment of the bag and keeps the mouth of the bag open to facilitate placement of the specimen within the bag. It has a three layer polymer laminate that is strong and resists rupture.

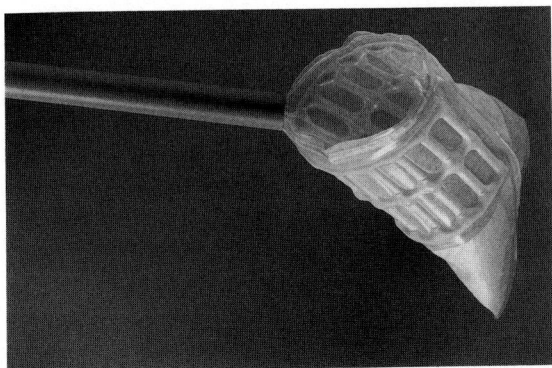

Figure 2.32. The eXtract specimen bag is noted to have inflatable "ribs." When air is injected the bag opens and allows easy placement of tissue to be extirpated. When the bag is closed and deflated it may be removed through a lateral port site, the umbilical area, or an opening in the cul-de-sac. This bag is strong and resists tearing despite a great deal of traction. (Courtesy of Advanced Surgical, Princeton, NJ)

Rectal and Vaginal Probes

Special probes have been designed for use in the rectum during dissection of the posterior cul-de-sac and for treatment of severe endometriosis or other severe adhesive pathology that obliterates this area.[21] The various shapes of the probe permit identification of the cul-de-sac in an attempt to reduce the possibility of inadvertent entry into the rectum during dissection.

Repair Instruments

As the use of operative laparoscopy has increased, the utilization of large trocars (11–13 mm) has also increased, as has the incidence of incisional hernia. Kadar et al. reported an incidence of 0.17% incisional hernias among 3560 operative laparoscopic cases, all occurring at the lateral ports (extraumbilical).[22] They found this incidence significantly higher when a 12 mm trocar was used than with a 10 mm trocar (3.1% versus 0.23%). These authors recommended that to prevent hernias it is necessary to close the fascia; and if the trocar is placed through, rather than lateral to, the rectus sheath, the peritoneum may also require closure. Such closure may be accomplished using traditional suturing methods. It is difficult to expose the fascia through such a small incision, and so several methods and instruments have been devised to accomplish this task.

1. Greis style needle is available in a reusable form or as a disposable product called the Endo Close (US Surgical). This instrument must be threaded intraabdominally by laparoscopic guidance, which may be a slight drawback to its use.
2. eXit™ puncture closure device (Figs. 2.33, 2.34) may be used to close the peritoneum and fascia at the same time with relative ease and safety. This innovative device is employed without needing to load the device with the suture intraabdominally. This instrument may be used for 10 or 12 mm puncture sites and is reusable except for the needle, which is designed for disposable use. It is slightly difficult to use but becomes easier with practice.

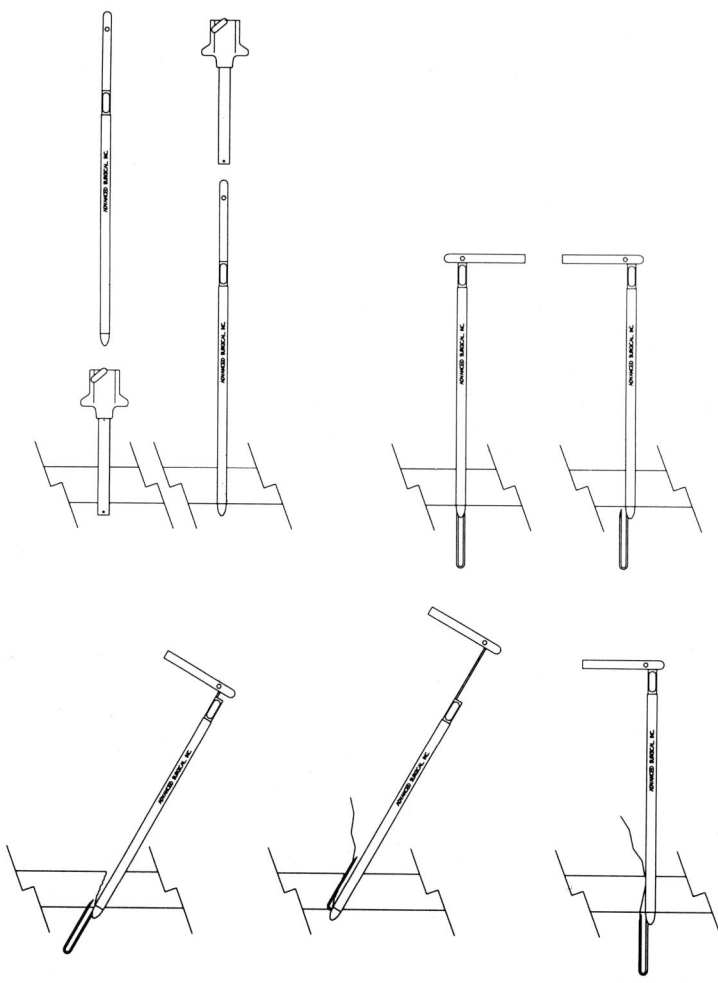

Figure 2.33. eXit™ puncture closure device is inserted through either a 10 or 12 mm trocar sheath, and the sheath is then withdrawn over the device. The handle is then pivoted and the needle advanced into the abdomen under direct vision. The entire instrument is then tilted, and the needle part alone is pulled up through the peritoneum and fascial layers, avoiding the skin. The needle is loaded with a ligature of either 0 monofiliment or a braided absorbable suture and pushed back into the abdomen, holding one end of the suture. (Courtesy of Advanced Surgical, Princeton, NJ)

3. A remarkably simple device that also closes 10 to 14 mm peritoneal and fascial incisions is the J-Needle (Unimar, Wilton, CT). This instrument comes in three sizes to meet various anatomic presentations. The needle is made of stainless steel, is reusable for a suggested 20 times, and is inexpensive. It must, however, be closely observed through the laparoscope to ensure that no injury occurs to the bowel.
4. A similar instrument that is completely disposable is the Endo-Judge (Synergistic Medical Technologies, Winter Park, FL).

Conclusion

In 1899 Charles H. Duell said, "Everything that can be invented has been invented." It is of course obvious that technical advancements have shown the folly of such a remark, and when one considers operative laparoscopy the proliferation of new ideas has been literally explosive. This rapid deluge of new instrumentation almost renders this chapter obsolete even before it is printed. Even so, we have endeavored to present material about basic instruments and some of the most current innovations. The utility and cost-effectiveness of many of these instruments may be debated, and surgeons may have their own prejudices or partiality against or for a particular implement without any solid basis. What seems inappropriate today may be the prototype for tomorrow's outstanding laparoscopic instrument.

The future will reveal many techniques for operative laparoscopy made possible by new instrumentation. The reader must be familiar

Figure 2.34. Entire eXit™ instrument is rotated 180° and again tilted, and the needle is pulled up through the tissues as before. The suture is removed from the needle eye and held while the needle is advanced back into the abdomen, rotated, resheathed, and the entire instrument withdrawn. When the suture is tied it encompasses all layers, precluding the occurrence of an incisional hernia.

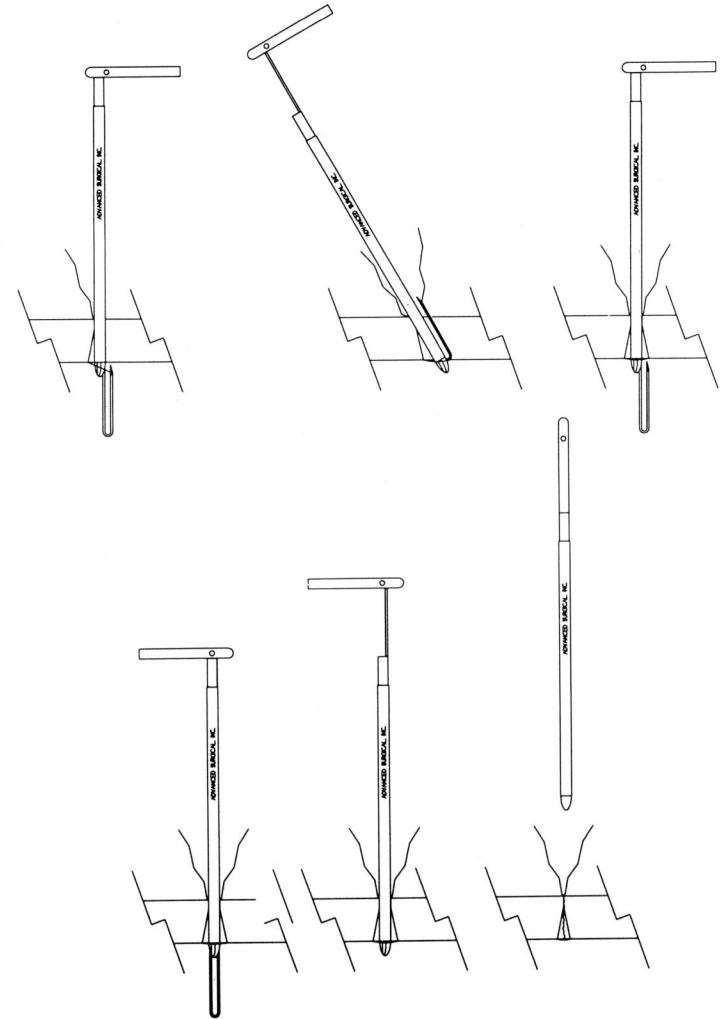

with the basic instruments so he or she is better able to judge the usefulness and application of the new ideas and equipment that will be propelling endoscopic surgery to new and more distant horizons in the exciting world of operative laparoscopy.

References

1. LEVINE RL: Economic impact of pelviscopic surgery. J Reprod Med 1985;30:655.
2. Handbook of Labor Statistics. Bulletin 2340. Washington, DC. US Department of Labor and Bureau of Labor Statistics, August 1989.
3. KLEPPINGER RK: Closed techniques for equipment insertion. In Manual of Endoscopy, Martin DC, Holtz GL, Levinson CJ, Soderstrom RM (eds). Santa Fe Springs, CA, AAGL, 1990, pp 15–22.
4. SEED RF, SHAKESPEARE TF, MULDOON MJ: Carbon dioxide hemostasis during anesthesia for laparoscopy. Anaesthesia 1970;25:223.
5. JANICKI TI: The new sensor-equipped Veress needle. J Am Assoc Gynecol Laparosc 1994;1:154.
6. LEVINE RL: Latest pelviscopic devices. Contemp Obstet Gynecol 1989(Oct);32:27.
7. HEALTH DEVICES: ECRI, 1992;(May)21:143.
8. HILL DJ, MAHER PJ, WOOD EC: Gasless laparoscopy: useless or useful? J Am Assoc Gynecol Laparosc 1994;1:265.
9. LEVINE RL: Disposable instruments for operative laparoscopy: pro and con. Infertil Reprod Med Clin North Am 1993;4:221.

10. CORSON SL, BATZER FR, GOCIAL B, MAISLIN G: Measurement of the force necessary for laparoscopic trocar entry. J Reprod Med 1989;34:282.
11. HASSON HM: Open laparoscopy. In Clinical and Diagnostic Procedures in Obstetrics and Gynecology (Vol 2), Symonds EM, Zuspan FP (eds). New York, Marcel Dekker, 1984, pp 309–318.
12. HURD WW, OHL DA: Blunt trocar laparoscopy. Fertil Steril 1994;61:1177.
13. DANIEL JF: Laparoscopic use of the argon beam coagulator. In Endoscopic Surgery for Gynaecologists, Sutton C, Diamond M (eds). London, Saunders, 1993, pp 71–76.
14. GALEN DI, JACOBSON A, WECKSTEIN LN: Argon beam coagulation rescue to correct bleeding during pelviscopy. J Am Assoc Gynecol Laparosc 1994;1:146.
15. SEMM K: Tissue-puncher and loop ligation: new aids for surgical therapeutic pelviscopy (laparoscopy) = endoscopic intraabdominal surgery. Endoscopy 1978;10:119.
16. LEVINE RL: Suturing and Ligation in Operative Laparoscopy: The Masters Techniques, Soderstrom RM (ed). New York, Raven Press, 1993, pp 129–135.
17. JOHNS DA: Reusable instruments for operative laparoscopy. Infertil Reprod Med Clin North Am 1993;4:233.
18. SEMM K: Morcellement and suturing using pelviscopy: not a problem any more. Geburtsh Frauenheilkd 1991;51:843.
19. STEINER RA, WRIGHT E, TADIR Y, HALLER U: Electrical cutting device for laparoscopic removal of tissue from the abdominal cavity. Obstet Gynecol 1993;81:471.
20. REICH H, MCGLYNN F, SEKEL L, TAYLOR P: Laparoscopic management of ovarian dermoid cysts. J Reprod Med 1992;37:640.
21. REICH H, MCGLYNN F, SALVAT J: Laparoscopic treatment of cul-de-sac obliteration secondary to retrocervical deep fibrotic endometriosis. J Reprod Med 1991;36:516.
22. KADAR N, REICH H, LIU CY, ET AL: Incisional hernias after major laparoscopic gynecological procedures. Am J Obstet Gynecol 1993;168:1493.

3
Lasers

Anthony A. Luciano

Surgical instrumentation and techniques undergo a process of continuous improvement as the scope and the goals of laparotomy and minimally invasive surgery expand. Perhaps this evolution is best exemplified in gynecology by the development of microsurgery, endoscopic surgery, electrosurgery, and laser surgery. Recognizing the importance of adhesion on the outcome of infertility surgery, the gynecologic surgeons developed more refined tools and techniques to minimize postoperative adhesion formation.[1,2] Having learned that the major contributing factors to adhesion formation include tissue trauma, drying of serosal surfaces, excessive bleeding, and tissue reaction,[3,4] reproductive surgeons developed the techniques of delicate tissue handling, constant irrigation, meticulous attention to hemostasis, and the use of fine instrumentation and less reactive suture material.[1,2] These important microsurgical principles are applicable not only to infertility procedures but to all gynecologic operations, especially when fertility potential is of paramount importance.[1]

Microsurgery has improved surgical results but the formation of postoperative adhesions has not been eliminated and surgical failures persist.[5-9] Thus the search for better instruments and better techniques continues.[10,11] Hoping to improve the surgical results, the CO_2 laser was introduced to gynecologic surgery during the late 1970s.[12,13] Before adequate trials had been conducted, unsubstantiated claims were propagated that the use of lasers resulted in shorter operating time, better hemostasis, less tissue trauma, less risk of infection, reduced postoperative adhesion formation, and improved pregnancy results.[12,14-17] Shortly thereafter the fiber-delivery lasers were introduced[18-20]; and because they are more selectively absorbed by pigmented tissue and yield better hemostasis, they were promoted to be better suited for the treatment of endometriosis, leiomyomas, and ectopic pregnancy, and for use in other procedures that involve vascular tissues.[18-21] Although none of these claims has been supported by experimental[22-29] or clinical[5,6,8,9,30,31] studies, the debate regarding the superiority of lasers versus electrosurgery or mechanical instruments continues. The relevant physics of the various lasers and their clinical application that enhances their safe and effective use in endoscopic surgery is conveyed in this chapter. In the last section, the benefits and limitations of available lasers are presented and their clinical application to the more traditional tools of electrosurgery or sharp dissection are compared, drawing on data from controlled animal and clinical studies.

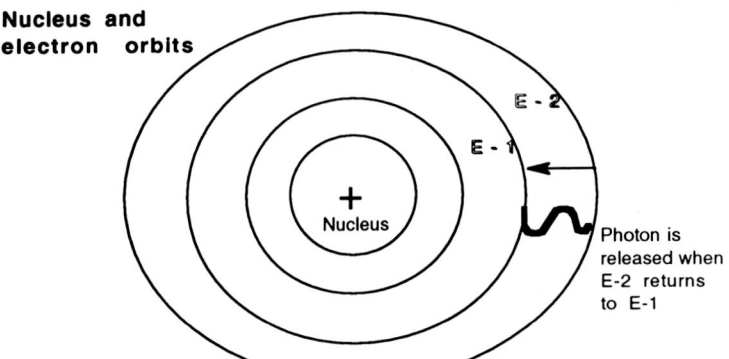

Figure 3.1. Photon emission. A photon (unit of laser energy) is released when an excited electron (E-2) circling the nucleus (+) returns to its resting state (E-1).

Physical Properties of Lasers

Laser is an acronym for light amplification by stimulated emission of radiation. It is a device that produces and amplifies light energy to create intense, coherent electromagnetic radiation. Unlike the ionizing radiation of x-rays and gamma rays, which result from nuclear destruction, the energy emitted by laser results from the release of photons, which occurs when stimulated electrons circling their nuclei return from their "excited" (E2) to their "resting" (E1) state, illustrated in Figure 3.1. These intermediate energy photons induce molecular vibration and create heat. Therefore although laser light is powerful and penetrating, it is neither mutagenic nor carcinogenic.[32,33]

Because each lasing substance has a unique atomic or molecular structure with its characteristic electron orbits, the wavelength, amplitude, and frequency of emitted photons are unique and uniform for each substance (e.g., CO_2, KTP, argon). Therefore laser light is *monochromatic,* consisting of a single wavelength that cannot be separated into any other components. Laser light contrasts with regular light, which can be separated into all colors of the spectrum when passed through a prism. When all the light waves are exactly in phase with each other the light is said to be *coherent,* and when all waves are parallel the light is *collimated.* Because the light waves of lasers have exactly the same length (*monochromatic*), are in phase with each other (*coherent*), and always run parallel (*collimated*), the laser can be precisely focused by lenses onto a small spot and can develop an extremely high power density (Figure 3.2).

Power Density

The amount of power delivered by lasers is measured in watts which may be adjusted at various settings by turning the power dial on the machine. The penetrating power of the laser depends mostly on the diameter of the laser beam reaching the tissue[20,32–34] because it is directly related to the wattage and inversely re-

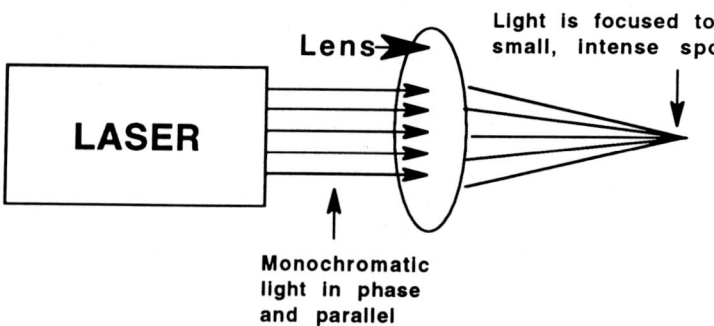

Figure 3.2. Light waves of laser energy are monochromatic, coherent, and collimated. Therefore laser energy can be precisely focused by lenses onto a small spot and can develop extremely high power density.

lated to the square of the spot size, as illustrated by the following formula:

$$\text{Power density (W/cm}^2) = \frac{\text{watts} \times 100}{\text{spot diameter}^2 \text{ (cm}^2)}$$

As the laser beam strikes the tissue, the cells at the site of impact are rapidly heated and vaporized, ablated, or coagulated, depending on the power density utilized. Power densities of less than 200 watts/cm^2 result in surface heating and serosal contraction. Such low power densities may be useful for denaturing or coagulating superficial endometriosis on bowel serosa, ureter, and bladder or may be useful to evert the ampullary stoma at salpingostomy. Power densities of 400–1200 watts/cm^2 result in superficial ablation with some hemostasis. Power densities of 1200–4000 watts/cm^2 result in wide vaporization and less hemostasis. Power densities greater than 4000 watts/cm^2 result in rapid, narrow vaporization with minimal coagulation or thermal damage. Although these general guidelines for power densities and tissue effects were developed for the CO$_2$ laser,[31] as summarized in Table 3.1, they can be equally applied to electrosurgery, radiosurgery, or other types of laser surgery.

Tissue effects

In addition to the power density, the other major determinants of tissue effects include the degree to which each laser is absorbed, refracted, or reflected by the impacted tissue.[26] For example, the CO$_2$ laser, which is not color-dependent, is fully absorbed by water. Because tissue is mostly water, all tissues regardless of color completely absorb the CO$_2$ laser energy, boil, and vaporize immediately. Argon, potassium, titanyl phosphate (KTP-532), and neodymium-yttrium-aluminum garnet (Nd-YAG) lasers are fully absorbed by pigmented tissues containing hemoglobin but are not absorbed by water or clear tissues. Consequently, the fiber lasers are much better for coagulating bleeding esophageal varices[35] or ablating pigmented tissue, such as endometrium[19,21] and vascular tumors[20]; they vaporize tissue less efficiently[35] and usually inflict greater tissue damage. This physical property of fiber lasers—to be refracted and not absorbed by clear tissues—has been successfully utilized to coagulate bleeding vessels on the retina of the eye without affecting the clear structures in front of it. Table 3.2 describes the commonly used lasers in gynecologic surgery, their physical properties, and their tissue effects.

Laser Components

The basic components of lasers consist of a pumping system, lasing medium, optical cavity, and operating system.

The *pumping system* is the power source that energizes the atoms or molecules of the lasing

Table 3.1. Tissue effects observed with the CO$_2$ laser at various power densities

Power density (watts/cm^2)	Tissue effects
200–400	Superficial desiccation and denaturation: mostly used to evert the ampullary stoma at salpingostomy by serosal desiccation.
401–1200	Superficial ablation with hemostasis: may be used to superficially ablate endometriosis on the bladder or in the cul de sac
1201–4000	Vaporization and minimal hemostasis: may be used to lyse vascular adhesions or dissect vascular planes (e.g., the adnexa from the pelvic side wall or from bowel)
> 4000 Continuous mode	Rapid vaporization and minimal coagulation: may be used to lyse avascular adhesions or excise endometriosis from the ovary or avascular planes
Superpulse/ultrapulse)	Rapid vaporization with minimal coagulation or charring: may be used for rapid vaporization and excision or for adhesiolysis and dissection of avascular planes with minimal tissue injury

Comparable tissue effects may result from fiber lasers or electrosurgery.

Table 3.2. Physical properties and characteristics of surgical lasers

Property	Laser			
	CO_2	Argon	KTP	Nd-YAG
Wavelength (nm)	10,600	488–514	532	1064
Color	Infrared	Blue-green	Green	Infrared
Delivery	Air or endoguide	Fiber	Fiber	Fiber
Absorption	All tissues and fluids	Color-dependent	Color-dependent	Color-dependent
Pass through fluids	No	Yes	Yes	Yes
Cutting	Excellent	Good	Good	Good
Coagulation	Fair	Good	Good	Excellent

medium to higher energy states. The ultimate power source of all lasers is the electrical outlet, which either stimulates the lasing medium directly or induces electrochemical reactions that in turn pump energy into the lasing medium to stimulate its electrons to higher energy levels.

The *lasing medium* consists of a selected assembly of atoms, molecules, or ions, which may be distributed in a solid crystal (ruby), a matrix (neodymium:yttrium aluminum garnet [Nd:YAG]), a gas (CO_2, helium-neon), or a liquid (gallium arsenide diode). As mentioned above, each lasing substance has a unique atomic or molecular structure with its characteristic electron orbits and energy levels. Thus the wavelength, wave amplitude, and frequency of photons emitted uniform and unique for each lasing substance, CO_2, KTP, YAG, and others.

The *optical cavity*, also referred to as a resonator cavity, consists of a tube with parallel mirrors on either side, which allow continuous reflection of photons back and forth in all directions as they strike other excited atoms to effect "stimulated emission of radiation." As the photons are repeatedly reflected back and forth between the parallel mirrors of the optical cavity they progressively accelerate, building in intensity until they finally flash out of the partially reflective mirror. This amplification is similar to the amplification in the resonator chamber of a musical instrument. At one end of the optical cavity, the mirror is only partially reflective, allowing escape of only those photons that are exactly in phase (coherent) and are traveling in the same parallel direction (collimated). Those photons that are transmitted to the partially reflected mirror provide the laser energy for use in surgical procedures (Fig. 3.3).

The *operating system* controls the delivery of laser energy to the tissue. It determines the power (watts) and the mode at which the laser is delivered from the unit. The power is adjusted by the power control knob. The mode of delivery of the laser energy may be continuous, pulsed, or super/ultra-pulsed (Table 3.3). In the *continuous* mode, the laser energy is delivered to the tissue without interruption for as long as the control pedal remains depressed. The *pulse*

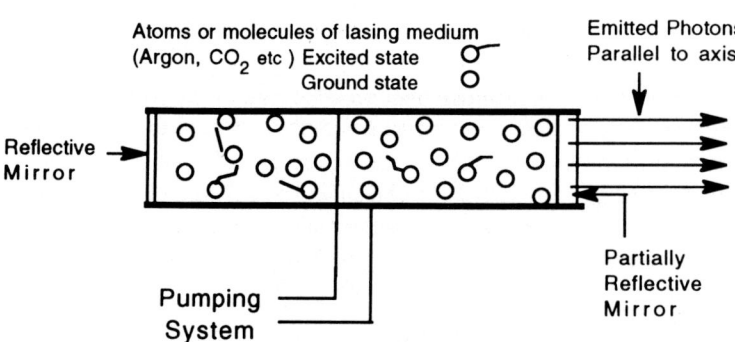

Figure 3.3. Generation of laser energy requires a power source (pumping system), an optical cavity, and the lasing medium.

Table 3.3. Delivery modes of the CO_2 Laser

Mode	Characteristics
Continuous	Uninterrupted delivery of laser energy, whose depth of penetration increases with power density. It may be used to ablate endometriosis on a large surface area. Usually associated with some charring and thermal damage.
Single pulse	Single burst of energy for a specified interval (0.05–0.50 second) used for precise, shallow ablation of endometriosis over the bowel or pelvic side wall to minimize the risk of perforating a viscus.
Repeated pulses	Repetitive pulses of laser energy delivered at specified intervals of variable duration with depth of penetration that vary according to the power density used. This method may be a safer alternative than the continuous mode for surgeons with limited experience.
Super/ultrapulse	Rapid pulses of high power energy alternating with refractory periods when the laser energy is not delivered. Use of the super/ultrapulse mode results in precise, rapid vaporization with decreased tissue smoke/plume and minimal carbonization or thermal injury. Best used to ablate avascular adhesions, adnexal adhesions, or along planes of dissection during ovarian cystectomy. Major advantages include minimal injury to adjacent structures and rapid vaporization. The main disadvantages include minimal hemostatic property and maximal depth of penetration.

mode may be in single or repeated pulses. With single pulses, the operating system releases one burst of energy for a specified interval (range 0.05–0.50 second) with every depression of the pedal. To discharge a second laser pulse, the pedal must be released and depressed again. The single pulse mode gives a controlled, precise penetration of the laser beam. It may be used to ablate endometriosis over the bowel to avoid perforating the bowel wall and on the pelvic side wall to avoid perforating the vascular structures and the ureter. The *repeat pulse* mode delivers intermittent bursts of laser energy of predetermined width and at specified frequency (number of pulses per second) for as long as the pedal remains depressed.

The *superpulse* mode of the CO_2 laser releases rapid pulses at short intervals, delivering extremely high peak power alternating with refractory, short periods when the laser energy is not delivered. By releasing "bursts" of peak power energy, the power density can be increased fourfold or more over the average obtained with continuous power output. The refractory periods between laser pulses allow heat to dissipate into the atmosphere rather than being conducted to adjacent tissue, thus minimizing thermal injury. The use of the superpulse mode results in precise, rapid vaporization with decreased tissue desiccation, carbonization, thermal injury, and smoke plume. Baggish and El Bakry[14] determined from animal studies that pulse intervals of 0.6–0.2 ms at rates below 700 pulses per second permit effective ablation with minimal thermal injury. Thus for the superpulse mode it is recommended that the pulse duration be set at 0.3 ms and the frequency should be 300 pulses per second. These high power densities are desirable when ablating or vaporizing avascular adhesions involving the ovaries or uterine tubes where thermal tissue injury should be minimized and coagulation effects of the laser are less critical. For vascular tissues, however, it may be desirable to use lower power densities to take advantage of the coagulation effects obtained.

The superpulse of the CO_2 laser is most effective when used with spot sizes of less than 0.75 mm. However, when used through the operative channel of the laparoscope and at high power settings, the CO_2 laser spot size becomes larger and the transmitted energy is reduced by the insufflating CO_2 gas by as much as 30–60%. This "blooming effect" at high power settings (60–100 watts), described by Reich et al.,[36] allows effective coagulation but slow cutting when used through the operating channel of the laparoscope. Unfortunately, the coagulating effects also cause thermal damage and should not be used on the uterine tubes or ovaries, where thermal tissue injury should be minimized. Therefore for endoscopy the full advantage of the superpulse mode may not be realized because the spot size usually exceeds 1.0 mm. The ultrapulse delivery mode of the CO_2 laser energy has been introduced and overcomes the blooming effect described above, keeping the spot size to a diameter of less than 0.75 mm.

Understanding Superpulse Versus Ultrapulse

Like the superpulse, ultrapulse delivers laser energy to tissue in a series of short, high power pulse intervals, instantaneously vaporizing a volume of tissue with little heating of the surrounding tissues. The delay between pulses increases the pulse energy and permits the minimal level of heat that has accumulated in surrounding areas to dissipate (cool down) before the next burst of laser energy is delivered. However, in comparison to superpulse, the ultrapulse mode delivers four to five times the energy per pulse, further enhancing its incising ability and further reducing thermal damage to adjacent tissues.

A cogent analogy that may facilitate understanding the difference between the continuous mode versus the superpulse/ultrapulse mode of CO_2 laser delivery may be made with the spray gun of a garden hose when it is continuously open versus when it is intermittently open. When the spray gun is continuously open (continuous mode) there is a steady stream of water that reflects the water pressure from the faucet (power setting in watts) and the size of the opening of the needle spray (spot size of the laser beam). When the spray gun is closed the water pressure from the faucet builds up exponentially and is stored within the wall of the hose. The longer the hose, the greater is the pressure that builds up behind the spray gun. When we fire the spray gun the initial spurt is extremely powerful because of the release of pressure from the faucet and the pressure stored along the wall of the hose. Thus when we intermittently open and close the spray gun (superpulse/ultrapulse), each spurt of water is sprayed much more forcefully than the stream when the gun is held continuously open. This analogy illustrates the difference between the continuous mode versus the superpulse mode. Ultrapulse differs from superpulse in that the ultrapulse mode delivers stronger pulses (spurts) of energy because the build up of power within the laser tube is greater (as if the hose were longer) and because the size of the spot (needle spray) is smaller. Therefore the ultrapulse delivers the highest power density available for CO_2 laser application through the laparoscope.

The blooming effect described by Reich et al.[36] is minimized with the use of carbon 13 (instead of carbon 12) isotope (most CO_2 lasers currently available) for generating of the CO_2 laser energy. The photons (laser energy) from $^{13}CO_2$ isotopes are not absorbed by the insufflation gas that is delivered through the same operative channel of the laparoscope. Therefore the blooming effect is less with the coherent ultrapulse laser, Coherent Medical Group, Palo Alto, CA, which uses the carbon 13 isotope to generate CO_2 laser energy. By keeping the spot size to a minimum and by providing stronger energy pulses, the ultrapulse operation system delivers the highest power density thus far available for CO_2 laser use at laparoscopy.

Delivery Systems

The CO_2 laser beam leaves the optical resonator and is delivered to the end of an articulated arm by several metallic mirrors precisely aligned to preserve the configuration and power of the beam as it leaves the generator. When it leaves the arm, the CO_2 laser beam and the helium-neon (He-Ne) beam are composed of parallel waves that need to be focused to increase the power density. Coupling lenses of various focal length are used to focus the beam at the end of either the hand-held probe or the laparoscope (Fig. 3.2). One type of coupling lens is a fixed lens that is easily assembled between the arm of the laser and the laparoscope. Its focal length may be set at 28 cm if the laser is delivered through the operating channel of the laparoscope or at 18 cm if the laser is delivered through a second puncture site to focus at the end of the shorter accessory trocar. For laparoscopic procedures the focal point is usually 2.0 cm from the tip of the laparoscope. Instead of a fixed lens, the laser couplers can have a galilean system with variable focal length that allows the surgeon to focus or defocus the laser beam to change the spot size by simply turning a knob on the coupler. This system allows the focal length to be adjusted between 100 to 315 mm and the spot size to be varied between 0.5 to 2.0 mm in diameter.

Wave Guides

It is obvious from the foregoing that the quality of the CO_2 laser output depends largely on proper alignment of the directing mirrors in the articulated arm of the laser, the quality and performance of the coupling lens, and the integrity of the operative channel of the laparoscope. A disturbance of any part of these three systems results in poor beam alignment and loss of laser power. To avoid this problem, rigid wave guides have been developed that guide the focused laser beam from the articulated arm through the operative channel of the laparoscope to its end, where it is always in perfect focus and in close proximity to the tissue to be lasered. The impact site of the beam lies immediately beyond the tip of the wave guide, which protrudes a few millimeters from the end of the laparoscope. Rigid wave guides are usually composed of ceramics with a high index of refraction so high power densities may be transmitted with less than a 10% power loss. A purge of continuous CO_2 of up to 1000 cc/min flows down the wave guide channel to keep it cool and clear of smoke. This CO_2 serves as an additional source of insufflation to replace the gas evacuated when the smoke is suctioned.

Fiber Lasers

The availability of fiber delivery systems is a major advantage of the argon, KTP, and Nd-YAG lasers. These quartz fibers are flexible, light, and thin. They can be delivered at a greater distance from the laser generator than the CO_2 laser, which needs to be close to the operative field because of its relatively short articulated arm. The laser beam is at maximal focus at the tip of the fiber, which may deliver the laser with or without contact with the tissue. By varying the diameter of the fiber or the distance between the fiber and the affected tissue, the power density of the argon or KTP lasers may be adjusted to vaporize, ablate, or coagulate. The Nd:YAG laser may be similarly modified with fibers or with sapphire tips of different size to effect variable degrees of coagulation or vaporization.

Surgical Lasers Used for Gynecology

The major lasers currently used for surgery are the CO_2, argon, KTP-532, and Nd-YAG. Ongoing developmental work involves use of the krypton, excimer, free electron, and tunable lasers, which may have surgical applications in the future.

Types of Laser

The CO_2 laser was the first laser to be used in our specialty. The CO_2 laser emits photons with a wavelength of 10.6 mm, which is within the infrared segment of the electromagnetic spectrum and therefore cannot be seen with the naked eye. Thus the CO_2 laser is delivered together with the visible He-Ne laser, which serves as the aiming beam. The CO_2 laser offers high power density and high efficiency, and it is ideally suited for incising and vaporizing tissue. It is highly absorbed by nonreflective solids and liquids, it is not dependent on the color of tissue for absorption, and it is not significantly scattered from the target point. Thus the impact of the laser is limited to the target tissue, sparing adjacent tissue layers. CO_2 laser cannot be delivered through a liquid medium, it is a poor coagulator, and it currently cannot be clinically delivered by fibers.[14] The wave-endo guide, described above, offers a fair alternative to reflective mirrors. By varying the output wattage or the diameter of the laser spot, a large range of power densities are available with the CO_2 laser. Low power densities, being more hemostatic, are used for the cervix and leiomyomas, where hemostasis is important and thermal damage is not a major concern. Higher power densities are preferred for reconstructive adnexal surgery where thermal damage must be minimized.

The *argon* and *KTP-532* lasers have similar characteristics and clinical applications, as they have similar wavelengths: 532 and 458–515 nm, respectively. Each releases a visible green light that travels through clear fluids and is absorbed by dark-pigmented tissue, and each can be delivered through flexible fibers, making them well suited for endoscopic use. Because they are not absorbed by clear fluids or unpigmented tissue, these lasers are ideal for coagulation of retinal bleeding or for ablation of peritoneal endometriosis where tissue coagulation can be effected without disrupting the "clear" overlying tissue.

The argon laser is available in two models, the 5 and 16 watt models, for abdominal and pelvic surgery. The more powerful model is more useful for reproductive surgery and ablation of endometriosis. This model requires high electrical current energy, triple phase, in excess of 200 volts at 60 amperes (amp). The laser fibers range in size from 300 to 600 µm in diameter and can be introduced through the small channels of the operating laparoscope or ancillary trocars; they can be steered toward the target with special bridges. The laser beam is maximally focused at the tip of the fiber. As the distance from the tissue is increased, the spot size increases (the beam diffuses) and the power density diminishes. Protective goggles for the specific laser wavelength are necessary when operating these lasers. When using the laser through the laparoscope, the operator may choose to cover the eyepiece of the laparoscope with the "monoshutter," an electronically triggered eyepiece that attaches to the laparoscope and interposes a protective filter between the operator's eye and the laparoscope when the laser is fired. The monoshutter may be used equally well with a videocamera for video-surgery and appropriate documentation.

The *Nd-YAG* laser is a crystal laser with an infrared wavelength of 1064 nm, in the near infrared spectrum. The YAG laser is invisible, is highly color-dependent, and passes through fibers and clear fluids. The YAG laser penetrates deeply into tissue, which is advantageous when coagulating tumors or hemorrhaging ulcers, or for endometrial ablation. Although it is an excellent coagulator, the YAG laser is a poor cutter unless used with sapphire tips to increase the power density and produce the ability to vaporize as well as ablate. The YAG laser is not a good choice for reconstructive procedures for adnexal disease because of the large amount of scatter and excessive thermal damage to tissue.[26]

Clinical Applications

Lasers have several unique characteristics that differentiate them from other devices used in medicine. The primary difference is that, with several exceptions, the tissue is not touched by surgical instruments but only by the laser beam. Thus the depth of the incision is not controlled by the pressure exerted on the tissue but by the power density and the length of time the laser is focused on any one spot. This "action at a distance" allows greater accessibility to the target tissue and perhaps less tissue trauma. When used at laparotomy the CO_2 laser may be delivered with a hand-held probe, or it may be attached to the operating microscope. The former has the advantage of a shorter focal distance and therefore a smaller spot size, which results in greater power density. This greater power density, as discussed above, yields much higher penetrating power and significantly less thermal damage to the contiguous normal tissue. The hand-held probe, however, is subject to hand tremor and less accurate beam delivery. Attaching the laser to the microscope increases precision owing to both the magnification and the absence of hand tremor; but because of the longer focal length, the spot size is larger. With more sophisticated lasers, high power density may also be achieved through the laparoscope using an endoguide at higher wattage (50–100 watts), with either the superpulse or ultrapulse mode, and with the use of $^{13}CO_2$ isotope as described above.

In experienced hands, each of the currently available lasers may be effectively used to ablate, coagulate, incise, or destroy tissue. Although each laser has its unique properties determined by the wavelength and tissue absorption, by varying the power density or mode of delivery (e.g., sapphire tips, fiber diameter) any desired tissue effect (ablation, coagulation, vaporization) may be achieved with most currently available surgical lasers.

Lasers Versus Electrosurgery

Comparative Studies of Tissue Effects, Incising Characteristics, Healing Patterns, Adhesion Formation

Since their introduction to pelvic reconstructive surgery, lasers have been proposed to be superior to the more traditional surgical tools of electrosurgery and scissors because they are allegedly less traumatic, more precise, and associated with reduced postoperative adhesion formation.[14–18] However, the results reported to date from experimental animal trials[22–29] and clinical trials[5,6,8,30,31] are controversial and do not support these claims. Because use of laser involves significant expense, not only for the purchase of the equipment but also for the numerous hours of required training, it is imperative that a definitive evaluation of lasers be carried out and that they be compared with the more traditional tools and techniques of electrosurgery and microsurgery so the role of laser in gynecologic surgery may be better defined.

The initial studies comparing tissue effects of electrosurgery versus laser surgery utilized electrosurgical generators and electrodes intended for electrocoagulation or tissue destruction.[16,22,28,31] Therefore some of these studies suggested that laser was superior to electrosurgery. More recent studies suggest that the two energy forms produce surprisingly similar tissue effects, healing patterns, and postoperative adhesion formation.[8,22,25–27,29] Some of the more current and better controlled animal studies are summarized in the following paragraphs and are compared to the clinical experience in the literature.

To help resolve the persisting controversy regarding the relative superiority and tissue effects of the CO_2 laser versus electrosurgery, randomized and controlled animal studies comparing the degree of thermal injury, healing patterns, and postoperative adhesion formation following CO_2 laser and microelectrosurgery on the reproductive tissue of rabbits were conducted.[25–28] In the first study, 20 sexually mature, female rabbits were subjected to the surgical procedure described later (Fig. 3.4). To ensure that each surgical tool was optimally utilized, similar power densities were used for electrosurgery and the CO_2 laser. Using standard microsurgical techniques with either the CO_2 laser or electrosurgery, each side of the reproductive tract underwent ovarian wedge resection and uterine segmental resection followed by microsurgical reanastomosis with 8-0

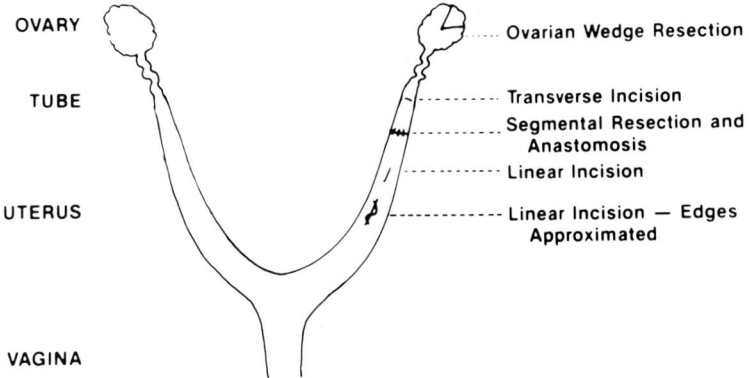

Figure 3.4. Operative procedure. The same procedure was carried out on both sides, using either CO_2 laser or electrosurgery as the only surgical instrument for each side, randomly, and at comparable power densities. (From Luciano et al.[25] Reproduced with permission of the American Fertility Society.)

Table 3.4. Depth of thermal injury on the ovarian and uterine tissues immediately following resection[a]

Procedure	Depth of thermal injury (mm)		p
	Ovary	Uterus	
CO_2 laser	0.041 ± 0.020	0.160 ± 0.040	0.007
Electrosurgery	0.041 ± 0.020	0.095 ± 0.010	< 0.050

[a]The depth of thermal injury (mean ± SD) was significantly greater in the uterus than in the ovary with both CO_2 laser and electrosurgery. No difference was observed in the extent of thermal damage between the CO_2 laser and electrosurgery in either ovarian or uterine tissue.
(From Luciano et al.[25] Reproduced with permission)

Vicryl sutures. The excised ovarian wedges and uterine segments were evaluated histologically to assess the extent of the acute thermal damage beyond the line of incision. Each uterine horn was further subjected to a single transverse and two longitudinal incisions, of which one was loosely approximated with 8-0 Vicryl sutures and the other left unsutured (Fig. 3.4). Four weeks later, at necropsy, the adhesions were blindly graded by the same observer on a scale of 0–3. To assess the extent of fibrosis 4 weeks postoperatively at the sites of injury with and without sutures after laser versus electrosurgery, histologic evaluation was performed blindly by the same observer, using a light microscope fitted with an optic micrometer with graduations of 0.01 mm when employing the 10× objective.

Tables 3.4, 3.5, and 3.6 summarize the results obtained from these studies. There was no difference in the depth of thermal damage, the extent of collagen deposition, or postoperative adhesion formation between CO_2 laser and electrosurgery at any of the several sites of surgical injury. These data support the concept that the power density is the major determinant of tissue penetration and thermal damage; hence when the power density for the CO_2 laser and electrosurgery is made comparable, similar results may be expected. Interestingly, it was noted that the thermal damage was significantly greater on the uterus than on the ovary for both the CO_2 laser and the electrosurgery sites, suggesting that ovaries are less susceptible to thermal injury than the uterine tissues, regardless of which energy source is used.

Ovarian Histology and Function After Surgery by Scalpel, CO_2 Laser, and Microelectrode

Racette et al.[37] reported that ovarian incision with CO_2 lasers inflicted significantly more damage to the oocyte than similar incisions made with either electrosurgery or scalpel. Because of the serious impact of germ cell damage on reproductive function, suggested by the report of Racette et al.,[37] studies to evaluate the relative damage to ovarian follicles and the conse-

Table 3.5. Width of fibrosis at the site of injury 4 weeks after operation

Site of injury	Width of fibrosis (mm)	
	CO_2 laser[a]	Electrosurgery[a]
Transverse incision	0.96 ± 0.25	0.97 ± 0.40
Site of anastomosis	1.73 ± 0.30	0.96 ± 0.30
Longitudinal incision		
With suture[b]	0.76 ± 0.40	0.80 ± 0.20
Without suture[b]	1.60 ± 0.40	1.60 ± 0.20

[a]No significant difference ($p > 0.05$) for laser versus electrosurgery for all sites.
[b]Statistically significant ($p < 0.05$). Wider areas of fibrosis appeared when edges were not approximated in both CO_2 laser and electrosurgery groups.
(From Luciano et al.[25] Reproduced with permission)

Table 3.6. Scores of postoperative adhesions at the site of surgery with CO_2 laser versus electrosurgery

Site of surgery	Adhesion score (mean ± SD)	
	CO_2 laser	Electrosurgery
Ovary	1.7 ± 1.3	1.6 ± 1.9
Transverse incision	1.8 ± 1.3	1.6 ± 1.9
Site of anastomosis	1.2 ± 1.1	1.75 ± 1.20
Longitudinal incision		
With suture	1.1 ± 1.0	1.2 ± 1.0
Without suture	1.7 ± 1.0	1.2 ± 1.0

(From Luciano et al.[25] Reproduced with permission)

quences on ovarian function when a surgical incision was made on the ovary with a scalpel, CO_2 laser, or microelectrode have been pursued.[27]

In one reported study, 30 sexually mature female rabbits were randomly assigned to one of three surgical groups. The injury consisted of a linear incision along the entire long axis of both ovaries, from the cortex to the hilum. One of the ovaries was removed and fixed immediately for histologic evaluation of the acute tissue damage to the follicular apparatus, oocytes, and stromal cells. The other ovary was left in situ to evaluate subsequent healing, steroidogenesis, folliculogenesis, ovulation, and ovum pickup. Blood samples were assessed weekly for estradiol and progesterone. Two weeks after operation the remaining ovary was removed from five animals of each group, cut in 10 μm sections, and evaluated histologically for stromal and follicular morphology. Five other animals were injected with human chorionic gonadotropin (hCG) and 18 hours later subjected to salpingo-oophorectomy to assess ovarian histology and to determine the number of corpora lutea and ovulated eggs.

Histologic evaluation revealed minimal (0.041 mm) but equal tissue damage along the incision made by the laser and microelectrodes. The laser and the electrical incisions were characterized by straight, sharp edges, in contrast to the jagged incision line made by the scalpel. No architectural disruption of the ovary was evident in either the acute or the healed specimens. The follicular apparatus and the oocytes, unless transected by the surgical instrument, did not appear to be particularly damaged and showed no differences among the three surgical groups. Postoperatively, the mean adhesion scores were the same for the three groups, and steroidogenesis was normal and similar as well. Table 3.7 summarizes the progesterone levels 8 hours after hCG administration, the number of antral follicles, corpora lutea on the remaining ovary, and the number of oocytes collected in the oviduct from each of the three study groups. Except for the higher number of oocytes identified in the oviduct of the electrosurgical group, there were no differences among the three surgical groups for any of the parame-

Table 3.7. Various measurements in the oviduct of animals from each surgical group

Measurement	Scalpel	CO_2 laser	Electrosurgery
Power density (W/cm^2)	—	58,964	88,888
Progesterone after hCG (ng%)	2.5 ± 5.0	1.9 ± 3.0	2.8 ± 6.0
No. of antral follicles in each ovary	33.0 ± 3.3	28.0 ± 3.3	32.0 ± 4.5
No. of corpora lutea in each ovary	4.4 ± 0.8	6.5 ± 0.8	6.8 ± 0.6
No. of ova in the tube	2.0 ± 0.8[a]	4.0 ± 0.8[a]	7.0 ± 1.2

[a] $p < 0.01$ between number of corpora lutea and the number of ova found in the ipsilateral oviduct.

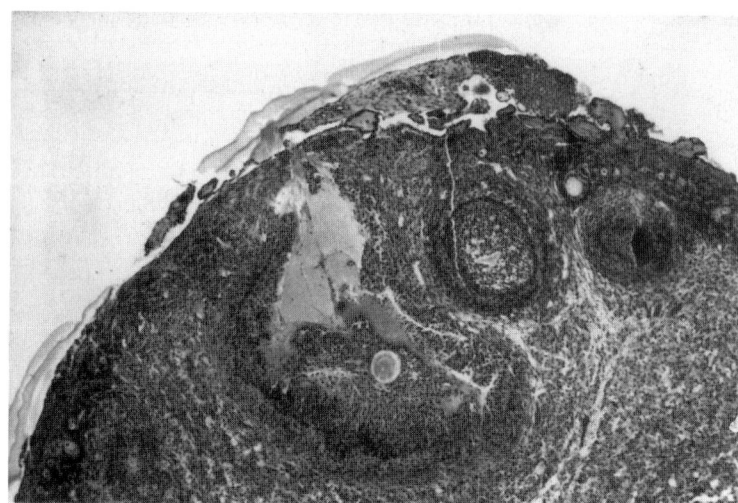

Figure 3.5. Photomicrograph of a luteinized follicle in which the oocyte had not been released. Note the thin layer of fibrous membrane covering the "stigma," suggesting that microscopic adhesions prevented release of the oocytes, entrapping them within the luteinized follicle. (From Luciano et al.[25] Reproduced with permission of the American Fertility Society.)

ters studied. The ova that did not appear in the oviduct were found at histologic evaluation to be entrapped in unruptured luteinized follicles, usually covered by thin, microscopic adhesions that had formed just above the ruptured, luteinized follicle with the entrapped oocyte (Fig. 3.5). These findings confirm that surgical trauma is, for the most part, well tolerated by the ovaries and suggests that the acute injury, subsequent healing, steroidogenesis, folliculogenesis, and ovum pickup by the oviduct do not differ following ovarian incision by microscalpel, CO_2 laser, or microelectrode. Moreover, the presence of entrapped oocytes within partially ruptured corpora lutea covered by microscopic adhesions underscores the role that periovarian adhesions may play in oocyte release and perhaps infertility (Fig. 3.5).

Comparative Studies of CO_2 Laser, Nd-YAG Laser, and Electrosurgery at Laparoscopy

The above summarized studies assessed the relative efficacy of the various surgical tools at laparotomy. Whether lasers offer any advantages over electrosurgical tools at operative laparoscopy is the next logical question. A study was designed using 30 rabbits that underwent surgical procedures to create extensive intraperitoneal adhesions.[26] The animals were then randomly assigned to undergo laparoscopic adhesiolysis utilizing electrosurgery, CO_2 or YAG laser exclusively for each assigned group. Each surgical tool was utilized at its optimal power density to achieve the best results (Table 3.8). In addition to evaluating the changes in adhesion scores and the depth of thermal injury in ovarian and uterine tissues for

Table 3.8. Operative factors for surgical modalities used at laparoscopy

Factor	Electrosurgery	CO_2 laser	Nd:YAG laser
Power density (W/cm^2)	66,666	6,000	75,000
Reduction of adhesions	61%	57%	44%
Depth (μm) of thermal injury			
Uterus	102.0 ± 11.3	109.9 ± 6.5	358.4 ± 42.0[a]
Ovary	43.7 ± 2.6	41.7 ± 4.1	175.6 ± 45.0[a]
Time (seconds) to transect uterine horn	1.5 ± 0.2	1.4 ± 0.2	2.6 ± 0.4[a]

[a] $p < 0.001$, indicating a significant difference compared to electrosurgery and CO_2 laser.

the three groups, the speed at which various segments of the uterine horn were transected by each of the three surgical instruments was also compared. All three modalites significantly and equally reduced intraperitoneal adhesions by approximately 50% (Table 3.8). The depth of thermal injury was threefold greater with the Nd-YAG laser than with either electrosurgery or the CO_2 laser in both ovarian and uterine tissues. The speed of transection across the uterine horn was significantly slower with the Nd-YAG laser than with the CO_2 laser or electrosurgery. The results obtained with operative laparoscopy are strikingly similar to those obtained at laparotomy, confirming the concept that the CO_2 laser and electrosurgery, when optimally used at comparable power densities, produce similar tissue effects.

Nd-YAG Laser: Greater Thermal Damage

Although the Nd-YAG laser was found to be equally effective at laparoscopic adhesiolysis, it caused significantly more tissue damage and was much less efficient at incising tissues than either the CO_2 laser or electrosurgery, despite application of the sapphire tip with a small diameter, yielding higher power density than either the CO_2 laser or electrosurgery. These findings suggest that, in contrast to the CO_2 laser and electrosurgery, the power density alone may not explain the different tissue effects of the Nd-YAG laser observed in this study. In research reported by Luciano et al.[26] and in a study by Joffe et al.[20] the extent of thermal damage was increased when the tissue was incised at slower speed. It is likely that these two phenomena are causally related and that the thermal damage may reflect the duration that the tissue is exposed to the laser energy. The slower incising efficacy of the Nd-YAG laser results in longer duration of tissue exposure to the laser energy, which results in greater thermal injury. This hypothesis is consistent with the decreased thermal effects associated with the superpulse/ultrapulse delivery of the CO_2 laser or the unblended (cutting) electrical current where the total duration the tissue is exposed to the laser or electrical energy is much less than the less efficient continuous or blended delivery mode.

The reason the Nd-YAG laser cuts less efficiently than either the CO_2 laser or electrosurgery may be explained by the fact that the Nd-YAG laser is selectively absorbed by pigmented tissues and only poorly absorbed by unpigmented (clear) tissues. The unpigmented tissue fibers transmit, rather than absorb, the laser energy and do not become vaporized or severed until heated by the adjacent pigmented tissue. This lower incising efficiency prolongs the contact of the laser energy with tissue and results in greater thermal damage.

Conclusion

The results from animal studies are consistent with most of those from the clinical studies published to date, which have reported no difference in the outcome of the treatment of periadnexal adhesions with CO_2 laser and electrosurgery.[5,6,8,9,31] Two studies from an "intra-abdominal laser study group," which included results from several gynecologic laser surgeons in North America, reported in 1984 that "nonlaser infertility surgery appeared to have equal or greater efficacy in the prevention of adhesion formation at most sites.[5,6] Thus the CO_2 laser does not appear to be a panacea for the treatment of tuboperitoneal causes of infertility."[5] The same group of laser surgeons reported in 1987 that "the use of CO_2 laser for neosalpingostomy at laparotomy with early secondlook laparoscopy provides a term pregnancy rate similar to that previously achieved by nonlaser microsurgical techniques."[6] Earlier studies by Bellina[15] and by Chong and Baggish[17] suggesting that the CO_2 laser may be more effective than electrosurgery for tubal reconstructive surgery and for endometriosis, respectively, were neither randomized nor controlled. On the other hand, Tulandi and Vilos[8,9] prospectively randomized infertile patients scheduled to undergo adhesiolysis and tuboovarian reconstruction to either CO_2 laser or electromicrosurgery at laparotomy. In these prospectively controlled studies, Tulandi found no difference between the CO_2 laser and electromicrosurgery groups in terms of either postoperative adhesion formation or pregnancy rate.[8,9]

Given the data from the controlled animal studies and most clinical reports, one may conclude that, when optimally utilized, lasers, microelectrodes, and mechanical instruments are equally effective in gynecologic surgery and perhaps in any surgery, whether performed via laparoscopy or laparotomy.[36-40] Yet the debate regarding the superiority of lasers versus electrosurgery or mechanical instruments continues, often misleading patients to develop unrealistic expectations from laser surgery or inducing hospitals to allocate otherwise needed resources to expensive laser instrumentation and training personnel in laser use and safety.

When considering these tools, surgeons do and should have preferences among them for particular applications. Given the objective evidence that the use of one particular tool yields no better results than the use of another, the choice and preference should be based on the surgeon's experience and skill with a tool for a particular procedure.

Even when optimally utilized, lasers, electrodes, or mechanical instruments appear to be equally effective in the surgical treatment of gynecologic diseases. These instruments are merely tools that are used to ablate, coagulate, incise, or dissect. No tool is more precise, faster, or safer, but the surgeon who uses it can be more precise, more efficient, and safer. In experienced surgical hands, each instrument can serve its function effectively and safely.

References

1. GOMEL V, MCCOMB P: Microsurgery in gynecology. In Microsurgery Silver JS (ed.). Baltimore, Williams and Wilkins, 1979, pp. 143–183.
2. GORDTS S, BOECKX W, BROSENS I: Microsurgery of endometriosis in infertile patients. Fertil Steril 1974;42:520.
3. Ellis H: The cause and prevention of postoperative intraperitoneal adhesions. Surg Gynecol Obstet 1971;133:497.
4. RYAN G, GROBETY J, MAJNO G: Postoperative peritoneal adhesions. A M J Pathol 1971;65:117.
5. DIAMOND MP, DANIEL JF, MARTIN DC, ET AL: Tubal patency and pelvic adhesions at early second look laparoscopy following intraabdominal use of the carbon dioxide laser: initial report of the intraabdominal study laser group. Fertil Steril 1984;42:717.
6. DIAMOND MP, DANIELL SF, FESTE J, ET AL: Adhesion reformation and de novo formation after reproductive pelvic surgery. Fertil Steril 1987;47:864.
7. TRIMBOS-KEMPER TCM, TRIMBOS JB, VAN HALL EV: Adhesion formation after tubal surgery: results of the 8 day laparoscopy in 188 patients. Fertil Steril 1985;43:395.
8. TULANDI T, VILOS GA: A comparison between laser surgery and electrosurgery for bilateral hydrosalpinx: a 2 year follow-up. Fertil Steril 1985;44:846.
9. TULANDI T: Salpingo-ovariolysis: a comparison between laser surgery and electrosurgery. Fertil Steril 1986;45:48.
10. DECHERNEY AH: The leader of the band is tired. Fertil Steril 1985;44:299.
11. LUCIANO AA, MAIER DB, NULSEN JC, ET AL: A comparative study of postoperative adhesion formation following laser surgery by laparoscopy versus laparotomy in the rabbit model. Obstet Gynecol 1989;74:220.
12. BRUHAT H, MAGE C, MANHES M: Use of the CO_2 laser via laparoscopy. In Laser Surgery III, Kaplan I (ed). Proceedings of the Third International Society for Laser Surgery, Tel Aviv, 1979, p 275.
13. TADIR Y, OVADIA J, ZUCKERMAN Z, ET AL: Laparoscopic application of the CO_2 laser. In Proceedings of the 4th Congress of International Society for Laser Surgery. Tokyo Japanese Society for Laser Medicine 1981, p. 25
14. BAGGISH MS, EL BAKRY MM: Comparison of electronic super pulsed continuous wave CO_2 laser in the rat uterine horn. Fertil Steril 1986;45:120.
15. BELLINA JF: Microsurgery of the fallopian tube with the carbon dioxide laser: analysis of 230 cases with a 2 year follow-up. Laser Surg Med 1983;3:255.
16. BELLINA JH, HEMMINGS R, VOROS IJ, ET AL: Carbon dioxide laser and electrosurgical wound study with an animal model: a comparison of tissue damage and healing patterns in peritoneal tissue. Am J Obstet Gynecol 1984;148:327.
17. CHONG AP, BAGGISH MS: Management of pelvic endometriosis by means of intraabdominal carbon dioxide laser. Fertil Steril 1984;41:14.

18. DANIELL JF, MILLER W, TOSH K: Initial evaluation of the use of the potassium-titanyl phosphate (KTP/532) laser in gynecologic laparoscopy. Fertil Steril 1986;46:373.
19. KEYE WR, HANSEN LW, ASTIN M ET AL: Argon laser therapy of endometriosis: a review of 92 consecutive patients. Fertil Steril 1987;47:208.
20. JOFFE SN, BRACKETT KA, SANKAR MY, DAIKUZONO N: Resection of the liver with Nd-YAG laser. Surg Gynecol Obstet, 1986;163:437.
21. SHIRK GJ: Use of Nd:YAG laser for the treatment of endometriosis. Am J Obstet Gynecol 1989;160:1344.
22. FILMAR S, GOMEL V, MCCOMB P: The effectiveness of CO_2 laser and electromicrosurgery in adhesiolysis: a comparative study. Fertil Steril 1986;45:407.
23. FILMAR S, JETHA N, MCCOMB P, GOMEL V: A comparative histologic study on the healing process after tissue transection. I. Carbon dioxide laser and electromicrosurgery. Am J Obstet Gynecol 1989;160:1062.
24. FILMAR S, JETHA N, MCCOMB P, GOMEL V: A comparative histologic study on the healing process after tissue transection. II. Carbon dioxide laser and surgical microscissors. Am J Obstet Gynecol 1989;160:1068.
25. LUCIANO AA, WHITMAN G, MAIER DB, ET AL: A comparison of thermal injury healing patterns, and postoperative adhesion formation following CO_2 laser and electromicrosurgery. Fertil Steril 1987;48:1025.
26. LUCIANO AA, FRISHMAN GN, KRATKA SA, MAIER DB: A comparative analysis of adhesion reduction, tissue effects, and incising characteristics of electrosurgery, CO_2 laser, and Nd-YAG laser at operative laparoscopy. J Laparoendosc 1993;2:305.
27. LUCIANO AA, MARANA R, KRAKTA S ET AL: Ovarian function after incision of the ovary by scalpel, CO_2 laser and microelectrode. Fertil Steril 1991;56:349.
28. MARANA R, LUCIANO AA, MARENDINO VE, ET AL: Reproductive outcome after ovarian surgery: microsurgery versus CO_2 laser. J Gynecol Surg 1991;7:159.
29. PITTAWAY DE, MAXSON WS, DANIELL JF: A comparison of the CO_2 laser and electrocautery on postoperative intraperitoneal adhesion formation in rabbits. Fertil Steril 1983;40:366,
30. LUCIANO AA, LOWNEY J, JACOBS SL: Endoscopic treatment of endometriosis-associated infertility: therapeutic, economic and social benefits. J Reprod Med 1992;37:573.
31. MAGE G, BRUHAT MA: Pregnancy following salpingostomy: comparison between CO_2 laser and electrosurgery procedures. Fertil Steril 1983;40:472.
32. MARTIN DC: Tissue effects of lasers. Semin Reprod Endocrinol 1991;9:118.
33. FULLER TA: Fundamentals of lasers in surgery and medicine. In Surgical Applications of Lasers, Dixon J (ed). Chicago, Year Book, 1983, pp 11–28.
34. MCKENZIE AL: How far does thermal damage extend beneath the surface of the CO_2 laser incision? Phys Med Biol 1983;28:905.
35. NEZHAT C, WINER WK, NEZHAT F: A comparison of the CO_2, argon, and KTP/532 laser in the videolaseroscopic treatment of endometriosis. Colposc Gynecol Laser Surg 1988;4:41.
36. REICH H, MACGREGOR TS III, VANCAILLE TG: CO_2 laser used through the operating channel of laser laparoscope: in vitro study of power and power density losses. Obstet Gynecol 1991;77:40.
37. RACETTE N, FILMAR S, JETHA N, ET AL: The viability of oocytes after incision of the ovary by CO_2 laser, microelectrode and scalpel. Presented at the 44th Annual Meeting of The American Fertility Society, Atlanta, October 1988. Program Supplement, p S50 (abstract PO-18).
38. NEZHAT C, CROWGEY S, NEZHAT F: Videolaseroscopy for the treatment of endometriosis associated infertility. Fertil Steril 1989;51:23.
39. FESTE JR: Laser laparoscopy: a new modality. J Reprod Med 1985;30:413.
40. MARTIN DC, VANDERZWAAG R: Excisional techniques for endometriosis with the CO_2 laser laparoscope. J Reprod Med 1987;32:753.

4
Electrosurgery

Roger C. Odell

Electrosurgical energy is without question the most common form of energy used for today's surgical procedures—both open (laparotomy) and closed (laparoscopy). It enhances dissection and helps to control bleeding. Unfortunately, the level of training for electrosurgery is often inadequate, and there are many misconceptions about the subject. With the shift from laparotomy to laparoscopy, surgical technique has become a subject for marketing and sales presentation, further complicating a topic that was not clearly understood from its inception.

Electrosurgical energy used during laparoscopy dates back to the mid-1960s when gynecologists began to perform surgery through a channel within the laparoscope (single puncture technique), subsequently multiple trocar techniques were developed. During the course of performing laparoscopic electrosurgery a number of "misadventures" occurred.[1] Investigation of these incidents led to a number of concerns regarding the use of electrosurgery, specifically about monopolar energy sources. Because of these problems monopolar electrosurgery has been discouraged in laparoscopic procedures beginning during the mid-1970s. One of the objectives of this chapter is to revisit these complications and explain the physics of how they occur. Ways to minimize the hazards of electrosurgery and the options available for eliminating them from being repeated in the future is of paramount importance. One other key objective is to explain the biophysics of electrosurgical energy utilized for laparoscopic dissection, fulguration, and desiccation.

Historical Perspective

The use of high frequency electrical energy for surgical application dates back nearly a century. Electrosurgery is defined as the generation and delivery of radiofrequency current between an active electrode and a dispersive electrode in order to elevate the tissue temperature for the purpose of cutting, fulguration, or desiccation. In contrast to electrocautery, the electrical current actually passes through the tissue. Harvey W. Cushing, with the assistance of William T. Bovie, were the first surgical team to document the principles regarding both the art and the biophysics of electrosurgery (1927). By no means did Cushing and Bovie invent electrosurgery: As early as the late 1800s the Germans and French (D'Arsonval and Jacques, 1891) documented the biophysics of electrosurgical current. A general surgeon, William L. Clark in Philadelphia, documented the removal of large benign and malignant growths of the skin, head, neck, and breast with electrosurgery (1910). It was Cush-

4. Electrosurgery

ing and Bovie's documentation, however, that changed the course of neurosurgery and expanded other surgeon's views on the ever-increasing potential uses of electrosurgical energy.

Temperature and Tissue

The first law of thermodynamics states that energy can be neither created nor destroyed, rather, it is converted to another form of energy. Electrosurgical energy is converted to heat at the active electrode target site and may be used for the purpose of vaporizing (cutting) and coagulation. An explanation of the correlation between temperature rise and tissue effect can help us to understand electrosurgery and its effects on tissues and blood vessels.

Mechanism of Electrical Energy Affecting Tissue Temperature

Three electrical properties cause a temperature rise.

Current (I): movement of electrons through a conductor in the same direction (direct current) or reversing at a particular frequency (alternating current)
Voltage (V): strength of the electrical force (volt)
Resistance or **impedance** (R): property of a substance that causes it to resist the flow of electrical current (ohms)

To help understand electrical energy terms and their meaning, a direct analogy to hydrostatic or hydraulic energy can be made. The water tower in Figure 4.1 represents a hydraulic energy source for the purpose of performing work. Figure 4.2 displays an equivalent electrosurgical tower equated with the electrical terms current, voltage, and resistance. This direct relation is important for understanding the mystique of electrosurgical units. One aspect worth mentioning is that the reader should understand that both the water tower and the electrosurgical energy source are operating with thousands of feet of head pressure and thousands of volts. This cardinal point must be recognized when performing electrosurgery. Water towers typi-

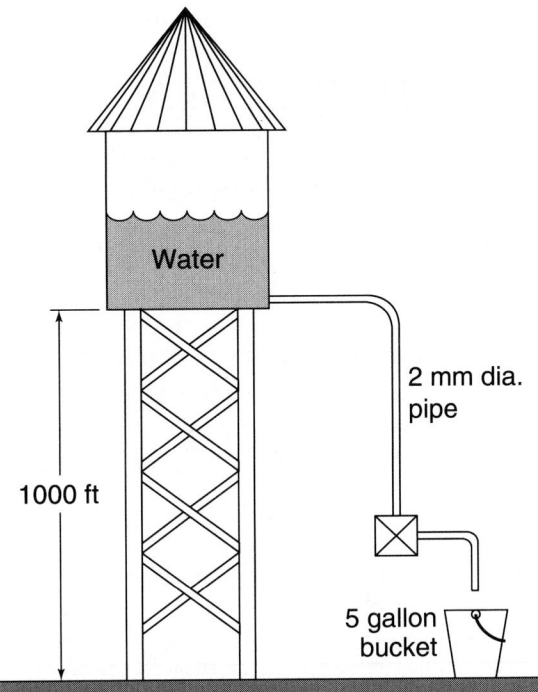

Figure 4.1. Hydraulic energy source. (Courtesy of Electroscope, Boulder, CO)

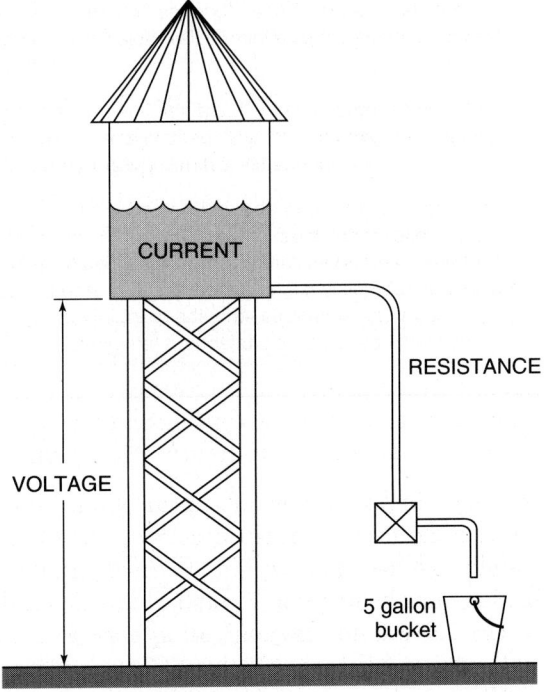

Figure 4.2. Electrical equivalents: terms. (Courtesy of Electroscope, Boulder, CO)

cally are 100 feet or so above the ground, and all our household appliances operate at 120 volts/60 cps. The voltages developed within an electrosurgical generator, in order to be effective for all aspects of electrosurgery, require ranges that exceed 7,000–10,000 volts peak to peak.

Other Factors

Ohm's Law

Ohm's law ($I = V/R$) describes the relation between the properties of electrosurgical energy.

Power Formula

Energy is expressed in AC watts, as in the formula $W = V \times I$, and it is imperative that we understand the three waveforms: those for cutting, fulguration, and desiccation. The voltage/current ratio of the electrosurgical waveform is primarily responsible for the effects on tissue observed when time and electrode size are equal.

Power Density

Power density = (current density)^2 × resistivity. Power density is the relation of the size of the active electrode in contact with the tissue and its effect on the tissue at a given energy setting. For noncontact modalities (i.e., cutting and fulguration) it would be equivalent to the sparking area between the active electrode and the tissue. With desiccation it is the surface area of the electrode in contact with the tissue of importance; here the power density can be *calculated*. During fulguration and cutting the electrode is not in contact; therefore the power density can only be *approximated*. It should be noted that with cutting and fulguration the electrode is in motion; hence the exact energy (in joules) is difficult to calculate at any given point. In general, the larger the electrode surface area, the lower is the power density; and the smaller the electrode surface area, the higher is the power density.

Time

Time is the primary component for depth and degree of tissue necrosis at a given energy setting. Many other components contribute, but time is extremely important, as discussed below.

Cutting, Fulguration, Desiccation

Three distinct therapeutic effects occur with electrical energy in the cutting, fulguration, and desiccation modes. Unfortunately, most electrosurgical units (ESUs) are labeled simply by two modes: "cut" and "coag." These terms do not help to alleviate the present confusion pertaining to the optimal use of the energy.

Cutting

During cutting a high current/low voltage (continuous) waveform that rapidly elevates tissue temperature (≤ 100°C) produces vaporization or division of tissue with the least effect of lateral thermal spread (coagulation, e.g., at the walls of the incision). An example of a cutting waveform with the ESU set at 50 watts is provided in Figure 4.3. During optimal electrosurgical cutting the current travels through a steam bubble between the active electrode and the tissue. Therefore it is important to recognize that electrosurgical cutting is a *noncontact* means of dissection. The electrode floats through the tissue, and there is little tactile response transmitted to the surgeon's hand. The dynamics (or velocity) of the electrode in association with the waveform have a profound effect on the depth

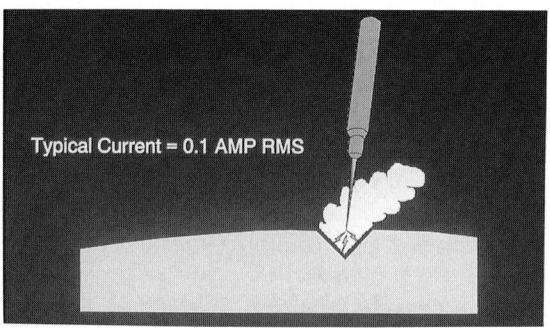

Figure 4.3. Electrosurgical cutting. Electrode is not in contact with tissue. (Courtesy of Electroscope, Boulder, CO)

and width of necrosis around an incision. A depth of necrosis of less than 100 μm is attainable with electrosurgical energy during dissection. The continuous waveform is analogous to a garden valve, fully opened, shown in Figure 4.1, that allows a constant even flow of water to be delivered. Because of the constant flow of current and the lowest possible voltage capable of dissection, the width and depth of necrosis at the walls of the incision are minimal. Therefore the high current/low voltage ratio within the waveform produces the desired effect: less necrosis or less coagulation. If the electrode is allowed to remain stationary or is slowed, the maximum temperature attained is increased as are the depth and width of thermal damage to the incision and the walls of the incision.

Modification of the cutting waveform ratio (i.e., change in the current or voltage product) by interrupting current and increasing the voltage causes the waveform to become noncontinuous, with a train of packets of energy consisting of higher voltage and reduced current per unit of time. Total energy remains the same, but the voltage/current ratio is modified to increase hemostasis (coagulation) during dissection with electrosurgical current (Fig. 4.4). This situation is analogous to a garden valve pulsing the water, with an increase in height to the water tower to compensate for the reduction of hydraulic energy as a result of reducing the time the water was allowed to flow. When utilizing the *blend modes* as well, the electrode should float through the tissue. The blend waveforms require a longer time to dissect the same length of incision than the cutting waveform because of the interrupted delivery of current at the same power setting. With this increased time comes an increase in thermal spread from the voltage component of the blend waveform. The latter enhances coagulation of small vessels during dissection. When indicated, blend modes are valuable options for controlling bleeding during dissection when it is encountered. On the other hand, an increase in the extent of necrosis may result in a high postoperative infection rate. Surgical planes are destroyed, and the amount of smoke plume is increased during the laparoscopy when using high blend or coagulation modes for dissection. Blend 1 is associated with slightly increased hemostasis, blend 2 with a moderate amount, and blend 3 results in a marked increase in hemostasis during dissection.

When dissecting tissue with a cut or blended mode, the ESU should be activated initially before the electrode touches the tissue. *Feathering*, or light stroking (similar to painting with a two-bristled brush for touch-up or fine detail work), should be simulated. This technique allows maximum power density as the electrode approaches the tissue just before contact. It results in vaporization or dissection of tissue. In theory and in practice with optimum technique and control setting, the force required to dissect tissue is zero grams of pressure between the electrode and the tissue. The key is not to allow the electrode to drag through the tissue.

Fulguration

Fulguration utilizes a high voltage/low current, noncontinuous waveform (highly damped) that is designed to coagulate by means of spraying long electrical sparks to the tissue. The coagulation (fulguration) waveform is set at 50 watts in Figure 4.5. The most common use of fulguration is when coagulation is indicated in an area that is oozing, such as in a capillary or arteriole bed where a discrete bleeder cannot be identified. The benefit of fulguration is its ability to arrest oozing emanating from a large area in an efficient manner. Cardiovascular, urologic, and general surgeons have relied on fulguration for their most demanding applications (e.g., hepatic resections, bleeding from a bladder tumor resection, surface bleeding on the heart).

A superficial eschar is produced with fulguration; hence the depth of necrosis is minimal as a result of the defocusing of the power density. By drawing the electrode away from the tissue, the power density decreases (defocusing the energy/current). Much of the energy is dissipated as it heats the air between the electrode and the tissue through which the current must pass.

Fulguration and electrosurgical cutting are noncontact modalities. Fulguration can be initiated in two ways: (1) by slowly approaching the tissue until a spark jumps to the tissue, after

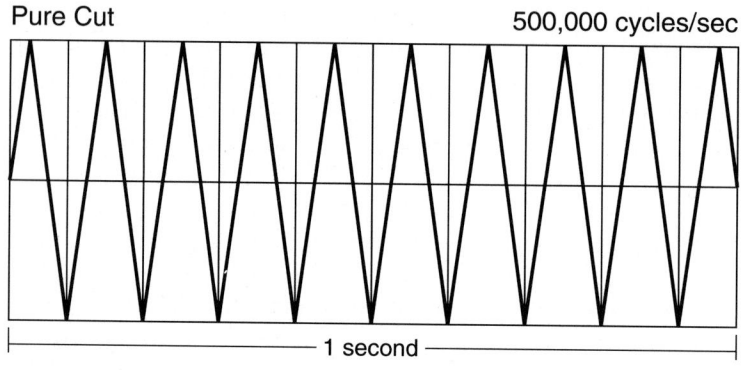
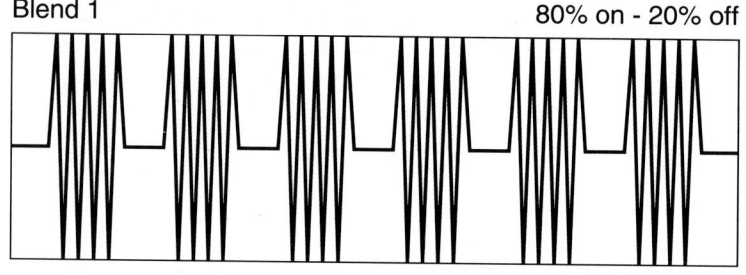
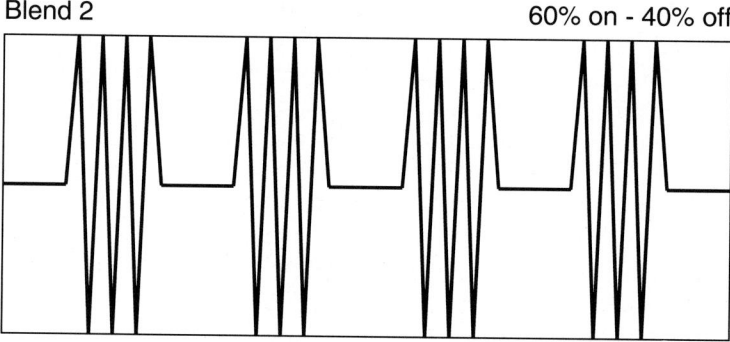
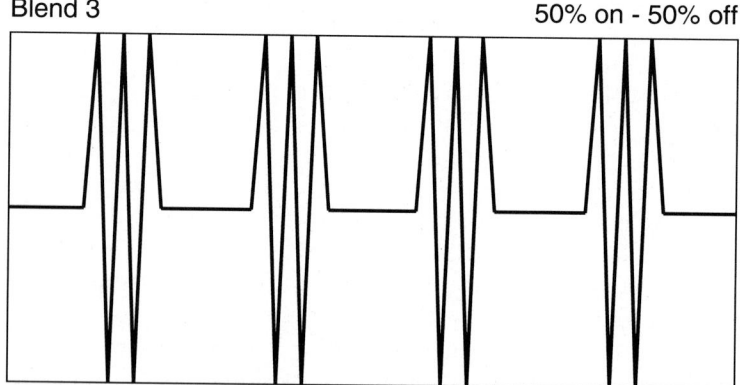

Figure 4.4. (A) Cut waveform. (B) Blend 1. (C) Blend 2. (D) Blend 3. (Courtesy of Electroscope, Boulder, CO)

4. Electrosurgery

Figure 4.5. Fulguration. Electrode is not in contact with tissue. (Courtesy of Electroscope, Boulder, CO)

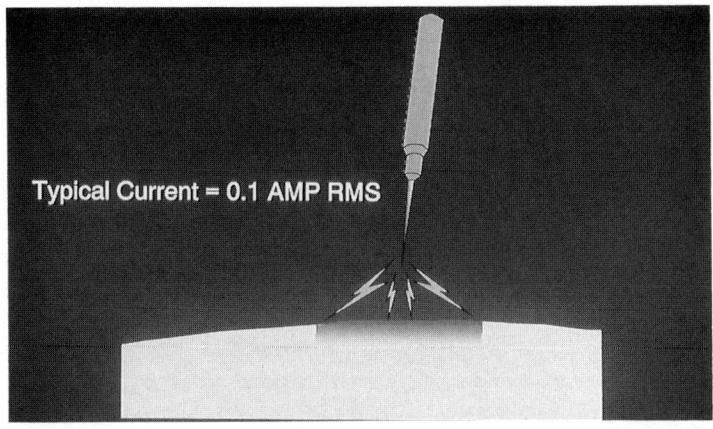

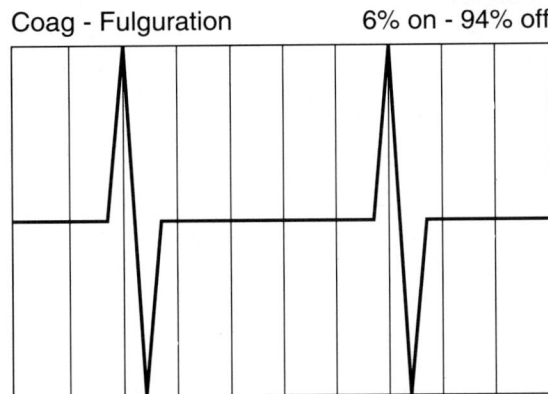

which a raining effect of sparks is maintained until such time as the electrode is withdrawn or the tissue is carbonized to the point where the sparks cease; (2) bouncing the electrode off the tissue, which results in a raining effect of sparks to the tissue without the painstaking effort to approach the tissue until a spark jumps without touching.

Electrosurgical fulguration is the most effective means to arrest capillary/oozing type of bleeding. Before applying fulguration it is of paramount importance to evacuate any blood or physiologic saline from the target site. Time and energy would be wasted sending sparks to these fluids. Evacuating or diluting the field with nonisotonic solutions such as glycine or sterile distilled water can clarify the target site and optimally deliver current to stop the bleeding most efficiently.

The depth of necrosis is in the range of 0.5 mm and may be up to 1–2 mm depending on how long the surgeon delivers sparks to the target site. The key is to stop the flow of energy the moment bleeding has stopped. The energy setting on the ESU multiplied by the time is critical for controlling the depth of necrosis.

Desiccation

Any waveform can cause desiccation because of direct contact of the electrode with the tissue (Fig. 4.6). Regardless of the current/voltage ratio, with the electrode in contact with tissue the magnitude of energy (wattage) is of the most importance.

Desiccation is another form of coagulation. Most surgeons do not make a distinction between fulguration and desiccation but refer to both as "coagulation." The application of elec-

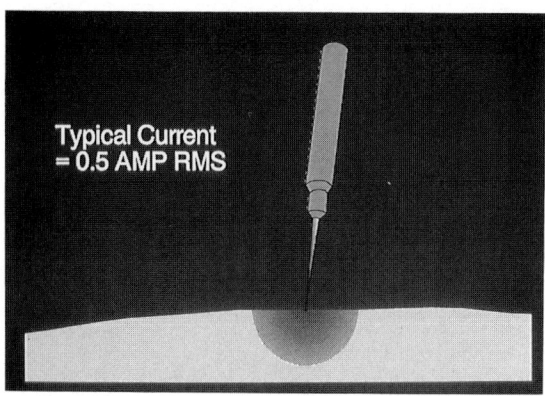

Figure 4.6. Desiccation. Electrode is in contact with tissue (no sparking between electrode and tissue). (Courtesy of Electroscope, Boulder, CO)

trosurgical current by means of direct contact with the tissue now results in all of the energy set on the ESU being converted to heat within the tissue. By contrast, with both cutting and fulguration a significant amount of the electrical energy is converted to heat and enters the atmosphere (air/CO_2) (between the electrode and the tissue). Therefore with contact coagulation/desiccation the increased energy delivered to the tissue results in deep and wide necrosis, as observed on the surface where the electrode makes contact (Fig. 4.6).

The most common application of desiccation is when a discrete bleeder is encountered during an open procedure. A hemostat is placed so as to occlude the vessel by mechanical pressure; and then electrosurgical energy is applied to the body of the hemostat. In this way the current must pass through the hemostat into the tissue grasped by the jaws and back to the electrode. The coaptation of vessels was noted[2] to produce a collagen chain reaction resulting in fibrous bounding of the dehydrated denatured cells of the endothelium. Because the electrode is in good electrical contact with the tissue the voltage/current ratio is not nearly as important as it is when cutting or fulgurating. In practical application the cut/blend waveforms are superior to the fulguration waveform for this application when desiccation is desired. The primary reason is that the fulguration waveform tends to spark through the coagulated tissue, resulting in voids in the bonding to the end of the vessel. Moreover, when sparks occur at the electrode in contact (or in near-contact) with the metal in the electrode it heats up rapidly, causing the tissue to adhere to the electrode when it is withdrawn from the target site. Bleeding thus continues each time the eschar is pulled off owing to adhesion caused by the heat within the electrode.

The waveform plays a far more important role with bipolar desiccation. Today, for the most part, the manufacturers have incorporated a continuous low voltage/high current waveform into the bipolar output to maximize the effect of desiccation. In the older models the manufacturer allowed the surgeon to select either a continuous cut, blend, or fulguration waveform when bipolar desiccation was required. The lack of understanding of the physician is due in part to the literature not being clear about the effect on tissue when bipolar desiccation was performed with these waveforms. Such confusion led to a number of associated documented problems. Therefore at this time the generally accepted waveform for bipolar desiccation is a continuous low voltage/high current waveform. When bipolar desiccation is critical, it is currently recommended that a newer model ESU with a dedicated continuous bipolar waveform be utilized. If the surgeon must use an ESU that allows selection, it is best to start with the pure cut (continuous) waveform. When performing desiccation, patience is the key to good results. Typically the power density is much lower when desiccating. The physical size of the active electrodes is therefore larger. The larger electrode or contact area to tissue requires longer activation times to attain the desired therapeutic effect. The introduction of high energy to speed up the desiccation process would likely be counterproductive. High energy levels increase the temperature in tissue adjacent to the electrodes, potentially forcing the current to spark through the necrosis, resulting in fulguration rather than desiccation. Fulguration, or sparking, immediately stops the deep heating process and starts carbonization of the surface of the tissue only. Therefore when sparking is observed during the process of desiccation, stop the process and reduce the power or pulse the current by keying the ESU on and off to overcome this natural tendency of the electrosurgical energy. Sparking is not necessary or desirable when desiccating. It causes tissue to stick and creates uneven necrosis; it may even compromise the intent to coapt the vessel. An ammeter (model EPM or EM-2; Electroscope, Boulder, CO) may be used during desiccation to determine the endpoint of the coagulation/desiccation. It helps confirm the visual effect noted by the surgeon. The ammeter shows current flow with both visual and audible indicators; and when the electrolyte fluid within the tissue is dehydrated, the meter reflects an absence of current flow. Total or complete desiccation occurs after dehydration has taken place.

Inherent Risks

Since the inception of monopolar electrosurgery, there have been three potential sites for patient burns due to the presence of the electrosurgical current—one intended and two unintended. The intended site is at the active electrode where the unit is used to cut, fulgurate, or desiccate the tissue during surgery. Because of its design, the active electrode has a high power density to heat tissue rapidly. If not attended to, this electrode can burn the patient severely. Therefore I strongly recommend that the active electrode, when not in use, be stored in an insulated holster or tray.

There are two unintended sites, the first being a consequence of current division. Current division to alternate ground points to the patient can occur only in ground-referenced electrosurgical units. Second, because of a fault at the site of the patient's return electrode (i.e., partial detachment or manufacturing defect) the current returning to the ESU is forced via a high current density. The patient may thus be burned. The patient return electrode (ground plate) has a surface area of approximately 20 in^2 or more when properly applied. Therefore little temperature rise occurs at this site under normal conditions. Both of these potential burn sites have now been eliminated by improved design of the electrosurgical instruments. (These safety circuits or features are available on most units sold since the mid-1980s.) The two major advancements in overcoming these risks are (1) isolated electrosurgical instruments and (2) contact quality monitors.

1. *Isolated electrosurgical instruments* were introduced during the early 1970s. Their primary purpose was prevention of alternate ground site burns due to current division. Today, with the introduction of isolated ESUs, the number of alternate site burns as a direct result of current division is essentially zero. A small number of hospitals still utilize ground-reference ESUs, however, so it would be wise to qualify the type of output with respect to the type of ESU that is in service at a particular hospital.

2. *Contact quality monitoring circuits* were introduced during the early 1980s, the primary purpose of which was to prevent burns at the patient return electrode site. The contact quality monitor incorporated a dual-section patient return electrode–circuit for the purpose of evaluating the total impedance of the patient return electrode during surgery. During the course of surgery, then, if the patient return electrode became compromised the contact quality circuit inhibited the electrosurgical generator's output based on this dual-section patient return electrode–circuit combination. This feature essentially eliminated unintended patient burns (i.e., those that appear at the site of the patient return electrode).

These two technologic advancements have reduced the potential for patient burns during classic open electrosurgical procedures. The improved features are now noted on equipment from major manufacturers of ESUs, such as Aspen, Birtcher, and Valleylab.

Laparoscopic Issues

The use of electrosurgery[4] during laparoscopy has been limited primarily to bipolar energy since the mid-1970s. With the flurry of changes in laparoscopic techniques for general, urologic, and other surgical disciplines, a major question of contention has arisen: Can monopolar electrosurgical energy be safely used during laparoscopy, compared to other energy sources? The purpose of this section is to address the issues pertaining to the safe use of this modality during laparoscopy. I address the potential hazards regarding the general use of electrosurgery during open surgery and the options available to minimize or eliminate the potential of unintended burns within the peritoneal cavity during laparoscopic surgery.

There are three potential hazards associated with the use of electrosurgical energy during laparoscopy, and they are a direct result of two factors. First is access to the peritoneal cavity through trocar cannulas, and second is that the laparoscopic view is less than 10% the size of the total electrosurgical device. When passing the electrosurgical active electrode through these access channels and viewing the tissues in such a fashion, there is a potential for unintended thermal burns as a result of stray energy.

In general, burn injuries are difficult to diagnose because they are usually not immediately obvious. Furthermore, the reporting of these injuries is incomplete because of the potential medical-legal implications.[5,6]

Insulation Failure

Most laparoscopic electrosurgical electrodes are approximately 35 cm long. The laparoscopic images viewed on the monitor show only a small portion, typically less than 5 cm of the distal end of the device. Therefore the active electrode used for delivery of electrosurgical energy has insulation covering most of the instrument (electrode) (Fig. 4.7A). Unfortunately, 90% or more of this insulated portion of the instrument is out of the viewing image. Therefore if an insulation breakdown occurs on the shaft of the electrode (out of view of the operator), a severe burn may occur to the bowel or other organs that are in close proximity to or touching the electrode (Fig. 4.7B). Insulation failures occur for several reasons, including normal wear and tear, handling by personnel, sharp edges on trocar cannula, and corona heating as a result of the high voltage frequency product.

These burns may not be noted during the course of surgery and can result in severe postoperative complications. It is most important to examine or have the biomedical staff set up a routine, periodic inspection of all electrodes. This practice can minimize, although not completely eliminate, this hazard. Some suggest that use of disposable devices eliminates insulation failure, but this practice cannot be relied on because the insulation typically found on disposable instruments is of a lower quality than that of reusable instrumentation.

Capacitative Coupling

The second hazard that exists is one of capacitively coupled energy. It occurs with metal laparoscopic instruments in a trocar cannula. Understanding how capacitance occurs requires a degree of understanding of electrical physics, which is beyond the scope of this text. Basically, 5–40% of the power the electrosurgical unit is set up to deliver can be coupled with or transferred to the standard 10 cm trocar cannula. This energy per se may not be dangerous, providing it is allowed to pass through a low power density pathway, such as the all-metal (conductive) trocar cannula inserted into the abdominal wall. This setup provides a conductive pathway and allows the current to return to the patient return electrode. Additional research is necessary to ensure that even small (3 and 5 mm) cannulas do not produce irreversible damage.

Capacitive coupling becomes a problem when this energy is allowed or made to pass through a high power density pathway (Fig. 4.8). For example, as with the part-plastic (nonconductive) and part-metal (conductive) trocar cannulas on the market. Some trocar manufacturers supply a plastic thread to the metal cannula tube to facilitate holding the cannula in the abdominal wall when the laparoscopic electrode is positioned in or out of the cannula port (Fig. 4.8). To avoid this hazard, use of all-metal or all-plastic trocar cannulas that enable the electrosurgical active laparoscopic electrode to be passed through is recommended. Capacitive coupling in conjunction with the use of suction irrigation devices has also been addressed,[7] where up to 80% of the energy was demon-

4. Electrosurgery

Figure 4.7. (A) Full view of electrosurgical accessory into the peritoneal cavity. (B) Full view of electrosurgical accessory with insulation failure. (Courtesy of Electroscope, Boulder, CO)

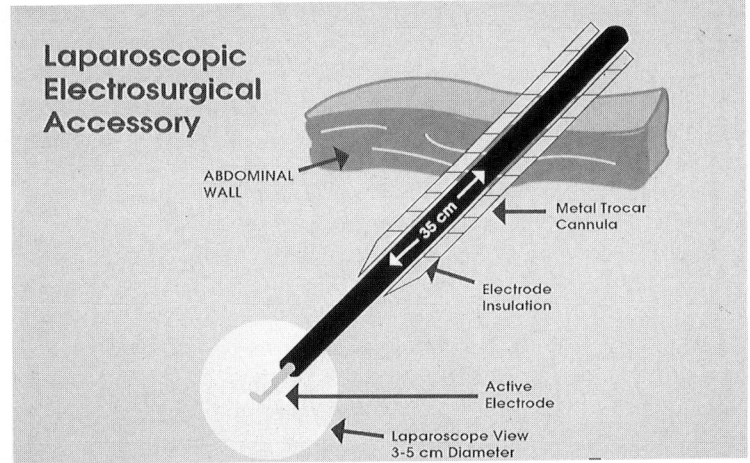

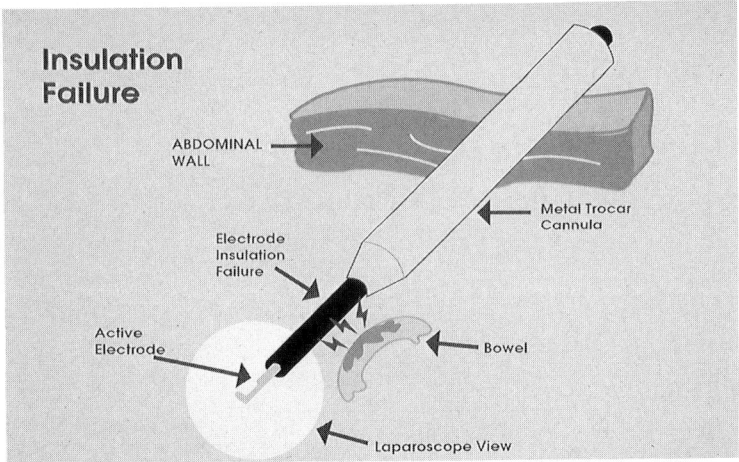

strated on commercially available devices. Capacitive coupling to a lesser degree can occur when "crossing" another laparoscopic instrument with the electrosurgical laparoscopic electrode within the peritoneal cavity (e.g., the atraumatic grasper). The energy transfer to these instruments can range from 1% to 10% of the power set on the electrosurgical unit. Some caution should be taken under these conditions, especially during periods of activation.

The issue of capacitive coupling was first determined during operative, single-puncture laparoscopic procedures.[8,9] These procedures required a long operating channel (30–40 cm) in order to pass various instruments. It was observed that when a plastic 10- to 12-mm cannula was used to pass the operating laparoscope through the distal end of the metal laparoscope, it could deliver a portion of the power (40–80%) set on the ESU, and burns to adjacent tissue were documented. Therefore during single-puncture operative laparoscopy where electrosurgery may be used, only an all-metal trocar cannula should be used to place both the laparoscope and electrosurgical electrode in the peritoneal cavity. There was a strong recommendation made by the U.S. Food and Drug Administration (FDA) to this effect.[10]

Accidental Power Transfer

The third potential hazard with the use of monopolar energy occurs when the active electrode is accidentally touched to the laparoscope

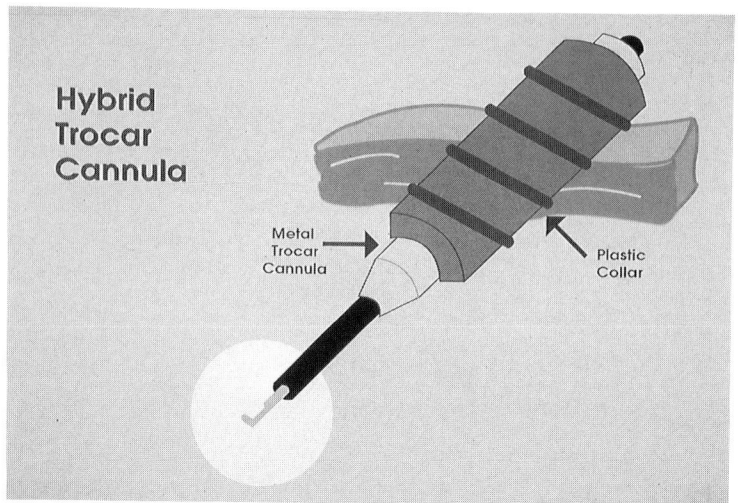

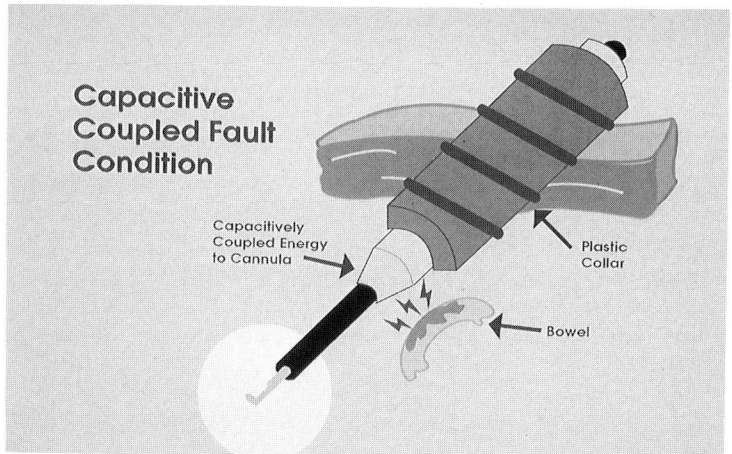

Figure 4.8. (A) Hybrid trocar cannula that blocks the capacitive current from the abdominal wall. (B) Capacitive coupling with dangerous stray pathway back to patient return electrode. (Courtesy of Electroscope, Boulder, CO)

or other conductive instruments such as during a traction/countertraction approach. Where does the current/energy go if contact is made? If an all-metal trocar cannula is used, this energy passes into the abdominal wall via a low power density pathway, thereby minimizing the potential for injury. If a plastic cannula is used, the current may exit to the bowel or other organs touching the laparoscope/device, out of the camera view. This situation is due to the plastic cannula blocking the directly coupled energy from being passed into the abdominal wall and back to the patient via the return electrode. Therefore it is strongly recommended to always use a metal cannula for the laparoscope port and other ports through which conductive instruments are inserted.

Solutions

To eliminate the first two hazards of the delivery of monopolar energy, one company (Electroscope) developed the Electroshield monitoring system, which is designed to actively monitor for insulation failure and excessive capacitive coupling that occurs out of the view of the laparoscope. The Electroshield system features either a reusable adaptive shield to the hospital's "existing" dissecting and coagulating laparoscopic electrodes (Fig. 4.9A) or a line of totally integrated 5 and 10 mm instrumentation (Fig. 4.9B), with the conductive shield built as a component of the device. These instruments are reusable or are of a limited use design. The Electroshield monitor EM-2 dynamically de-

4. Electrosurgery

Figure 4.9. (A) Electroshield: a conductive shield that surrounds existing laparoscopic electrosurgical instruments. (B) Integrated shielded electrode. (Courtesy of Electroscope, Boulder, CO)

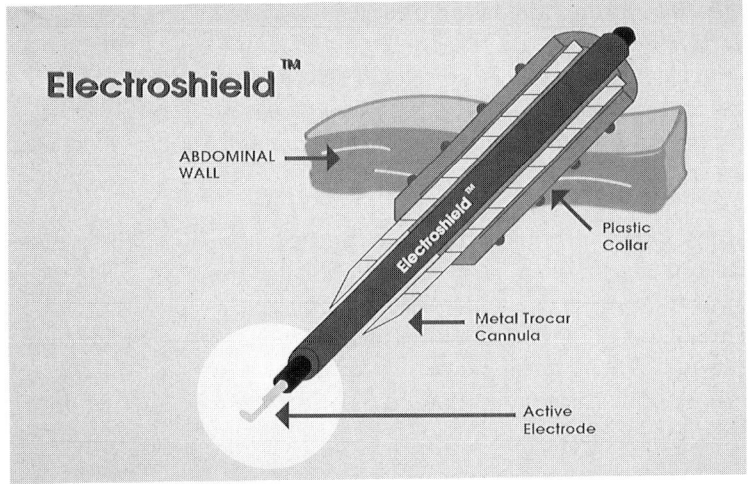

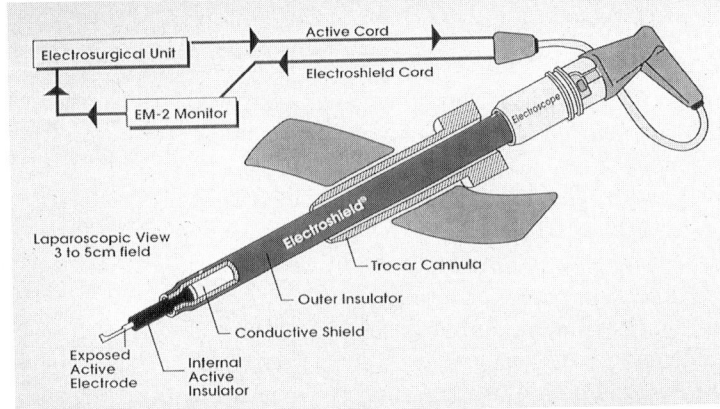

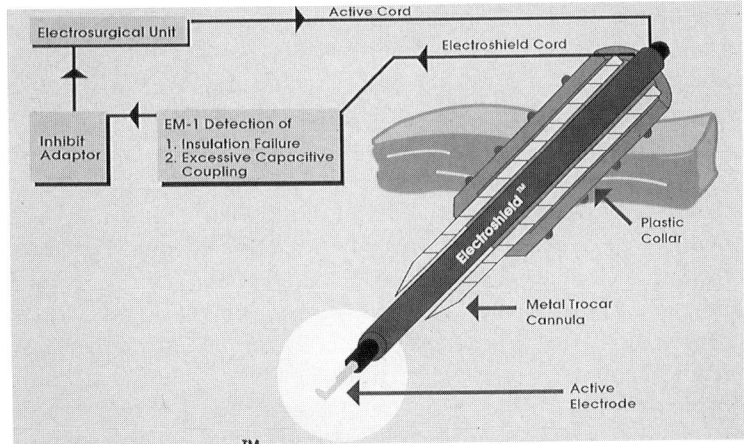

Figure 4.10. Electroshield monitoring system: dynamically detects any insulation faults and shields against capacitive coupling. (Courtesy of Electroscope, Boulder, CO)

tects any insulation faults and shields against capacitive coupling[11] (Fig. 4.10). If an unsafe condition exists, the Electroshield system automatically deactivates the electrosurgical unit before a burn occurs. This technologic "fail-safe" advancement allows the surgeon to use monopolar electrosurgical energy for laparoscopic procedures with the same degree of confidence as for open procedures. The shielding system controls the potential hazard of stray energy out of view of the laparoscope, which is the fundamental difference in the delivery of this energy during laparoscopy compared to that during laparotomy.

Misconceptions

There are two misconceptions that must be addressed in regard to the delivery of monopolar electrosurgical energy during laparoscopy.

First, the electrosurgical current, when delivered at the target site, has the potential to behave differently during laparoscopy versus open surgical procedures. There have been statements to the effect that the current is delivered to one site and then mysteriously exits to an adjacent site, burning the patient at the exit/entry point during laparoscopic procedures. The biophysics are identical with regard to the path the current takes en route to the patient return electrode during open or laparoscopic procedures. Again, the key point is from the target site (i.e., the point at which the active electrode delivers the current—commonly understood as the path of least resistance).

There are a number of known reported complications associated with the use of monopolar energy, such as with procedures where a pedicle of tissue is created by putting tissue on traction and the current is reconcentrated through this narrowed cross section of tissue. This technique results in a temperature rise in the tissue. Such a problem may occur during open or laparoscopic procedures. The interesting point, after thoroughly examining these incidents, is that the surgical technique could have avoided the complication if the surgeon had had a better understanding of the biophysics of delivering the energy.

Second, the voltages necessary to perform monopolar (coagulation) electrosurgery are known to be on the order of 3000–5000 volts (peak) at maximum control settings (120 watts). Therefore normal operating settings (20–50 watts), coagulation mode, or control settings of 3–5 may produce voltages of 1,500–3,000 volts (peak).

There have been statements to the effect that in a closed peritoneal cavity (during laparoscopy) the humidity level and other factors suggest that uncontrollable sparks may occur but would not occur when delivering monopolar energy during an open procedure. Therefore monopolar electrosurgery is not suitable for laparoscopy. Principles of physics indicate that it takes 30,000 volts to spark 1 inch in air under the best conditions.[12,13] Hence in a CO_2 atmosphere it takes roughly 30% more voltage to spark 1 inch, or 39,000 volts, when compared to that in normal air. Humidity levels do not appear to play a significant factor. Hence with operative laparoscopy, sparking from the active tip of the electrode can be controlled better during laparoscopy than during open procedures.

Conclusion

The use of monopolar electrosurgical energy has been the "gold standard" for the past half-century.[14] Its utility is widely diverse (fulguration, precise vaporization, coaptation of large vessels) compared to other energy sources. The technologic advances in performance and safety[15] have positioned this device as one of the most useful tools in a surgeon's armamentarium. The adaptation of active monitoring for stray energy as a result of insulation failure or capacitive coupling and the use of all-metal trocar cannulas will increase the confidence of the surgeon in that "what you see is what you get." As with any surgical tool or energy source, education and skill are required. This introduction on the principles of the biophysics of the interaction of electrical energy and tissue, as well as its safety considerations, is a step toward furthering one's understanding of this powerful surgical tool in an effort to advance the art.

References

1. PETERSON HB, ORY HW, GREENSPAN JR, TYLER CW: Deaths associated with laparoscopic sterilization by unipolar electrocoagulating devices, 1978 and 1979. Am J Obstet Gynecol 1981;139:141.
2. SIGEL B, DUNN MR: The mechanism of blood vessel closure by high frequency electrocoagulation. Surg Gynecol Obstet 1965;121:823.
3. SODERSTROM RM: Refinements in laparoscopic sterilization equipment. Contemp Obstet Gynecol 1980;16:121.
4. RIOUX JE: Laparoscopic tubal sterilization: sparking and its control. Vie Med Can Fr 1973;2:760.
5. WILSON PD, MCANENA OJ, PETERS EE: A fatal complication of diathermy (electrosurgery) in laparoscopic surgery. Minimally Invasive Ther 1994;3(1):19–20.
6. BERRY SM, OSE KJ, BELL RH, FINK AS: Thermal injury of the posterior duodenum during laparoscopic cholecystectomy. Surg Endosc 1994;8(3):197–200.
7. VOYLES CR, ET AL: Unrecognized hazards of surgical electrodes passed through metal suction-irrigation devices. Surg Endosc 1994;8:185–187.
8. CORSON SL: Electrosurgical hazards in laparoscopy. JAMA 1974;227:1261.
9. ENGEL T: Electrosurgical dynamics of laparoscopic sterilization. J Reprod Med 1975;15(1):33–37.
10. Federal Registry 1980;45:12701.
11. LUCIANO AA, SODERSTROM RM, MARTIN DC: Essential principles of electrosurgery in operative laparoscopy. 1994;1:189–195.
12. GALLAGHER TJ, ET AL: High Voltage Measurements Testing and Design. New York, Wiley, 1983, pp 44–56.
13. PEARCE JA: Electrosurgery. New York, Wiley, 1986, pp 60–90.
14. VOYLES CR, TUCKER RD: Education and engineering solutions for potential problems with laparoscopic monopolar electrosurgery. Am J Surg 1992;164:57–62.
15. TUCKER RD, VOYLES CR, SILVIS SE: Capacitive coupled stray currents during laparoscopic and endoscopic electrosurgical procedures. Biomed Instrum Technol 1993;26:303–311.

5
Documentation

John M. Leventhal

> The historian, essentially, wants more documents than he can really use.
> HENRY JAMES

Although Henry James may not have considered the prospect, the physician, in a very real sense, has always been a historian. Whether physicians have *wanted* more documents or have just been forced by the litigious world in which we live to produce them is a moot question. In any case it is probable, as James predicted, that often there are more than can be used.

The primary objective of every endoscopic procedure is success of the operation. On initial consideration, documentation of the procedure may seem to contribute little to that objective. Deeper reflection, however, reveals to the thoughtful reader many areas in the overall evaluation of the patient and perhaps the surgical procedure itself, to which one type of documentation—specifically visual imaging—is capable of lending clarity and continuity not otherwise attainable. Such understanding, gained by reviewing the visual record, often contributes significantly to the success of treatment and to better comprehension of the problem by both physician and patient.

Few would argue that the explosion in imaging technology since the mid-1970s has not changed the fabric of our daily lives or the way we practice medicine. Most, however, would quickly admit to a lack of expertise in technologies not immediately concerned with our ever-narrowing spheres of specific medical interest. The result has been a decreasing ability to distinguish between aspects of the expanding technology that are most applicable to our practice, and therefore helpful in the treatment of our patients, and those that are merely interesting or even exciting. The connection between the technologic achievement of today and the application to the practice of medicine is not always clear, even to the most sophisticated. Who, for instance, could have equated Neil Armstrong's "small step for man" on the moon in 1969 with a two-ounce digital videocamera for endoscopy in 1995? Yet we all appreciate now that the camera and the generation of equipment that goes with it are indeed the direct result of the technology that made that "step" possible. Examples of such areas of technology that touch the realm of endoscopic surgery include the charge-coupled device (CCD), digital archiving, freeze-framing, and nonsilver photography. These terms, long familiar to the imaging engineer, have worked their way into our own lexicon and along with a host of others demand assimilation and understanding by today's endoscopic surgeon.

In this chapter we explore the technology of photographic and electronic imaging as applied

5. Documentation

to visual documentation of gynecologic endoscopic procedures. We attempt to bring some order to the profusion of terms and try to define clearly those aspects of modern documentation technology that can be most useful to the endoscopic surgeon.

What is Documentation?

Documentation is simply the recording of observed phenomena. It is the legally mandated duty of every physician to record in one way or another the observations and procedures he or she performs during the practice of medicine. Most often this recording takes the form of written notes and diagrams, but increasingly in today's technical milieu it consists of radiographs, photographs, and electronic images. In each instance the recording involves an attempt to preserve what is observed or thought about during the care of the patient. The purpose is not, as it often seems, to satisfy the requirements of the hospital record room or to protect against litigation; rather, it is to assist in solving a problem, arriving at a diagnosis, or recording the specifics of treatment for future reference. Every form of documentation is therefore important to the physician in his or her role as a health problem-solver. The more traditional forms of documentation, such as written or dictated records, are to a greater or lesser degree *subjective*. They often reflect as much of the background and prejudice of the observer as they do the object of observation. They are at best interpretive of what is observed or, put in the vernacular of modern technology, not *transportable* as truly objective representations. Although it is probably true that no two individuals observing the same occurrence "see" it the same way, it is also true that the act of "seeing" is the event from which most of the recorded interpretations flow. To observe, however, is to sample with *all* of the senses. Visual observation alone is only one of the bases for conclusions about the observed phenomenon. Consistency, odor, sound, and sometimes even taste are also important in directing the physician to correct interpretations and conclusions.

However, visual and audio observations are the most easily preserved. It has long been said that "seeing is believing," and in most cases we do indeed rely principally on what we see. The audiotape recording of an interview with a patient may be of maximal interest to a psychiatrist conducting the interview. To another psychiatrist, however, not present at the original interview the inability to associate the recorded voice with the patient's facial expressions and body movements might lead to an incorrect interpretation of the data. To the laparoscopic surgeon, primarily concerned with problems of anatomic structure and function, visualization is the key element when formulating a correct and useful interpretation.

Documentation, then, as we discuss it here, means the acquisition, transportation, and storage of visual images in such a manner as to make them available to a number of secondary observers, providing each with the fresh opportunity to draw conclusions based on the closest possible approximation of the "raw" observed material. Our discussion includes some of the underlying principles of various methods of visual documentation and provides the reader some practical suggestions for recording and preserving gynecologic endoscopic procedures.

Types of Documentation

The recording of what has occurred during a surgical procedure can take many forms and involve a variety of technologies, from simple handwriting to electronic recording. It is important to remember that each form may or may not be ideally suited to a particular application but may represent the best available at a particular time to any one physician or in any one institution. This chapter champions electronic documentation, but it should not be necessary to emphasize that *any* form of documentation, so long as it represents the surgeon's best effort to be accurate, is better than none at all.

Written Documentation

Operative dictation is the form of recording most familiar to the surgeon. Its primary purpose is to provide for the patient's permanent hospital record an account of the details and findings of the operative procedure performed. It is intended to inform future readers of the dictation exactly what was seen and done. For many reasons, however, it usually falls short of its intended task. Not infrequently, particularly in teaching institutions, the dictation is left to the junior member of the operating team whose lack of experience often results in the omission of critical observations and many times becomes only a recitation of the details of the technique, with little regard to, or recognition of, the importance of the findings. Far too often, for one reason or another, the dictation is completed long after the operation when it is impossible to remember the findings accurately or sometimes even exactly what was done.

It has been suggested by some that the operative report should be complemented by a drawing of the operative site(s), identifying abnormalities and lesions.[1] Unfortunately, the wide range of artistic talent found in any group of surgeons makes this potentially useful addition to the record variable in its accomplishment and its value.

In today's litigious climate, the operative report, with or without an accompanying sketch, often assumes more importance for the medical record librarian and attorneys than it does for the medical care of the patient. It is unfortunate because, at its best, it is only an *interpretation* of the findings and therefore always a subjective form of documentation.

Visual Documentation

Visual documentation, on the other hand, is usually objective. As applied to operative endoscopy, it is accomplished by any one or a combination of three technical modalities: (1) still photography; (2) cinematographic photography; and (3) electronic (video) imaging. A photograph, movie, or videotape of the findings at surgery represents a much more objective form of documentation than the dictated narrative or crude sketch. Although it is true that the subjectivity of the observer enters into the choice of what to record, those events that *are* recorded most often speak for themselves and present essentially the same view to the secondary observer as they did to the surgeon at the time of the procedure. Although it is true that the surgeon has the advantage of using other sensory input for the interpretation of findings, the recorded visual images present the next best approximation of the original data. Most importantly, they allow accurate fresh interpretation by each subsequent viewer. Inasmuch as the surgeon's simultaneous description can greatly assist the secondary viewer in understanding the original findings, visual documentation is best accompanied by a contemporaneous audio recording on the same tape or disk. If audio recording is used, extreme care must be taken by all members of the operating team to refrain from irrelevant conversation or inappropriate remarks during the procedure.

Before discussing the various types of visual recording in detail it is valuable to review the basic principles of light and lenses that underlie all three forms of documentation. The physician for whom these remarks are intended need not be an engineer to have a good grasp of the optics and electronics of the imaging systems employed. However, the clinical value of the document produced in any procedure is usually directly proportional to the surgeon's knowledge of, and willingness to apply, these basic principles.

All imaging involves recording an observed image on some light-sensitive medium. The medium may be sensitive to light directly (e.g., silver halide photographic film), may be reacted on indirectly by light-dimensioned changes in magnetic fields (e.g., magnetic videotape), or may be altered physically by light-controlled electrical signals (e.g., digital disks, optical laser disks). The quantity of light required in any system depends on the recording medium utilized. For example, in general more light is required for photographic recording than for electronic imaging, which means that even "fast" film is usually not as sensitive to light as the electronic light sensors of a microprocessor chip. In any case, it is the resultant image that is important. The desired result is an image that is reproduced in a manner that renders it recognizable to the observer and is accurately representative of the original object observed.

5. Documentation

Achievement of the desired result implies that illumination of the object was within the threshold of sensitivity of the system and medium employed. With all three modalities of imaging used for endoscopic surgery, illumination of the object is provided by a separate light source designed to work with the endoscope system in use. In all cases of electronic imaging (video) the light source used for documentation and to illuminate the field are the same. Still photographic imaging, however, usually requires an electronic flash as well in order to obtain good color images.

The optical axis, through which light must travel to the subject and return to the sensitized medium in the camera, is composed of the lens systems of the camera (if the camera has a lens) and the endoscope to which it is attached. Because the interface of these two systems is a source of light attenuation, the imaging assemblage should have a close, well aligned coupling at each lens–lens junction. The optical characteristics of these combined systems are subject to many factors that directly influence the amount of light available for imaging and image quality. An understanding of the interdependence of these factors contributes significantly to consistently useful visual documentation of the highest quality.

Adequate illumination is the key to useful imaging and is dependent on four variables: (1) sensitivity of the recording medium; (2) light transmission efficiency of the lens system used; (3) illuminating power of the light source (usually expressed in lumens); and (4) size of the exposed image.

Figure 5.1. Charge-coupled device microprocessor chip used in video cameras.

trical changes brought about in a semiconductor microprocessor chip by light striking its surface. The most common microprocessor chips in current use in video cameras designed for endoscopic imaging in medicine are of the *charge-coupled device* (CCD) type (Fig. 5.1). It is not the purpose of this chapter to detail the electronics involved in the conversion of light energy to electrical impulses or to discuss the advantages and disadvantages of the various types of microprocessor chips (e.g., CCD, CCD-FIT, MOS). It is sufficient to remind the reader that it would be wise to update knowledge in this rapidly changing field at the time of purchase decisions for new equipment. It is important for the surgeon personally to evaluate a number of video imaging systems on the market before making the expensive commitment to buy.

Sensitivity of the Recording Medium

In the case of film, sensitivity is expressed as "film speed," or ASA rating. The higher the ASA rating the "faster" the film and the more sensitive it is to light. The chemical reaction involves a silicon halide salt, layered on film, which is dissolved to a greater or lesser degree in a developing solution depending on the quantity of light striking the emulsion at the time of exposure.

Based on an entirely different set of physical principles, *electronic imaging* depends on elec-

Light Transmission Efficiency

The quantity of light transmitted through a lens system is a function of the light transmission efficiency of each lens comprising the system. All endoscopic imaging involves several lens systems (i.e., lenses of the camera, the endoscope, and sometimes the fiberoptic light bundle). Light passing through any lens is attenuated to some degree, so the attenuation in overall illumination transmitted back to the recording medium through multiple lenses is additive. In addition, the quantity of light varies directly with the diameter of the fiberoptic light bundle carrying the illumination, so documentation is always better accomplished through large-diameter endoscopes.

The surgeon can be easily misled when making a valid judgment about the lighting requirements in a particular imaging situation, as the human eye and its attendant system of central interpretation are capable of managing a wide range of light intensity almost instantaneously. The eye therefore defines detail in both bright and dark areas at practically the same time. In contrast, microprocessor chips used in today's video cameras have narrower ranges of sensitivity, forcing darker areas to be black if the camera is adjusted for detail in bright areas and bright areas to be "washed out" if adjustment is made for detail in shadows. It is therefore important when contemplating the purchase of a video system to select a camera with the broadest dynamic range possible. For the most part, with almost all modern systems, what the eye can discern is usually captured clearly and accurately by the video camera. For this reason there is little to be gained by the surgeon looking directly through the endoscope before attaching the videocamera—or, for that matter, at any time during the case. It is not to say that clarity and resolution are not better under direct vision, only that the difference is usually unimportant. The view on the video monitor is exactly the same quality as that being recorded and has the advantage of making the case visible to all members of the surgical team. Fortunately, when using today's highly automated video imaging systems, it is seldom necessary to make image lighting decisions. Exposure and lighting are also automated in most current imaging systems when taking still 35 mm color slides utilizing synchronized flash. Strobe flash is usually necessary for proper illumination and accurate color rendition for 35 mm still photographic documentation.

Illuminating Power of the Light Source

High quality documentation requires adequate illumination for whatever type of recording equipment is being employed. The modern endoscopic light source, utilizing either xenon or osram as the illuminating element, provides excellent illumination of the operative field and adequate light for imaging. The light produced is a high intensity light in the color temperature range of about 6000°K, approximating the temperature of outdoor lighting and allowing the use of outdoor film for still pictures. Many endoscopic light sources are equipped with electronic strobe flash for use with still photography, although this feature becomes less important with the increased utilization of video freeze-framing equipment.

Size of the Image

With photographic recording, adequate illumination is inversely related to the size of the projected image on the film. If the image area projected onto the film is small (e.g., the frame size of 8 mm movie film), the quantity of light for correct exposure is less than that required for a single 35 mm slide (which has an area approximately 87 times that of an 8 mm frame). This phenomenon explains why the light source alone, without electronic flash, provides inadequate illumination for proper exposure of 35 mm slide film but is adequate for 8 or 16 mm movie recording.

Static Recording

Static imaging can be accomplished photographically or electronically. In either case the product is a "snapshot" of a single moment in the endoscopic procedure. The moment captured and reproduced can be used for a variety of purposes, such as (1) demonstration of a specific part of the surgical procedure for teaching or referral purposes or (2) representation of the "before" and "after" for the benefit of the patient's understanding of the surgery. It is often desirable to make a series of pictures to demonstrate the details of a particular technique or the overall progression through an entire procedure. Sometimes even a single picture of an observed abnormality obtained at diagnostic laparoscopy is useful for planning a subsequent operative procedure designed to correct the abnormality. Still pictures are particularly

5. Documentation

informative to a referring physician and encourage further referrals.

Photographic Recording

Traditional photography with a 35 mm single-lens reflex camera probably remains the least expensive, and perhaps the simplest, method of visual documentation of endoscopy. Still photographs can be obtained in a number of formats. The most common is the conventional (noninstant) 35 mm color transparency used for slides. Furthermore, 35 mm print film and instant formats (i.e., Polachrome, Polaroid Corporation, Rochester, N.Y.) are available and make readily accessible hardcopy of observed findings for records, patient viewing, and inclusion in correspondence. The almost universal availability of rapid 1-hour film processing in most areas makes it possible to have prints or slides the same day as the operative procedure and makes the use of instant film less attractive.

Reduced to the barest essentials, the only equipment necessary in the operating room for documentation is a camera and an adequate light source. However, considering the problems usually encountered when adapting the camera and lens system to the endoscope, it is best to consider the purchase of a dedicated still photography system. Most endoscope manufacturers offer complete systems for still photographic recording of findings using distal strobe flash and automatic exposure control (Fig. 5.2). For all of its simplicity and lower cost, however, the conventional camera-generated photograph is slowly yielding to electronic freeze-frame technology, which is capable of producing static images of nearly comparable quality.

Electronic Frame-Grabbing

The ability to take an electronic "snapshot" of a single video frame has developed to the point where today the hardcopy picture produced has almost the same clarity and resolution as that of a conventional photograph. The obvious advantage to the surgeon is elimination of the conventional camera. The picture is obtained electronically from the videocamera by taking the digital information in a single frame directly from the microprocessor chip and printing it on a sensitive hardcopy medium. It is done with no noticeable interruption in the video recording and, most importantly, can be done "on the fly" by the surgeon without pausing during the performance of the operation. Any chosen single moment or any series of moments demonstrating an important aspect of the procedure can be documented in this fashion by simply pressing a button on the videocamera or by stepping on a foot pedal. Although considerably more expensive than photographic systems, freeze-framing

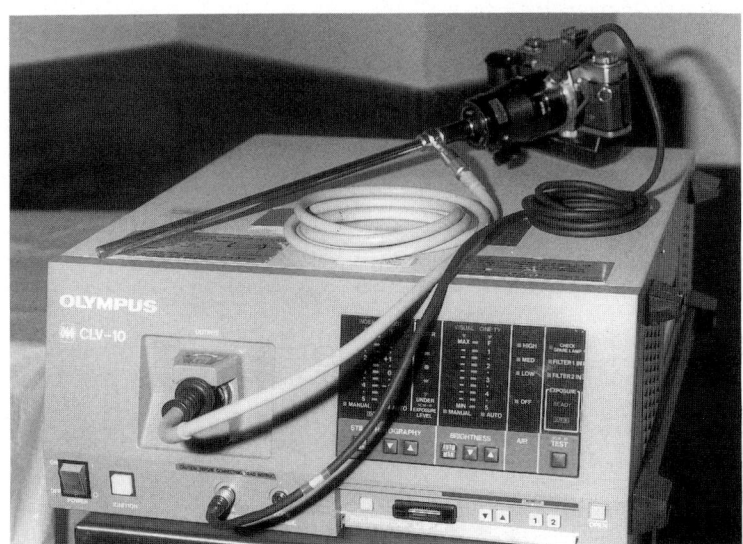

Figure 5.2. A 35 mm single lens reflex camera and electronic strobe flash system for endoscopic recording. (Courtesy of Olympus Corporation)

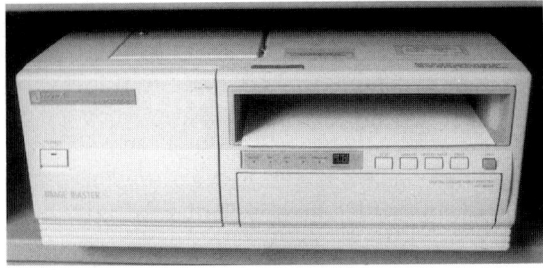

Figure 5.3. Electronic digital freeze-frame printer. (Courtesy of Dyonics Corporation)

systems are available from most endoscope manufacturers and are becoming a standard of the industry (Fig. 5.3).

Dynamic Recording

If the ancient Chinese adage that a picture is worth more than 10,000 words is true, a continuous series of pictures (e.g., cine or video) is thus worth infinitely more. The most useful record of any endoscopic procedure is a *dynamic* one. Whether recorded photographically (cine) or electronically (video), the "live" moving record of the procedure makes the documentation significantly more meaningful to the subsequent viewer.

Cinematography

Because they contributed significantly to the teaching of endoscopy, traditional film motion pictures warrant brief mention. Before the advent of video imaging for endoscopic procedures, cinematography was the only form of dynamic imaging available. Because the film format used was usually 16 mm color, the equipment necessary was cumbersome, heavy, and expensive, placing such documentation beyond the means (and usually the interest) of the average endoscopic surgeon. When produced professionally, with the expenditure of considerable time, money, and talent, there is little question that films produced for wide distribution for teaching are of outstanding quality and value. Some smaller, lighter-weight, 8 mm movie cameras became available during the early 1980s, including an instant 8 mm film cassette system by Polaroid Corporation.[2] Arriving at about the same time as videocameras, however, they enjoyed a short life before giving way to electronic imaging. Modern digital technology has, for all practical purposes, completely replaced film as the medium for dynamic imaging. Not just in medicine but everywhere in today's world, the movie and the heavy projector have given way to the videotape and videocamera recorder (VCR).

Electronic Imaging

It was predictable that the introduction of electronic imaging to medicine during the 1970s would darken, restrict, and eventually completely replace silver halide technology for dynamic imaging. For the reasons discussed above and many others as well, movie-making simply proved too much trouble for practical application in endoscopic surgery. The inevitable application of increasingly efficient, smaller microprocessors to videocamera design starting during the 1980s has resulted in small, lightweight cameras with light sensitivities and image resolution comparing favorably with film. As an illustration of how fast this technology has grown, the National Library of Medicine during late 1994 listed more than 2000 references on video applications in medicine.

The marriage of the videocamera and the endoscope was a natural one from the beginning. First to utilize the video camera on a regular basis in the operating room were the orthopedic surgeons. Video visualization of arthroscopy became *de rigueur* during the mid-1980s. Today it is literally unheard of for the arthroscopist to view the field in any other way than from the video monitor. Diagnostic and operative laparoscopy lend themselves equally well to this "all video" approach. Although acceptance of video technology has spread slowly among gynecologic endoscopists, the general surgeon, relatively new to the laparoscopic approach, learned from the beginning to depend entirely on the video monitor to view the operative field.

With the ability to achieve extreme miniaturization, the newest technical development in video imaging has been to mount the camera itself at the distal end of the endoscope, thereby eliminating the need for lenses entirely. This technique, which has been termed *direct video endoscopy*, found application initially in flexible gastrointestinal endoscopes but was quickly adapted by a highly competitive industry to rigid endoscopes as well. Satava's comparison of direct and indirect video endoscope systems with respect to resolution, brightness (luminosity), and color intensity (chroma) revealed that the direct system produces the best overall video image.[3] At this writing, the direct video system has found little application in gynecologic endoscopy, although at least one manufacturer is offering the equipment.

Video Imaging

It is clear that the videocamera system coupled to the endoscope represents the best method for visual documentation. Nothing comes without a price, however, not only from the financial standpoint but from the educational viewpoint as well. The complexity that makes modern video imaging so useful demands that the endoscopic surgeon, in today's world of ever-tightening budgets, be conversant, at least in a basic sense, with the underlying technology of video imaging. Appropriate decisions with regard to purchasing and utilization of expensive imaging equipment depend on knowledge of the basics of modern video technology. It is pertinent therefore to discuss some of the principles and terminology in common use and briefly review the principles on which video documentation is based.

Basic Principles of Video Imaging

The videocamera used for endoscopy today is based on the solid-state microprocessor chip. One or more of such chips are employed with or without an optical lens system. There are a number of electronic variations of microprocessor chips in use, but because all behave in essentially the same way with respect to image handling, this discussion does not attempt to characterize the internal differences but concentrates on describing what happens to the viewed image in its pathway to the observer's eye and to the recording medium employed.

Each chip is divided into an array of *pixels* (*pic*ture *el*ements), which sense light and cause changes in the electrical resistance of a metallic or silicon oxide ion depending on the intensity of light striking the surface of the array. The pixels are arranged in groups of three in single-chip cameras, each assigned one of the primary colors: red, green, or blue (*RGB*). Unable to distinguish color, only the intensity of light, each of the three pixels is covered by a filter that allows only the assigned color to pass to the element. Videocameras used for broadcast television have three solid-state chips assigning a primary color to each entire array with appropriate filters. This technique greatly increases the number of pixels available, resulting in images of higher resolution. Although not yet commercially available, this three-chip videocamera, with increasing miniaturization, undoubtedly will be refined for endoscopic use in the near future.

The electrical signals produced by the pixels are stored in what is called the *image register*. The circuitry controlling the microprocessor chip allows rapid sequential "sweeping" of the signals (image information) stored in the image register to temporary storage in the *storage register*, freeing the pixels for the next fragment of light stimulation. The rate at which this transfer occurs is known as the *frame rate*, measured in images per second. The electronic signal itself, as stored in the storage register, consists of three components corresponding to the three primary colors. An increasing number of video monitors provide for separate inputs for each component and accept the separated RGB signal. Most monitors and VCRs provide for only a single input signal for the entire video image. Such devices require that the three separate signals be mixed into a single composite video signal. The method by which this mixing is accomplished is termed *encoding* and involves creating a mixed signal consisting of luminance (black and white), chrominance (color), blanking pulses, sync pulses, and color burst; these parts are then transmitted in a time-phased manner. Unfortunately, despite numerous international meetings, as we approach the first decade of the next millennium, there is still no universal standard for this encoding process and no single accepted format. Knowledge of this reality is important to the physician who wishes to make a video presentation in Europe with a videotape produced in the United States. In North America, parts of South America, Japan, and parts of Asia the National Television Standards Committee (NTSC) format is in general use. In most of Europe and Australia the phase alternation by line (PAL) format is usually standard, whereas the French and some countries of the Middle East and Eastern Europe including Russia use séquential couleur à mémoire (SECAM).

In all formats the process of encoding the RGB signal into a single composite signal results in some degree of degradation of the image. The different formats represent differing ways to decrease this degradation. An interim solution to the problem has been the development recently of what is called a Y/C output from the storage register of the camera controller. This output consists of separate Y (luminance) and C (chrominance) transmitted separately at different phase frequencies. Some of the newer monitors and VCRs accept this Y/C input, which markedly enhances edge sharpness and reduces the tendency seen in the single composite image for colors to "bleed" into one another (Fig. 5.4).

The quality of the final image from the recording seen by the surgeon at operation or subsequently by a secondary observer depends on a number of additional factors, not the least of which is the subjective evaluation of the observer. There are, however, some readily detectable differences between images at hysteroscopy and those at laparoscopy. With the former, with distances short and colors grouped around the same frequency, the range of brightness of the image is less important than with laparoscopy, where the white reflection of the ovary is contrasted to the dark reflections of recesses in the cul-de-sac.

Resolution capability of the camera is often used as the sole criterion for evaluating a video system. The camera is only a part of the resolution question, and image resolution is only a part of the larger question of image quality. Resolution is a measure that indicates to what extent details can be distinguished on the monitor and is generally called *horizontal resolution*. It represents the maximum number of vertical lines that can be seen to be clearly separated with the naked eye as measured on standard test patterns (Fig. 5.5). Resolution in the range of 450–500 lines for single-chip cameras used for medical endoscopy is rapidly improving with advancing technology but has not yet approached that of commercial cameras, which can resolve as many as 750 lines. Because chip resolution is directly related to the number of pixels, the extremely small size required for endoscopic surgical applications restricts this number. Evolving technology to increase the density of pixel placement serves to improve the situation. It must be remembered that the monitor used must be capable of resolving at least the same number of lines as are produced by the camera. Most high quality monitors are configured such that in general the monitor is more than adequate with respect to resolution.

Important also to the quality of the image is the signal-to-noise (S/N) ratio. The S/N ratio, which is the ratio of noise to total signal, indicates how much higher the signal level is than the level of noise. It is expressed in decibels (dB). The larger the decibel value, the more crisp and clear are the picture and sound. Video noise appears as "snow" and appears to degrade the

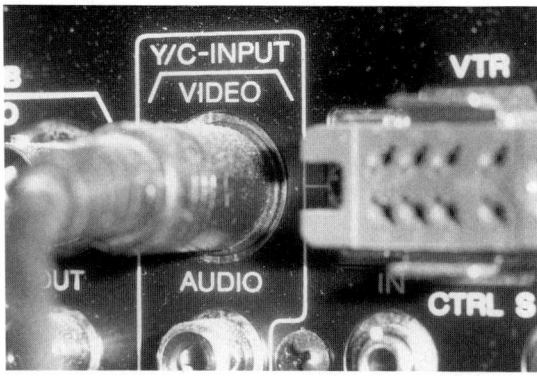

Figure 5.4. Y/C input for video monitor. (Courtesy of Sony Corporation, New York, NY)

5. Documentation

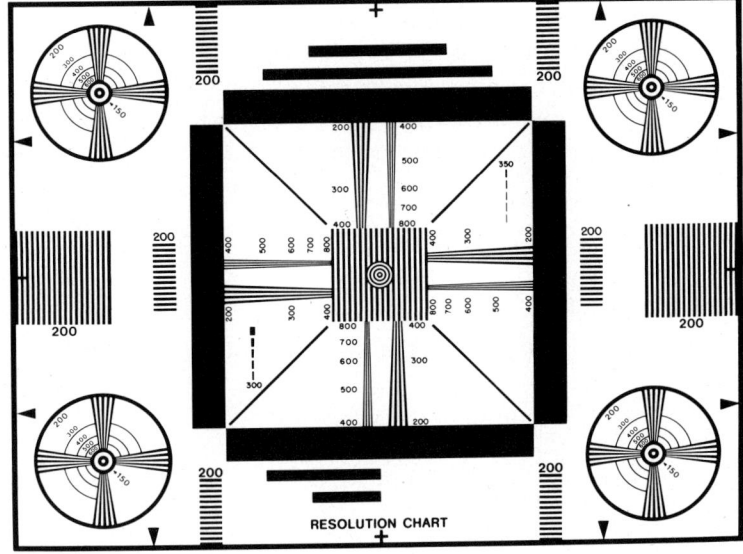

Figure 5.5. Video resolution chart. The resolution represents the maximum number of lines that can be seen to be clearly separated with the naked eye. (Courtesy of Comprehensive Video Supply Corp., Northvale NJ)

crispness of the image on the monitor screen. S/N ratios can be calculated separately for the luminance signal, the chrominance signal, and if appropriate the audio signal. Unfortunately, for the recording of endoscopic procedures, the noise is greatest in the red spectrum, so attention to the specification sheet is critical when considering purchase of a camera. S/N ratios in the range of 45–50 dB are available with endoscopic cameras and range up to 70+ dB with higher quality commercial units.

Video Documentation of Endoscopic Surgery

The modern use of video for endoscopy calls for the videocamera to be attached directly to the eyepiece of the endoscope and for all observations to be made from the video monitor(s). A typical operating room setup for laparoscopy, utilizing continuous video control of the operation, is depicted in Figure 5.6. Orientation to this "indirect" viewing technique takes some practice, but the skill is quickly acquired by

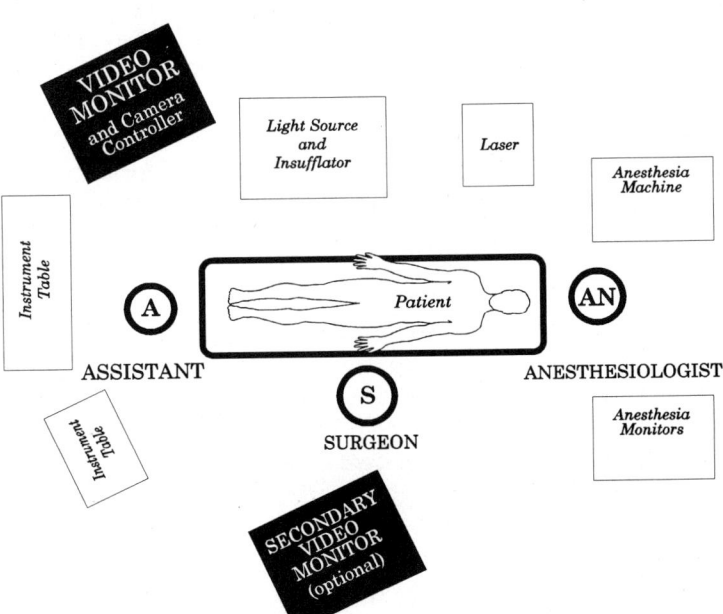

Figure 5.6. Operating room set up for gynecologic video-controlled laparoscopy.

most endoscopists. Hand–eye coordination is particularly important in the case of laparoscopy because of the offset placement of ancillary instrumentation. Observation by way of the monitor is somewhat more straightforward in the case of hysteroscopy, requiring a greater degree of hand–eye coordination in the case of laparoscopy. Continuous video monitoring offers a number of benefits that more than compensate for the inconvenience of learning to manipulate instruments from the monitor screen. Perhaps the greatest benefit has less to do with documentation than it does with providing the opportunity for the operating team to have the same view of the operative field as the surgeon. When all members of the team are working from the monitor screen(s), the surgeon can count on informed assistance in holding instruments and manipulating tissue. Additionally, with the operation "open" to observation by more than the surgeon, there is less chance that subtle abnormalities or potential dangers are missed.

An additional, probably underutilized advantage of video imaging is its ability to combine simultaneous video and audio signals on the same recording medium. A small lapel microphone attached to the surgeon's gown or an overhead microphone, found in some operating rooms, makes commentary during the operation easy. If used, the surgeon can comment in detail on findings and specifics of the operative procedure. This nonvisual aspect of the documentation lends another dimension whereby the viewer is better able to appreciate the thoughts and interpretations of the surgeon at the time of surgery.

In addition to providing a clear visual record of the operation for purposes of review and perhaps the teaching of colleagues, the video record serves to educate the patient concerning her condition better than any other form of documentation. Few would argue the importance of having an informed patient. No medium could be better for informing the patient of the details of her condition and the specifics of the operative treatment than video documentation. The necessary time should be taken postoperatively to sit down with the patient (and appropriate others) to review the videotape. If the anatomy in any particular case is so grossly distorted it makes understanding the normal situation difficult, a videotape of a normal pelvis can be used to demonstrate and compare. Despite early criticism by colleagues, there has not been an instance in 26 years of visually documenting endoscopic procedures when I have had a patient who objected to this method of becoming informed. On the contrary, most patients are enthusiastic about viewing their operative findings.

Storage and Archiving

Visual documents of endoscopic surgery, like written documents, must be conveniently stored and easily retrieved if they are to be useful to others. The best storage in the case of still photographs might well be in the patient's record. Videotapes and movies, however, create more of a problem.

As soon as possible after the procedure and after patient review, the video document must be stored. I believe that videotapes should be stored in unedited form, although it is sometimes useful for purposes of teaching or clarity to make an edited second-generation tape. If the tape is used for teaching, the patient's permission must be obtained and all identifying information edited out. The surgeon would be well advised to use the expertise and facilities of the hospital's audiovisual department (if available) for the dubbing and editing of videotape. If this option is not available, the simple use of two VCRs can do a creditable job.

The storage of documentation materials presents some problems in terms of space. Color slides can be kept most simply in plastic slide sheets (20 to a page) in three-ring binders or, more conveniently if somewhat expensively, in special storage cabinets (Fig. 5.7). Ideally, film is stored in a cool, dry place. On the other hand, the accumulation of VHS videotapes soon becomes a space problem. It is important to establish criteria for the destruction or reuse of tapes based on storage for a finite length of time. I save videotapes (and inactive patient records)

5. Documentation

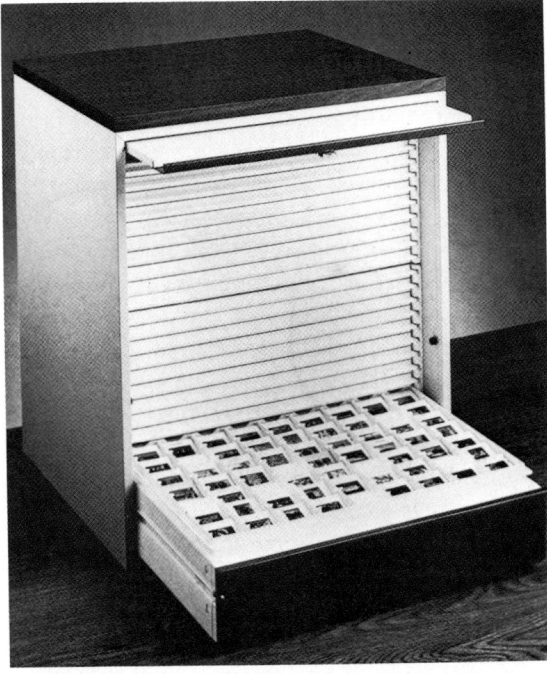

Figure 5.7. A 35 mm transparency storage cabinet with lighted tray for previewing. (Courtesy of Multiplex, Fenton, MO)

for 7 years. At the end of that interval, videotapes are returned to the hospital for erasure and reuse.

Whatever the method of physical storage, it is critical that all documentary materials are organized for quick identification and retrieval. For many years we have used a simple system in which slides, films, and videotapes are assigned consecutive four-digit numbers preceded by "S" for slide, "F" for cine film, and "V" for videotape (e.g., V1234) In the case of slides, as soon as they are returned from the processor the unusable slides are discarded, and a numbering machine is used to number consecutively each slide retained. The identifying number and data on any of the three types of media are then entered in a simple computer database system using the following fields.

Document number
Hospital number
Date of procedure
Diagnosis(es)
Patient name
Age
Operation
Key words

The database can be sorted in a variety of ways to access groups of records of particular interest, or a single record can be retrieved within minutes by simple reference to one of the above fields. Each videotape, slide, or film is stored numerically. Nothing else need be considered. It is vital, however, that documents removed for review be returned to storage in the correct numeric order. This system makes it easy to organize presentations for teaching or conferences and makes a considerable body of experience immediately available.

Legal Aspects of Video Documentation

Because the VCR can be switched on and off without interrupting the monitor picture, any or all parts of the procedure can be recorded at the discretion of the surgeon. This capacity offers a considerable degree of flexibility when deciding what is placed in the visual record, but unfortunately in today's world it brings up the subject of the legal status of the document produced. From the standpoint of legal accountability, all the reasons for documentation are important. However, in the United States and abroad, the legal status of video documentation of endoscopic procedures is vague and has seldom been addressed by legislative bodies or the courts. Critical questions remain largely unanswered. Is the videotape an official part of the medical record? Whose record? Where should it be maintained and for how long? Does the videotape belong to the patient, the doctor, or the hospital? Can the tape be edited during or after the procedure? Can the surgeon tape only those portions of the procedure he or she believes significant? Few courts in the United States charged with interpreting statutes have rendered decisions relating to video documentation or have attempted to answer these questions.[4]

In Massachusetts in 1990, lawyers for a Boston hospital held that declaring the videotape to be a part of the hospital record made the hospital responsible for its storage and preservation—and made it discoverable in any action brought against the institution. It was therefore the opinion of the attorneys that any video record made by a physician should belong to, and be kept by, the physician. They further advised that copies (never the *original*) of the videotape be given to the patient *only* if requested and signed for. This example brings to light possible conflicts of interest between the physician and the hospital and demonstrates the dilemma that stems from the inability of law-making bodies to keep pace with rapid advancements in medical documentation technology. Although it should never be forgotten that the video record of the procedure can be helpful to a defendant physician involved in litigation, it must also be remembered that it is a potential source of trouble as well. If we are to use the video document as the preferred medium for recording endoscopic procedures, the eventual legal decisions must take into account the protection and interests of both the patient and the physician.

The Future

The pace with which imaging technology is advancing makes it difficult to foretell what direction and with what technology endoscopic documentation will proceed. Certainly, equipment and techniques not even dreamed of today will be commonplace before our grandchildren finish their schooling. New equipment for documentation appears on the scene only slightly less rapidly than new endoscopic instrumentation, and with each step forward visual documentation of endoscopy becomes more efficient and easier to achieve.

Videodisk Recording

There is little question that the archiving medium of choice in the near future will be laser-recorded optical disks.[5-10] Similar to the now ubiquitous compact disk (CD), optical disks are rugged, long-lived, and capable of storing enormous quantities of data. For example, Panasonic produces a single rewritable double-sided disk cartridge capable of storing 72,000 still color images ("slides") or 40 minutes of video motion. Any combination of still images and motion can be mixed on the disk. Each "slide" in storage is a digitized representation of the original, stored in a computer database exactly as any compressed file would be in a home computer. As such it is immediately retrievable in exactly the same way a bank balance might be retrieved from a computer. A logbook describing each slide briefly and identifying it by a unique bar code can make retrieval possible by just running a bar code reader pen over the entry. The accessed "slide" appears immediately on the computer screen and can be projected if desired. Because the "slide" is stored as digital information it lends itself to long distance transmission by modem like any other data. In fact, connected by modems and telephone lines or satellite it is possible for someone lecturing on the East Coast to show the "slides" from a colleague's library in California without having any actual slides.

Until recently laser-recordable optical disks have been of the write-once-read-many (WORM) type. Because pits are burned into the disk by laser during the process of recording, the medium is permanently altered and cannot be changed. However, a burgeoning variety of new technologies that allow rewriting to optical disks has completely transformed image archiving. A technique developed by Sony Corporation (New York, NY) uses what is known as Langmuir-Blodgett (LB) thin-film technology.[11] LB films are extremely thin with 2.5- to 10.0-nm layers (virtually (10–40 molecules in thickness) of phthalocyanine. Mixtures of organic dyes in the film absorb light by predictable laser-induced disordering of their structure. By this process the laser writes information to the LB layer on the disk. The light-absorbing spots created in the LB film assume the same role as the pits in conventional laser recording and can be read by low intensity laser scanning. Erasure of the information on the disk is made possible by subjecting the LB layer to suitable temperature and humidity, which reverses the disordering and restores the layer to its original condition.

Using the same LB thin-film technology, Sony has developed a process to lay down multiple

LB films sensitive to different absorbing frequencies of light, making it possible for a disk to hold several images separately accessed by lasers of different colors. Methods designed to achieve similar results are emerging almost daily, with the consequence that the storage capacity of single optical disks has increased sufficiently to make practical the storage of dynamic images such as long sequences from videotapes or segments of digital imaging recorded directly onto the optical disk in the operating room. The latest innovation, known as RAID (redundant arrays of independent disks), combines a bank of optical disk drives by connecting or grouping two or more disks into an array that appears to the user as a single mass storage device. This technique has allowed Tektroniks to place in the market a digital disk recorder with 24 drives totaling a capacity of 96 gigabytes, thus storing 480 minutes of dynamic recording, or more than 800,000 still color images.[12] Applied to endoscopic documentation, such technology allows the recording, archiving, and virtually instant retrieval of entire surgical procedures.

The interactive nature of videodisks, now with the added ability to be erased and rewritten, has made this medium an ideal teaching tool in almost all fields of medicine.[13-19]

It seems inevitable that digital archiving, in one of its mass storage forms or another, will become routine in medicine as it already is in the imaging industry. Physical storage requirements will shrink to a small fraction of that required by older technologies, and both local and remote retrieval will be almost immediate.

Digital Signal Processing

Digital signal processing (DSP) technology is possibly the most exciting development in imaging in decades. DSP advances camera design far ahead of other cameras currently on the market and results in the camera of the future. In the DSP camera the analog signal from the pickup device is converted to a digital signal, processed digitally for signal separation, proper bandwidth setting, and signal adjustment, and then converted back to the analog as NTSC video. As video recording moves steadily into the digital domain, DSP cameras are designed to be easily converted to digital by simply changing the encoder board. These cameras, presently available for commercial applications only, were developed by Matsushita Electric Industrial, Panasonic's parent company. Because of their light weight, small size, and vastly superior image handling, it should not be long before DSP technology finds its way to the endoscopy operating room where it will allow a significant advance in visual documentation.

Conclusion

Visual documentation, and in particular video documentation, plays a vital role in both the evaluation and treatment of the patient. Acquiring skill in documentation techniques should therefore be an integral part of training for gynecologic endoscopy. The significant advances in electronic imaging technology have provided the endoscopic surgeon with an impressive array of documentation equipment with which to record and store operative findings and procedures. So rapid is the technologic pace that almost every month sees an incremental advance in electronic imaging. In any institution, however, there is no need (and especially no financial ability) to constantly update equipment and facilities to match the cutting edge of development. Documentation objectives should be discussed and decided on, and then the minimum amount of quality equipment that can be afforded and is capable of fulfilling the objectives should be obtained and used to its full potential until it no longer satisfies the requirements of that setting.

References

1. YUZPE AA, GOMEL V, TAYLOR PJ, RIOUX JE: Endoscopic documentation. In Laparoscopy and Hysteroscopy. Chicago, Year Book, 1986.
2. LEVENTHAL JM: Documentation of laparoscopy with Polaroid cinematography. J Reprod Med 1981;26:5.
3. SATAVA RM: A comparison of direct and indirect video endoscopy. Gastrointest Endosc 1987;33:69.

4. GREEN HD JR: Medical technology vs. the law. Professional Med Monitor 1991;1:7.
5. The preservation of archival material. J Audiov Media Med 1986;9:43 [editorial].
6. FRIEDMAN RB: Interactive video. MD Comput 1984;1:64.
7. JONES RR, WOODS JW, TOWBIN JA, ET AL.: Use of the interactive videodisk to teach pathology: a preliminary report. J Biocommun 1986;13:22.
8. MORTON R: Image permanence: the videodisk, a hope for the future. J Audiov Med 1986;9:5.
9. SCROGGIE IP: Videorecording and high-definition television systems for the late 1980s: a review. J Audiov Media Med 1986;9:91.
10. WIGTON RS: The new knowledge bases: CD-ROM and medicine. MD Comput 1987;4:34.
11. MANNHEIM LA: Thin-film for erasable disks. Funct Photog 1987;22:49.
12. GREEN H: Magnetic storage for imaging: latest in RAIDs/recorders/tape. Advanced Imaging 1994; 9:32.
13. BLACKMAN JA, ALBANESE MA, HUNTLY JS, LOUGH LK: Use of computer-videodisc system to train medical students in developmental disabilities. Med Teach 1985;7:89.
14. FASEL J, SIEBER R, ROHR HP: Laservision-disk and computer-assisted medical learning. J Audiov Media Med 1986;9:15.
15. HARLESS WG, ZIER MA, DUNCAN RC: A voice-activated, interactive videodisc case study for use in the medical school classroom. J Med Educ 1986;61:913.
16. JAMESON D, ROBERTS L: Interactive video: a new approach to training. Occup Health (Lond) 1987;39:88.
17. LARDENNOIS B, ADNET JJ, OISMAYO C, ET AL: The storing of medical images on videodisc lasers: presentation of the first instructional videodisc in urology. Acta Urol Belg 1987;55:113.
18. TEMPLETON AC: Videodisc-computer technology in the teaching of pathology. Physiologist 1985; 28:432.
19. THURSH DR, MABRY F, LEVY AH: Computers and videodiscs in pathology education: ECLIPS as an example of one approach. Hum Pathol 1986; 17:216.

Section III
Laparoscopic Techniques

6
Laparoscopic Myomectomy

Harrith M. Hasson

It is well known that uterine leiomyomas occur in every four to five women of premenopausal age. They are the most common indication for hysterectomy in the United States. During 1988–1990 a total of 570,000 procedures were performed for leiomyomas. These procedures accounted for one-third of all hysterectomies.[1] Another 33,000 abdominal myomectomy procedures were performed in the United States in 1988.[2] With the current increase of women in the population approaching menopause, any change in the operative approach to treating leiomyoma, from standard laparotomy to operative laparoscopy, may have a significant impact on the quality of life for the increasing number of women who are treated.

A review of the literature suggests that much is unknown regarding the etiology of leiomyomas. These benign tumors arise from a single neoplastic cell derived from the smooth muscle elements of arterioles as well as directly from the myometrium. Their growth is apparently influenced by various factors including increased estrogen.[3] Approximately one-fourth of leiomyomas produce symptoms, the severity of which are due to size and location. Such symptoms include menstrual abnormalities, infertility, and pain.[4]

When compared to standard laparotomy, operative laparoscopy offers several potential advantages, including reduced intra- and postoperative morbidity, shorter hospital stay and recovery time, less bleeding, earlier return to normal activities, fewer postoperative adhesions, less disfiguring cosmetic scars, and improved documentation than traditional abdominal myomectomy.[5-7]

For laparoscopy, access is accomplished through several small incisions, in contrast to the large, retracted incision required for laparotomy. Tension from the distending CO_2 gas, the Trendelenburg position, and occasional manipulation with probes provide the exposure, whereas with laparotomy the bowel is packed away by surgical sponges and retracted by metallic devices. With laparoscopy the viscera are not dried out by exposure to room air or manipulated grossly by the human hand as is the case with laparotomy. There has been less operative bleeding since the development and use of video; moreover, laparoscopy provides some magnification, which permits precise microsurgical dissection of tissue planes and accurate identification of intact blood vessels. It also provides a certain degree of intraabdominal pressure that compresses veins and minimizes venous bleeding if such vessels are cut before they are occluded. Video documentation of the operative procedure provides an opportunity for laparoscopic surgeons to analyze and improve their technique, educate their patients, and provide objective follow-up.

Despite its advantages, the role of laparoscopy in the management of uterine leiomyomas remains controversial.[8] This controversy is the combined result of a fear of intraoperative complications and technical difficulties; apprehension concerning the ultimate status of the uterine scar; uncertainty about the extent of postoperative adhesions, reproductive outcome, and operative efficiency relative to relief of symptoms; and doubt concerning recurrence and reoperation. The fact that laparoscopic myomectomy is sometimes performed by those who do not have sufficient knowledge or experience and do not follow the basic surgical principles that optimize safety and efficacy of the procedure contributes to this controversy. Surgeons who are well trained and skilled in the procedure have an opportunity to diminish these fears and improve the quality of life for their patients with this cost-effective, beneficial treatment.

Indications, Contraindications, and Preoperative Assessment

Myomectomy can be a challenging procedure to perform laparoscopically. However, when a patient is chosen carefully and the procedure is performed within the appropriate guidelines, the benefits are significant.

Myomectomy by laparoscopy is indicated if the myoma is associated with infertility, recurrent abortion, bleeding, pain, or pressure symptoms of significant nature and duration in patients who want to preserve their uterus. It is also appropriate if the size of the pelvic mass is more than 12 gestational weeks or if the dominant myoma is larger than 7 cm or growing rapidly.

Laparoscopic myomectomy is contraindicated when it is inadvisable for the patient to be maintained in the Trendelenburg position with a distended abdomen for a long time, the uterus is larger than 18 gestational weeks, or the dominant myoma is larger than 15 cm. It is relatively contraindicated when the patient has advanced disease with diffuse leiomyomatosis or more than six significant myomas 3 cm or larger, or the lesion is submucous and protrudes more than 50% into the endometrial cavity.

Leiomyomas are evaluated by pelvic examination. Confirmation is usually accomplished by ultrasonography, although this evaluation is not accurate in patients who have marked uterine enlargement, submucous lesions,[9] congenital uterine anomalies,[10] or excessive obesity.[11] In these cases, magnetic resonance imaging (MRI) appears to be more reliable.[9] This type of radiologic imaging has been used successfully to differentiate between leiomyomas and adenomyosis.[12] For most patients, MRI is not cost-effective. It is important to evaluate the endometrial cavity with hysteroscopy, ultrasonography, or hysterosalpingography prior to surgery. The endometrium is sampled as deemed necessary.

Instrumentation

Laparoscopic myomectomy requires the availability of an appropriate videocamera system and laparoscope, an electronic high-flow insufflator, and an electrosurgical unit. Alternative energy sources may include the CO_2 or neodymium-yttrium-aluminum garnet (Nd:YAG) laser, the Harmonic ultrasonic scalpel, and endocoagulation according to Semm.

Instruments required for this operation include cannulas to secure stable access to the operative field, such as the Laparosac ballooned cannula (Marlow Surgical Technologies, Willoughby, OH). This cannula, which protrudes minimally into the abdomen, offers optimal stability during tissue manipulation and instrument exchanges and eliminates the occurrence of subcutaneous emphysema (see Figure 2.10). Appliances for uterine elevation and tools for incision, cutting, grasping, manipulation, and suturing are also necessary. Preferred implements include a bulldog grasper (Linvatec, Largo, FL) or a forceps with spike to hold tissues securely and the myoma drill (Resnick Instrument Co., Skokie, IL) to fix and manipulate the tumor. A vaginal speculum with attached

6. Laparoscopic Myomectomy

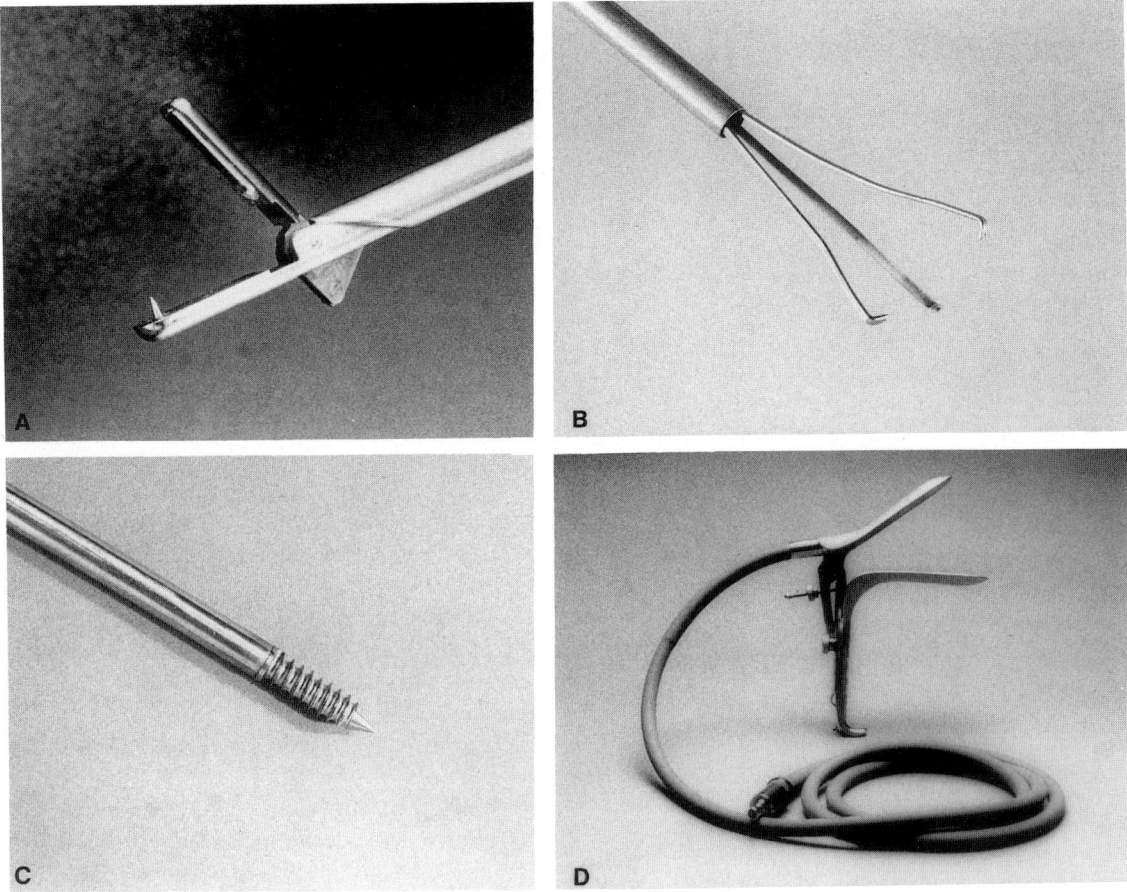

Figure 6.1. Special instruments for laparoscopic myomectomy. (A) Toothed forceps. (B) Bulldog grasper. (C) Myoma drill. (D) Vaginal speculum with fiberoptic light. (From Hasson et al.[5] Reprinted with permission from *Obstetrics and Gynecology*)

fiberoptic light source is useful for furnishing enhanced illumination of the vaginal apex during vaginal extraction (Fig. 6.1).

Preoperative Preparation

Preoperative medical therapy is usually limited to patients with leiomyomas larger than 6 cm. Gonadotropin-releasing hormone agonists (GnRH-a) have effectively replaced earlier drug therapies. Medical treatment with GnRH-a is prescribed to: (1) reduce the volume and vascularity of myomas and the host uterus; (2) relieve associated symptoms; (3) reduce intraoperative blood loss; and (4) facilitate removal of the tumor masses during laparoscopic surgery. By inducing an anovulatory hypoestrogenic state, shrinkage of the uterine volume was reported to result in a 36% mean decrease in size at 12 weeks and 45% at 24 weeks,[6,13] with a range of 35–57%.[14] However, GnRH-a may have an additional inhibitory role on the growth of leiomyomas through direct action on specific GnRH binding sites in the leiomyomas.[15]

Vasomotor flushes, insomnia, mood changes, headache, and vaginal dryness are a number of the unpleasant side effects of the induced hypoestrogenic state,[13,14] as is the potential for trabecular bone loss with long-term administration. For these reasons preoperative GnRH-a therapy is limited to 6 months, especially as it has been shown that maximal benefits are essentially achieved by 12 weeks.[13]

The primary inhibitory effect of GnRH-a on myomatous tissue and the reduced blood supply to the tumor that is secondary to the hypoestrogenic state may cause intense degenerative changes in large myomas, which may lead to difficult enucleation of affected tumors during laparoscopic myomectomy and difficult microscopic evaluation of the excised tissues.

Patients who undergo laparoscopic myomectomy receive cleansing enemas or a Golytely (Braintree Laboratories, Braintree, MA) bowel preparation prior to surgery. Prophylactic antibiotics are also routinely administered.

The patient is placed in the lithotomy position following adequate anesthesia. The legs are placed into stirrups (e.g., Allen Universal Stirrups; Allen Medical Systems, Cleveland, OH) with the thighs roughly parallel to the floor and the feet resting comfortably in the footrests of the boot. The patient's toe, knee, and opposite shoulder are aligned in a straight line. Jelly pads are placed between the boot of the stirrup and the leg of the patient to prevent inappropriate pressure points. A suitable uterine elevator is placed in the uterus to allow satisfactory uterine manipulation and orientation. A Foley catheter is placed in the bladder and left in-dwelling.

Surgical Technique

A capable associate surgeon or assistant is indispensable, as many of the steps of the operation require movements that must be precisely coordinated between two knowledgeable and able individuals. After establishing laparoscopic access, the procedure consists of three distinct steps: (1) disengaging the myoma from its uterine bed; (2) managing the uterine defect; and (3) removing the myoma from the abdomen.

Access and Evaluation

In addition to a laparoscope port, three secondary access cannulas at points drawn along the line of an imaginary Pfannenstiel incision are placed for operative manipulation. The level of the secondary access points varies with the size of the uterus.

After exploration of the pelvic organs and upper abdomen, associated conditions are evaluated and treated, such as endometriosis, adhesions, or an ovarian cyst. The laparoscopic procedure should be terminated and converted to standard laparotomy if the extent of the disease is beyond the scope of the procedure's selection criteria or the operative capacity of the surgical team.

Disengaging the Leiomyoma(s)

The surgeon begins by injecting dilute vasopressin, 10 U in 50 ml of saline, subserosally along the site of incision and into the myometrium at the base of the myoma (Fig. 6.2). Pedunculated myomas at the base of the pedicle are excised. A vertical incision is made into the pseudocapsule down to the characteristically pearly white substance of the tumor. Either unipolar small surface electrodes, CO_2 laser beam, the YAG laser or the ultrasonic Harmonic Scalpel is used for this purpose. More than one myoma can be removed from the same vertical incision. All dissections are performed inside the pseudocapsule of the myoma. Leiomyomas should not

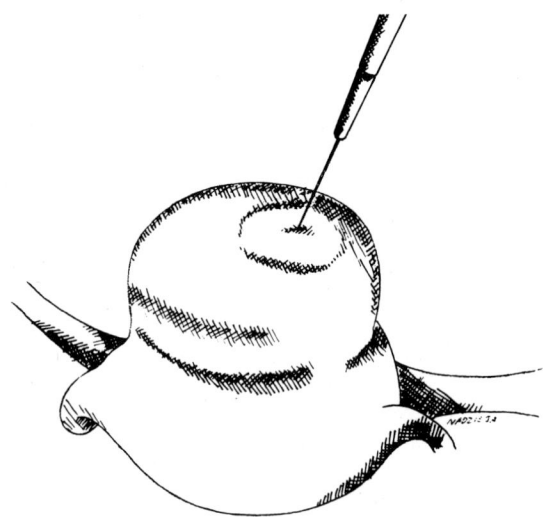

Figure 6.2. Vasopressin injection over incision site. (From Hasson.[6] Reprinted with permission from Raven Press)

6. Laparoscopic Myomectomy

be resected en masse with the surrounding myometrium because it would invariably cause bleeding and lead to weakness of the uterine wall, which predisposes the uterus to dehiscence and fistula formation.

The largely avascular tissue plane that separates the tumor from its uterine bed should be located and any connecting bridges sought. The arrangement is somewhat analogous to an onion; the space between two layers of an onion is similar to the avascular plane. These bridges consist of connective tissue and blood vessels of varying size that feed the tumor. Video magnification allows accurate identification of the tissue planes and the blood vessels. The next step is to develop the cleavage plane between the myoma and its pseudocapsule by cutting the connecting bridges. It is accomplished, as with any other surgical procedure, by applying traction on the myoma and countertraction on the cut edge of the pseudocapsule (Fig. 6.3). Do not dissect haphazardly in vascular planes, as it would lead to excessive bleeding. The vessels must be coagulated before they are incised. Capture large vessels on two sides between the jaws of an instrument that carries an energy source. This instrument provides effective hemostasis and seals the blood vessels prior to cutting. Attempting coagulation from just one side of the vessel may prove ineffective, as coagulation may not be complete and the compro-

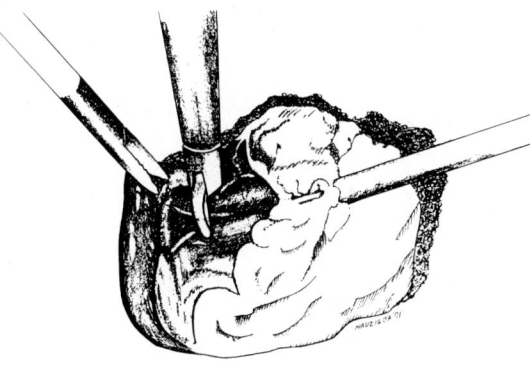

Figure 6.3. Exposure of connective tissue bridges between the myoma and the pseudocapsule with traction and countertraction and cutting of the bridges. (From Hasson et al.[5] Reprinted with permission from *Obstetrics and Gynecology*)

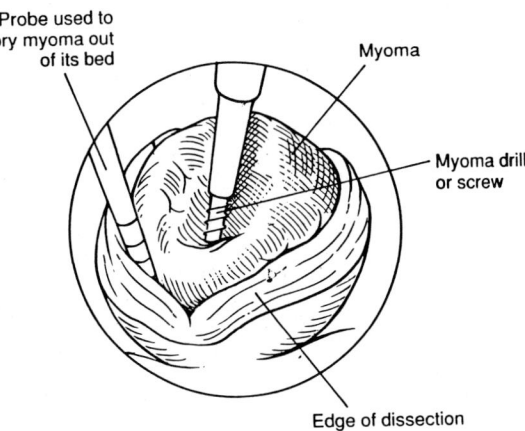

Figure 6.4. Prying technique. The myoma is fixed and manipulated with a myoma drill and pried out of its bed with a probe placed in the cleavage plane. (From Hasson.[7] Reprinted with permission from Raven Press)

mised vessel may retract, continue bleeding, and become difficult to identify and control. The application of sutures or staples is effective but not practical.

A myoma drill is helpful for manipulation and traction. The next step requires the "prying method" for blunt dissection by placing a probe (or any instrument that functions as a probe) in the cleavage plane to leverage the tumor against the uterine wall and pry it out of its bed (Fig. 6.4). This step should be done firmly but gently to avoid shearing large vessels and subsequent bleeding. Once the myoma is substantially excised from its bed, the myoma drill is replaced by the bulldog grasper, and strong traction is applied in various directions to expose any remaining bridges as well as the primary vascular pedicle. When the proper technique is used, dissection proceeds with surprising ease and little or no bleeding. Once the vascular pedicle is identified, it is coagulated thoroughly with bipolar cautery and cut with sharp scissors to free the myoma (Fig. 6.5).

Occasionally the findings are those of adenomyosis; soft spongy tissue having the appearance of altered myometrium (adenomyoma) or of a homogeneous degenerating mass of tissue. Degeneration may result from benign conditions that diminish blood supply to the tumor

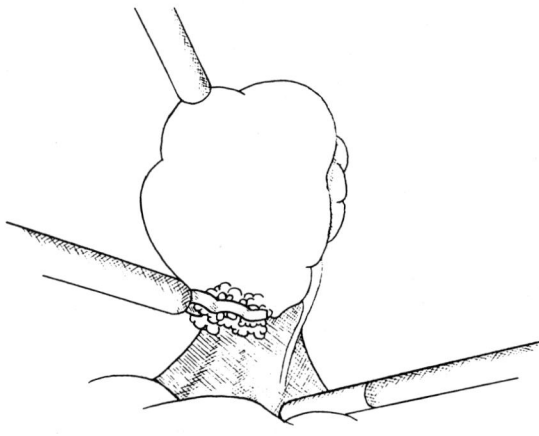

Figure 6.5. Bipolar coagulation of the vascular pedicle. (From Hasson.[6] Reprinted with permission from Raven Press)

(e.g., rapid growth), use of GnRH-a, or malignant transformation. Unfortunately, benign degeneration cannot be clearly differentiated from sarcomatous change by gross examination[16] or even by intraoperative frozen sections.[17] The operative management of adenomyosis includes simple biopsy and subsequent conservative medical therapy or definitive surgery, wedge resection of the lesion and closure of the uterine defect, and at times myolysis.

Managing the Operative Defect

Close the uterine surgical defect in layers. The cut muscles of the myometrium tend to retract and maintain the surgical gap on a permanent basis unless they are connected by sutures that support uterine healing and remodeling. Although correct approximation and scaffolding of the myometrial edges is essential, the use of many layers of constricting sutures is not. In fact, excessive use of tight hemostasic sutures in the myometrial bed may be harmful.

The operative defect is managed according to the following guidelines.

1. *Pedunculated, subserosal, and intraligamentary leiomyomas.* It is important to coagulate the edges of the operative site to achieve meticulous hemostasis; as it prevents postoperative hematomas and mitigates against adhesion formation. The site may be covered with a tissue barrier, although this measure is not usually necessary.

2. *Superficial intramural tumors.* Achieve hemostasis of the wound edges and then approximate the uterine defect with one continuous "baseball"-type stitch that includes the serosa (Fig. 6.6). The needle-through-the-noose knot secures the beginning of the suture[18] (Fig. 6.7), and the half-hitch end knot secures the end[19] (Fig. 6.8).

3. *Deep intramural myomas* (with or without a submucous component). Add one or more interrupted sutures to close the myoma bed. Use a 122 cm (48 inches) Gore-Tex (W. L. Gore and Associates, Flagstaff, AZ) or other non-absorbable suture, size 0, on a large straight or ski needle to make a "belt" stitch—a vertical mattress that approximates the uterine muscles at a deep and more superficial level. Enter the uterus with a needle from outside in through the serosa and emerge at the surgical bed. Grasp the needle, reapply it, and go through the opposite uterine wall from inside out. When the needle clears the uterine wall, grasp it and reapply in a reverse fashion at a more superficial level to complete the vertical mattress suture. Bring the needle end of the suture out of the 5 mm cannula, tie a Roeder loop knot extracorporeally, and bring it down into the abdomen to cinch the stitch. Apply a staple on the long suture strand

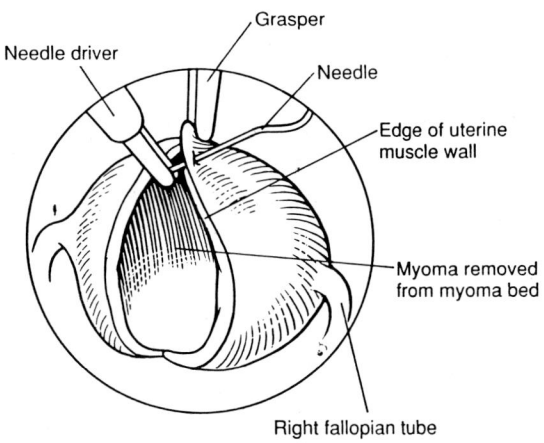

Figure 6.6. Beginning of a baseball stitch to close a superficial uterine defect. (From Hasson.[7] Reprinted with permission from Raven Press)

6. Laparoscopic Myomectomy

Figure 6.7. Sequence for securing the beginning of a continuous suture using the needle through the noose knot. (A) Noose loop resting on one side of the incision. (B) Needle pulled through the noose loop. (C) Noose loop tightens over the enclosed suture. (D) Knot is formed. (From Hasson.[19] Reprinted with permission from *Obstetrics and Gynecology*)

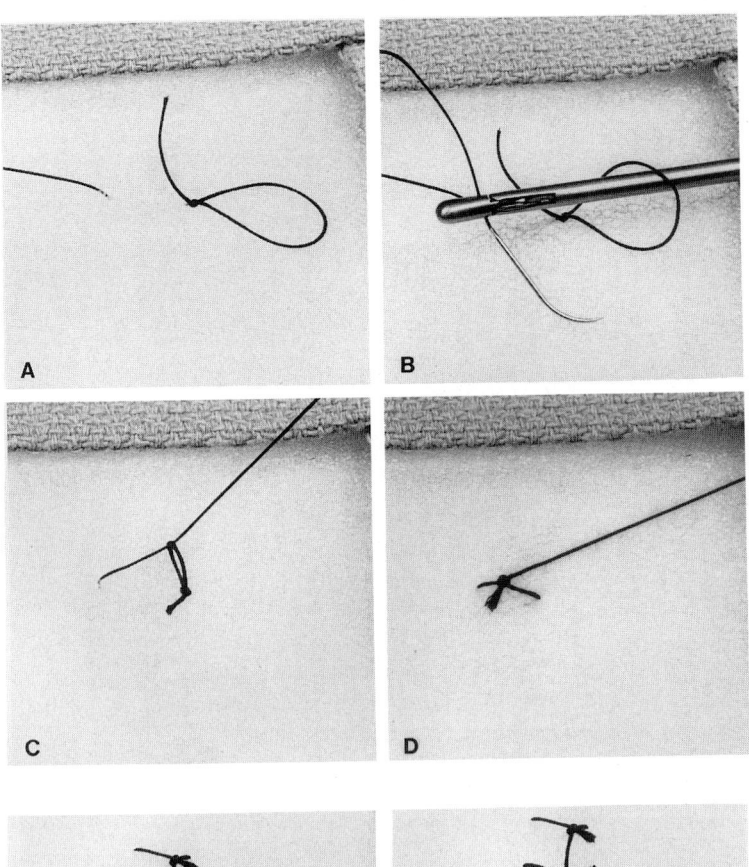

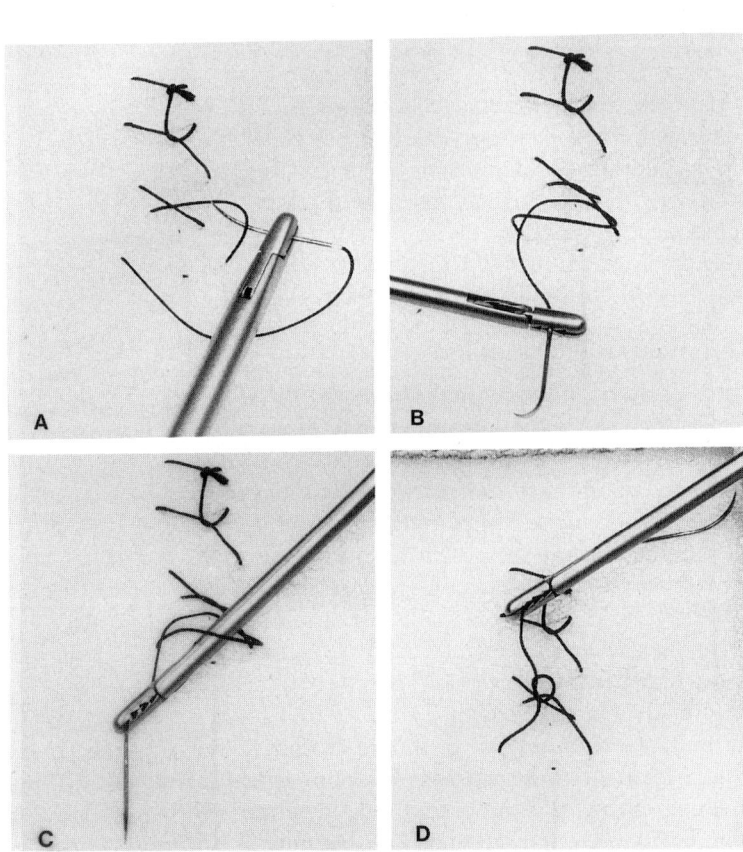

Figure 6.8. Sequence for completing a continuous suture using the half-hitch end knot. (A) Needle is passed under the loop of the last stitch. (B) Second loop is formed within the remaining suture. (C) Knot-forming end of the suture is pulled into the loop. (D) Knot-forming end is pulled out of the loop to tighten the sliding knot over the enclosed suture. (From Hasson.[19] Reprinted with permission from *Obstetrics and Gynecology*)

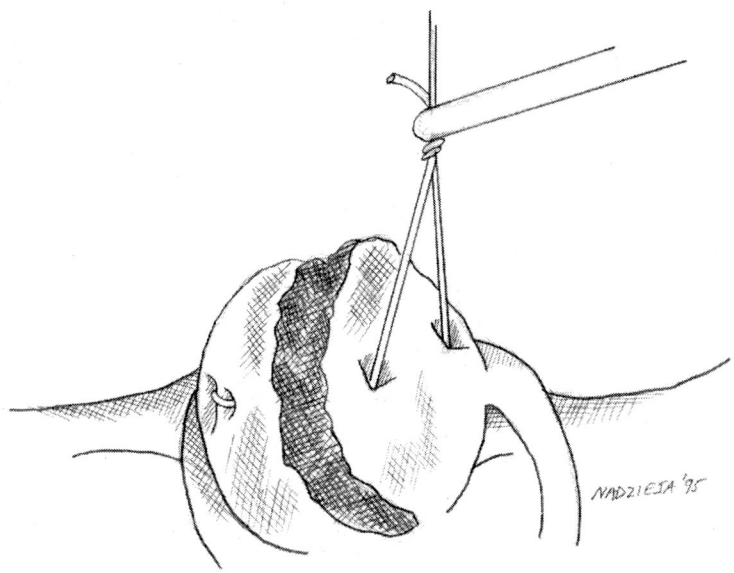

Figure 6.9. Belt stitch. A vertical through-and-through mattress suture is used to close the uterine defect at a deep level and at a more superficial level.

over which the loop slides to secure the knot (Fig. 6.9). Alternatively, secure the Roeder loop knot by forming another knot between the two suture loops.

Tissue barriers such as expanded polytetrafluoroethylene (ePTFE; Gore-tex membrane; W. L. Gore and Associates, Flagstaff, AZ) or Tc7 (Interceed; Ethicon, Somerville, NJ) may be useful for preventing or minimizing the formation of adhesions. Staples may be used as markers for subsequent evaluation of the uterine scar by hysterosalpingogram.[20] Alternatively, the scar may be evaluated by ultrasonography or MRI.

Removing the Myoma(s)

After excision individual myomas are stored in the cul-de-sac or the left upper quadrant. It is preferable to excise the myoma intact from the uterine wall and then morcellate it. At times the tumor can be incised after bulging out and cut down the middle, or a central portion is removed to facilitate dissection of each half. At other times, when the myoma is soft and degenerated, it can be sliced transversely to debulk it and to facilitate exposure of the vascular pedicle. Remove the myomas through a 10 or 12 mm cannula, a colpotomy, or a minilaparotomy incision. Morcellation according to Semm, posterior colpotomy and the orange peel technique[5] (Fig. 6.10), bisection, and minilaparotomy with

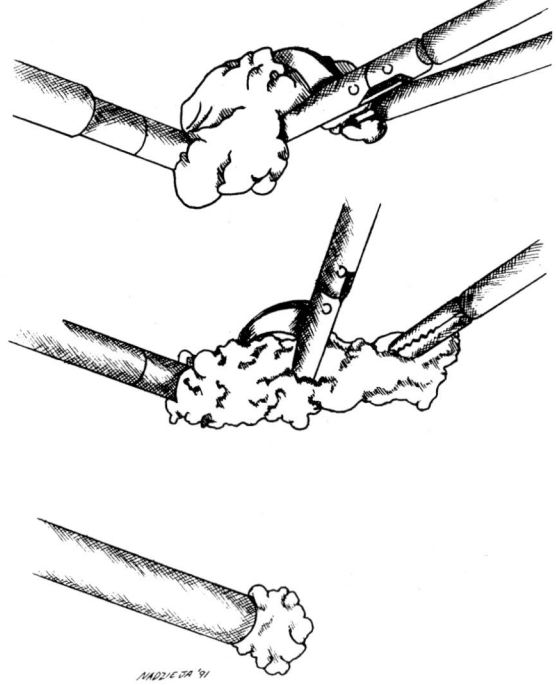

Figure 6.10. Converting a myoma into a narrow strip of tissue with the "orange-peel technique." (From Hasson et al.[5] Reprinted with permission from *Obstetrics and Gynecology*)

externalization of morcellation outside the abdomen[21] are effective techniques for removal, but they are cumbersome and time-consuming.

A simplified laparoscopic abdominal morcellation (SLAM) technique has been developed (C. Rotman, personal communication) that is much easier and faster to perform. The specimen is held securely from both sides and sliced longitudinally with a sharp knife. The slices are removed through a slightly enlarged incision following removal of the suprapubic cannula. The orange peel technique using a sharp knife or scissors complements the SLAM technique. Instruments and methods for the SLAM technique are currently being researched.

Clinical Experience and Comparison

The results of 110 procedures performed over the last 6 years confirm the safety and efficacy of laparoscopic myomectomy. My initial experience with 56 cases[5] in conjunction with that from nine other studies on myomectomy by laparotomy or laparoscopy[22-30] (Table 6.1) revealed a lower estimated blood loss and shorter length of stay with laparoscopy than laparotomy. Our operative time diminished as our experience and technique improved (currently it is 1–2 hours depending on the size, location, and number of leiomyomas and the extent of associated adhesions and other lesions). In the reported series, 34% of the patients had associated pelvic adhesions, 27% had endometriosis, and 4% had ovarian cysts. Other investigators have reported similar observations.[24,28,29]

Complications

There have been few complications in the 110 patients evaluated. To date, no blood transfusion or return to surgery has been required. One patient developed febrile morbidity associated with an upper respiratory tract infection and subcutaneous emphysema. Five patients developed subcutaneous emphysema (this complication was no longer seen after the ballooned stable access cannula was introduced for operative access). All postmyomectomy vaginal and abdominal deliveries were uncomplicated. At cesarean section the uterine scar was inspected in four patients and found to be intact.

Nezhat et al.[28] reported six uterine fistulas after laparoscopic removal of deep intramural fibroids. However, the authors either did not suture the uterine defect or simply approximated the uterine serosa. Harris[32] reported a case of uterine dehiscence at 34 weeks' gestation in a patient who conceived 3 months after laparoscopic excision of a 3 cm myoma. The myoma was resected from the posterior uterine wall with electrocautery after retraction with a myoma screw. The serosa of the resulting uterine defect was reapproximated with 4-0 interrupted polyglycolic sutures. Appropriate layer closure of the surgical defect appears to be essential. Excessive simultaneous use of electrocautery and the CO_2 laser should be avoided, as it may result in serious complications, such as uterine decapitation.[33]

Postoperative Adhesions

Approximately two-thirds of the patients in the above reported laparoscopic myomectomy series who underwent second-look procedures had postoperative adhesions. All of the patients who had undergone abdominal CO_2 laser myomectomy followed by second-look procedures had postoperative adhesions.[27] There appears to be an association between the site of the myomectomy incision and the occurrence of postoperative adhesions. Tulandi et al.[34] performed 26 second-look laparoscopies after abdominal myomectomy and found that incisions on the posterior uterine wall were associated with significantly more adnexal adhesions than those on the fundus or anterior uterine walls. We have noted similar findings in 28 patients with second-look procedures. Adhesions were associated with 80% of posterior wall incisions, 20% of anterior or fundal incisions, 44% of single incisions, and 86% of multiple incisions. Adhesions were seen in 25% of patients with "dry" wound edges and 80% of patients with "wet" edges, which underscores the important value of hemostasis.

Postoperative adhesion formation is a complex, multifactorial phenomenon that involves genetic predisposition and immunologic considerations, as well as surgical technique. The laparoscopic approach does not prevent postoperative adhesions, although measures such as complete hemostasis and the use of adhesion-preventing membranes to cover exposed sutures may be of value. We strongly advocate the use of second-look laparoscopy within 3 weeks after laparoscopic myomectomy to clear adhesions in reproductive-age patients. Studies based on third-look laparoscopy confirm the benefit of second-look laparoscopic adhesiolysis in terms of improving the ultimate outcome.[35,36]

The integrity of the uterine scar should be evaluated in infertility patients before they are allowed to conceive. I routinely perform these evaluations at approximately 4 months after myomectomy. Data developed through ultrasonographic assessment of uterine volume following myomectomy tend to support this concept. Beyth et al.[37] demonstrated a gradual decrease in uterine volume during the first 6 months after surgery in all patients, with the most remarkable change in size occurring during the initial 2–3 months. The authors suggested that the period of uterine shrinkage may represent the time of healing, during which conception should be prevented.[37]

Reproductive Outcome

Myomectomy appears to have a positive effect on fertility enhancement despite the recognized high potential of postoperative adhesion formation. Adhesions that do not involve the adnexa may not compromise reproductive performance. In our updated series, the conception rate in infertile patients was 71% and the live birth rate 59%.[7] These rates remained substantially representative of subsequent experience and may be compared to a conception rate of 40% following abdominal myomectomy in 1202 infertile patients as reviewed by Buttram and Reiter in 1981.[38] In a more recent review of six studies of abdominal myomectomy in 132 infertile patients, Verkauf[39] found a conception rate of 58%.

Table 6.1 shows the reproductive performance after myomectomy in infertile patients in individual studies. According to a personal communication, the low conception rate initially reported by Nezhat et al.[28] was significantly improved upon later follow-up. Tulandi and associates[34] reported a pregnancy rate of 66.7% at 12 months among 26 infertile women who had abdominal myomectomy procedures followed by second-look laparoscopy with adhesiolysis.

Uterine Sarcoma

Opinions differ regarding the number of mitotic figures that justify the diagnosis of leiomyosarcoma: from 5 per 10 high power fields (hpf)[16,40] to 10 per 10 hpf[16,41] to 2 per any hpf.[42] The degree of malignancy is directly related to the number of mitotic figures per high power field. Tissue examinations of the leiomyomas in our series revealed various benign degenerative changes in about 30%, adenomyosis in 7%, and calcification in 5% of cases. These findings are similar to those reported earlier by Ranney and Frederick.[23] There were no leiomyosarcomas in either series.

Uterine leiomyosarcomas may arise within a myoma or de novo from the myometrium.[42] The incidence increases steadily from the fourth to the sixth decade of life.[16,43] The mean age at diagnosis in one study was 56 ± 14 years with a range of 30–83 years.[17] The incidence of sarcomatous degeneration in surgically removed leiomyomas is between 0.07%[44] and 0.50%.[43] Parker et al.[44] reported a 0.27% incidence of sarcoma among patients who had surgery for a rapidly growing tumor, but they found no sarcomas among patients who met the published criteria of an increase of 6 weeks gestational size over a 1 year period.[38] Patients with lesions arising in leiomyomas have significantly better prognosis than those with primary myosarcoma.[42] Patients younger than 50 years of age have a significantly better prognosis than older patients.[40,42]

GnRH-a has a variable effect on sarcomatous lesions. The uterine mass may not change in size,[45] or it may enlarge.[46] Additionally, abnormal uterine bleeding may occur during treat-

Table 6.1. Comparison of studies on myomectomy

Study and approach	Year	No. of cases	Tumor size (cm)	Solitary (%)	Total removed	EBL (ml) Range	EBL (ml) Mean	LOS (days)	Conception (%)	Variable pregnancy (%)
Conventional laparotomy										
Babaknia et al.[22]	1978	46	—	—	—	—	—	—	—	—
Ranney & Frederick[23]	1979	51	1–12	76	—	—	—	—	46	42
McLaughlin[24]	1985	9	—	—	—	—	311	—	—	—
Rosenfeld[25]	1986	23	3–14	35	—	—	—	—	—	—
Smith & Uhlir[26]	1990	63	—	—	—	200–400	300	4	65	56
CO_2 laser laparoscopy										
McLaughlin[24]	1985	18	1–10	56	42	—	200	—	—	—
Starks[27]	1988	32	4–18	16	—	50–400	150	—	63	53
Operative laparoscopy										
Nezhat et al.[28]	1991	154	2–15	48	347	100–600	—	1	16	11
Dubuisson et al.[29]	1991	43	1–11	—	92	—	—	2.8	—	—
Daniell & Gurley[30]	1991	17	3–7	—	—	5–200	78	1	—	—
Hasson et al[5]	1992	56	3–16	38	144	10–400	75	1	64	50

Reprinted from ref. 31, with permission from Churchill Livingstone.
EBL, estimated blood loss; LOS, length of stay in hospital (mean).

ment.[46,47] Therefore, lack of a shrinkage response, the presence of a paradoxical growth response, or the occurrence of abnormal uterine bleeding during GnRH-a treatment of a leiomyoma suggests the possibility of malignancy and calls for further evaluation and prompt surgical management. Schwartz et al.[17] reviewed a 10-year experience with 21 patients with uterine leiomyosarcomas and reported that leiomyosarcoma was either the largest or the only mass in all patients except one; it was limited to one mass in all the patients except one; and it had no preferential type or uterine location. The authors suggested close monitoring of the largest myoma during conservative management with GnRH-a therapy.[17]

Unsuspected leiomyosarcoma in a laparoscopic myomectomy specimen in a patient who wishes to conceive poses a therapeutic dilemma. Hysterectomy is a safer approach, but preserving the uterus may be a viable option if the patient accepts and understands the risk. Only one of six patients who had myomectomy alone for leiomyosarcoma arising in a myoma developed recurrence.[42]

Myolysis

Laparoscopic myolysis is a technique of coagulating leiomyomas to effect devascularization and subsequent shrinkage of the tumors. It is modeled after a similar hysteroscopic procedure.[48] Early experience with this technique using the Nd:YAG laser showed a 41% mean reduction in myoma size after 6 months and 1 year.[49] However, when second-look laparoscopy was performed 6 months after the myolysis, all of the patients had dense fibrous adhesions between the treated myomas and the bowel. The authors concluded that because of this risk additional studies were required.[49]

Goldfarb[50] suggested the use of bipolar needles and combined his procedure with endometrial ablation in most of the patients. He did not report second-look procedures, and so the incidence of postoperative adhesions is not known. Furthermore, combining uterine coagulation from outside in (myolysis) and inside out (ablation) potentially poses additional problems.

Recurrence and Reoperation

The rates of recurrence and reoperation after laparoscopic myomectomy are expected to be similar to those noted after abdominal myomectomy. In their 1981 review of 3206 abdominal myomectomies, Buttram and Reiter[38] recorded a recurrence rate of 15% and a retreatment rate of 10%, which included reoperation and radiation therapy. In a more recent review of seven studies totaling 185 patients, Verkauf[39] reported a recurrence rate of 8% and a reoperation rate of 7%. Smith and Uhlir[26] reported on recurrence and reoperation in 62 patients who underwent abdominal myomectomy. One had recurrence at 4 years and three had recurrence after 5 years that led to repeat myomectomy in one, hysterectomy in two, and expectant management in one. Candiani et al.[51] found the cumulative 10-year recurrence rate after abdominal myomectomy to be 27% by life table analysis. Clinically significant recurrences usually occurred 3 years or more after surgery.[51]

Studies that report on ultrasonographic recurrence of uterine myomas after abdominal myomectomy yield higher rates. Most of the patients with recurrent myomas did not have clinical symptoms at the time of ultrasonic evaluation.[52] The recurrence rate increased with time: The cumulative 3-year ultrasonographic recurrence rate was 20%, and the 5-year value was 51%.[53] There was no significant relation between the number or the site of the myomas removed and the risk of recurrence. The 5-year recurrence rate was 38% in women with one myoma, 70% in women with two or three tumors, and 52% in women in whom four or more tumors were removed.[53] Friedman et al.[52] reported a significantly higher ultrasonographic recurrence rate for surgically treated patients with more than three leiomyomas when they were followed for 27–38 months.

Currently, there are no published data regarding recurrence and reoperation after laparoscopic myomectomy. Although the follow-up in our series is not complete because of the patients who had been referred from other physicians, the rate of ultrasonographically detected recurrence appears to be low. Two of our patients had repeat surgical procedures. One had a supracervical laparoscopic hysterectomy 3 years after laparoscopic myomectomy for recurrent menometrorrhagia. The pathology report identified adenomyosis and two minute myomas. The second had another laparoscopic myomectomy for recurrent leiomyomas. We generally try to limit laparoscopic myomectomy to patients with four or fewer significant myomas (> 3 cm).

These data confirm the benefit of myomectomy in preserving the reproductive organs of symptomatic patients.

Conclusion

Laparoscopic myomectomy requires the combined skills of two surgeons or a surgeon and a well trained assistant. Regardless of surgical skill and experience, the laparoscopic approach is not suitable for patients with advanced disease and multiple lesions; these patients require laparotomy.

When proper technique and appropriate patient selection criteria are employed, the procedure is at least as effective as myomectomy by laparotomy in terms of reproductive outcome and relief of symptoms. When compared to laparotomy, myomectomy by laparoscopy is associated with less blood loss, fewer complications, shorter hospital stay and recovery time, fewer adhesions, better documentation for future follow-up, and a better cosmetic scar.

To optimize the safety and efficacy of the procedure, it is essential to adhere to certain basic surgical principles: (1) dissecting exclusively inside the pseudocapsule of the leiomyoma; (2) finding the avascular tissue planes and connecting bridges; (3) coagulating large vessels with suitable means before incising them; (4) closing the uterine surgical defect in layers; and (5) achieving hemostasis.

References

1. WILCOX LS, KOONIN LM, POKRAS R, ET AL: Hysterectomy in the United States, 1988–1990. Obstet Gynecol 1994;83:549.
2. National Center for Health Statistics: Vital Health Statistics. National Hospital Discharge Survey. Series 13, No. 108. Washington, DC, NCHS, 1989.
3. ROBBINS SL, COTRAN RS: Leiomyoma. The Pathogenic Basis of Disease. Philadelphia, Saunders, 1984, p 1136.
4. LEVINE RL: Myomectomy. In Operative Gynecologic Endoscopy, Sanfilippo JS, Levine RL (eds). New York, Springer-Verlag, pp 133–139.
5. HASSON HM, ROTMAN C, RANA N, ET AL: Laparoscopic myomectomy. Obstet Gynecol 1992;80:884.
6. HASSON HM: Laparoscopic myomectomy. In Operative Laparoscopy, The Master's Techniques, Soderstrom RM (ed). New York, Raven Press, 1993, pp 137–142.
7. HASSON HM: Laparoscopic myomectomy. In Endoscopic Management of Gynecologic Diseases, Adamson GD, Martin D (eds). New York, Raven Press (in press).
8. American College of Obstetricians and Gynecologists (ACOG): ACOG Technical Bulletin: Uterine Leiomyomata. N. 192. Washington, DC, ACOG, 1994.
9. ZAWIN M, MCCARTHY S, SCOUTT LM, ET AL: Highfield MRI and US evaluation of the pelvis in women with leiomyomas. Magn Reson Imaging 1990;;4:371.
10. HRICAK H, TSCHOLAKOFF D, HEINRICHS L, ET AL: Uterine leiomyomas: correlation of MR, histopathologic findings and symptoms. Radiology 1986;158:385.
11. DUDIAK CM, TURNER DA, PATEL SK, ET AL: Uterine leiomyomas in the infertile patient: preoperative localization with MR imaging versus US and hysterosalpingography. Radiology 1988;167:627.
12. TOGASHI K, OZASA H, KONISHI I, ET AL: Enlarged uterus: differentiation between adenomyosis and leiomyoma with MR imaging. Radiology 1989;171:531.
13. FREIDMAN AJ, HOFFMAN, DI, COMITE F, ET AL: Treatment of leiomyomata uteri with leuprolide acetate depot: a double-blind placebo-controlled multicenter study. Obstet Gynecol 1991;77:720.
14. ROCK JA: Gonadotropin-releasing hormone agonist analogs in the treatment of uterine leiomyomas. J Gynecol Surg 1991;7:147.
15. WIZNITZER A, MARBACK M, HAZUM E, ET AL: Gonadotrophin-releasing hormone specific binding sites in uterine leiomyomata. Biochem Biophys Res Commun 1988;152:1326.
16. LEIBSOHN S, D'ABLAING G, MISHELL RD, ET AL: Leiomyosarcoma in a series of hysterectomies

performed for presumed uterine leiomyomas. Am J Obstet Gynecol 1990;162:968.
17. SCHWARTZ LB, DIAMOND MP, SCHWARTZ PE: Leiomyosarcomas: clinical presentation. Am J Obstet Gynecol 1993;168:180.
18. HASSON HM: Suture loop techniques to facilitate microsurgical and laparoscopic procedures. J Reprod Med 1987;32:765.
19. HASSON HM: Half-hitch knot for securing the end of continuous sutures. Obstet Gynecol 1992; 80:724.
20. BEYTH Y, OHEL G: Postmyomectomy evaluation of uterine scar: a new hysterographic method. Fertil Steril 1983;39:564.
21. HASSON HM, ROTMAN C, RANA N, ET AL: Experience with laparoscopic hysterectomy. J AAGL 1993;1:1.
22. BABAKNIA A, ROCK JA, JONES HW: Pregnancy success following abdominal myomectomy for infertility. Fertil Steril 1978;30:644.
23. RANNEY B, FREDERICK I: The occasional need for myomectomy. Obstet Gynecol 1979;53:437.
24. MCLAUGHLIN DS: Metroplasty and myomectomy with CO_2 laser for maximizing the preservation of normal tissue and minimizing blood loss. J Reprod Med 1985;30:1.
25. ROSENFELD DL: Abdominal myomectomy for otherwise unexplained infertility. Fertil Steril 1986; 46:328.
26. SMITH DC, UHLIR JK: Myomectomy as a reproductive procedure. Am J Obstet Gynecol 1990;162: 1476.
27. STARKS GC: CO_2 laser myomectomy in an infertile population. J Reprod Med 1988;33:184.
28. NEZHAT C, NEZHAT F, SILFEN SL, ET AL: Laparoscopic myomectomy. Int J Fertil 1991;36:275.
29. DUBUISSON JB, MANDELBROT L, LECURU F, ET AL: Myomectomy by laparoscopy: a preliminary report of 43 cases. Fertil Steril 1991;56:827.
30. DANIELL JF, GURLEY LD: Laparoscopic treatment of clinically significant symptomatic uterine fibroids. J Gynecol Surg 1991;7:37.
31. HASSON HM: Laparoscopic myomectomy. In Operative Laparoscopy and Hysteroscopy, Cohen SM (ed). New York, Churchill Livingstone (in press).
32. HARRIS WJ: Uterine dehiscence following laparoscopic myomectomy. Obstet Gynecol 1992;80: 545.
33. BARLET E, GRIFFIN WT: Uterine decapitation resulting from laparoscopic laser myomectomy. Presented at the 48th Annual Meeting of the American Fertility Society, New Orleans, November 1992.
34. TULANDI T, MURRAY C, GURALNICK M: Adhesion formation and reproductive outcome after myomectomy and second-look laparoscopy. Obstet Gynecol 1993;82:213.
35. JANSEN RP: Early laparoscopy after pelvic operations to prevent adhesions: safety and efficacy. Fertil Steril 1988;49:26.
36. PEREZ RJ: Second-look laparoscopy adhesiolysis: the procedure of choice for preventing adhesion recurrence. J Reprod Med 1991;36:700.
37. BEYTH Y, JAFFE R, GOLDBERGER S: Uterine remodelling following conservative myomectomy: ultrasonographic evaluation. Acta Obstet Gynecol Scand 1992;71:632.
38. BUTTRAM VC, REITER RC: Uterine leiomyomata: etiology, symptomatology and management. Fertil Steril 1981;36:433.
39. VERKAUF BS: Myomectomy for fertility enhancement and preservation. Fertil Steril 1992;58:1.
40. KAHANPAA KV, WAHLSTROM T, GROHN P, ET AL: Sarcomas of the uterus: a clinicopathological study of 199 patients. Obstet Gynecol 1986;67:417.
41. BERCHUCK A, RUBIN S, HOSKINS WJ, ET AL: Treatment of uterine leiomyosarcoma. Obstet Gynecol 1988;71:845.
42. DINH TV, WOODRUFF JD: Leiomyosarcoma of the uterus. Am J Obstet Gynecol 1982;144:817.
43. VOLLENHOVEN BJ, LAWRENCE AS, HEALY DL: Uterine fibroids: a clinical review. Br J Obstet Gynaecol 1990;97:285.
44. PARKER WH, YAO SF, BEREK JS: Uterine sarcoma in patients operated on for presumed leiomyoma and rapidly growing leiomyoma. Obstet Gynecol 1994;83:414.
45. MEYER WR, MAYER AR, DIAMOND MP, ET AL: Unsuspected leiomyosarcoma: treatment with a gonatropin-releasing hormone analogue. Obstet Gynecol 1990;75:529.
46. LOONG EPL, WONG FWS: Uterine leiomyosarcoma diagnosed during treatment with agonist of luteinizing hormone releasing hormone for presumed uterine fibroid. Fertil Steril 1990;54:530.
47. HITTI IF, GLASBERG SS, MCKENZIE C, ET AL: Uterine leiomyosarcoma with massive necrosis diagnosed during gonadotrophin-releasing hormone analog therapy for presumed uterine fibroid. Fertil Steril 1991;56:778.
48. DONNEZ J, GILLEROT S, BOURGONJON D, ET AL: Neodymium:YAG laser hysteroscopy in large submucous fibroids. Fertil Steril 1990;54:999.
49. NISOLLE M, SMETS M, MALVAUX V, ET AL: Laparoscopic myolysis with the Nd:YAG laser. J Gynecol Surg 1993;9:95.

50. GOLDFARB HA: Removing uterine fibroids laparoscopically. Contemp Obstet Gynecol 1994;39:50.
51. CANDIANI GB, FEDELE L, PARAZZINI F, ET AL: Risk of recurrence after myomectomy. Br J Obstet Gynaecol 1991;98:385.
52. FRIEDMAN AJ, DALY M, JUNEAU-NORCROSS M, ET AL: Recurrence of myomas after myomectomy in women pretreated with leuprolide acetate depot or placebo. Fertil Steril 1992;58:205.
53. FEDELE L, VILLA L, BOCCIOLONE L, ET AL: Risk of recurrence after myomectomy: a transvaginal ultrasonographic study. Presented at the 49th Annual Meeting of the American Fertility Society, Montreal, October 1993.

7
Ovarian Surgery

Ronald L. Levine

One of the most common sites of gynecologic surgery is the ovary. A 1990 survey of the American Association of Gynecologic Laparoscopists revealed that 13,739 operative laparoscopies were performed for ovarian masses by the respondents.[1]

In 1979 Semm, from Kiel, Germany, reported on new approaches to adnexal surgery,[2] and in 1980 Semm and Mettler reported on laparoscopic oophorectomy using the loop ligature.[3] In 1985 Levine published the first American report of a bilateral oophorectomy that was performed laparoscopically.[4] Since then numerous reports of many techniques using a variety of modalities have been published regarding laparoscopic ovarian surgery.

Laparoscopic procedures have been developed and described for treating most types of ovarian pathology, ranging from treatment of some developmental anomalies such as excision of ovarian streaks[5] to extirpation of low grade ovarian malignancies[6] and ovarian remnants.[7]

Oophorectomy

Indications

The indications for operative laparoscopic oophorectomy are much the same as for open laparotomy with a few exceptions. The indications include the following:

1. Benign neoplasms such as an endometrioma in a patient not interested in fertility, or where the ovary may be so involved with pathology as to be unsalvageable.
2. Benign teratomas or cystadenomas. These tumors may necessitate oophorectomy if the ovary is destroyed by the disease process or if the patient is close to or at menopausal age.
3. Chronic pelvic inflammatory disease or severe ovarian adhesions that are producing symptoms and have not responded to previous surgery.
4. Palpable ovary syndrome and prophylactic removal in a patient who has completed her child-bearing with at least two first-degree relatives with ovarian cancer.

In a study of laparoscopic surgery in women over 40 years of age the most common postoperative diagnoses were adhesions, endometriosis, and functional cysts; 45.5% of the surgical procedures included oophorectomy.[8]

Diagnosis

In view of the possibility of ovarian malignancy, adequate screening must be performed to decrease the likelihood that an ovarian lesion may subsequently be found to be malignant, especially in postmenopausal women. The problem of spillage of a malignant ovarian cyst has been addressed by several authors, and the use of laparoscopy was decried by Maiman et al.[9] because of the potential of ovarian cyst rupture and the consequent effect on prognosis. They concluded that the presence of so-called benign characteristics did not preclude malignancy. Their study involved 42 cases of mismanagement of ovarian malignancy; in particular, they cited long delays from the discovery of the malignancy to definitive surgery and therapy. This problem obviously was not the fault of the procedure; rather, it is a sad commentary on the experience and knowledge of the laparoscopic surgeon. Dembo et al.[10] questioned the effect of spillage, showing that the only factors that influenced the ultimate rate of relapse and survival were the tumor grade, the presence of dense adhesions, and the presence of a large volume of ascites. When these factors were accounted for, the rate of relapse and prognosis were not influenced by the rupture of the tumor. Cristalli et al.,[11] from France, concluded that operative laparoscopy can be used in nearly 90% of cases of ovarian tumors that are thought to be benign. They also claimed that this type of surgery is safer for the diagnosis and treatment of ovarian tumors during pregnancy. Shalev et al.,[12] using the criteria of a normal serum CA-125 and the appearance of a simple cyst on vaginal ultrasonography, performed laparoscopic bilateral oophorectomy in 55 postmenopausal women, all of whom had benign pathology. They compared these patients to 75 women in whom the ovaries were the same size as the first set, but this group underwent laparotomy because the cyst was complex or the CA-125 was elevated. In the second group 23 patients had malignant tumors. They therefore had a positive predictive value of 100% and a negative predictive value of 30.7%. Using this rationale, if the indicators for a possible malignancy are present, the choice of surgical approach is obviously laparotomy.

If the significance of rupture of an ovarian mass is still controversial, it is apparent that the surgeon should do whatever is necessary to avoid the laparoscopic approach in the presence of a frank malignancy and to use whatever techniques are possible for total extirpation without spillage in all cases, including laparoscopy. Patients with low grade ovarian malignancies that are removed intact may be followed without additional treatment.[13] It is therefore important to determine whether an ovarian mass is benign or malignant preoperatively. The workup should consist of the following steps.

1. *Adequate history and physical examination.* It must include family history and a thorough pelvic examination including a rectovaginal component. The history should include a complete investigation of previous abdominal surgeries and diagnostic workups.

2. *Tumor markers.* The CA-125 antigen is not completely specific, although more than 80% of ovarian cancer patients have levels higher than 35 U/ml. A number of benign conditions can also produce elevated CA-125 levels, including pregnancy, endometriosis, pelvic inflammatory disease, and peritonitis. The CA-125 is not elevated in patients with nonepithelial ovarian cancers and may not be elevated in those with mucinous histology.[14] This test is most useful in the postmenopausal patient and probably is not as helpful in patients under 40 years of age due to a relatively high false-positive rate. Other cancers, such as fallopian tube carcinoma, colon cancer, and hepatic tumors, may also cause CA-125 elevation. Another limitation to the use of CA-125 as a screening tool may be cost. Recent developments that may be helpful in improving the specificity and predictive value of the tumor marker CA-125 have been described.[15]

3. *Transvaginal ultrasonography.* This modality provides a close look at the ovary and is particularly useful with cystic ovarian pathology. A high frequency transducer is placed in the vagina, permitting closer positioning of the transducer in relation to the intrapelvic structures. There are several advantages over the use of a transabdominal transducer, including better imaging in obese patients and elimination of the need to fill the bladder. Sassone et al.[16] described a scoring system based on the ultrasonographic character of the ovary. The system uses the presence of septa, wall thickness, and

Table 7.1. Ultrasonographic scoring system

Score	Inner wall structure	Wall thickness (mm)	Septum (mm)	Echogenicity
1	Smooth	Thin (< 3 mm)	No septum	Sonolucent
2	Irregularities (< 3 mm)	Thick (> 3 mm)	Thin (3 mm)	Low echogenicity
3	Papillations (> 3 mm)	Not applicable, mostly solid	Thick (> 3 mm)	Low echogenicity with echogenic core
4	Not applicable, most solid			Mixed echogenicity
5				High echogenicity

Adapted from Sassone et al.[16] Reprinted with permission of *Obstetrics and Gynecology*.

echogenicity to develop a score. They used a score of 9 as the threshold to indicate if a mass is malignant (Table 7.1). We have used a simplified approach that evaluates the presence or absence of papillations and the presence or absence of thick septa. As transvaginal ultrasonography is rapidly becoming standard in many gynecologist's offices, the cost of this type of screening has become economically feasible.

Other modalities for evaluation have been described, such as colorflow and duplex Doppler,[17] but they are not universally available and have not received as much clinical recognition. The theory of this technique is based on visualizing the ovarian mass; the characteristics of the blood flow are assessed and low resistance blood vessels that theoretically are characteristic of malignant tumors are detected. Some authors have stated that Doppler ultrasonography with color flow imaging can determine whether a tumor is benign or malignant more accurately in some difficult cases than tumor markers or ultrasonography.[18] Other imaging methods, such as computed tomography (CT) and magnetic resonance imaging (MRI) are expensive and not as easily available; moreover, CT is often less accurate than simple vaginal ultrasonography.

If the preoperative workup as described above shows a low risk of malignancy, the operative laparoscopic approach may be considered. Even if all aspects are negative for malignant potential, the aim should be, if possible, to remove tissue in such a manner as to obviate intraperitoneal rupture and dispersion of tissue or fluid from the mass. As noted previously, laparoscopic oophorectomy or salpingo-oophorectomy have the same indications as laparotomy and frequently involve a cystic mass rather than a solid one. Indeed, a solid ovarian mass may well contraindicate the laparoscopic approach unless one can be assured of intact removal, such as through the cul-de-sac.

Operative Techniques

The patient is positioned in a semilithotomy position using Allen Stirrups (Allen Medical Systems, Cleveland, OH). It is important that there is little flexion of the thigh on the trunk in order to eliminate interference with the movement of instruments in the lower ports. The same positioning is utilized in all of the subsequently described surgical procedures. If the uterus is intact, a good uterine manipulator is needed. We prefer the Endopath Uterine Manipulator, or a Semm-type vacuum cannula. The patient is catheterized, prepared, and draped.

Laparoscopic ovarian surgery must be performed in the same fashion, regarding basic techniques, as open laparotomy. Exploration of the peritoneal cavity is mandatory, and if any question of possible malignancy exists pelvic washings with heparinized saline must be carried out. The washings are sent for a cell block study at the termination of the case. The abdomen is explored in a standard fashion, in a set pattern. I start at the bladder area and then progress to the right adnexa, right ovarian fossa, appendix and cecum, right gutter, right lobe of the liver and gallbladder, right hemidiaphragm, left hemidiaphragm, left lobe of the liver, omentum, sigmoid colon, left adnexa and

Figure 7.1. A loop ligature is passed over the infundibulopelvic ligament and uteroovarian ligament. It may be necessary to skeletonize the vessels first if there is too much tissue to encompass and ligate safely. Most often the first loop ligature acts to compress the tissue, and subsequent loops ensure hemostasis.

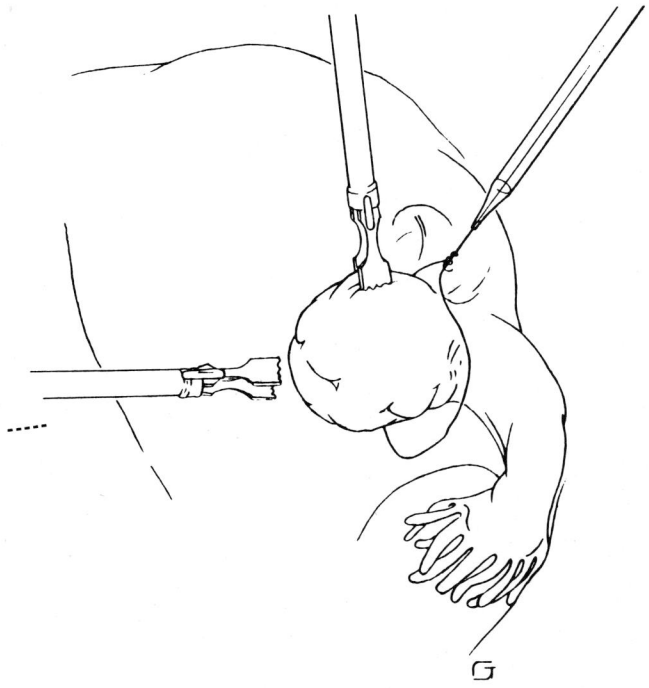

ovarian fossa, uterus, cul-de-sac, and uterosacral ligaments. The exploration is carried out after a secondary puncture site is made in the low midline to accommodate a 10 mm trocar sheath with a 5 mm step-down converter. This technique allows the use of a blunt probe, an irrigating sleeve, or an atraumatic grasper to mobilize bowel, omentum, and adnexa for adequate visualization. Only with the use of a secondary instrument can an adequate exploration be accomplished. If all the areas are clear, the other secondary puncture sites may be placed as required. Most commonly, lateral 5 mm trocar sheaths are placed at or slightly higher than the hairline and lateral to the inferior epigastric vessels. The secondary puncture sites are always placed under direct vision so the inferior epigastric artery can be identified even without transillumination.

If the classic approach, described by Semm, is used, only 5 mm trocar sheaths are needed at first. The loop ligature may be used and passed down the lateral port on the same side as the pathology and advanced over the ovary onto the infundibulopelvic ligament. The ureter must always be identified and can usually be traced from the pelvic brim if necessary. Often a bit of patience is needed while observing for peristalsis, but it is sometimes necessary to open the peritoneum in order to trace the course of the ureter. At least two and preferably three loop ligatures are passed on to the ligament and set into place (Figs. 7.1, 7.2, 7.3). The ovary is freed, but it is often helpful to have placed a fourth ligature distally and then incise the pedicle proximal to this ligature. It is then possible to use this length of suture to pull the mass either into a pouch or into an opening in the cul-de-sac for extirpation. If the mass is cystic it may be drained from below (Fig. 7.4). By draining with this technique intrapelvic spillage may be avoided. Some authors consider the loop ligature approach poor technique and prefer either a suture method, electrodesiccation of the blood supply, or use of a stapling device.[18]

If the stapling device is utilized a 12 mm trocar sheath must be used and should usually be placed at a higher site, almost lateral to the umbilicus. Such placement allows a perpendicular approach to the infundibulopelvic ligament. The ligament should be isolated to be sure it is clear of the ureter. The amount of tissue encom-

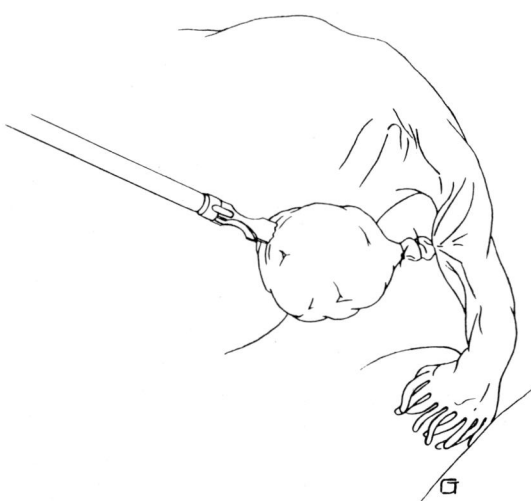
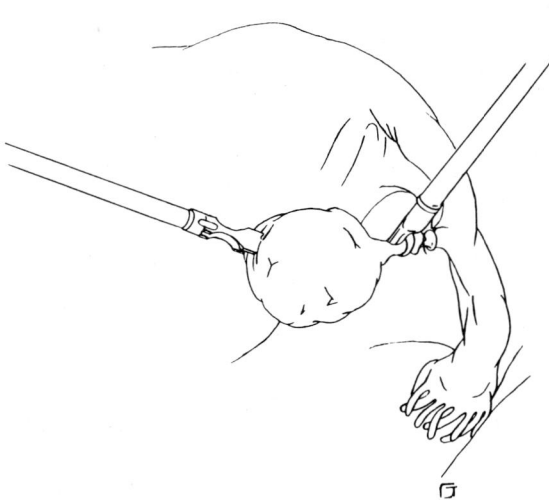

Figure 7.2. A second and then a third loop ligature is passed with some space between them. It is frequently helpful to have a fourth ligature as the most distal one and to leave a long tail on that ligature.

Figure 7.3. Ovary may be cut free but it is advantageous to have a fourth ligature left on the free ovary to facilitate subsequent removal.

passed by the jaws of the stapling device should be as little as possible, but it is not necessary to skeletonize the vessels. An alternative technique is to place a 12 mm trocar at the initial umbilical port and then use the lower midline port as the site for the 10 mm sleeve for the laparoscope. This option decreases the number of large lateral incisions with the possibility of subsequent incisional hernias.

The other alternative approach to oophorectomy is the use of electrodesiccation of the blood supply. The 10 mm laparoscope is placed through the intraumbilical incision, and then two 5 mm trocar sheaths are placed laterally as previously described. It is mandatory to visualize the ureter during this technique, as injury by electrosurgery is more likely than by other techniques owing to the spread of the electrothermal energy. The ovarian artery and vein may be isolated and then coapted using a Kleppinger-type bipolar forceps. It is important to use the ammeter on the electrosurgical unit to be sure that complete desiccation has occurred. The

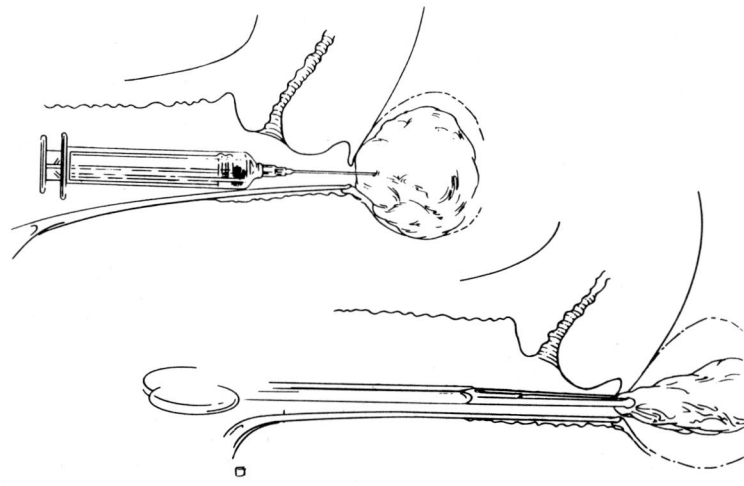

Figure 7.4. Cystic mass may be removed through the posterior cul-de-sac by grasping either the ligature or the capsule through a colpotomy incision. Keeping the mass tight against the incision maintains the pneumoperitoneum. An 18 gauge spinal needle and syringe are used to drain the mass as traction is applied, thereby precluding intraabdominal spill and permitting removal of the mass intact. The incision is easily closed through the vagina.

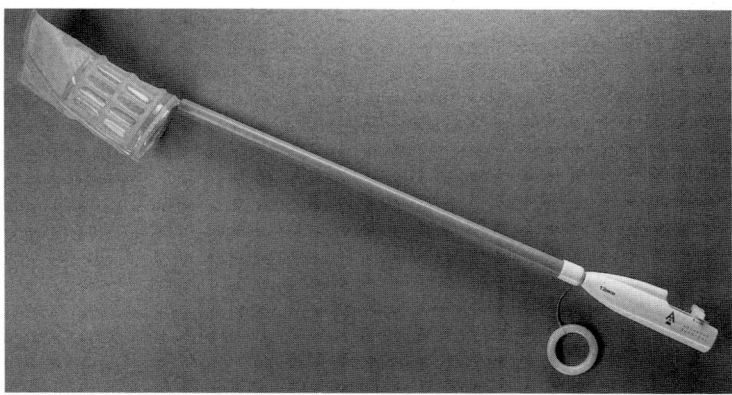

Figure 7.5. One type of sack is illustrated. When the sack is deployed as shown, the tissue may be placed within it and the sack closed by pulling a string. The limiting factor in this type of sack is the size of the opening.

uteroovarian ligament is also coagulated and then incised. At times it is useful to use a scissors with unipolar current to cut this area, as it is thicker than the skeletonized infundibulopelvic ligament and there may be a small amount of bleeding because of incomplete desiccation.

The ovary, once free from all of the connective tissues and blood supply, must then be removed. The ability to remove bulky tissue intact remains the "Holy Grail" of laparoscopy. Several methods are available, and all should avoid if possible morcellation of the ovary freely within the abdominal cavity. There are several types of sacks or bags described to remove tissue from the abdomen, all having some good and bad points. Most are commercially available specifically for laparoscopy (Fig. 7.5); others are food bags such as Ziploc sandwich bags that have been gas-sterilized, rolled up, and introduced into the abdomen. Regardless of the receptacle utilized, the opening must be closed to prevent spillage and the sack then delivered outside the abdominal cavity. An incision may be made into the cul-de-sac and the mass removed intact, drained, or even morcellated within the sack and the entire sack removed. The colpotomy incision can then be closed transvaginally, or closure can be accomplished laparoscopically depending on the skill of the surgeon. The sack can also be brought up through a 12 mm trocar site, either at the umbilicus or any other 12 mm port. The incision may be enlarged as necessary.

At the end of the procedure, the pelvis is flooded with irrigation solution, and all the pedicles and operative areas are examined under the fluid to ensure hemostasis. Approximately 300–500 ml of fluid is left in the pelvis. The irrigating solution may be lactated Ringer's solution, sterile water, or glycine. The incisional sites are sutured after the remaining gas is removed. Small incisions for 5 mm or smaller trocars may be closed with subcuticular stitches; larger trocar sites ideally should have the fascia closed with 2-0 or 0 synthetic absorbable suture in the standard manner or with some type of laparoscopic closure device (see Chap. 2).

The method of oophorectomy seems to make little difference. Daniell et al.[19] compared the three techniques (staples, ligatures, coagulation) and found all three methods to be effective with similar operative times and good results for all 65 patients in their study.

Ovarian Cystectomy

Surgery for ovarian cysts is one of the most common procedures performed by the gynecologist. Most ovarian cysts are benign[20] and may easily be treated by the laparoscopic approach. Many papers have now been published addressing the technique and the concerns regarding potential malignancy.[8,11,21–23] As noted previously, even if malignancy is unlikely, it is necessary that the surgeon be as careful as one would be during open surgery and attempt to remove a mass intact without rupturing the cyst capsule if possible. Seltzer et al.[24] addressed the problems of potential malignancy in ovarian cysts and made several recommendations for the laparoscopic approach to this pathology. Their suggestions covered preoperative evaluation and preparation, including the use of tumor markers and ultrasonography. They encouraged extirpation of the mass intact if possible. They recommended the following whenever laparoscopy was used as the surgical approach to an ovarian cyst: (1) Peritoneal washings should be obtained. (2) The upper abdomen should be explored and biopsy performed on any abnormal area. (3) The pelvis should be explored; if there is any finding suggestive of malignancy a laparotomy should be performed. (4) If any external excrescences are identified on the ovary, immediate laparotomy should be performed. (5) High quality frozen sections should be prepared and examined. (6) The mass should be removed intact if possible. (7) If malignancy is encountered, it is optimal to proceed with immediate laparotomy; if a delay is necessary, the delay to open surgery should be as short as possible.

If the laparoscopic approach to an ovarian cyst is considered, it may be desirable to use a 12 mm trocar for the initial umbilical port, as it provides a large portal for the subsequent extirpation of tissue if necessary. After the laparoscope is placed, a thorough evaluation of the abdomen and pelvis is carried out. If even a slight suspicion of a possible malignancy exists, washings with heparinized saline should follow. The secondary ports are placed in much the same fashion as during oophorectomy.

The question frequently arises as to whether to puncture and aspirate the ovarian cyst. The external cyst wall should first be closely examined to be sure there are no excrescences present. If it is clear, should the next step be a puncture? If the cyst is benign in a young patient, should she just have a cyst aspiration? It has long been accepted that aspiration of ovarian cysts have no lasting therapeutic value.[25] Hasson[21,26] addressed the problem of using needle aspiration and concluded that there is little if any danger when using fine-needle aspiration to inspect the contents of an ovarian cyst. Vancaille[27] agreed that puncture of an ovarian cyst subsequently found to be malignant should not lead to an upgrade of the tumor stage from Ia to Ic. If the ovary is to be preserved and a cystectomy is the operation of choice, needle aspiration may help to define the etiology of the cyst with little if any risk. If the fluid is clear, it is likely that one is dealing with a simple cyst. Often the surgeon can tell from the preoperative sonogram whether the probable pathology is an endometrioma, or a benign teratoma, a serous cystadenoma, or a mucinous cyst.

The ovary is easily stabilized with an atraumatic grasper holding the uteroovarian ligament. The surgeon must then make a choice of performing the cystectomy with the cyst intact or by evacuating the cyst fluid first. In the case of a serous cyst, aspiration of the cyst contents is easily accomplished. If a teratoma is diagnosed, one must definitely attempt to remove the cyst intact. Because benign ovarian teratomas are rarely malignant in women under age 40[28] laparoscopic removal in the hands of an experienced laparoscopist is both safe and effective.[29] A cystectomy with the cyst either completely evacuated or even partially drained is easier than an intact cystectomy. If the contents of a dermoid cyst spills into the pelvic cavity, the patient should be placed immediately into a reverse Trendelenberg position. The pelvis must be copiously irrigated until the fluid is clear with no fat droplets visualized.

The ovarian capsule may be incised in a variety of ways, but whatever the mode of incision the initial incisional line is performed on the antimesenteric side of the ovary. A laser may be used, but it is expensive and may be disadvantageous as it can easily penetrate the capsule deeper than one would desire and enter the cyst directly. The same is true for the unipolar needle, but I believe that the needle is easier to control. Another approach is to incise the capsule with a Harmonic Scalpel (UltraCision, Smithfield, RI) and then use the Harmonic energy to dissect the capsule back. Even simpler and certainly less expensive is the use of a sharp laparoscopic scissors. The incision is carried out only over the cortex covering the cyst, trying to avoid incising normal ovarian cortex (Fig. 7.6). The cortex is then peeled from the cyst using a traction and countertraction technique. Each side of the incision is held with a grasper and

7. Ovarian Surgery

Figure 7.6. Capsule of the cyst may be incised with a laser, electrosurgical needle, Harmonic Scalpel, or simply with a scissors as shown. The incision is made away from the tubal fimbria and from the base of the ovary. Some care must be taken to avoid entry into the cyst proper and to find the correct plane of dissection.

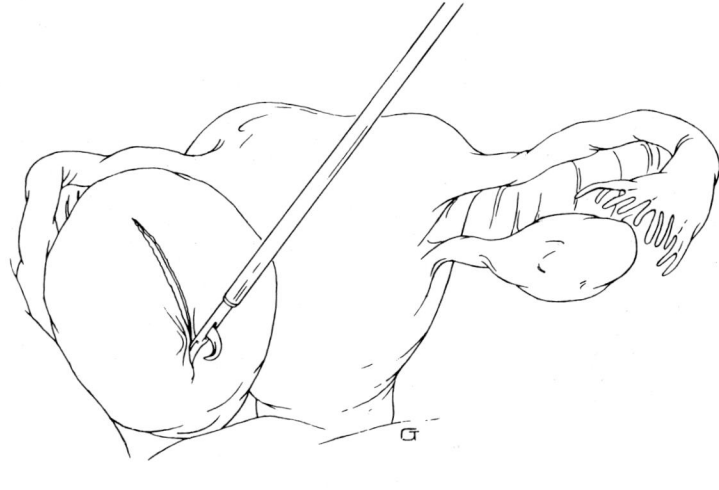

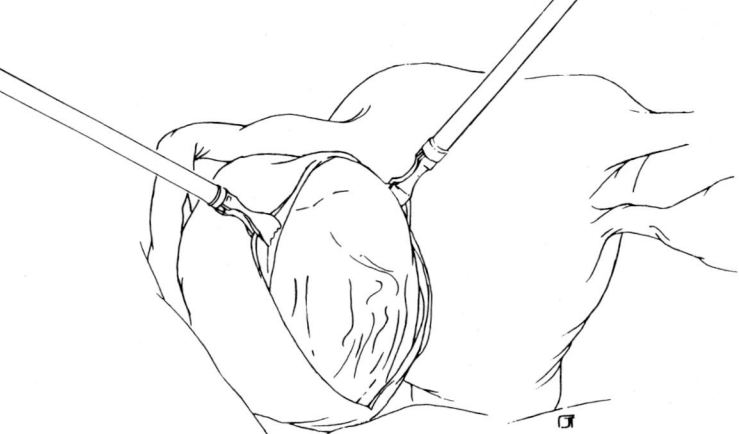

Figure 7.7. Cyst capsule is dissected back mainly by a traction–countertraction maneuver, and the capsule is stripped away.

Figure 7.8. Wall of the cyst may be grasped to facilitate stripping of the capsule, and the graspers are frequently moved close to each other to maximize the traction. When the base of the cyst is reached, a bipolar forceps may be used to coagulate the blood supply to the cyst. After removal of the cyst it is usually not necessary to suture the capsule.

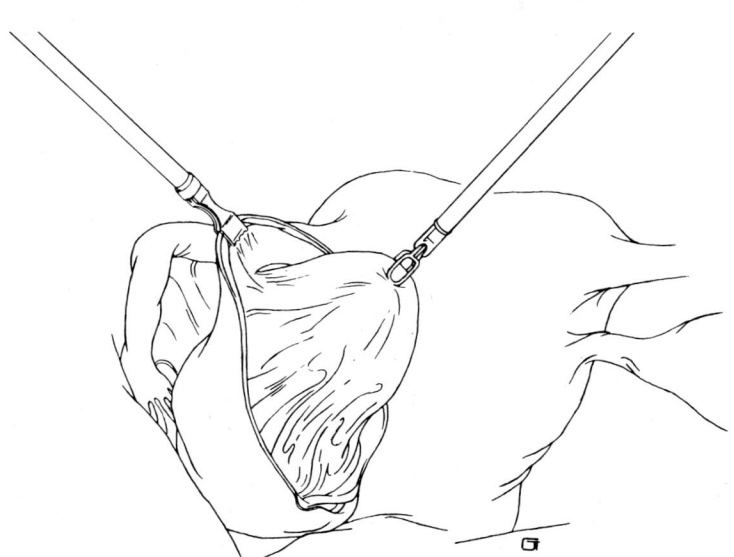

slowly peeled back (Fig. 7.7). The site of the graspers must be moved frequently to achieve better purchase and traction. It may be necessary to grasp the cyst directly, but when that technique is needed it is almost always necessary to at least partially empty the cyst so adequate traction can be applied (Fig. 7.8). As the base of the cyst is approached it is imperative to begin to control potential sites of bleeding—best accomplished with bipolar coagulation. When the cyst is removed there is frequently some bleeding from the cyst bed, which can be controlled with judicious use of bipolar coagulation. This situation is an excellent place to utilize the Argon Beam Coagulator or the ball tip of the Harmonic Blade System (UltraCision).

The cyst, if removed intact, may be placed in the cul-de-sac while preparations are made for removal. The cystic mass is best extirpated intact, which can be accomplished in one of several ways. It can be removed intact through the cul-de-sac via a culdotomy incision performed transvaginally or laparoscopically, or it may be removed using a bag or sack through the umbilical port or other trocar site as described for oophorectomy.

The remaining ovarian capsule usually does not require suturing for closure. It is sometimes necessary to coagulate the base as noted, and sometimes the edge of the capsule requires bipolar coagulation; most often nothing further needs to be done. The area should be well irrigated, and the ovary may then be inspected under fluid. One may use either lactated Ringer's as an irrigating solution, sterile water, or glycine. When the operative site is viewed under the irrigating solution, bleeding may be noted and subsequently coagulated with one of the previously mentioned modalities. The ovarian capsule most frequently falls together and does not require sutures. If for some reason the capsule does not seem to fall together, it may be reapproximated by sutures, but the fewer sutures used the better. Usually one suture of 2-0 or 3-0 synthetic absorbable material suffices. The suture is usually tied with an extracorporeal knot that is placed with a Clarke-Reich Knot Pusher (Marlow Surgical Technology, Willoughby, OH). The pelvis is irrigated to clear it, and 300–500 ml of solution (lactated Ringer's) is left in the pelvic cavity for flotation in an attempt to minimize adhesion formation.

The material that is removed is sent for frozen section; and if any malignancy is reported, laparotomy may be performed immediately, providing the patient has been properly counseled and informed. The consent should include mention of a midline incision and a total abdominal hysterectomy, bilateral salpingo-oophorectomy, and omentectomy.

Ovarian Drilling

Polycystic ovarian disease (PCOD) was treated in the past with laparotomy and wedge resection, but postoperative adhesions often resulted in continuing infertility.[30] As early as 1983 there were descriptions of a positive response to operative laparoscopic surgery. The early reports described using a technique of multiple biopsies.[31] Electrocautery was described by Gjonnaess, who postulated a theory for the use of this technique.[32] He assumed that ovulation was elicited by either nonspecific ovarian stromal destruction or extensive capsular destruction resulting in the release of the contents of subcapsular follicular cysts.

The hormonal changes associated with ovarian drilling are still poorly understood, but most likely there is a temporary reduction of ovarian steroid production with a persistent decrease in testosterone.[33] Current management of this syndrome is generally with medical therapy (clomiphene citrate alone or in combination with dexamethasone, human chorionic gondotropin, or gonadotropins). If the patient fails to respond to conventional medical treatment, ovarian drilling might be considered. This therapy was first described by Daniell and Miller[34] using both CO_2 and later the fiber lasers (KTP and argon). Within 6 months of laser drilling 56% of the patients conceived. Adhesions with this technique are highly possible,[35] so there must be concern and close follow-up of these patients. Gurgan et al.,[36] however, reported only minimal and mild adhesions with Nd:YAG laser photocoagulation that they contend did not hamper ovulation or oocyte pickup.

The operative technique involves the following steps: The laparoscope is placed through the umbilical port, with a secondary 5 mm port placed in the midline; if needed, secondary 5 mm ports are placed in the usual lateral areas. If the drilling is performed with a CO_2 laser or fiber laser, one may use either a secondary port or a laser laparoscope. The ovary is stabilized with a 5 mm atraumatic grasper holding the uteroovarian ligament. It is best to use a high power density so the capsule is well penetrated. Multiple punctures are made—up to 30 or more—so that at completion of these multiple firings the ovary has the appearance of a golf ball.

A similar result can be obtained using an electrosurgical needle, making multiple punctures with a high energy cutting current at 30–60 watts. All of the punctures should avoid the area near the hilum so as to decrease the possibility of trauma to an ovarian blood vessel with its concomitant heavy bleeding, which could jeopardize the ovary.

Following the multiple puncturing, especially when using the laser, the entire surface of the ovary must be thoroughly irrigated to remove any carbon particles that may be present. It is important to leave a large amount of fluid in the abdomen in an attempt to deter the formation of adhesions, one of the more serious complications of the procedure as previously noted.

Ovarian Torsion

Ovarian torsion is relatively uncommon, although it is estimated to account for 3% of gynecologic operative emergencies.[37] If the patient is young, as is often the case, conservative surgery using laparoscopy has become increasingly more acceptable using a detorsion technique. The risk of thromboembolism is only theoretic.[38]

The laparoscope is inserted through the usual 10 mm intraumbilical port. Two 5 mm ports are placed, one in the midline in the suprapubic area and the other on the same side as the pathology, lateral to the inferior epigastric vessels as in the previously described technique. A blunt probe and an atraumatic grasper are passed through the 5 mm ports. The uteroovarian ligament may be gently grasped with the atraumatic grasper and the adnexa gently untwisted with the blunt probe. One must recognize the direction of the twist, but usually the adnexa rotates toward the uterus (clockwise for the left and counterclockwise for the right) After slowly untwisting the adnexa, it is observed and evaluated; and depending on the recovery, one must make a decision as to whether the adnexa should be left in situ or removed. Bruhat[38] described a system that categorizes the damage to the adnexa into three types: mild, severe, or irreversible torsion (Table 7.2). Using their criteria they suggest that only the irreversible lesion necessitates salpingo-oophorectomy, and the surgeon should tend to be conservative, particularly in young patients. If the etiology of the torsion appears to be due to a cyst, it should be resected after detorsion in a manner as previously described. If the torsion has occurred in a postmenopausal patient, salpingo-oophorectomy is performed. If the etiology is an ectopic pregnancy, it may be dif-

Table 7.2. Adnexal torsion

Adnexal torsion	Before detorsion	After detorsion
Mild		
Ovary	Increased volume	Almost normal
Tube	Congested	Almost normal
Severe		
Ovary	Enlarged	Slow recovery
Tube	Dark red or purple—distended	Recovery quicker
Irreversible		
Adnexa	Black, friable, enlarged	No improvement

Adapted from Bruhat et al.[38] Reprinted with permission of McGraw-Hill.

ficult to diagnose and salpingectomy may be necessary.

Following detorsion, the area should be well irrigated and the adnexa observed to see if it appears to be improving. The surgeon may then conclude the surgical procedure. Bruhat's group in Clermont-Ferrand, France has had one of the largest series (38 cases), and on the basis of this experience they recommended a second-look laparoscopy to evaluate the affected adnexa.[38]

Conclusion

Laparoscopic ovarian surgery has progressed from "trick" surgery, as performed by only a few surgeons during the early 1980s, to accepted procedures added to the armamentarium of most gynecologic surgeons. With the increased use of markers and ultrasonography to decrease the possibility of inappropriate surgery, combined with more refined extirpation techniques, the interest in laparoscopic ovarian surgery is burgeoning. This interest may be illustrated by the fact that an entire European congress on the management of adnexal cysts, primarily by laparoscopy, was held in Clermont-Ferrand, France in September 1992, and a number of the reports from that congress were gathered into a book of more than 250 pages.[39]

The ability to perform safe and effective ovarian surgery is the benchmark of a competent gynecologic surgeon. With proper training and practice the modern gynecologist can utilize operative laparoscopy to achieve the same therapeutic effect while enabling the patient a more rapid return to her normal life style with less pain and inconvenience.

Figures 7.1–7.4 and 7.6–7.8 from Levine, Operative Laparoscopy, in Telinde's Operative Gynecology Update, Vol. 1, No. 3, 1992, Thompson JD, Rock JA (eds.). Philadelphia, Lippincott. Reprinted with permission.

References

1. HULKA JF, PARKER WH, SURREY MW, PHILLIPS JM: Management of ovarian masses. AAGL 1990 survey. J Reprod Med 1992;37:599.
2. SEMM K: New methods of pelviscopy (gynecologic laparoscopy) for myomectomy, ovariectomy, tubectomy, and adenectomy. Endoscopy 1979;2:85.
3. SEMM K, METTLER L: Technical progress in pelvic surgery via operative laparoscopy. Am J Obstet Gynecol 1980;138:121.
4. LEVINE RL: Economic impact of pelviscopic surgery. J Reprod Med 1985;30:655.
5. SHALEV E, ZABARI A, ROMANO S, LUBOSHITZKY R: Laparoscopic gonadectomy in 46XY female patient. Fertil Steril 1992;57:459.
6. REICH H, MCGLYNN F, WILKE W: Laparoscopic management of stage I ovarian cancer: a case report. J Reprod Med 1990;35:601.
7. NEZHAT F, NEZHAT C: Operative laparoscopy for the treatment of ovarian remnant syndrome. Fertil Steril 1992;57:1003.
8. LEVINE RL: Pelviscopic surgery in women over 40. J Reprod Med 1990;35:597.
9. MAIMAN M, SELTZER V, BOYCE J: Laparoscopic excision of ovarian neoplasms subsequently found to be malignant. Obstet Gynecol 1991;77:563.
10. DEMBO AJ, DAVY M, STENWIG AE, ET AL: Prognostic factors in patients with stage I epithelial ovarian cancer. Obstet Gynecol 1990;75:263.
11. CRISTALLI B, CAYOLA A, IZARD V, LEVARDON M: Benefit of operative laparoscopy for ovarian tumor suspected of benignity. J Laparoendosc Surg 1992;2:69.
12. SHALEV E, ELIYAHU S, PELEG D, TSABARI A: Laparoscopic management of adnexal cystic masses in postmenopausal women. Obstet Gynecol 1994;83:594.
13. YOUNG RC, WALTON LA, ELLENBERG SS, ET AL: Adjuvant therapy in stage I and stage II epithelial ovarian cancer: results of two prospective randomized trials. N Engl J Med 1990;322:1021.
14. BAST RC, KLUGG TL, ST. JOHN E, ET AL: Radioimmunoassay using a monoclonal antibody to monitor the course of epithelial ovarian cancer. N Engl J Med 1983;309:883.
15. HOSONO MN, ENDO K, SAKAHARA H, ET AL: Different antigenic nature in healthy women with high serum CA-125 levels compared with typical patients with ovarian cancer. Cancer 1992;70: 2851.
16. SASSONE A, TIMOR-TRITSCH I, ARTNER A, ET AL: Transvaginal sonographic characterization of ovarian disease: evaluation of a new scoring system to predict ovarian malignancy. Obstet Gynecol 1991;78:70.
17. KURJAK A, ZULAD I, ALFIREVIC Z: Evaluation of adnexal masses with transvaginal color ultrasound. J Ultrasound Med 1991;10:295.

18. KAWAI M, KANO T, KIKKAWA F, ET AL: Transvaginal Doppler ultrasound with color flow imaging in the diagnosis of ovarian cancer. Obstet Gynecol 1992;79:163.
19. DANIELL JF, KURTZ BR, LEE JY: Laparoscopic oophorectomy: comparative study of ligatures, bipolar coagulation, and automatic stapling devices. Obstet Gynecol 1992;80:325.
20. SCHWARTZ PE: An oncologic view of when to do endoscopic surgery. Clin Obstet Gynecol 1991;34:467.
21. HASSON HM: Laparoscopic management of ovarian cysts. J Reprod Med 1990;35:863.
22. MECKE H, LEHMANN-WILLENBROCK E, IBRAHIM M, SEMM K: Pelviscopic treatment of ovarian cysts in premenopausal women. Gynecol Obstet Invest 1992;34:36.
23. JOHNS A: Laparoscopic oophorectomy/oophorocystectomy. Clin Obstet Gynecol 1991;34:460.
24. SELTZER VL, MAIMAN M, GOLDSTEIN S, ET AL: Laparoscopic surgery in the management of ovarian cysts. The Female Patient vol 17, Jun 92 pp 19.
25. KLEPPINGER RK: Ovarian cyst fenestration via laparoscopy. J Reprod Med 1978;21:16.
26. HASSON HM: Ovarian surgery. In Operative Gynecologic Endoscopy, Sanfilippo JS, Levine RL (eds). New York, Springer-Verlag, 1989, pp 97–98.
27. VANCAILLE TG: The role of laparoscopy in the surgical treatment of ovarian cysts. Infertil Reprod Med Clin North Am 1993;4:305.
28. RICHARDSON G, ROBERTSON DI, O'CONNOR ME: Malignant transformation occurring in mature cystic teratomas of the ovary. Can J Surg 1990; 33:499.
29. LABASTIDA R, LLUECA JA, GOMEZ T, ET AL: Laparoscopic removal of dermoid cysts. Gynaecol Endosc 1994;3:9.
30. WEINSTEIN D, POLISHUK WS: The role of wedge resection of the ovary as a cause for mechanical sterility. Surg Gynecol Obstet 1975;141:417.
31. CAMPO S, GARCEA N, CARUSO A, SICCARDI P: Effect of celioscopic resection in patients with polycystic ovaries. Gynecol Obstet Invest 1983;15:213.
32. GJONNAESS H: Polycystic ovarian syndrome treated by ovarian electrocautery through the laparoscope. Fertil Steril 1984;41:20.
33. KOVACS G, BUCKLER H, BANGAH M, ET AL: Treatment of anovulation due to polycystic ovarian syndrome by laparoscopic ovarian electrocautery. Br J Obstet Gynaecol 1991;98:30.
34. DANIELL JF, MILLER W: Polycystic ovaries treated by laparoscopic laser vaporization. Fertil Steril 1989;51:232.
35. DABIRASHRAFI H, MOHAMAD K, BEHJATNIA Y, MOGHADAMI-TABRIZI N: Adhesion formation after ovarian electrocauterization on patients with polycystic ovarian syndrome. Fertil Steril 1991;55:1200.
36. GURGAN T, URMAN B, AKSU T, ET AL: The effect of short-interval laparoscopic lysis of adhesions on pregnancy rates following Nd-YAG laser photocoagulation of polycystic ovaries. Obstet Gynecol 1992;80:45.
37. ADELSON MD, ADELSON KL: Miscellaneous benign disorders of the upper genital tract. In Textbook of Gynecology, Copeland LJ (ed). New York, Saunders, 1993, pp 865–866.
38. BRUHAT MA, MAGE G, POULY JL, ET AL: Adnexal torsion. In Operative Laparoscopy. New York, McGraw-Hill, 1992, pp 205–215.
39. BRUHAT MA (ED): The Management of Adnexal Cysts. London, Blackwell Scientific, 1992.

8
Laparoscopic-Assisted Hysterectomy: American Perspective

C. Y. Liu and D. Alan Johns

Hysterectomy is one of the most frequently performed gynecologic surgical procedures in the United States, with more than 650,000 hysterectomies performed at an annual cost of more than $3 billion. Approximately 70% of hysterectomies are performed abdominally and 30% vaginally. It is predicted that as the number of women in the population increases in the near future, so will the number of hysterectomies. With the current rate of 6.7 per 1000 women, it is estimated that the number of hysterectomies will rise to 783,000 in 1995 and 824,000 in the year of 2005.[1]

From 1965 to 1987 the five most common indications for hysterectomy in the United States, according to a report of a major insurance company,[2] were for leiomyomas (30%), endometriosis (19%), genital prolapse (16%), gynecologic malignancy (10%), or endometrial hyperplasia (6%). The remaining 19% were due to other causes, such as dysfunctional uterine bleeding or adnexal diseases. The objectives of a hysterectomy can be categorized into three groups: (1) to save a life; (2) to improve the quality of life by relieving symptoms; (3) to restore normal anatomy and function. The surgical procedure chosen for a particular patient, whether it be performed vaginally, abdominally, or laparoscopically, should fulfill at least one of these objectives. The method chosen should always be that which is in the best interest of the patient. Consideration must be given regarding the surgeon's experience and competence when the method of hysterectomy is chosen, as well as operating time, cost of equipment, length of hospitalization, recuperation period, and complication rate. Without a large abdominal incision, vaginal hysterectomy has the advantage of shorter operative time, more comfortable and quicker recovery period, and fewer complications; it is also cosmetically appealing to the patient. Vaginal hysterectomy is more cost-effective, but it may be more difficult and in some cases is even contraindicated. Some of the negative conditions include the following:

1. Lack of mobility of the uterus.
2. Contracted pelvis
3. Leiomyomatous uteri larger than 18 weeks' gestational size
4. Extensive pelvic endometriosis involving the cul-de-sac and the rectovaginal septum and space
5. Adnexal mass in which malignancy is suspected
6. Congenital anomalies, such as didelphic uterus, double cervix, and double vagina
7. Multiple previous major pelvic surgical procedures or a history of pelvic inflammatory disease

With advanced technologic development in laparoscopic instruments and improved skill in performing operative laparoscopy, the gynecologist, when in doubt about the feasibility of a vaginal hysterectomy, may first evaluate the patient laparoscopically, prior to embarking upon laparotomy. In most cases, with the aid of operative laparoscopy a difficult or contraindicated vaginal hysterectomy can often be converted to a routine vaginal hysterectomy.[3] The number of abdominal hysterectomies will be drastically reduced in the years to come. However, enthusiasm for the new must be tempered with surgical common sense. The patient's best interests and the cost-effectiveness of the procedure must be the primary concern of the surgeon, rather than flaunting a new surgical technique.

The media had introduced the advantages of minimally invasive surgery to a responsive consumer market. Patient demand may tempt some gynecologists to perform laparoscopic hysterectomies for which they may not have been properly trained. It is important to remember that laparoscopic-assisted hysterectomy is not intended to replace vaginal hysterectomy but is an alternative to abdominal hysterectomy, converting what would have been a difficult vaginal hysterectomy or abdominal hysterectomy into a routine vaginal hysterectomy.

Laparoscopic-assisted vaginal hysterectomy (LAVH) offers patients the advantage of conversion from what would otherwise be an abdominal operation to a vaginal procedure. If this conversion is associated with minimal or no additional risk, shorter recovery, and costs no more than abdominal hysterectomy, the benefits are unquestionable. Unfortunately, LAVH is often performed when vaginal hysterectomy is not only possible but preferable. Prolonged operating time, expensive disposable equipment, and significant complications combine to make LAVH the most expensive hysterectomy.[4] However, when good endoscopic skills are combined with adequate and inexpensive equipment, the properly selected patient benefits with minimal additional risk.

LAVH is not a substitute for lack of skill in vaginal surgery. To complete LAVH in the patient who is truly not a candidate for vaginal hysterectomy, considerable skills in vaginal and laparoscopic surgery are required. If the surgeon is uncomfortable with a difficult vaginal hysterectomy, problems are compounded during the difficult LAVH. Laparoscopic techniques simply allow completion of those portions of the procedure that would otherwise be impossible with a vaginal approach. In addition, LAVH adds the risks associated with laparoscopy to those of hysterectomy (vaginal or abdominal).

Complications of laparoscopic surgery, though uncommon, tend to be major: bowel perforation, major vessel injury, ureteral injury, and delayed bowel injury (usually thermal). None of these risks is commonly associated with abdominal or vaginal hysterectomy, as neither of these procedures commonly require a trocar. If these risks are to be added to those of hysterectomy, they must be offset by significant benefits to the patient.

The patient must be informed of the potential risks associated with laparoscopic surgery, regardless of the endoscopic procedure planned. The patient should agree that the potential advantages of the endoscopic approach to her hysterectomy is worth the risks associated with laparoscopy. The patient must make the decision to assume that added risk, not the doctor.

Definition and Classification

The definition of LAVH is difficult to establish. Clinics use the same term to describe a number of completely different procedures. They describe operations from minimal surgery performed laparoscopically followed by a fairly standard vaginal hysterectomy[3] to procedures in which most or all of the hysterectomy is accomplished via the laparoscope, with a minimal vaginal component.[5-9] The problem appears to lie in assessing statistical results and complication rates. A generally accepted definition and classification of the LAVH must be standardized.

Garry and colleagues[10] proposed the following classification system. If the laparoscopic

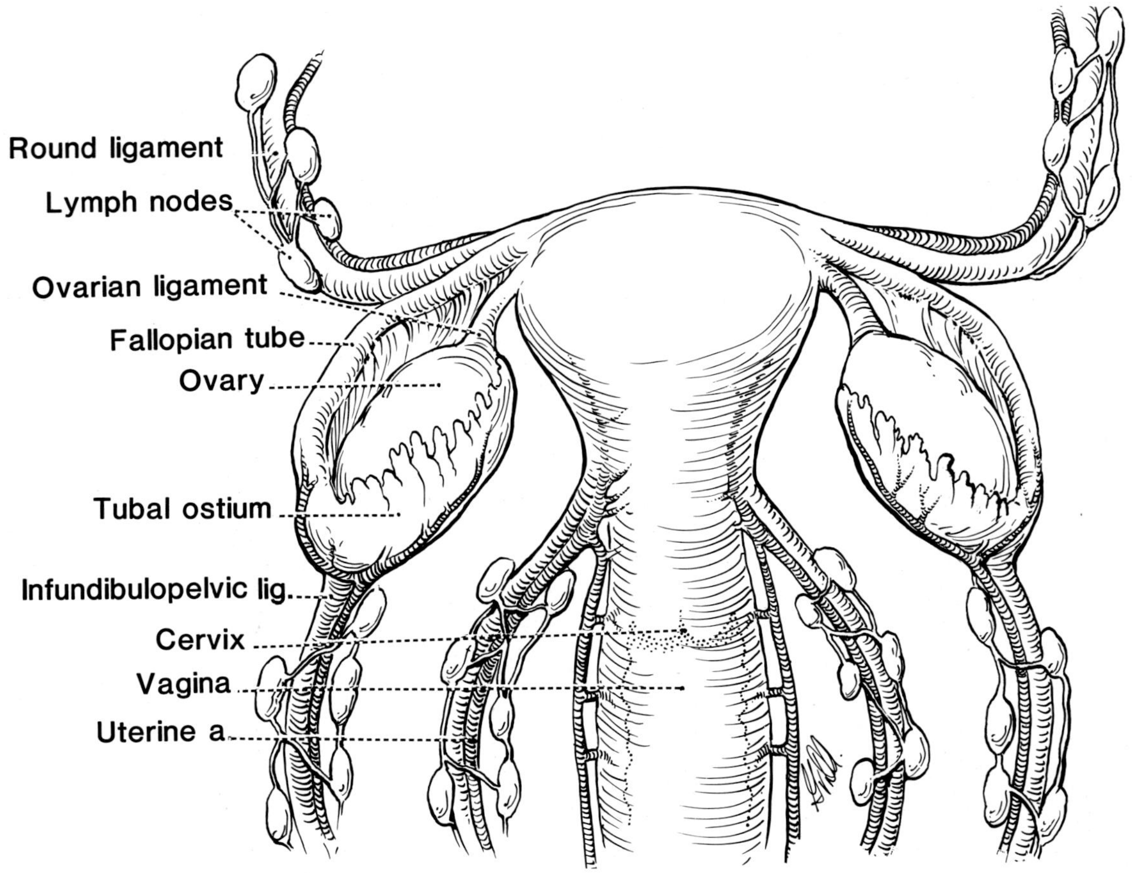

Figure 8.1. Pelvic structures that are amenable to laparoscopy. (a = artery.)

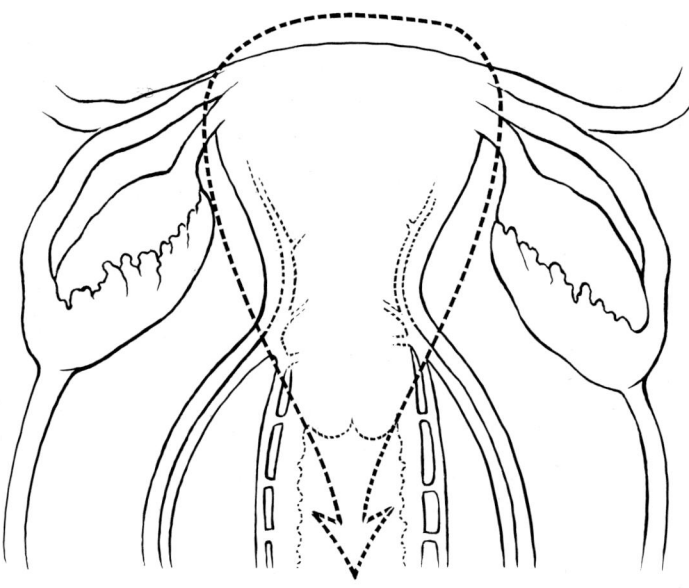

Figure 8.2. Standard vaginal hysterectomy following a diagnostic laparoscopy. (- - - represents vaginal surgical approach; —— represents laparoscopic surgical approach.)

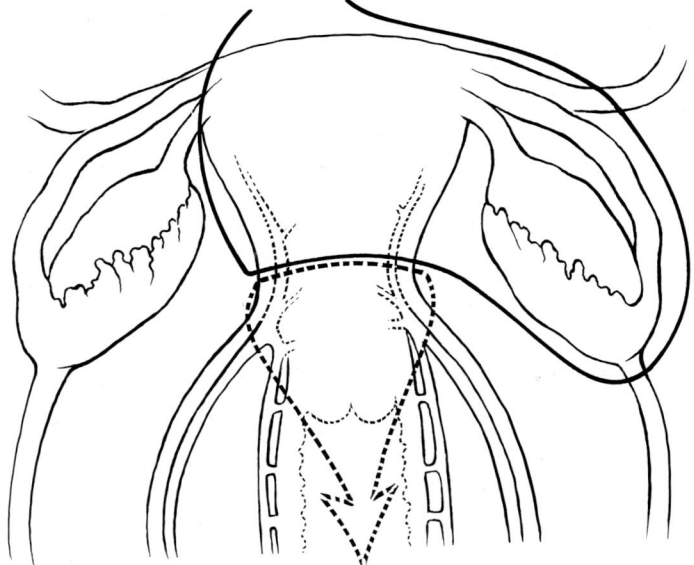

Figure 8.3. Total laparoscopic-assisted vaginal hysterectomy (LAVH).

component of the operation is completed above the uterine vessels, which are subsequently secured by the vaginal route, such a procedure should be called an LAVH. If the uterine vessels are secured laparoscopically, the procedure should be termed a laparoscopic hysterectomy (LH). If the uterosacral and cardinal ligaments are also secured by laparoscopic technique, the procedure is analogous to a total abdominal hysterectomy and should be called a total laparoscopic hysterectomy (TLH). The complete descriptive classification is shown in Figures 8.1 through 8.7.

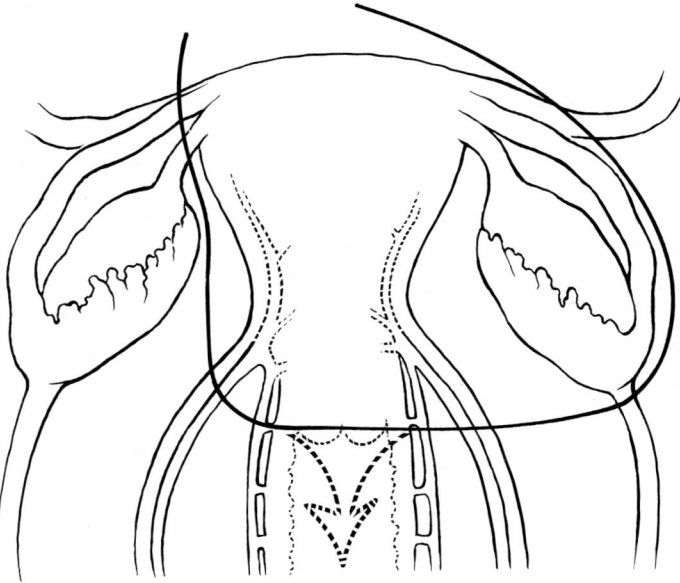

Figure 8.4. Total laparoscopic hysterectomy. This procedure includes complete mobilization of the uterus laparoscopically including the uterosacral and cardinal ligaments combined with laparoscopic opening of the anterior and posterior cul-de-sacs. The uterus, cervix, and adnexum are removed vaginally.

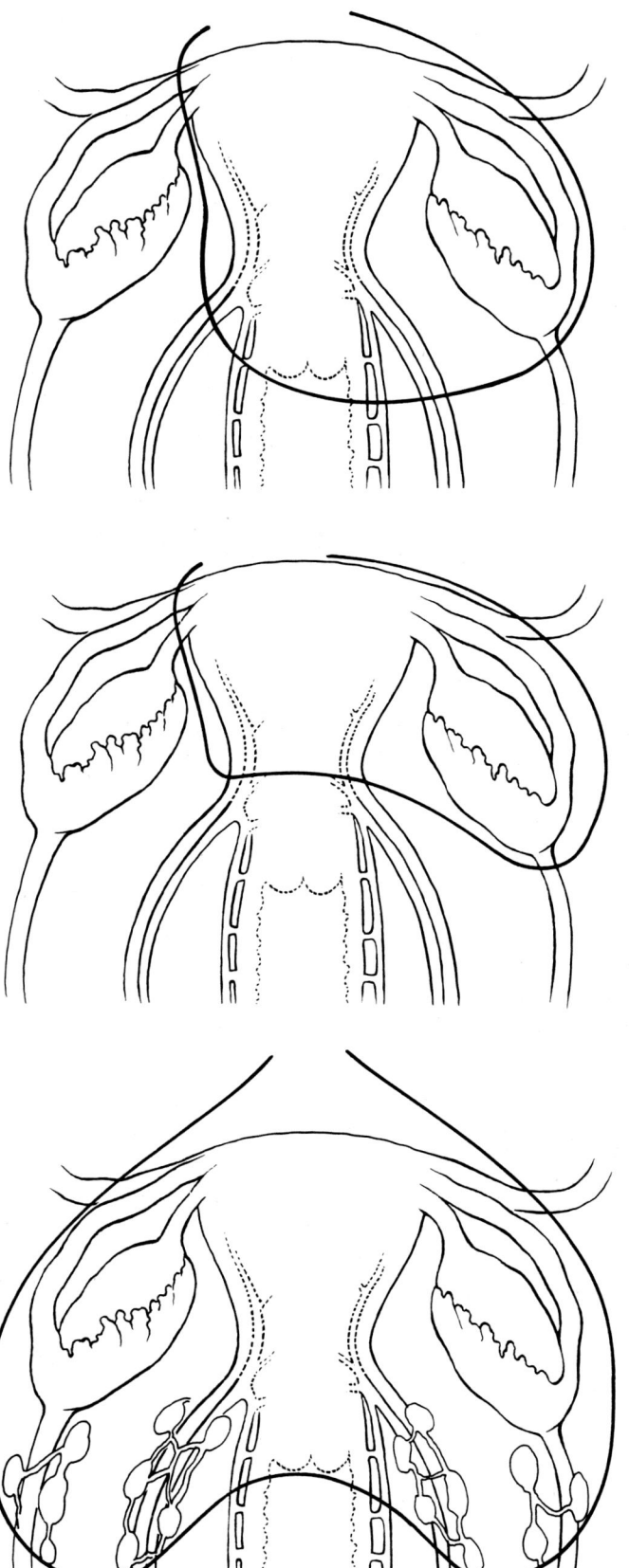

Figure 8.5. Total laparoscopic hysterectomy.

Figure 8.6. Laparoscopic supracervical hysterectomy. The adnexa and infundibulopelvic ligaments are mobilized laparoscopically, and the uterine fundus is removed from the cervix at the level of the internal os.

Figure 8.7. Radical laparoscopic hysterectomy. Wertheim's type of hysterectomy with full bilateral pelvic lymph node dissection and wide removal of the adnexae is performed entirely with laparoscopic techniques.

Surgical Technique

After induction of general anesthesia with endotracheal intubation, the patient is placed in dorsolithotomy position with both legs and feet supported by Allen Stirrups (Allen Medical Systems, Mayfield, Ohio) (Plate 1). Inadequate positioning of the patient for laparoscopic surgery often engenders a frustrating experience for the entire operating room team. The patient must be optimally positioned for each segment of the procedure (endoscopic and vaginal). One position usually does not suffice. Operative laparoscopy requires the patient to be in the dorsal lithotomy position with both legs positioned low (the thigh level with the abdominal wall). Vaginal surgery requires the patient to be positioned with the legs high and lateral, allowing maximal room for the assistant to work.

When the position of the patient on the operating table causes the surgeon to struggle, time is lost and mistakes may occur. Begin the endoscopic portion of the operation with the patient in the ideal position for laparoscopic surgery. Once the endoscopic portion of the procedure is completed, take the time (usually no more than 5 minutes) to position the patient as you would for vaginal hysterectomy. This small investment in time is offset by facilitating the vaginal portion of the LAVH.

A single dose of prophylactic antibiotic is administered.[11] The bladder is catheterized, and 30 ml of concentrated indigo carmine dye is instilled as a precautionary measure to facilitate recognition of any potential bladder injury during the procedure. A uterine sound is inserted into the uterine cavity and secured to two single-toothed tenaculums, which are attached to the (anterior and posterior) cervix. The sound serves as a uterine manipulator. A 10 mm laparoscope is inserted through a 12 mm trocar sleeve in a vertical intraumbilical incision. Four 5 mm puncture sites are established in the lower abdomen, all being placed lateral to the deep inferior epigastric vessels and the rectus abdominis muscles (Fig. 8.8). The location of these sites varies with the size of the uterus and the pathology in the pelvis. The internal organs are carefully inspected, and biopsies are performed if needed; pelvic pathology including adhesions, endometriosis, and ovarian cysts can be excised laparoscopically. The CO_2 laser is delivered into the abdominal cavity through a 10 mm operative laparoscope.

As with any other surgery, the operative technique may vary from case to case. The following description outlines one technique.

1. Both pelvic ureters are identified and dissected to the ureteric canal, where the uterine artery crosses above the ureter and the cardinal ligament lies below the ureter; *if necessary the ureteric canal can be opened and the ureteral dissection carried further. Positive identification of both ureters avoids injury (thermal and mechanical) to them during the procedure.* This step is accomplished by opening the peritoneum covering the ureter with the CO_2 laser or scissors. If pelvic side wall pathology exists, such as ovarian endometrioma or other adnexal mass or dense tuboovarian adhesions, the ureteral dissection must start at or above the pelvic brim. This usually is easier on the right side, where the ureter can be readily visualized just underneath the bifurcation of the iliac artery. It is more difficult to identify the ureter on the left side, where its course is usually obscured by the sigmoid colon. The colon should be freed and reflected from the left iliac fossa to expose the ovarian and mesenteric vessels and the iliac artery. In most cases the left ureter is located above the internal iliac artery while the right ureter is beneath it in the area of the upper pelvic side wall. The uterosacral ligaments also should be dissected away from the ureters. If the adnexal structures are densely adherent to the pelvic side wall, a retroperitoneal approach allows the peritoneum to be stripped from the side wall with the ovary remaining attached. This technique should also decrease the risk of leaving behind an ovarian remnant.

2. Reflect the bladder all the way to the upper part of the vagina by first making a transverse incision on the vesicouterine peritoneal fold. The upper junction of the uterovesical fold appears as a white line when viewed laparoscopically (Plate 2). The peritoneum attaches tightly to the broad ligament above this white line, but the peritoneum is loosely attached to

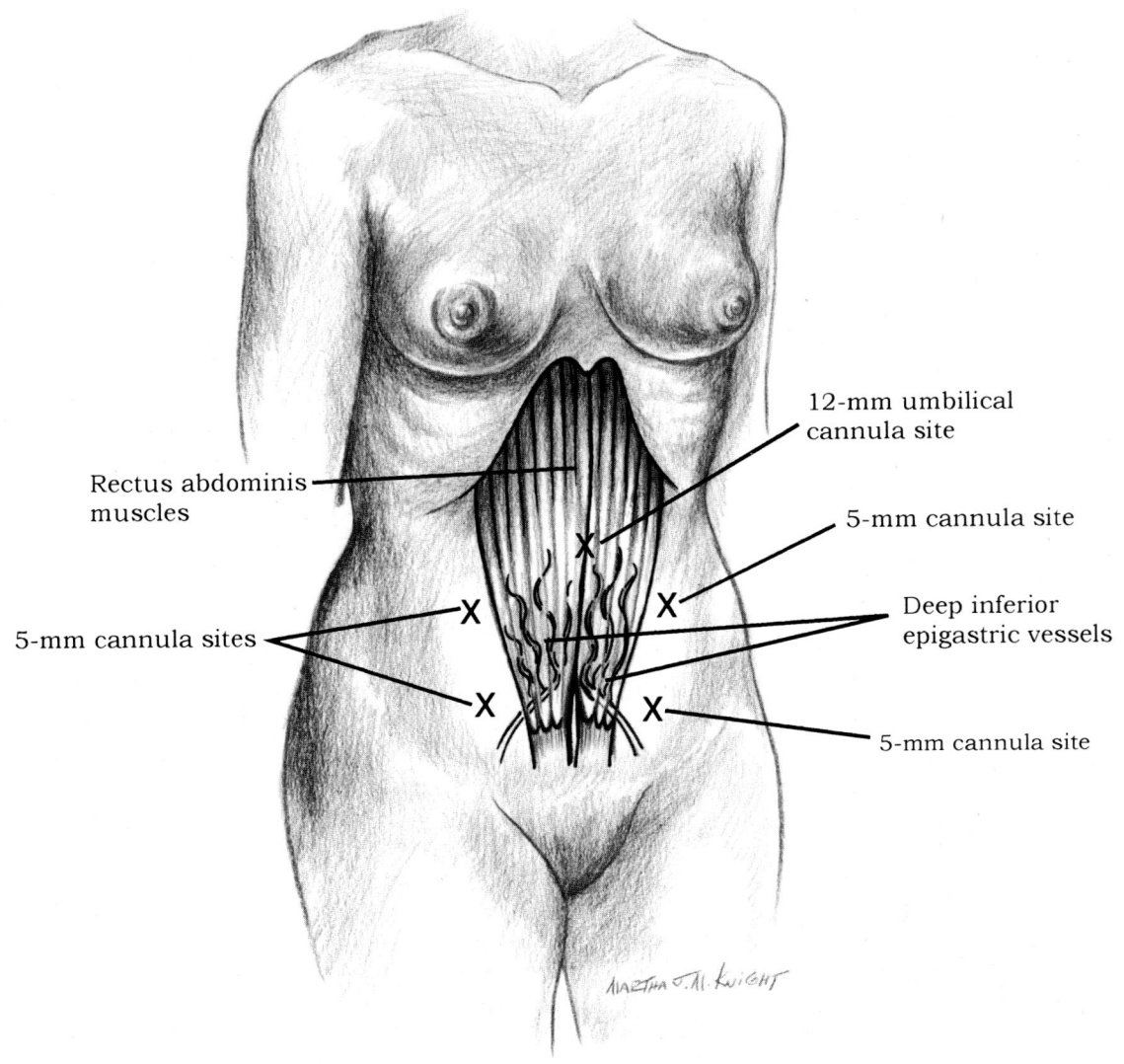

Figure 8.8. Trocar entry sites for laparoscopic hysterectomy.

the cervix for a distance of 2.0–2.5 cm between the white line and the dome of the bladder. This structure is the vesicouterine pouch. The initial incision should be made below the white line to avoid difficult and bloody dissection of the bladder. After the transverse incision below the white line is made, the peritoneum below the incision is lifted up, exposing three "condensations" of connective tissues. The middle *bands* of the loose connective tissue are the vesicocervical ligaments, which are relatively avascular and can thus be divided with minimal blood loss. The vesicocervical space with its characteristic glistening white surface is then entered. The lateral bands of connective tissue on both sides of the cervix are the bladder pillars, which are part of the endopelvic fascia and extend from the cardinal ligaments to the pubovesical ligaments. The bladder pillars secure the bladder to the cervix and contain the blood vessels from the cervix. These pillars are coagulated with bipolar electrodes (Plate 3) and divided with scissors or laser, after which the bladder can be easily dissected down to the upper part of the vagina pulling the ureters laterally away from the cervix (Plate 4). If the cul-de-sac is obliterated partially or completely because of endometriosis or previous pelvic inflammatory disease, the rectosigmoid colon is dissected away from the cervix, and any endometrial nodules present in the area are resected.

3. Both round ligaments are coagulated with bipolar Kleppinger forceps (Richard Wolfe, Rosemont, IL) about 2–3 cm from the uterus and then divided. The anterior leaf of the broad ligament is opened downward toward the cervix, and the uterine artery is identified. An opening is usually made on the avascular segment of the posterior leaf of the broad ligament above the uterine vessels.

4. If the fallopian tube and ovary are to be removed, the infundibulopelvic ligament is first mobilized; bipolar forceps may be used to compress and desiccate the vessels (Plate 5), which are then divided sharply. This step should be done with direct visualization of the ureter. The mesosalpinx and mesoovarian structures are desiccated and divided. If the ovary is to be preserved, the uteroovarian ligament and mesosalpinx are desiccated with bipolar forceps and then divided.

The automatic laparoscopic stapling device (Multi-Fire Endo GIA-30, US Surgical Corp., Norwalk, CT; or Linear Cutter-35, Ethicon, Somerville, NJ) is especially time-saving for this portion of the procedure. The automatic laparoscopic stapling device can be inserted into the peritoneal cavity through a 12 mm umbilical trocar sleeve and guided by a 5 mm laparoscope inserted in the left upper 5 mm port. This step can also be achieved by passing ligatures through the opening of the broad ligament and tying the infundibulopelvic ligament or the uteroovarian junction *with extracorporeal knot tying, using the laparoscopic knot pusher.*

5. Most gynecologists with expertise in vaginal surgery are comfortable controlling the uterine artery vaginally. It is a rare patient in whom the surgeon is unable to safely place a clamp across the cardinal ligament (including the uterine artery) transvaginally. Because ureteral injury commonly occurs at the level of the uterine artery, common sense dictates that the surgeon should use those techniques most familiar to him or her to avoid such injuries. The hysterectomy, at this point, should be completed vaginally.

If the surgeon has determined that the uterine arteries must be controlled endoscopically, careful dissection and isolation of these vessels permit their safe electrosurgical coaptation. Laparoscopic suturing may also be effective but requires considerable skill and patience. At this point the posterior leaf of the broad ligament is divided to the level of the uterine artery, which is then skeletonized laterally to the ureteric canal, where the uterine artery crosses above the ureter (Plate 6). With the ureter in direct view, the uterine artery is desiccated with bipolar forceps and divided. Alternatively, the uterine artery can be secured using a suture technique with O Vicryl on a CT-1 needle (Plate 7). An automatic laparoscopic stapling device can also be used effectively for this step (Plate 8).

6. While directly visualizing both ureters, the remaining cardinal ligament and both uterosacral ligaments are desiccated with bipolar forceps and divided with scissors or laser. *The uterus and lower uterine segment must be pushed up toward the patient's head and retracted away from the pelvic side wall to safely accomplish this step.*

7. At this point the surgical assistant puts a wet 4 × 4 sponge on a forceps and places it in the anterior vaginal fornix, tenting the vagina from below. The anterior culdotomy is performed laparoscopically using electrosurgical or laser techniques. With the sponge in the vagina as a guide and the suction-irrigator probe as the backstop, circumferential culdotomy is performed, and the cervix is completely detached from the vagina. Careful coordination between surgeon and assistants is required, as the CO_2 gas begins to leak rapidly as soon as the anterior cul-de-sac is opened. This step can be performed more easily by removing the uterine manipulator from the cervix as soon as the anterior culdotomy is done. A small sponge pad in a surgical glove placed inside the vagina can maintain the pneumoperitoneum. The cervix is then grasped with toothed grasping forceps laparoscopically, and the circumferential culdotomy can be performed using scissors. The uterus is then pulled or pushed into the vagina to maintain the pneumoperitoneum (Plate 9).

For the large fibroid uterus, morcellation can be done through the vagina.

8. The vagina is then closed transversely or vertically, with special emphasis on suturing both uterosacrocardinal ligaments to the vaginal vault to ensure good vaginal support. Three interrupted figure-of-eight sutures with O Vicryl are used to close the vaginal cuff laparoscopically. Under direct visualization of the left ureter, a suture is placed deeply through the left uterosacrocardinal ligament and into the vagina, exiting out the vagina through the anterior vaginal wall including both the rectovaginal and pubocervical fascia. The suture is then placed through the same structures again to ensure that the vaginal angle is closed, and the suture is tied with an extracorporeal knot-tying technique using a knot pusher. The same procedure is then performed on the right side of the vaginal cuff. An additional figure-of-eight suture is placed between these two lateral sutures to close the middle portion of the vagina (Plate 10). The entire pelvic cavity is then carefully inspected laparoscopically and irrigated with copious amounts of Ringer's lactate solution. All debris and blood are removed, and endoscopic underwater viewing of the pelvis is done to ensure satisfactory hemostasis. Both ureters are inspected carefully. If ureteral injury is suspected, 5 ml of indigo carmine dye and 20 mg of *furosemide (Lasix)* are injected intravenously, and a cystoscopic examination is performed. Visualization of the normal peristalsis of the intramural portion of the ureter and observation of the indigo carmine dye from the ureteral orifice is reassuring.

Results and Discussions

Total laparoscopic hysterectomy has been evaluated in 518 patients.[12] The patients' ages, weights, uterine weights, operation times, hospital stays, and blood losses are conveyed in Table 8.1. The pathologic findings and indications are provided in Table 8.2, and the procedures performed concomitantly with these hysterectomies are shown on Table 8.3. The overall complication rate was 5.7%. One patient, a heavy smoker, developed bilateral pneumonia on the third postoperative day after an otherwise uncomplicated hysterectomy. She subsequently developed adult respiratory distress syndrome and expired 9 days after her operation. At autopsy her death was attributed to massive bilateral pneumonia. Complications included febrile morbidity (2.1%), injury to the urinary tract system (1.3%), injury to bowel (1.1%), vaginal cuff bleeding (0.5%), unanticipated blood transfusions (0.3%), and pulmonary embolism (0.2%) (Table 8.4). Four patients developed pelvic hematoma with associated postoperative fever, two required second-look laparoscopy to evacuate the hematoma,

Table 8.1. Characteristics of 518 laparoscopic hysterectomies and concomitant surgeries

Characteristics	Mean	Range
Age (years)	42	26–79
Body weight (pounds)	142	106–328
Uterine weight (g)	175	48–1000
Operating time (minutes)	120	45–390
Hospital time (days)	1.4	1–7
Blood loss (ml)	115	25–1000

Table 8.2. Pathology of 518 laparoscopic hysterectomies and comcomitant surgeries

Pathology	No. of patients
Leiomyoma	289
Endometriosis[a]	211
Adenomyosis	185
Ovarian cysts (> 6 cm)[b]	7
Postmenopausal uterine bleeding with endometrial polyps/submucosal fibroids[c]	5
Benign pathology[d]	37
Endometrial adenocarcinoma (stage I)	5
Ovarian cancer (stage I)	2
Cervical cancer (stage I)	2
Total	743

[a]By the American Fertility Society classification 58 patients had stage IV endometriosis, and 49 patients had stage III.
[b]Five cysts were hemorrhagic, one was a benign teratoma, one was a benign serous cystadenoma.
[c]All five patients had had previous major pelvic surgery.

Table 8.3. Procedures performed concomitantly with 518 laparoscopic hysterectomies[a]

Procedure	No. of patients
Vaporization/excision of endometriosis	210
Lysis/excision of adhesions	240
Appendectomy	158
Retropubic colposuspension (Burch procedure)	58
Repair of bowel injury[b]	4
Repair of bladder injury	5
Pelvic lymphadenectomy	3
Lymphadenectomy and omentectomy	2
Radical hysterectomy with lymphadenectomy	2
Total	682

[a]Procedures exclude salpingo-oophorectomy.
[b]Two small bowel injuries, two rectal injuries.

and the other two hematomas resolved with conservative measures. An automatic laparoscopic stapling device, Multi-Fire Endo GIA-30 was used with each hysterectomy. When an automatic stapling device is used, careful underwater examination of the staple line for complete hemostasis at the completion of surgery after discontinuation of the pneumoperitoneal pressure is important for hematoma prevention; any bleeding detected at this time requires bipolar coagulation behind the stapler line. No hematoma formation occurred in either group using electrosurgery or suturing for large-vessel hemostasis. Six bladder injuries occurred in the reported series, five were detected intraoperatively and successfully repaired. Routine installation of concentrated indigo carmine dye into the bladder preoperatively facilitates early recognition of bladder injury during sur-

Table 8.4. Complications of 518 laparoscopic hysterectomies and concomitant surgeries

Complication	No. of patients	Rate[a]
Febrile morbidity ($m = 11$)		2.12
Pneumonia[b]	1	0.19
Pelvic hematoma[c]	4	0.77
Dehydration	1	0.19
Transient febrile episodes	5	0.96
Urinary tract system ($m = 7$)		1.35
Bladder injury	5	0.96
Vesicovaginal fistula	1	0.19
Ureterovaginal fistula	1	0.19
Intestinal complications ($m = 6$)		1.15
Small bowel enterotomy	2	0.38
Thermal injury of sigmoid colon	1	0.19
Partial bowel obstruction	1	0.19
Richter's hernia[d]	2	0.38
Vaginal cuff bleeding	3	0.57
Unanticipated blood transfusion	2	0.38
Pulmonary embolism	1	0.19
Total	30	5.76

[a]Rate per 100 women who underwent hysterectomy and concomitant surgical procedures.
[b]This patient later developed adult respiratory distress syndrome and expired.
[c]Two of the patients had second-look laparoscopy and evacuation of hematoma.
[d]Richter's hernia occurred at the 12 mm trocar puncture sites.

gery. One patient developed a vesicovaginal fistula 4 weeks postoperatively; this late occurrence was unusual. The operative videotape was reviewed, and no evidence of bladder injury was noted. The fistula formation might have been due to a suture penetrating the bladder wall during vaginal cuff closure. One case of ureterovaginal fistula occurred early in the series, and the ureteral injury was not recognized intraoperatively. Subsequently, routine identification and dissection of the ureters prior to the hysterectomy ensured that no additional ureteral injuries occurred. Ureteral identification is critically important before laparoscopic ligation of the uterine artery and cardinal ligaments. On more than one occasion the ureter was inside the jaws of the automatic stapling device and would have been injured if the ureters had not been completely dissected before applying the stapling device. On many occasions the ureters were noted to be in close proximity to the cervix. When a hysterectomy is performed laparoscopically, the surgeon must rely on ureteral visualization to avoid injury. Two patients developed Richter's hernia at the 12 mm trocar sites. Closure of the fascia is now recommended for a trocar size exceeding 10 mm.[13–15]

Bowel injury during hysterectomy is usually associated with extensive adhesions and endometriosis.[16–] In reported series, two small bowel injuries occurred during enterolysis due to extensive adhesions. If laparoscopic repair of the small bowel laceration is intended, special care must be taken to avoid narrowing the intestinal lumen and compromising the vascular supply.[19, 20] Two intentional rectal wall resections were performed because of full-thickness infiltration of the endometriosis, and the rectal defect was repaired laparoscopically.[20–22] It is important to perform a bowel preparation in all patients suspected of having cul-de-sac pathology. Our suggested regimen for bowel preparation is erythromycin 250 *mg every 6 hours and neomycin 18 mg every 4 hours orally* starting 48 hours preoperatively, clear liquid diet for at least 36 hours before surgery, and *Golytely* 4 L by mouth beginning the afternoon prior to surgery.

Conclusion

After reviewing the literature and from our own experience in performing laparoscopic hysterectomies, we conclude that even in the hands of experienced laparoscopic surgeons laparoscopic hysterectomy is not an innocuous procedure. Gynecologists who are interested in performing laparoscopic hysterectomy must know their limits and select patients accordingly. The high cost of laparoscopic-assisted hysterectomy has been criticized.[4] Exclusive use of disposable instruments and the surgeon's inexperience in performing the surgery (which prolongs the operating time) are the two main causes of increased operative cost. It is imperative that gynecologists become as cost-effective as possible without compromising safety or efficacy. The transition from open surgery to video-guided laparoscopic surgery requires considerable adjustment for novices. The surgeon must have knowledge of laparoscopic instrumentation, suturing techniques, the physics and clinical application of electrosurgery and laser energy, and must be able to avoid and manage laparoscopic complications. Assisting and training with surgeons proficient in laparoscopic hysterectomy is critical, as we are convinced that one cannot learn the operation outside the operating room. Conversion to abdominal hysterectomy should never be considered a complication; rather, it is a prudent surgical decision when the surgeon becomes uncomfortable with the laparoscopic approach.

References

1. US Bureau of Census: Projection of the Population of the United States, by Age, Sex, Race: 1983–2080. Current Population Reports Series P-25.
2. POKRAS R: Hysterectomy: past, present, and future. Stat Bull Metrop Insur Co 1989;70:12.
3. KOVAC SR, CRIKSHANK SH, RETTO WF: Laparoscopic assisted vaginal hysterectomy. J Gynecol Surg 1990;6:185.
4. BAGGISH MS: The most expensive hysterectomy. J Gynecol Surg 1992;8:57.

5. LIU CY: Laparoscopic hysterectomy, a review of 72 cases. J Reprod Med 1992;37:351.
6. LIU CY: Laparoscopic hysterectomy: report of 215 cases. Gynecol Endosc 1992;1:73.
7. LUI CY: Laparoscopic hysterectomy. Gynecol Endosc 1993;2:73.
8. REICH H: Laparoscopic hysterectomy. Surg Laparosc Endosc 1992;2:85.
9. REICH H, MCGLYNN F, SEKEL L: Total laparoscopic hysterectomy. Gynecol Endosc 1993;2:59.
10. GARRY R, REICH H, LIU CY: Laparoscopic hysterectomy—definitions and indications. Gynecol Endosc 1994;3:1 [editorial].
11. HIRSCH HA: Prophylactic antibiotics in obstetrics and gynecology. Am J Med 1985(Suppl 6B); 78:170.
12. LIU CY, REICH H: Laparoscopic hysterectomy in 518 cases—analysis of complications. Gynecol Endoscopy 1994;3:203–207.
13. KADAR N, LIU CY, REICH H, GIMPELSON R: Incisional hernias following major laparoscopic gynecological procedures. Am J Obstet Gynecol 1993;168: 1493.
14. SCHIFF I, NAFTOLIN F: Small bowel incarceration after uncomplicated laparoscopy. Gynecology 1974;43:674.
15. BOURKE JB: Small intestinal obstruction from a Richter's hernia at the site of a laparoscope. BMJ 1977;2:1993.
16. AMIRIKIA H, EVANS TN: Ten-year review of hysterectomies: trends, indications, and risks. Am J Obstet Gynecol 1978;134:431.
17. CHRYSSIKOPOULOS A, LOGHIS C: Indications and results of total hysterectomy. Int Surg 1986;71:188.
18. WINGO PA, HUEZO CM, RUBIN GL, ET AL: The mortality risk associated with hysterectomy. Am J Obstet Gynecol 1985;152:803.
19. WHEELESS CR JR: Gastrointestinal injuries associated with laparoscopy. In Endoscopy in Gynecology, Phillips JM (ed). Downey, CA, AAGL, 1978.
20. REICH H: Laparoscopy bowel injury. Surg Laparosc Endosc 1992;2:74.
21. REICH H, MCGLYNN F, BUDIN R: Laparoscopic repair of full thickness bowel injury. J Laparoendosc Surg 1991;1:119.
22. HARDER F, VOGELBACH P: Single layer end-on continuous suture of colonic anastomosis. Am J Surg 1988;155:611.

9
Pelviscopic Intrafascial Hysterectomy Without Colpotomy

Paul F. Vietz

Hysterectomy is often considered by the gynecologic surgeon to be the conclusion of a logical progression of therapeutic steps. The decision often has a profound psychologic effect on a woman's feeling of femininity. It is estimated that in the United States more than 600,000 hysterectomies are performed annually.[1] Since the mid-1980s this operation has become second only to cesarean section with respect to all surgical procedures in women.[2] It is estimated that most hysterectomies (ca. 90%) are performed for benign disease to improve the quality of life rather than to treat life-threatening conditions such as malignancy.

Advances in anesthesia, blood banking, infection control, and operative techniques, such as operative laparoscopy,[3] (pelviscopy) and the development of medical and surgical alternatives have led to reevaluation of hysterectomy. Health care costs are certainly a concern.

We live during an era in which basic surgical skills and competence are of great importance. At the same time, cost-effectiveness demands the shortest hospitalization and conduct of the safest, most uncomplicated procedure possible. The availability of a safe, simplified, cost-effective alternative procedure to the classic total abdominal or vaginal hysterectomy is of paramount importance. CISH [classic intrafascial SEMM (serrated edge macromorcellator) hysterectomy] appears to fulfill these requirements.[4]

Historical Perspective

Table 9.1 presents a historical perspective of significant events concerning hysterectomy. From 1900 to the 1940s in the United States subtotal hysterectomy was most often performed. The technique was considered simpler, safer, and associated with lower morbidity and less blood loss than total abdominal hysterectomy. During the 1940s and 1950s, however, a great debate ensued at national and international meetings about the wisdom of removing the cervix at the time of hysterectomy as prophylaxis against cervical cancer. A number of studies reported an incidence of cervical stump cancer that ranged from 0.3% to as high as 10.7%.[16-21] Opponents to cervicectomy argued that removal of the cervix with transection of the uterine vessels bilaterally, the cardinal and uterosacral ligaments, and the paracervical nerves would lead to destruction of the pelvic floor topography, resulting in weakened support, urinary and bowel dysfunction, and a change in the sexual response of both partners.[21-25] With the philosophy "cancer kills, a

9. Pelviscopic Intrafascial Hysterectomy Without Colpotomy

Table 9.1. Historical perspective of hysterectomy

Author	Date	Event
Soranus of Ephesus	2nd century AD	First hysterectomy for prolapse, gangrenous uterus
Giaccorne Berengario DaCapi	1480–1550	Altered sex life following vaginal hysterectomy for gangrenous uterus
Reported mortality rate	—	90% Unlikely to survive hysterectomy
Semmelweiss and Lister	—	Antiseptic techniques reduced morbidity and mortality
Heath (Manchester, England)	1843	First successful subtotal hysterectomy
Burnham (Lowell, MA)	—	15 Cases of successful abdominal hysterectomy
Alexander Freund (Breslau, Germany)	1878	First refined standardized reproducible "simple" abdominal hysterectomy
Poro (Milan, Italy)	1876	First hysterectomy for gravid uterus
Schauschartd (Germany)	—	Refined radical hysterectomy for uterine cancer
Wertheim (Austria)	—	Refined radical hysterectomy for uterine cancer
Cervical stump cancer	1940–1950	Reported incidence 0.3–10.7% ($m = 10$–15)
	1936–1985	Procedures resulting in destruction of pelvic floor topography
Palmer	1940s	Introduction of laparoscopy
Rauramo	1949	
Ries	1961	Transvaginal electroconization
Aldridge and Meredith	1964	Resolved dilemma by excising cervical canal at supracervical hysterectomy
Frangenheim	1950s/1960s	Minimally invasive, organ-preserving endoscopic surgery replaces laparotomy
Semm (Kiel, Germany)	1987	Marked advance with operative laparoscopy
Reich	1989	First laparoscopy-assisted vaginal hysterectomy

prolapse can be corrected," by the 1960s total abdominal hysterectomy was universally recommended and found wide acceptance (Figs. 9.1, 9.2). Cervical cancer prevention became the sole reason for removing the cervix. Rauramo[10] and Aldridge and Meredith[11] tried to resolve the dilemma by excising the cervical canal at supracervical hysterectomy, but the operation was fraught with complications. Ries[12] recommended transvaginal electroconization but had little success because of bleeding and infection.

During the mid-1980s up to 80% of gynecologic surgery was performed by operative laparoscopy. The technique enjoyed worldwide

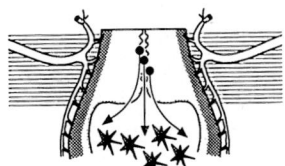

subtotal hysterectomy

Figure 9.1. Hysterectomy complex factors for subtotal hysterectomy.

Problems:

Psychic +
Cyclic +
Bacteriologic +
Oncologic +
Colposcopic +

Urologic ø
Proctologic ø
Pericervical ø

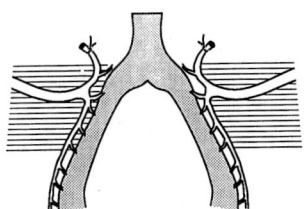

Hysterectomy Complex

Problems:

Urologic ø
Proctologic ø
Pericervical ø
Cyclic ø
Bacteriologic ø
Oncologic ø

Figure 9.2. Hysterectomy complex factors for CISH.

acceptance following its introduction in the United States. It was then only a matter of time before an attempt at endoscopic hysterectomy would be tried.

Principle of CISH

By 1991 a woman for whom there was an indication for hysterectomy had three choices of procedure: (1) subtotal/total abdominal hysterectomy; (2) vaginal hysterectomy; (3) laparoscopic-assisted vaginal hysterectomy (LAVH). If indicated, vaginal hysterectomy was preferable to total abdominal hysterectomy, as the operative time, postoperative recovery, and length of hospitalization were shortened. Moreover, cosmetically there are minimal scars. When there were special contraindications to vaginal hysterectomy (i.e., suspected or known pelvic abnormalities), LAVH was a welcomed alternative, as many total abdominal hysterectomies could be transformed into vaginal hysterectomy with its described benefits. The uterus and particularly large leiomyomas had to be removed through the vagina or through a small incision in the abdominal wall after morcellation.

To some purists these procedures were not compatible with the concept of minimally invasive and organ-preserving surgery, as proposed by Semm. A way had to be found to allow the abnormal uterus and other pelvic tumors to be removed from the closed abdominal cavity without colpotomy or creation of an abdominal incision. For this purpose, Semm developed special instrumentation: (1) The SEMM (*s*errated *e*dge *m*acro*m*orcellator) set (Fig. 9.3), consisting of a large claw forceps and a metal cylinder with a serrated edge of 10, 15, or 20 mm diameter. (2) The CURT (*c*alibrated *u*terine *r*esection *t*ool) set, consisting of an 80 cm long guide rod, a stabilizer, and a 15, 20, or 24 mm morcellator (Fig. 9.4). The guide rod is introduced through the cervix and corpus uteri, perforating the fundus and creating a straight uterine cylinder. The morcellator then cores out the cervical/endocervical region and a significant amount of corporeal tissue. A fibromuscular shell of cervix remains, leaving the pelvic topography intact with its ligaments, vessels, and nerves.

In view of the fact that cervical carcinoma over the past 40 years has decreased from the

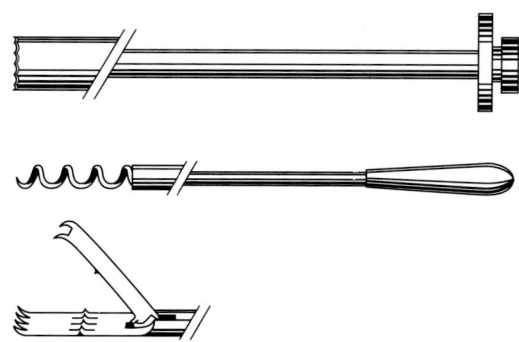

Figure 9.3. Serrated Edge Macro Morcellator (SEMM Set).

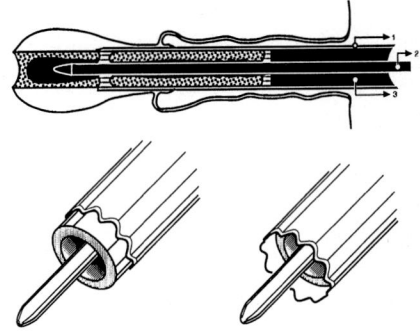

Figure 9.4. Calibrated Uterine Resection Tool (CURT).

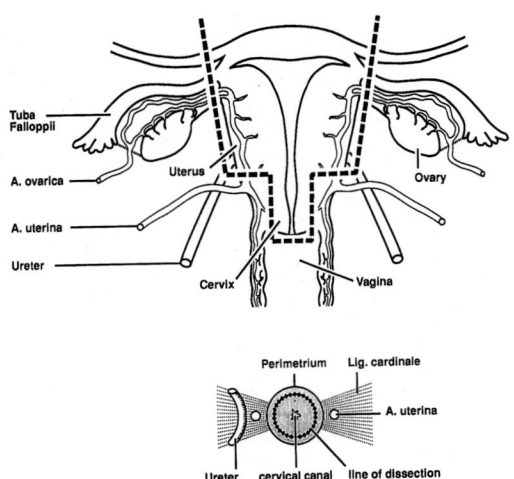

Figure 9.6. CISH technique.

most frequent to the third most frequent pelvic malignancy (after carcinomas of the endometrium and ovary),[26] perhaps it is less than justified to remove the cervix for cancer prophylaxis, especially when the functional cervical/endocervical tissue has been removed. The incidence of cervical stump cancer can thus be reduced to 0.02%.[27] What Aldridge and Meredith[11] and Reis[12] tried to achieve may now be accomplished safely and accurately (Figs. 9.5, 9.6). CISH is the synthesis of three well established modalities: (1) supracervical amputation of the corpus uteri; (2) conization of the cervix; and (3) operative laparoscopy.

The first CISH was successfully performed by Semm in Kiel, Germany on September 7, 1991.[28] The first CISH in the United States was performed on December 26, 1991.[29]

Patient Selection and Preparation

Since the introduction of CISH, selection of the type of hysterectomy has been simplified. CISH has completely replaced total abdominal hysterectomy for benign pelvic disease in my practice. Even in cases of mild to moderate uterine descensus, we prefer CISH, as the topography after amputation of the corpus lends itself to pelvic floor suspension and repair with additional vaginal repair if needed. Cervical and endometrial pathology (i.e., cervical dysplasia or atypical endometrial hyperplasia) are contraindications. Abnormal tissue should not be morcellated; therefore vaginal hysterectomy or LAVH may be performed in these cases. Previous cervical intraepithelial neoplasia is not considered a contraindication provided cone margins have been free of disease and subsequent Papanicolaou smears are consistently normal.

After obtaining a thorough history and undergoing physical examination, the patients are informed about the various types of hys-

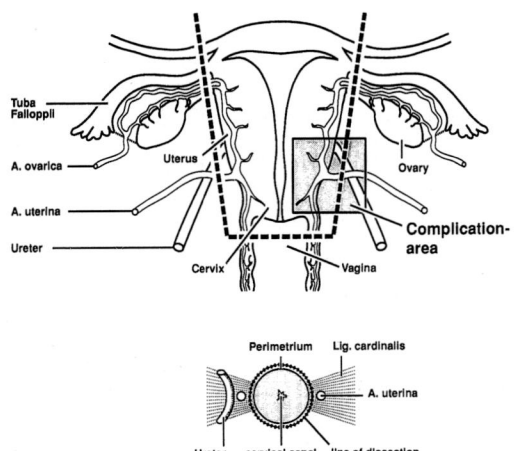

Figure 9.5. Hysterectomy: traditional technique.

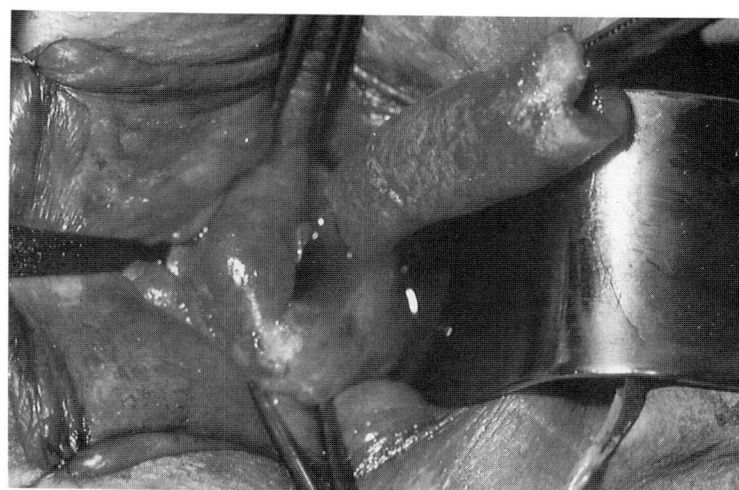

Figure 9.7. Removal of cervical core at time of vaginal CISH.

terectomy and their indications, advantages and disadvantages, and risks/benefits. The patient is involved in the decision-making process.

A consent is obtained for possible laparotomy in every case. The switch from operative laparoscopy to laparotomy is not considered failure of the procedure. CISH can be performed by laparotomy as well as vaginally (Fig. 9.7). Physical preparation is simple: Cervical cytology and the endometrial sampling must be normal, the latter with abnormal bleeding. (Endometrial biopsy and pelvic sonography are performed when appropriate.) A CBC, urinalysis, and, as indicated, chemistry profile, electrocardiography, and chest radiography satisfy preadmission testing. Additional laboratory work and consultation(s) are obtained if indicated. In the case of large leiomyomas encroaching on the pelvic brim, the patients are treated preoperatively with gonadotropin-releasing hormone (GnRH) agonists, usually leuprolide acetate (Lupron) 3.75 mg IM for three months.

The day before surgery the patient is requested to take a bottle of citrate of magnesia, and she must remain NPO after midnight. She is admitted during the morning for surgery. If bowel complications are anticipated, a bowel preparation is prescribed.

Apparatus and Instrumentation

Safety, efficiency, competence, simplicity, and cost-effectiveness are the keys to endoscopic surgery. To achieve these goals, the following approach is recommended.

Apparatus

A cart (model Kiel; Wisap, Sauerlack, Germany) is required with the following equipment (Fig. 9.8).

1. CO_2 electronic high flow insufflator with insufflation pressure read-out
2. Endocoagulator for hemostasis (monopolar or bipolar current, lasers, harmonic scalpel, clips, or staples may be used at the discretion of the surgeon but does not contribute to enhanced patient safety or cost containment)
3. Light source with camera and audiovisual system, printer
4. Irrigation and suction system
5. Warm solutions for irrigation

Instruments

About 100 instruments must be at the disposal of the gynecologic surgeon for a laparotomy. Similarly, the same complement of instruments must be available for endoscopic surgery. Reusable, stainless steel instruments are prefera-

9. Pelviscopic Intrafascial Hysterectomy Without Colpotomy

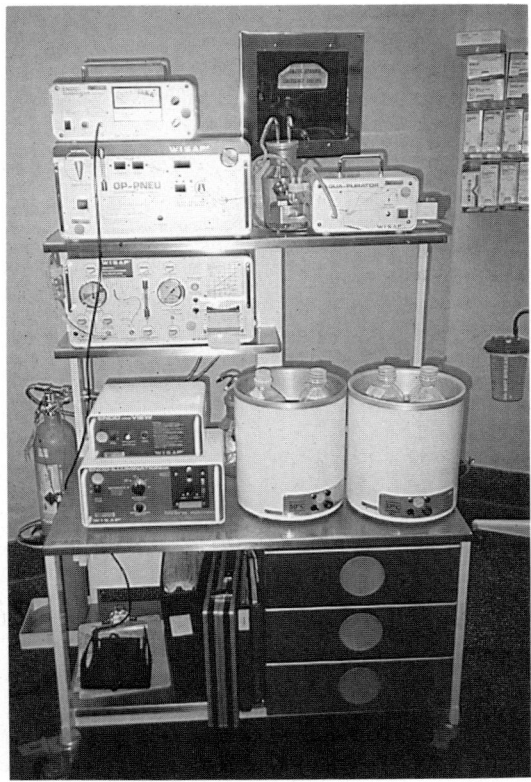

Figure 9.8. Equipment cart for the CISH procedure.

ble, especially in an effort to contain cost. All trocars have a conical tip with beveled sleeves. The instrumentation for CISH includes the following.

Conical trocars, 5 mm (4)
Conical trocars, 10 mm (3)
Conical trocar, 15 mm (1)
Conical trocar, 20 mm (1)
Biopsy forceps, 5 mm (3)
Hook scissors, 5 mm (1)
Peritoneal scissors, 5 mm (1)
Dilatation set, from 5 to 10 mm with reducer (1)
Dilatation set, from 5 to 15 mm with reducer (1)
Dilatation set, from 5 to 20 mm with reducer (1)
Sponge holder, 10 mm (1)
Needle holder, 3 mm (1)
Needle holders, 5 mm (2)
Pitressin application set (1)
SEMM sets: 10, 15, 20 mm diameter
CURT sets: 15, 20, 24 mm diameter

Vaginal speculum
Hegar dilators
Single-tooth tenacula (2)
Ring forceps (1)
Syringes: 10 and 35 cc
Injection needle, 22 gauge
Sponges
Surgicel (Johnson and Johnson Medical Inc., Arlington, TX)
Band-Aids
Skin clips
Pitressin solution (5 units in 100 ml Nacl)
Roeder loops: 0 PDS and 0 catgut, plain and chromic
Ligatures and sutures for extracorporeal knot-tying: 0 Vicryl

Operating Room Setup

The operating room setup is relatively simple and efficient. The patient is placed in modified lithotomy position with her thighs as flat as possible. With CISH there is no need to change the patient's position intraoperatively. The left arm is tucked in, and the right arm is positioned on an arm board. A metal bridge crosses the patient's chest for the surgeon and the assistant to lean on. The surgeon stands to the left of the patient with the apparatus cart on the side. The assistant surgeon stands opposite, cephalad to the arm board. The scrub nurse stands next to the assistant surgeon with a small instrument table in front and the ancillary equipment beside him or her. A small instrument tray is placed between the patient's thighs, as is the television monitor. A small tray with instruments for the vaginal part of the CISH, is ready, placed away from the table. A circulating nurse is available at all times. A well trained, well rehearsed team is indispensable for a safe, smooth, efficient CISH.

CISH Technique

Cervical Preparation

Preoperative preparation includes cytologic studies, possibly colposcopy, and establishment of a normal flora. Vaginal ultrasonography and digital examination are performed to determine the diameter of the calibrated uterine resection tool needed (15, 20, or 24 mm diameter). Intraoperative preparation includes dilatation with a No. 5 Hegar dilator, followed by sounding the uterus and inserting the uterine manipulator of choice.

Operative Laparoscopic Steps

The success of a CISH procedure depends on creation of an adequate pneumoperitoneum (at least 12 mm Hg). Injury to the abdominal wall, large vessels, bowel, or ureters is a constant concern, particularly in patients with a previous laparotomy.[3]

After general anesthesia with endotracheal intubation, the patient is placed in a modified lithotomy position. She is prepared vaginally and abdominally, and sterile drapes are placed. We then proceed as follows.

1. *Palpation of the aorta:* The aorta and its bifurcation are palpated through the umbilicus, if possible. The location and distance from the abdominal wall are appreciated.

2. *Needle flow test:* Patency, functionality of the snap mechanism, and the flow resistance of the inflow tube and needle system are determined, with the CO_2 gas flow set at 1 L/min. The gas flow resistance should not exceed 6–8 mm Hg. This pressure must be the same after the needle has perforated the parietal peritoneum.

3. *Snap test:* While inserting the Veress needle vertically into the umbilicus, one can observe the snap mechanism three times: at the skin, the fascia, and the parietal peritoneum. If the needle is introduced at 45°, the snap mechanism cannot function optimally and the needle tip works like a scalpel.

4. *Hiss test:* If the needle is placed correctly and the abdominal wall is elevated, air is brought through the needle, causing a hissing sound. The insufflator then indicates negative abdominal pressure.

5. *Aspiration test:* Saline solution 5 ml is injected through the needle and aspirated. If fluid is not aspirated, the surgeon may be sure that the needle lies properly (otherwise blood or bowel content is immediately visible). With the

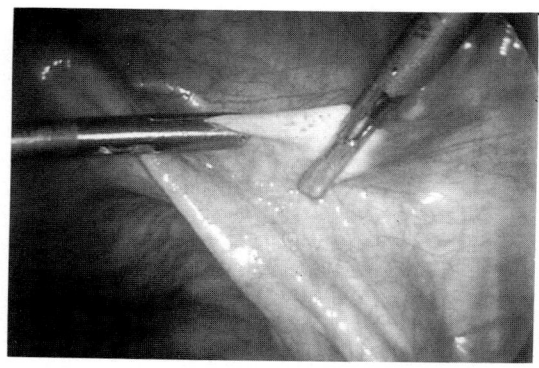

Figure 9.9. Endocoagulation of round ligament prior to division.

needle safely in place, CO_2 gas is insufflated until an intraabdominal pressure of 12 mm Hg is reached and the insufflator shuts off.

6. *Sounding test:* Once the pneumoperitoneum has been established, a sounding needle (150 mm long and 0.8 mm thick) can be inserted 2–3 cm below the umbilicus and slowly advanced. When aspirating gas through a small column of saline in a syringe, gas bubbles through the fluid if the needle tip is free, otherwise bubbling stops, indicating the interference of underlying structures, such as bowel or adhesions. The needle is advanced in different directions, looking for a free space above the contents of the abdomen into which a trocar is to be inserted.

7. *Trocar insertion:* Having established an adequate pneumoperitoneum, a small vertical intraumbilical incision is made through the skin. A 5 mm conical trocar is inserted in a Z fashion through the rectus muscle avoiding the linea alba. Care is taken to not damage the fascia, thereby avoiding possible hernia formation at the end of the procedure. The incision closes in different layers to prevent omental or intestinal prolapse.

A complete 360° abdominopelvic inspection is carried out. The diagnosis and indication for surgery are confirmed. Dilation is accomplished with trocars of 5 mm to 11 mm and a 10 mm laparoscope inserted. Three 5 mm ancillary trocars are inserted subrapubically in Z fashion

9. Pelviscopic Intrafascial Hysterectomy Without Colpotomy

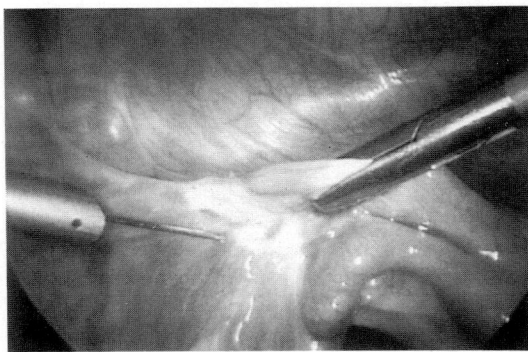

Figure 9.10. Injection of dilute pitressin for hemostasis and aquadissection prior to division.

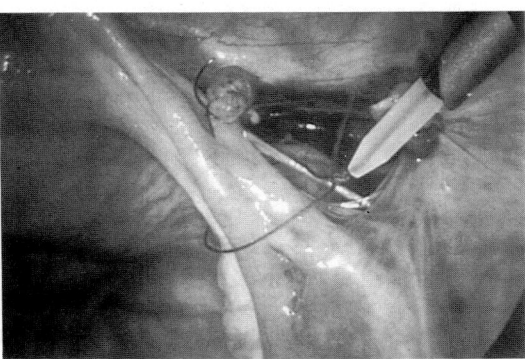

Figure 9.12. Creation of "window" in broad ligament and ligation of utero-ovarian ligament with ramus tubarius of uterine artery.

under direct visualization: two lateral to the deep epigastric vessels and one off-center through the left or right rectus muscles.

The patient is placed in a 15° Trendelenburg position. The bowel is displaced cephalad out of the pelvic cavity. The CISH can now be safely started. The uterus and adnexa are isolated from adhesions by adhesiolysis, as indicated.

If the adnexae are to be removed with the uterus, we proceed as follows: The round ligament is grasped with a biopsy forceps close to the fundus and endocoagulated with a crocodile clamp at 110°C for 20 seconds (Fig. 9.9). Vasopressin with chlorobutanol (Pitressin; Parke-Davis, Morris Plains, NJ) 5 units in 100 ml of saline solution, is injected into the ligament and under the anterior and posterior leaf of the broad ligament (hemostasis and aquadissection). The ligament is divided with hook scissors (Figs. 9.10– 9.12). Roeder loops are placed over the pedicles for security. The posterior leaf of the broad ligament is identified and widely incised with blunt dissection. Large uterine vessels and the ureter are clearly visible at the caudal and lateral border of the peritoneal window. An endoligature is passed through the window in the broad ligament with 3- and 5-mm needle holders. An extracorporeal sliding knot is tied, and the ligature is placed over the infundibulopelvic ligament. A second ligature is placed over the proximal portion of the adnexa. The infundibulopelvic ligament is divided with laparoscopic scissors and the pedicle secured with two additional Roeder loops (Figs. 9.13–9.16).

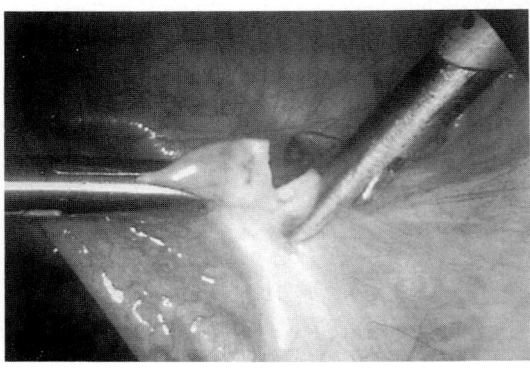

Figure 9.11. Bloodless division of round ligament.

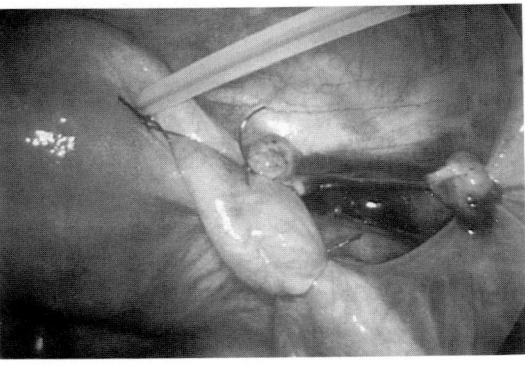

Figure 9.13. Placement of proximal ligature around utero-ovarian ligament.

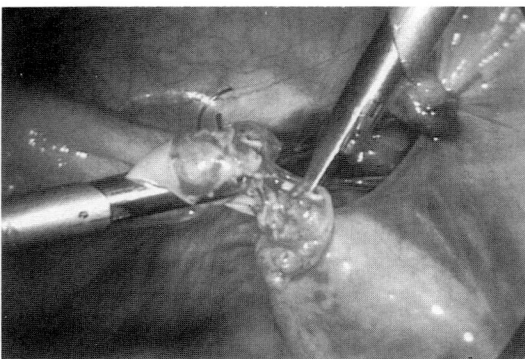

Figure 9.14. Bloodless division of utero-ovarian ligament.

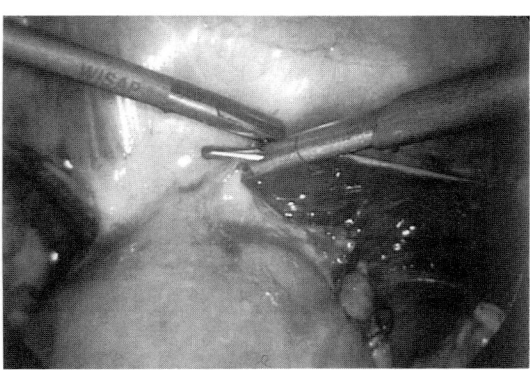

Figure 9.17. Sharp dissection of bladder flap to expose isthmic portion of cervix.

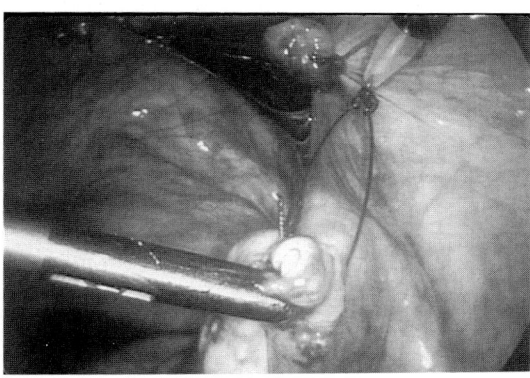

Figure 9.15. Securing utero-ovarian pedicles with additional PDS and catgut Roeder loops.

If the adnexae are to be left in situ, ligatures are placed around the uteroovarian ligament and a cut is made between them. The pedicles are secured with additional Roeder loops. The uterus is now freed to the level of the large vessels. The bladder peritoneum and posterior broad ligament are injected with a dilute solution of vasopressin with chlorobutanol (5 U/100 ml saline solution) (Fig. 9.17). Blunt and sharp dissection exposes the bladder, uterine vessels, and ureters (Fig. 9.18). With the isthmus portion of the cervix exposed, a Roeder loop or endoligature is placed over the cervicocorporeal junction, at the level of the uterosacral ligaments (Fig. 9.19).

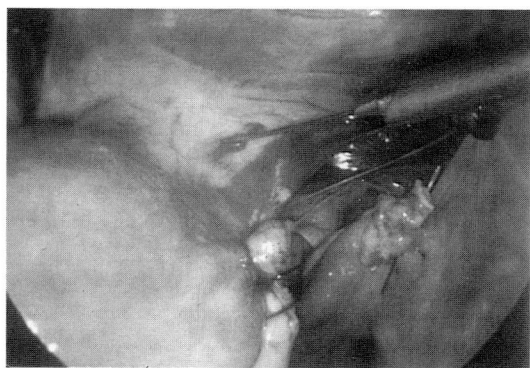

Figure 9.16. Injection of dilute pitressin solution under bladder serosa for hemostasis and aquadissection.

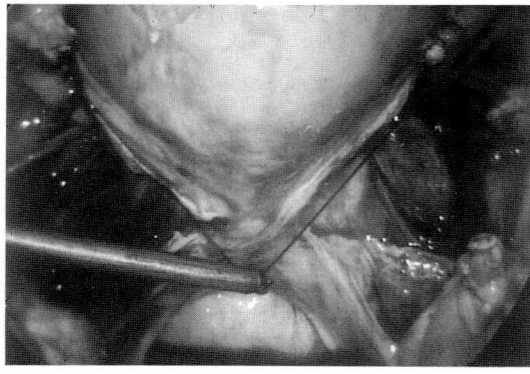

Figure 9.18. Placement of PDS Roeder loop around isthmic portion of cervix in level of uterosacral ligaments.

9. Pelviscopic Intrafascial Hysterectomy Without Colpotomy

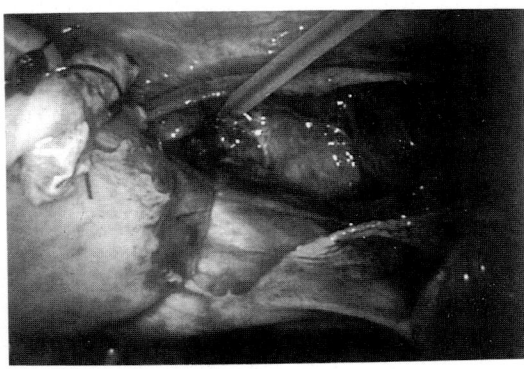

Figure 9.19. Occlusion of ascending branch of uterine artery with Roeder loop. Ureter is safely out of the operating field.

Vaginal Steps

The manipulator is removed, and single-tooth tenacula are placed at the 9 and 3 o'clock positions. The cervix is infiltrated with dilute vasopressin with chlorobutanol solution (5 U/ 100 ml saline solution) (Figs. 9.20). A Schiller test is performed to demonstrate the squamocolumnar junction (Fig. 9.21). If the morcellator does not include the squamocolumnar junction, cold knife conization or loop electrosurgical excision should be performed. The guide rod of the calibrated uterine resection tool is inserted through the cervical canal, and the fundus is perforated under laparoscopic guidance to create a straight

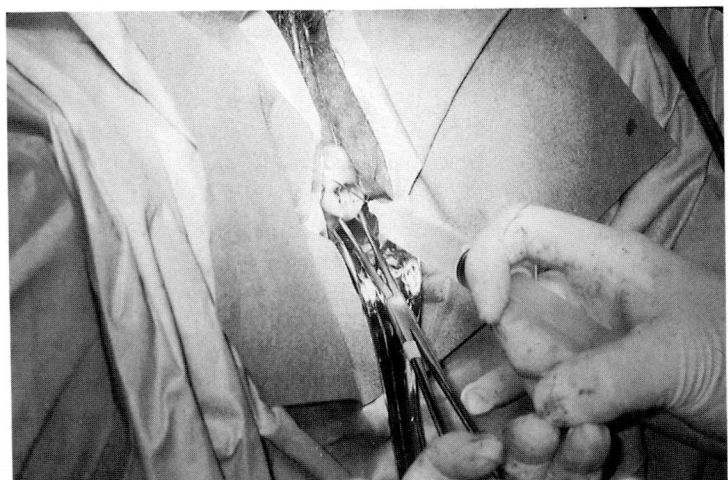

Figure 9.20. Infiltration of cervix with dilute pitressin for hemostasis.

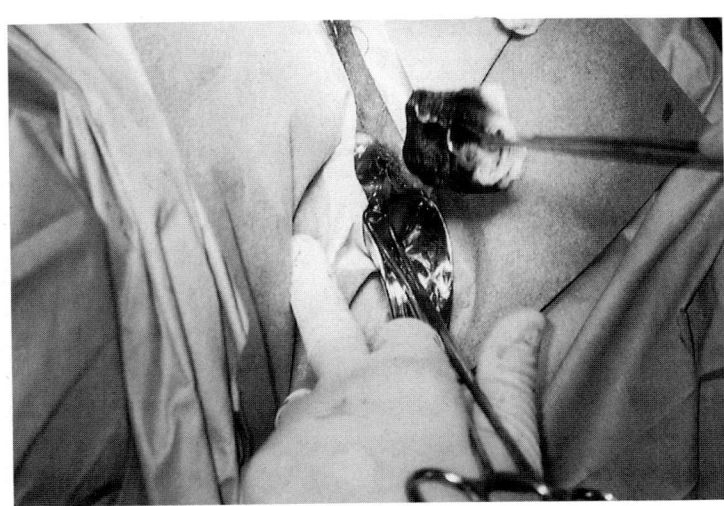

Figure 9.21. Schiller test to demonstrate the squamocolumnar junction.

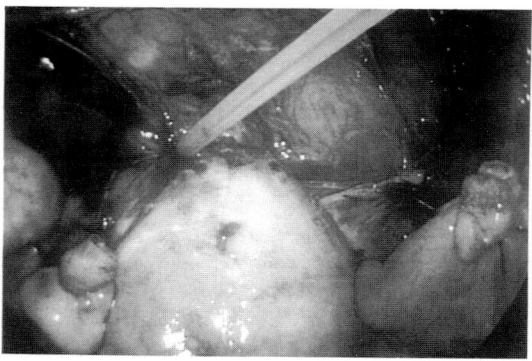

Figure 9.22. Closure of cervical canal and occlusion of ascending branches of uterine artery.

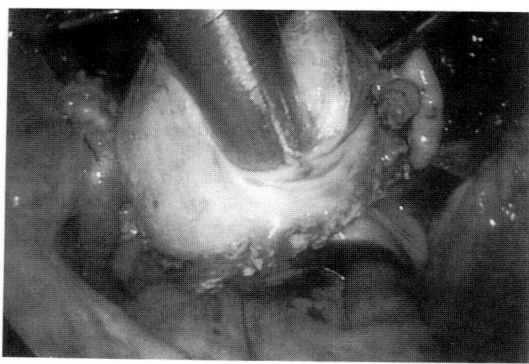

Figure 9.24. Morcellation of amputated uterus out of closed abdominal cavity.

cervicocorporeal axis. The morcellator of the calibrated uterine resection tool is placed over the stabilizer and is used to core out a tissue cylinder from the squamocolumnar junction of the exocervix to the fundus (Plates 11, 12). As the tissue cylinder is removed, the preplaced Roeder loop or endoligature is quickly and securely tied (Fig. 9.22). This maneuver prevents loss of the pneumoperitoneum and possible CO_2 embolization. Both ascending branches of the uterine artery are safely occluded.

Abdominal Steps

After two additional Roeder loops are placed around the cervical isthmus, the corpus is amputated with hook scissors, and a fourth catgut loop is tied for enhanced hemostasis (monofilament sutures tend to slip) (Fig. 9.23). The middle suprapubic 5 mm trocar is dilated to 15 or 20 mm. The amputated uterus with or without adnexae are morcellated and removed using the serrated-edge macromorcellator (Fig. 9.24). The remaining cervical stump and pedicles are treated with the point coagulator at 120°C to minimize postoperative adhesions, sterilize the cervical remnant, and ensure that all remaining endometrium is destroyed. The cervical stump is ideally suited for suspension by the round ligaments. An incidental enterocele can also be repaired at this time. The remaining raw surface is peritonealized by bringing the anterior bladder flap to the posterior aspect of the cervical stump

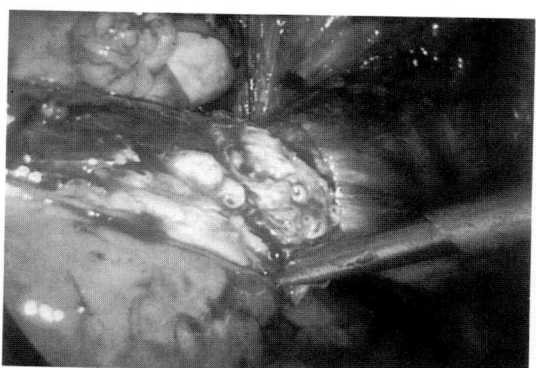

Figure 9.23. Amputation of uterine fundus with hook scissors.

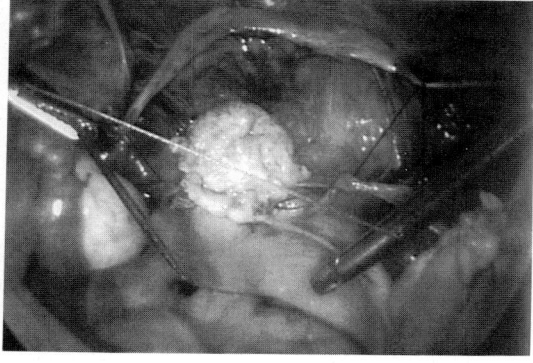

Figure 9.25. Peritonealization of pelvic floor with one O-vicryl suture.

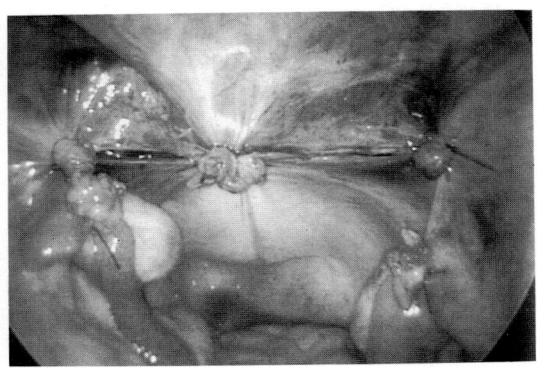

Figure 9.26. Final view after CISH.

Figure 9.2. Characteristics of patients

	CISH		
Characteristic	Without BSO[a]	With BSO[b]	Combined[c]
No. of patients	98	81	179
Age (years)	38 (24–53)	46 (29–59)	41
Weight (lb)	151.1 (106–246)	152.0 (91–259)	151.5
Parity			
Nullipara	4	9	
Para 1	16	12	
Para 2	57	32	
Para > 2	14	17	

BSO, bilateral salpingo-oophorectomy.
[a]Average parity = 1.9.
[b]Average parity = 2.0.
[c]Average parity = 1.94.

in the midline with an endosuture (Fig. 9.25). The pelvis is thoroughly irrigated with Ringer's solution. After complete hemostasis is confirmed, all trocars are removed under direct visualization (Fig. 9.26).

Results

From December 1991 to December 1994, a total of 179 operative laparoscopic intrafascial hysterectomies were performed. Table 9.2 conveys information regarding the patient population. Table 9.3 provides the main indications and histopathologic diagnoses, and the outcomes of the operations are shown in Table 9.4. Average hospitalization was 50.6 hours. Operating time ranged from 2 hours 20 minutes to 5 hours 10 minutes. Blood loss was consistently lower than at conventional abdominal or vaginal hysterectomy. All patients had hemoglobin determinations before and after surgery, with levels ranging from 0.4 to 3.6 g% (average 2 g%). No patient required a blood transfusion. In most cases blood loss averaged about 100 ml, but there were losses as high as 300–350 ml. Initially our operating time ranged from 2 hours 20 minutes to 5 hours 10 minutes. More recently the total operating time was 2–3 hours, and by improving the setup we have been able to reduce the operating time even further to 1.5–2.0 hours.

Potential complications include the following: (1) Intraoperatively: excessive bleeding that requires transfusion, injury to neighboring organs, laparoscopy-related complications, and anesthesia-related complications. (2) Immediately postoperatively: febrile morbidity, urinary tract infections, ileus, pulmonary complications, and hemorrhage. (3) Late postoperatively: wound infection, late bleeding, and readmission because of complications related to the procedure.

Table 9.3. Postoperative pathologic diagnosis

	CISH (no. of patients)		
Pathologic diagnosis	Without BSO	With BSO	Combined
Uterine leiomyomas	43	58	101
Adenomyosis	32	33	65
Endometriosis	32	31	63
Intractable uterine bleeding	24	3	27
Benign ovarian cysts	8	7	15
Endometrial hyperplasia	5	1	6
Endometrial polyp	1	1	2
CIN I	2	0	2
Uterine prolapse	2	2	4

Note: Some patients have more than one diagnosis.
BSO, bilateral salpingo-oophorectomy; CIN I, cervical intraepithelial neoplasia, grade I.

Figure 9.4. Outcomes of operations

Parameter	CISH	
	Without BSO (mean)	With BSO
Operating room time[a] hours: minutes	1:40–5:10 (3:5)	2:00–6:07 (3:20)
Hemoglobin changes[b]	0.1%–4.4%	0.6%–3.8%
Hospitalization duration		
24 Hours	5	2
48 Hours	83	56
72 Hours	6	11
Average (days)	2.01	2.13

The values in parentheses represent averages.
BSO, bilateral salpingo-oophorectomy.
[a]Operating room time was from the time the patient moved into the operating room to the time the patients left the room.
[b]Change from preoperative to postoperative values.

There were no major complications in our series. Six patients had transient lower urinary tract infections that were quickly resolved with antibiotics. Occasionally, we saw a patient whose maximum temperature was 101°F while still hospitalized.

Conclusion

In this author's opinion, CISH has completely replaced total abdominal hysterectomy and, in many instances, vaginal hysterectomy for benign pelvic disease. LAVH has limited indications. CISH may be an option instead of total abdominal hysterectomy when there is a contraindication to vaginal hysterectomy and LAVH, such as uterine size or absence of descensus, suspected or known pelvic pathology, or a surgeon's inexperience. CISH safely meets the objectives of minimal invasion and organ preservation. Patient acceptance is excellent, as there are only four small abdominal surgical sites without visible scarring. The pelvic floor is completely intact with no disruption of the cervicovaginal complex (Fig. 9.2). Pain is apparently markedly reduced, and recovery is rapid, as only the four small pedicles, serosa, and cervical facial sheath must heal. Blood loss has been minimal. With CISH, there is only an intrauterine wound. The large denervation zone of total hysterectomy or LAVH does not exist.

Since the introduction of CISH three questions have been repeatedly asked: (1) Does CISH prevent cancer of the cervical stump? (2) Are there enough data to support the statement that there is less chance of pelvic relaxation and prolapse? (3) Does the patient have less psychosexual dysfunction?

First, the incidence of cancer of the cervical stump was about 0.3–1.9%.[16–21] Semm's group[27] studied 254 cases and indicated that the epithelium of the transformation zone was removed in 100% of these women. In only six of the women did a possible risk of cervical glands remain, which indicates a potential incidence of cancer of 0.02%, or one in 5 million. In our opinion, patients should continue to have sporadic Papanicolaou smears as appropriate. Second, there is ample literature[23, 24] to support the fact that severing the cardinal and uterosacral ligaments, paracervical nerves, and uterine vessels weakens the pelvic floor support, leading to cystorectoenterocele formation and vaginal wall prolapse. CISH eliminates these risks, as none of these structures is severed. On the other hand, the "male effect" is often ignored. Third, the importance of the uterus as a psychosexual organ varies from woman to woman.[30] Some look at it as "a child-bearing organ, an excretory organ, a regulator and controller of body process, a sexual organ, a source of female competence, a reservoir of strength and vitality and a maintainer of youth and attractiveness."[30] Hysterectomy is viewed by some women as a "threat to her health, vitality, and ability to function and she may experience psychologic problems, such as depression, anxiety and sexual dysfunction."[30]

Additional studies are required to elaborate on these points. With our present knowledge, the gynecologic surgeon should strive to treat and cure pelvic disease with minimum invasion and trauma and maximum organ preservation.

References

1. GRAVES EJ: National Center for Health Statistics. National Hospital Discharge Survey: Annual Summary, 1990. Vital and Health Statistics. Series 13, No. 112. DHHS publ (PHS)92-1773. Washington, DC, Government Printing Office, 1992.
2. POKRAS R: Hysterectomy: past, present and future. Stat Bull Metrop Insur Co 1989;70:12.
3. SEMM K: Atlas of Gynecologic Laparoscopy and Hysterectomy. Philadelphia, Saunders, 1977.
4. SEMM K: Operative Manual for Endoscopic Abdominal Surgery. Chicago, Year Book, 1987.
5. BENRUBI GI: History of hysterectomy. J Fla Med Assoc 1988;75:553.
6. THOREK M: Modern Surgical Technique. Philadelphia, Lippincott, 1949.
7. MATTHIEU A: History of hysterectomy. West J Surg Obstet Gynecol 1934;42:1.
8. RICCI JV: One Hundred Years of Gynecology. Philadelphia, Blakiston, 1945.
9. SPEERT H: Obstetrics and Gynecology in America: A History. Baltimore, Waverly Press, 1980.
10. RAURAMO M: On excision of the cervical canal in conjunction with uterus amputation. Acta Obstet Gynecol Scand 1949;28:381.
11. ALDRIDGE AH, MEREDITH RS: Complete abdominal hysterectomy. Am J Obstet Gynecol 1950; 59:748.
12. RIES J: Individuelle Indikation zur Art der Myomoperation. Arch Gynakol 1961;195:225.
13. PALMER RA-M, DOURLEN ROLLIE A, AUDEBERT R, GERAUD: La sterilisation voluntaire en France et dans le monde. Masson, Paris, 1981.
14. FRANGENHEIM H: Die Laparoskopie bei der Diagnostik und Therapie maligner und benigner Tumoren im Genitalbereich. In Fortschritte der Endoskopie, Rosch W (ed). Erlangen, Straube, 1976, pp 203–208.
15. REICH HJ, DECAPRIO J, MCGLYNN F: Laparoscopic hysterectomy. J Gynecol Surg 1989;5:213.
16. MILLER BE, COPELAND LJ, HAMBERGER AD, ET AL: Carcinoma of the cervical stump. Gynecol Oncol 1984;18:100.
17. KHINT EK, BOKHMAN YV, VEL'RE RJ, ET AL: Prophylaxis and treatment of cervical stump cancer. Vopr Onkol 1975;21:83.
18. WOLFF JP, LACOUR J, CHASSAGNE D, ET AL: Cancer of the cervical stump: a study of 173 patients. Obstet Gynecol 1972;39:10.
19. MAGGI R, BORTOLOZZI G, MAGIONI C, ET AL: Residual cervical stump cancer (true cancer) and residual cancer of the cervical stump (coincident cancer): statistics and therapeutic results in the period 1955–1979. Eur J Gynaecol Oncol 1985; 2:92.
20. PRATT JH, JEFFERIES JA: The retained cervical stump. Obstet Gynecol 1976;48:711.
21. RIVA HL, HEFNER JD, MARCHETT AA, ET AL: Prophylactic trachelectomy of cervical stump: two hundred and twelve cases. South Med J 1961; 54:1082.
22. BAKER HW: Selective indications for subtotal abdominal hysterectomy. J Ky Med Assoc 1985; 7:355.
23. JASZCZAK SE, EVANS TN: Intrafascial abdominal and vaginal hysterectomy: a reappraisal. Obstet Gynecol 1982;59:435.
24. MENGERT WF: Mechanics of uterine support and position. Am J Obstet Gynecol 1936;31:775.
25. KILKKU P, GRONROSS PM, HIRVONEN T, RAURAMO L: Supravaginal uterine amputation vs hysterectomy: effects on libido and orgasm. Acta Obstet Gynecol Scand 1983;62:147.
26. HERBST AL: Cervical intraepithelial neoplasia. Yearbook of OB/GYN, 1994. St. Louis, Mosby-Yearbook, 1994.
27. ALVAREZ-RODAS E, METTLER L, CASTRO E, ET AL: Histologic features of the CISH procedure. J Am Assoc Gynecol Laparosc 1994;2(1):37.
28. SEMM K: Hysterektomie per laparotomiam oder per pelviskopiam. Geburstsh Frauenheilkd 1991; 51:996.
29. VIETZ PF, AHN TS: A new approach to hysterectomy without colpotomy: pelviscopic intrafascial hysterectomy. Am J Obstet Gynecol 1994;170: 609.
30. BACHMANN GA: Hysterectomy, a critical review. J Reprod Med 1990;35:839.

10
Vaginal Prolapse and Bladder Suspension: Role of Endoscopic Surgery

C. Y. Liu

The goal of laparoscopic treatment for vaginal prolapse and bladder suspension is to restore normal anatomy by repairing pelvic floor defects. When a defect in the pelvic support system is of such magnitude that it requires the patient to undergo reparative surgery for symptomatic enterocele, rectocele, cystocele, urinary or fecal incontinence, or uterovaginal or rectal prolapse, the defect in the pelvic floor usually involves other components as well. Therefore surgery for vaginal prolapse, urinary incontinence, or any other pelvic floor defect must not be thought of as an isolated procedure. Restorative surgery for urinary continence, for example, changes the direction of force vectors to the remaining pelvic floor so a slight deficiency in another compartment existing at the time of the urinary incontinence surgery may become a marked deficiency postoperatively, necessitating further surgery. Up to 28% of patients undergoing a Burch colposuspension develop middle or posterior compartment deficiency (or both) and subsequently manifest enterocele, rectocele, and vaginal vault prolapse, which require additional surgery.[1] Therefore the entire pelvic floor supporting system must be thoroughly investigated before surgery, reconfirmed during surgery, and all the defects reconstructed concurrently.

There are three important anatomic structures with which every pelvic surgeon must be familiar.

1. *Endopelvic fascia*. The endopelvic fascia is one continuous body of connective tissue that contains a considerable quantity of smooth muscle. The uppermost portion of the endopelvic fascia is composed of cardinouterosacral ligaments that are incorporated into pubocervical fascia and bladder pillars caudally. They suspend the upper part of the vagina and cervix to the pelvic side walls through their attachment to the pericervical ring. The midportion of the vagina comes in closer contact with the pelvic walls than the upper portion, which is suspended by the cardinouterosacral ligaments. This portion of the vagina attaches to the arcus tendineus fascia of the pelvis (white line) on both sides through the pubocervical fascia in the front and through the rectovaginal septum in the back. The rectovaginal septum contains an abundance of fibromuscular tissue, which lies ventral to the rectovaginal space. Superiorly, it blends with the cardinouterosacral ligaments, and inferiorly it fuses with the perineal body and levator ani muscles. Laterally it attaches to the superior fascia of the pelvic diaphragm.

2. *Levator ani muscle*. The levator ani muscle consists of both pubococcygeus and ilio-

coccygeus muscles. It is often referred to as the levator plate or pelvic diaphragm. The pubococcygeus muscle begins at the inner portion of the pubic bone, passes downward into the anus between the internal and external sphincters, circles around the dorsal parts of the anorectal junction, and finally returns to the other side of the pubic bone. The iliococcygeal muscle emerges from the arcus tendineus fascia of the levator ani of the fascia of the obturator internus muscle. The two sheets of the iliococcygeal muscles from either side are joined in a midline raphe just above the anococcygeal raphe. The levator ani muscle forms the shelf on which rests the pelvic viscera.

3. *Urogenital diaphragm.* The urogenital diaphragm is frequently referred to as the perineal membrane. It spans the anterior portion of the pelvic outlet and connects the perineal body to the ischiopubic rami. The bulbocavernosus, ischiocavernosus, and superficial transverse perineal muscles and the anal sphincter muscles form the floor that seals off the lower aspect of the pelvic cavity.[2]

Preoperative Evaluation of the Pelvic Floor Support

There are many and varied clinical classification systems used by pelvic surgeons to describe the severity of the pelvic floor defect. Each system describes criteria for grading the degree of the supporting defects, comparing preoperative with postoperative, patient with patient, and series with series support status to determine the therapeutic results. There is still no consensus among gynecologists, however, as to which system best serves the purpose.

In our practice, we divide the pelvic floor defects into three compartment categories; each compartment connects and supports one another. The urethrocele and cystocele belong to the anterior compartment defect; and the enterocele and rectocele belong to the posterior compartment defect. Preoperatively, we map out and describe each compartment defect in detail, using the posterior half of a bivalve vaginal speculum for retracting the anterior and posterior vaginal wall and using the hymenal ring as the zero point. The patient reclines 45°–60° on the examination table with both legs bent and resting on the footings of the table. The table then is raised to avoid straining the examiner's neck and back (an electrically powered table is helpful). The degree of prolapse with the patient at rest and at maximum strain is observed and described (e.g., the cervix is 2 cm above the hymenal ring at rest and 1 cm below the hymenal ring with maximum strain). Next, the posterior half of a vaginal speculum is inserted deep into the vagina, retracting the posterior wall of the vagina, in order to evaluate the anterior compartment defect. The location of the urethrovaginal crease and the pattern of the vaginal rugal fold are especially important. The distinction must be made between the central fascial defect (distention cystourethrocele) and the lateral fascial defect (displacement cystourethrocele), so proper treatment can be planned. The half-speculum is then turned 180° to retract the anterior vaginal wall upward, and the posterior compartment defect is evaluated. The defects in this compartment are sometimes difficult to assess, especially between the enterocele and the high rectocele, which coexist in most cases. When the posterior vaginal wall is observed to be descending below the hymenal ring, a significant posterior compartment defect exists. It may be caused by a rectocele, an enterocele, or both. Two hands rectovaginal examination with the index finger of the dominant hand inside the rectum and the index and third fingers of the other hand inside the vagina, palpating the entire posterior vaginal wall is the best way to identify the posterior compartment defects. Enteroceles usually appear as a distinct bulging sac above the rectocele and are especially notable when patient is performing the Valsalva maneuver during the rectovaginal examination. Examination of the perineal body is important to rule out pseudorectocele, which is caused by a deficiency in the perineal body, allowing the normal rectum to bulge into the vagina.[3,4]

The severity of the middle compartment defect is determined by the location of the cervix or the apex of the vagina in patients who have had a previous hysterectomy. When the uterus is in place, the position of the cervix serves as a marker for poor support of the upper vagina. However, descent of the vaginal apex is often missed in cases of posthysterectomy vaginal prolapse when a large cystocele or rectocele is present. In these cases, if the vaginal vault is not suspended or if only the anterior and posterior compartment defects are repaired, the operation fails and the prolapse recurs.

Because defects in pelvic support frequently occur in more than one compartment, careful assessment of these defects preoperatively followed by intraoperative confirmation is critical. With increased pressure of the pneumoperitoneum during laparoscopic surgery, the pelvic floor support defects can be easily confirmed and treated.

Laparoscopic Bladder Neck Suspension

Many patients with urinary incontinence can be managed satisfactorily with nonsurgical treatment. When surgery is necessary, however, choosing the procedure most appropriate for the given patient's condition is crucial. Currently more than 150 surgical procedures have been reported in the medical literature for treatment of urinary stress incontinence in women. It is important to understand that in most patients with genuine stress urinary incontinence the intrinsic sphincteric mechanism is intact but functioning poorly because of displacement of the ureterovesical junction and the proximal part of the urethra as a result of loss of fibromuscular support. For these patients the ultimate goal of surgery is to restore the normal anatomic position of the ureterovesical junction and the proximal part of the urethra for proper functioning of the urethral sphincter. Objectives of antiincontinent surgery include the following.

1. To elevate and maintain the ureterovesical junction within the abdominal zone of pressure, thereby allowing equal transmission of the pressure to the ureterovesical (U-V) junction and the proximal part of the urethra
2. To allow posterior rotational descent of the bladder base
3. To preserve the pliability and compressibility of the urethra
4. To avoid compromising the urethral sphincteric mechanism[5, 6]

For patients with an intact urethral sphincter and hypermobility of the U-V junction, there are currently three surgical operations available.

1. Retropubic urethropexy, such as the Marshall-Marchetti-Krantz procedure, Burch colposuspension procedure, or paravaginal suspension
2. Needle bladder neck suspension procedure, such as the Raz, Stamey, modified Pereyra, or Gattis procedure
3. Suburethral sling procedure

The needle bladder neck suspension provides a simple, rapid way to suspend the U-V junction. Evidence suggests, however, that long-term results with needle suspension procedures are not as good as with retropubic urethropexy. Furthermore, the high incidence of postoperative urinary retention secondary to the suburethral sling procedure makes it a poor choice if the patient is unwilling, or unable, to perform intermittent self-catheterization. Both operations also have an increased incidence of postoperative uterovaginal prolapse and enterocele formation. In recent years there seems to be a consensus, especially among gynecologists, that retropubic colposuspension (Burch procedure) is the surgical treatment of choice for patients with genuine urinary stress incontinence who have an intact urethral sphincter but a displaced U-V junction. For patients who have a poor urethral sphincteric mechanism, a suburethral sling procedure, periurethral injection (e.g., GAX collagen, Teflon paste), or implantation of an artificial urinary sphincter is more appropriate. This chapter addresses only the laparoscopic treatment of urinary stress incontinence with Burch colposuspension.

Evolution of the Procedure

In 1949 Marshall, Marchetti, and Krantz reported their results of vesicourethral suspension on 50 patients (5 men, 45 women) with stress urinary incontinence. They sutured the periurethral fascia to the back of the symphysis pubis and reported an 82% success rate; 7% more improved, and 11% were failures.[7] This retropubic suspension of the bladder neck (called the MMK procedure) has since undergone many modifications. In 1961 Burch (Nashville, Tennessee) reported a modified MMK procedure, using Cooper's ligament instead of the periosteum of the pubic bone so as to avoid the occasional complication of osteitis pubis and to obtain more secure points of urethrovaginal fixation. All 53 patients in his initial series were relieved of their incontinence. In 1968 he reported a subsequent series of 143 patients, with an overall success rate of 93%; a rare recurrence appeared after 20 months of follow-up. Because his most frequent complication was the development of enterocele (7.6%), he emphasized the need for obliteration of the cul-de-sac.[8] In 1976 Tanagho modified the Burch procedure by advocating no dissection within 2 cm of the urethra or vesical neck and removing the fatty tissue lateral to this area to stimulate fibrosis and fixation to the retropubis.[9] He noted that the sutures must be tied without undue tension to avoid necrosis and breakdown at the suture placement site and to avoid compressing or kinking the proximal part of the urethra. It is not necessary to bring the anterior vaginal wall all the way to meet Cooper's ligaments. Instead of using No. 1 chromic catgut, as in original Burch procedure, Tanagho used two delayed absorbable sutures (No. 1 Dexon): one placed at the midurethral level and the other at the U-V junction on both sides of the urethra.[9] In 1979 Cardozo et al. reported that 18% of patients who underwent retropubic urethropexy developed detrusor instability. Potential etiologic factors include sutures through the bladder, vesical neck obstruction, and extensive surgical dissection around the U-V junction.[10] This report supports the important surgical principles outlined by Tanagho. The Tanagho modification of the Burch colposuspension is widely accepted and has become the standard today.

With advanced technologic development of laparoscopic and video equipment and improved skill in performing operative laparoscopy, we have no difficulty applying the important surgical principles for retropubic colposuspension to laparoscopy. In some cases we even improve on traditional surgery by meeting the stringent surgical criteria for the Burch procedure: adequate exposure with good visibility of the operative field, accurate dissection of the retropubic space, perfect hemostasis, precise placement of paraurethral sutures, and approximation of tissue without undue tension.

Preoperative Evaluation

Prior to surgery the diagnosis of genuine stress urinary incontinence must be confirmed and differentiated from other causes of incontinence, such as detrusor instability and overflow incontinence. The preoperative evaluation includes a complete history and physical examination with particular emphasis on neurologic history and current medication. Urinary incontinence questionnaires and the patient's voiding diary (urolog) can provide invaluable information. The lower neurologic examination, with emphasis on the sensory and motor dermatome pattern of S_2, S_3, and S_4, are important. Pelvic examination to assess the concomitant pelvic floor defects as previously described is crucial for avoiding additional surgeries.

Other office tests include urinalysis and urine culture, a stress test, and a Q-Tip test, as well as simple office cystometry and measurement of residual urine. If there is any deviation in these tests or if the patient is frail and old (age > 60) or has had previous unsuccessful antiincontinence surgery, she should undergo more sophisticated multichannel urodynamic studies before treatment is rendered (Table 10.1).

Table 10.1. Patients requiring multichannel urodynamic studies

Age > 60
Previous unsuccessful antiincontinence surgery
Any deviation in the office tests
Continuous or unpredictable leakage

Operative Technique

Under general anesthesia with endotracheal intubation, the patient is placed in a low dorsolithotomy position with both legs supported in Allen's Universal Stirrups (Edgewater Medical System, Cleveland, OH). A 20F Foley catheter with 30 ml balloon tip is then inserted into the bladder. After the bladder is emptied, 50 ml concentrated indigo carmine dye is instilled into the bladder and the Foley catheter clamped. Accidental penetration of the bladder during the procedure is immediately recognized by the escape of blue dye. A 10 mm laparoscope is inserted through a vertical intraumblical incision, and four 5 mm puncture sites are made in the low abdomen. The lower pair of puncture sites is made lateral to the deep inferior epigastric vessels, and the upper pair is placed lateral to the abdominis rectus muscle at about the umbilical level. The internal viscus is carefully inspected after which the patient is placed in a 20° Trendelenburg position and the pelvic organs meticulously examined. All visible pathology, such as adhesions and endometriosis, are excised using the appropriate laparoscopic instrument. Additional procedures, such as adnexectomy and hysterectomy, vaginal vault suspension, or repair of the enterocele and rectocele, are performed if indicated. The cul-de-sac is obliterated using 2-0 permanent sutures with modified Moschcowitz technique[11] through the laparoscope. More than one purse-string suture may be needed to obliterate the cul-de-sac. It is important to obliterate the channels on either side of the sigmoid colon to prevent future enterocele formation.

A transverse incision is made on the parietal peritoneum about 1 inch above the symphysis pubis between two umbilical ligaments with laparoscopic scissors. The anterior peritoneum is dissected away from the anterior abdominal wall toward the pubic bone, and the retropubic space is entered and dissected with scissors. Note that no dissection is carried out within 2.0–2.5 cm of the urethra.

Anatomic landmarks such as the obturator canal, aberrant obturator vein, arcus tendineus fascia of the obturator interna, and arcus tendineus fascia of the levator ani are identified. As much retropubic fat as possible is removed to promote fibrosis and scar formation in the paravaginal area. The bladder is mobilized; and the pearly white, glistening appearance of the paravaginal fascia should be identified on both sides of the urethra. During retropubic dissection and bladder mobilization, the paraurethral vascular plexus frequently is injured, causing bleeding, which is sometimes troublesome. Hemostasis can always be achieved by bipolar electrocoagulation, sutures, or both. Four sutures of nonabsorbable material, such as No. 2 Gore-Tex, are used to raise and pull the anterior vaginal wall forward and upward to Cooper's ligaments. A pair of sutures is placed at the level of the midurethra and the U-V junction, inserted at least 2 cm from the urethra and the U-V junction. A double bite of the whole thickness of the anterior vaginal wall, avoiding the vaginal canal, is obtained and is then passed through Cooper's ligament on the ipsilateral side at a level immediately above the location of the anterior vaginal wall suture (Plates 13–15; Fig. 10.1). During suture placement, the assistant (or preferably the operating surgeon) places his or her middle and index fingers at the level of the U-V junction with the tips of the fingers at the junction of the Foley catheter balloon and the drainage tube. The assistant should wear protective devices on the fingertips to prevent accidental needle prick. Tenting of the anterior vaginal wall in this manner facilitates correct placement of the sutures. Once the sutures are placed, they can be tied using the extracorporeal knot-tying technique with the Clarke-Reich knot pusher. Tying is facilitated if the assistant pushes the finger in the vagina up toward Cooper's ligament (Plate 16). The procedure is then repeated on the contralateral side. During the knot tying particular care must be taken to avoid tying the knots too tightly. It is not necessary to have the vaginal wall in direct contact with Cooper's ligament (Plate 17). Adequate support is obtained if the sutures are tied without undue tension; excessive tension compresses or kinks the urethra and may produce necrosis at the suture sites, possibly resulting in suture release and surgical failure. The retropubic space is then irrigated with copious amounts of Ringer's lactate solution. Any bleeders are coagulated with

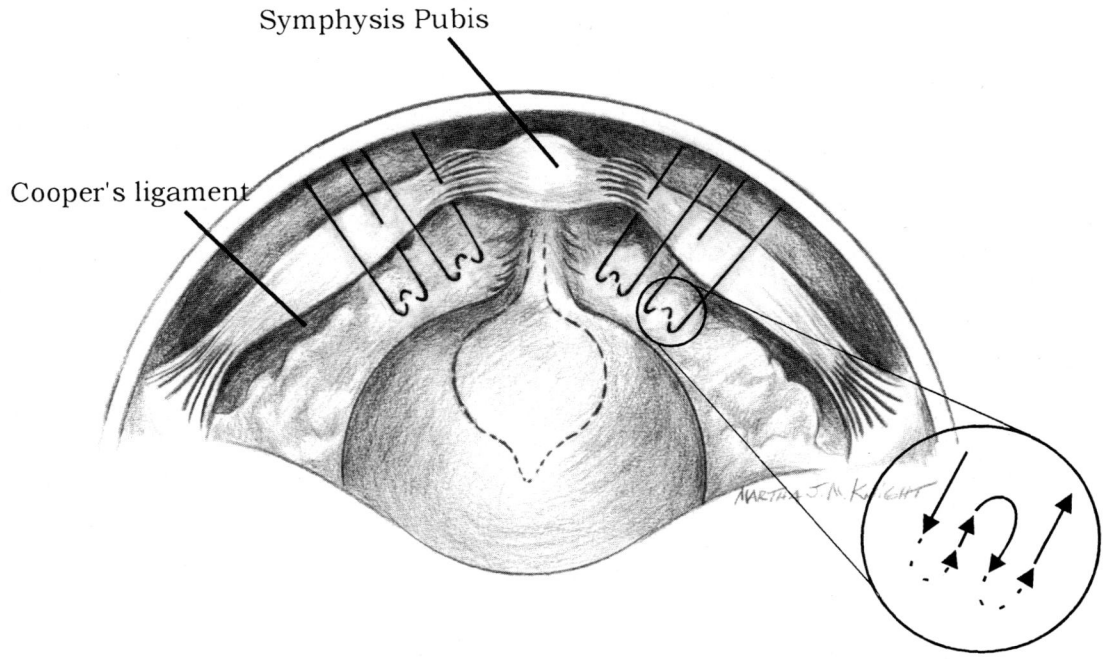

Figure 10.1. Two sutures are placed on each side of the urethra. The first suture is placed at the mid-urethral level and the second at about the U-V junction. Both sutures are placed at least 2 cm from the urethra and then through Cooper's ligament on the ipsilateral side.

bipolar forceps and occasionally sutures. A suprapubic catheter is inserted into the bladder under direct visualization (Plate 18), and the peritoneal defect is closed with 2-0 absorbable sutures. No drain is necessary in the retropubic space, as adequate hemostasis can always be obtained laparoscopically. Cystoscopic examination is then performed to ensure that no suture material has penetrated through or on the bladder wall. Indigo carmine dye (5 ml) and 20 mg of furosemide (Lasix) may then be injected intravenously to confirm the integrity of the ureters. The peristalsis and ejection of dye from ureteral orifices can be clearly observed cystoscopically.[12, 13]

Laparoscopic Retropubic Colposuspension

Laparoscopic retropubic colposuspension is an alternative to laparoscopic bladder neck suspension. Some investigators use synthetic mesh, stapling one end of the mesh to the anterior vaginal wall and the other end to Cooper's ligament to suspend the anterior vaginal wall and elevate the U-V junction. Others use a combined laparoscopic and vaginal approach.

The retropubic space is approached extraperitoneally; and under laparoscopic guidance the Pereyra needle with suture on it is used to puncture Cooper's ligament and go through the anterior vaginal wall. The needle is then reversed, passing through the anterior vaginal wall and Cooper's ligament again. The sutures are tied on Cooper's ligament laparoscopically. The shortcomings of the extraperitoneal retropubic colposuspension include an inability to inspect and detect any unsuspected abdominal and pelvic pathology and an inability to repair the concomitant middle and posterior compartment defects simultaneously.

Postoperative Care

The postoperative care is similar to that after any major laparoscopic surgical procedure. Most patients can be discharged from the hospital within 24 hours of the surgery with mild analgesic medication. Others are discharged with an indwelling suprapubic catheter that can be removed when the residual urine measures 50 ml at three consecutive voidings.

All patients are allowed to drive and return to work within 2 weeks of the surgery, providing their jobs require little physical exertion. Patients are instructed in detail regarding their postoperative physical activities. They are told to limit their activities for at least 3 months after surgery to allow the formation of strong fibrotic and scar tissues in the retropubic area. No heavy lifting, pushing, stooping, bending, or reaching should be undertaken during this time. Strong scar tissue ensures a better long-term result from the surgery.

Complications

The complications associated with traditional abdominal retropubic colposuspension are intraoperative urethral and bladder injury, ureteral kinking and obstruction, retropubic hematoma and abscess, urinary tract infection, urinary retention, postoperative detrusor instability, enterocele, genital prolapse, and sexual dysfunction. In our series of 132 laparoscopic retropubic colposuspensions, the overall complication rate was 9.8% (Table 10.2); there were no conversions to laparotomy. Four of our patients had intraoperative bladder injuries, all of which occurred on the dome of the bladder during the initial entry into the retropubic space. The bladder injuries were recognized and repaired laparoscopically. Four patients developed postoperative voiding difficulty with urinary retention and required prolonged catheterization for more than 10 days. Three patients developed de novo detrusor instability; all improved with the administration of oxybutynin (Ditropan) and bladder retraining. One patient developed a right ureteral obstruction postoperatively; a second-look laparoscopy and cystoscopy, performed 10 days after the initial surgery, revealed a kinked right ureter, which was relieved laparoscopically by releasing the retropubic colposuspension sutures on the right side. Another patient had gross hematuria that derived from the suprapubic catheter site, which required a second cystoscopic examination. The suprapubic catheter was removed and the bleeder coagulated cystoscopically. No other complications, such as retropubic hematoma, abscess, or urinary fistula, occurred in our series.[14,15]

Summary

There are two distinctive types of urinary stress incontinence. With one, the intrinsic sphincteric mechanism of the urethra is intact but there is poor fibromuscular support of the urethra and the U-V junction. With the other, urethral sphincter dysfunction is present. The Burch procedure can only elevate the bladder neck and restore its normal anatomic position; it cannot correct the urethral sphincteric dysfunction. A displaced and hypermobile bladder neck and proximal portion of the urethra are a result of the defect in the pelvic supporting system. After Burch colposuspension, the vaginal axis is altered. Pulling the anterior vaginal wall up to high retropubic position may cure the stress incontinence, but it also pulls the posterior vagina upward, resulting in a wide open cul-de-sac with increased chance of enterocele formation and uterovaginal prolapse. Up to 28% of patients undergoing a Burch colposuspension develop middle and posterior compartment deficiency, and they subsequently manifest enterocele, rectocele, and vaginal vault prolapse.[1] Therefore the entire pelvic floor function must be thoroughly investigated and considered before and during any reconstructive surgery.

Table 10.2. Complications in 132 laparoscopic retropubic colposuspensions

Complication	No. of patients	Rate
Bladder injury	4	3.0
Urinary retention	4	3.0
Ureteral obstruction	1	0.7
Detrusor instability	3	2.3
Gross hematuria[a]	1	0.7
Total	13	9.8[b]

[a] Gross hematuria was secondary to insertion of a suprapubic catheter.
[b] Rate per 100 women undergoing the laparoscopic Burch procedure.

Increased intraabdominal pressure during laparoscopy facilitates the identification of pelvic floor defects. Concomitant repair of such defects must be carried out laparoscopically or vaginally at the time of laparoscopic retropubic colposuspension.

Although most failures of antiincontinence surgery occur within the first 2 years after the procedure, the failure rate increases with time. The main causes of immediate surgical failure are not placing the anchoring sutures deep enough and not incorporating a sufficient amount of the anterior vaginal wall. Placing the sutures in a figure-of-eight fashion is helpful. The outcome of the repair depends on anchoring this suture securely into the paraurethral tissues around the bladder neck. The strength of this suture should be tested by pulling on it forcefully to make sure it is anchored in the tissue before attaching it to Cooper's ligament.

The laparoscopic approach to retropubic colposuspension provides better visualization of the space of Retzius than the traditional laparotomy. It facilitates dissection of the retropubic space and mobilization of the bladder. With greater magnification from the video display system, the important anatomic landmarks and the vessels are more easily visualized, thus contributing to more accurate placement of sutures, decreased blood loss, and the avoidance of drains. I have been performing laparoscopic retropubic colposuspensions for 3 years at the time of this writing. Although my series is still small and the follow-up time is short (Table 10.3), I am encouraged by the results. Of 132 patients, 127 have been satisfied with the surgery. Patients who have had a laparoscopic retropubic colposuspension experienced less discomfort, much shorter hospital stay, and a quicker recovery than patients treated with a similar procedure through an abdominal incision. I believe laparoscopic retropubic colposuspension is a satisfactory alternative to abdominal retropubic colposuspension in well selected patients.

Laparoscopic Rectocele and Enterocele Repair

Rectocele and enterocele repairs are almost always combined with concomitant repair of other coexisting pelvic floor defects, such as cystocele, uterovaginal prolapse, or urinary stress incontinence caused by anterior compartment defect. Large, low rectocele repair frequently involves reattaching the rectovaginal septum and urogenital diaphragm to the perineal body, and it is best approached vaginally. A perineorrhaphy usually is also necessary in this situation.

The patient is placed in low dorsolithotomy position with both legs supported by Allen's Universal Stirrups. A 10 mm laparoscope is inserted into the peritoneal cavity through an umbilical trocar sleeve. Four additional 5 mm trocar sleeves are placed in the abdomen, two of which are at about the umbilical level lateral to the rectus muscle and the other two in the lower abdomen lateral to the deep inferior epigastric vessels. The patient's position and trocar placement are exactly the same as described previously for the laparoscopic technique of retropubic colposuspension. In addition to the regular laparoscopic equipment, a rectal probe and vaginal manipulator, which is a wet 4 × 4 sponge on the tip of a sponge forceps (Plate 19), are important instruments when performing laparoscopic rectocele and enterocele repairs.

During the laparoscopic examination the important anatomic landmarks, such as the ureters and uterosacral cardinal ligaments, are identified. The high rectocele and the enterocele are carefully evaluated. Inserting the vaginal manipulator into the vagina with a gentle upward push and placing a rectal probe inside the rectum provide much better assessment of the enterocele (Plate 20). A transverse incision is made

Table 10.3. Length of follow-up (as of August 1993)

Follow-up	No. of patients
> 6 Months	31
6 Months to 1 year	36
1 to 2 Years	55
> 2 Years	10
Total	132

between the insertion of the two uterosacral ligaments; the peritoneum covering the anterior portion of the enterocele is excised and the rectovaginal space entered. Dissection of the rectovaginal space is carried downward as far as possible toward the perineum. The dissection also continues laterally on both sides to identify the rectal pillars. Often the dissection is difficult owing to obliteration of the rectovaginal space, which is caused by adhesion formation between the rectum and the rectovaginal septum. Interrupted sutures with 2-0 delayed absorbable sutures are then placed through the pararectal fascia, which includes both rectal pillars and the medial fascia of the levator ani on both sides. These sutures are tied transversely with either extracorporeal or intracorporeal instrument ties, bringing both rectal pillars and medial fascia of the levator ani together in the midline anterior to the rectum. After the rectocele is repaired, the enterocele is repaired with the modified Moschcowitz procedure. One or more purse-string sutures with 2-0 permanent material are used. First, the suture is placed through the left uterosacral ligament and then through the posterior vaginal wall on the apex after several bites of the posterior vagina, and finally to the right side of the uterosacral ligament. The suture then catches the peritoneum of the right gutter of the rectum; it passes through the serosal layer of the rectal wall and peritoneum of the left side of the gutter of the rectum, and then back through the left uterosacral ligament. The suture is then tied with an extracorporeal knot-tying technique. Care must be taken to avoid leaving any peritoneal gap while tying the sutures, which may cause recurrence of the enterocele. In most cases vaginal vault suspension is performed at the same time.

Vaginal Vault Prolapse

Basically there are two important supporting systems that maintain the upper part of the vagina: (1) the uterosacrocardinal ligament complex of the endopelvic fascia; and (2) the levator plate on which the upper vagina and rectum rest. Increased intraabdominal pressure results in posterior (rather than inferior) displacement of the upper vagina. This supporting system maintains the upper half of the vagina in a nearly horizontal position. A defect in the supporting system causes the vagina to prolapse.

A universal classification of the severity of vaginal prolapse has not been adopted, and we use the following system. The patient is examined in the resting state and with the Valsalva maneuver.

Grade 1: Vaginal apex is above the hymenal ring at rest and descends to the hymenal ring during strain.
Grade 2: Apex of the vagina reaches the introitus at rest and protrudes through the introitus with strain.
Grade 3: Apex of the vagina extends outside the introitus, and the vaginal vault is totally everted.

Laparoscopic Surgery

Any reconstructive surgery should return the upper vagina to the normal, nearly horizontal position. It should also repair any coexisting pelvic floor defects. Because there is no single operation that corrects all the pelvic defects that might be present, a combination of surgical procedures is often needed. Vaginal vault prolapse is frequently associated with defects in the urogenital diaphragm and perineal body. These defects can best be repaired vaginally.

With grade 1 vaginal vault prolapse, the cardinal uterosacral ligaments can be shortened and used to suspend the vault of the vagina, providing satisfactory results. For grades 2 and 3, there are three alternative ways to suspend the vagina.

1. Sacral colpopexy: The vaginal vault is suspended to the hallow of the sacrum with synthetic graft materials such as Gore-Tex or Marlex grafts.
2. High McCall-type suspension. The vaginal vault is attached to the uterosacral ligaments close to their origin from the sacrum.
3. Sacrospinosus suspension. The vaginal vault is suspended to the sacrospinosus ligament.

Laparoscopic sacropexy of the vaginal vault is technically difficult. It involves placing a graft in the hollow of the sacrum below the promontory, which may result in life-threatening hemorrhage when the graft is sutured to the anterior longitudinal ligaments of the bony sacral promontory. Infection and graft rejection have been reported even years after the surgery. Our preference is to perform either a high McCall-type vaginal suspension or sacrospinosus vaginal vault suspension. The sacrospinosus ligament can be easily accessed by laparoscopy; and so long as the sutures are placed away from the ischial spine, the danger of bleeding or nerve injury is minimal. The sacrospinosus ligament and the coccygeus muscle are basically the same structure, extending from the ischial spine on each side to the lower portion of the sacrum and coccyx, where it attaches to the sacrotuberous ligament.

Patients with an anthropoid or android type of pelvis are not good candidates for sacrospinosus suspension because of the short distance between the sacrospinosus ligaments and the introitus. Sacrospinosus vaginal suspension in those patients would result in a shortened vagina. High McCall-type vaginal vault suspension is preferable for these patients.

Surgical Technique

The patient's position and the laparoscopic trocar placement sites are the same as for the laparoscopic Burch procedure and for enterocele and rectocele repair.

High McCall Vaginal Vault Suspension

After the vaginal probe is inserted into the vagina, the enterocele is repaired first, as described previously. The uterosacral ligaments on both sides are identified and traced all the way to the presacral region. Such tracing can be accomplished even in an obese patient by pulling the sigmoid colon back toward the upper abdomen. With a gentle upward push of the vaginal probe toward the sacrum, the level of the presacral uterosacral ligaments reached by the vaginal vault is noted. The uterosacral ligament on the left side is then sutured through with No. 2 Gore-Tex suture about 1.5 cm above the enterocele suture; a second bite is taken through the same structure about 1 cm toward the cul-de-sac. The suture is then passed through the posterior wall of the vagina but not into the vaginal canal, with several bites reaching the right uterosacral ligament. Double bites of the right uterosacral ligament are also taken. The suture is then passed through the peritoneum on both channels of the rectosigmoid colon and returned to the left uterosacral ligament, making a purse-string suture. The suture is then tied using the extracorporeal knot-tying technique with a knot pusher. Care must be taken not to leave a peritoneal gap, which may result in future enterocele formation. A second suture using the same suture material is placed in the same fashion through the uterosacral ligaments at the level the tip of the vagina can reach. Usually two or three sutures are needed to complete the high McCall suspension. Both ureters must be carefully monitored during the procedure.

Laparoscopic Sacrospinous Vaginal Vault Suspension

After the rectal probe is placed in the rectum and rectum is pushed toward the left side of the pelvis, the operator places his or her fingers inside the vagina and palpates the right ischial spine and the sacrospinosus ligament. This maneuver helps identify the location of the sacrospinosus ligament laparoscopically. The right pararectal space is entered and dissected downward and toward the sacrum. After the sacrospinosus ligament has been identified, the enterocele is repaired as described previously. A No. 2 Gore-Tex suture with a C-V 2 needle is used to suture through the sacrospinosus ligament. It is important to place the suture deep into the sacrospinosus ligament. The strength of this suture should be tested by pulling on it forcefully to make sure it is indeed deep in the ligament (Plate 21). The suture must be placed away from the ischial spine and close to the sacrum. A double bite is taken, and the suture is passed through the tip of the vagina twice, avoiding the vaginal mucosa. The suture is then tied with extracorporeal knot-tying technique using a knot pusher (Plate 22). Special attention is given to avoiding the appearance of a gap between the sacrospinosus ligament and the vagina.

References

1. WISKIND AK, CREIGHTON SM, STANTON SL: The incidence of prolapse after the Burch colposuspension. Am J Obstet Gynecol 1992;167:399.
2. DELANCEY JOL, RICHARDSON AC: Anatomy of genital support. In Female Pelvic Floor Disorders: Investigation and Management, Benson TJ (ed). New York, Norton, 1992, p. 19.
3. NICHOLS DH, RANDALL CL: Significance of restoration of normal vaginal depth and axis. Obstet Gynecol 1970;36:251.
4. NICHOLS DH, RANDALL CL: Vaginal Surgery (3rd ed). Baltimore, Williams & Wilkins, 1989.
5. HERTOGS K, STANTON SL: Lateral bead-chain urethrocystography after successful and unsuccessful colposuspension. Br J Obstet Gynaecol 1985;92:1179.
6. HERTOGS K, STANTON SL: Mechanism of urinary continence after colposuspension: barrier studies. Br J Obstet Gynaecol 1985;92:1184.
7. MARSHALL VF, MARCHETTI AA, KRANTZ KE: The correction of stress incontinence by simple vesicourethral suspension. Surg Gynecol Obstet 1949;88:509.
8. BURCH JC: Cooper's ligament urethrovesical suspension for stress incontinence. Am J Obstet Gynecol 1968;100:764.
9. TANAGHO EA: Colpocystourethropexy: the way we do it. J Urol 1976;116:751.
10. CARDOZO LD, STANTON SL, WILLIAMS JE: Detrusor instability following surgery for genuine stress incontinence. Br J Urol 1979;51:204.
11. MOSCHCOWITZ AV: The pathogenesis, anatomy, and cure of prolapse of the rectum. Surg Gynecol Obstet 1912;15:7.
12. ST LEZIN MA, STOLLER ML: Surgical ureteral injuries. Urology 1991;38:497.
13. SYMMONDS RE: Ureteral injuries associated with gynecological surgery: prevention and management. Clin Obstet Gynecol 1976;19:623.
14. LIU CY: Laparoscopic retropubic colposuspension: a review of 58 cases. J Reprod Med 1993;38:526.
15. LIU CY, PAEK WS: Laparoscopic retropubic colposuspension (Burch procedure). J Am Assoc Gynecol Laparosc 1993;1:31.

11
Ectopic Pregnancy

Harry Reich and Dwight Pridham

One of every 66 pregnancies in the United States is an ectopic gestation. The success of laparoscopic management of ectopic pregnancy has been well documented (Table 11.1).[1-19]

An ectopic pregnancy can be tubal (ampullary, isthmic, or infundibular), interstitial, angular, ovarian, cervical, or abdominal and can be present in more than one location or with an associated intrauterine pregnancy. It is usually located within the lumen of the ampullary tube (67%) or in its extraluminal space between the serosa and muscularis mucosa.[20,21] The ectopic gestation may be leaking blood through the distal tubal ostium, may be in the process of rupturing, or may be frankly ruptured with varying degrees of intravascular volume compromise. Distal tubal abortion may be in progress or completed. The ectopic pregnancy may be viable with a fetal heartbeat noted on ultrasonography or nonviable with surrounding blood clot in various states of organization. The American Society for Reproductive Medicine has provided a classification scheme for tubal pregnancies (Fig. 11.1).

A number of laparoscopic techniques can be used to treat tubal ectopic pregnancy. With the use of sensitive radioimmunoassays for the β-subunit of human chorionic gonadotropin (β-hCG) and high-resolution ultrasonography, most tubal gestations frequently remain unruptured at diagnosis. Laparotomy with salpingectomy was the "gold standard" for treatment of tubal pregnancy earlier this century. Today laparoscopy is supplanting laparotomy. This chapter discusses the relative merits of a conservative approach (salpingotomy or partial salpingectomy) versus radical treatment (salpingectomy or salpingo-oophorectomy). Nonsurgical management is evaluated because of its potential as an adjunct to laparoscopic surgery and as definitive therapy per se.

The major advantages of the laparoscopic approach are reduced hospital stay, return to full activity generally within 1 week of surgery, and good prognosis with respect to subsequent intrauterine pregnancy. The average hospital stay after laparotomy is 5.2 days, whereas a laparoscopic approach frequently results in hospitalization of less than 24 hours.[22] Laparoscopy apparently prevents drying of the parietal and visceral peritoneum, and it may limit the risk of infection, both of which advantages may result in avoidance of the postoperative adhesions commonly associated with laparotomy. Blood loss and cutaneous scarring associated with an abdominal incision are also avoided.

The term *salpingotomy* is used throughout this chapter to describe conservative removal of products of conception through an incision in the fallopian tube, whether the tube is left to

Table 11.1. Reported success of laparoscopic salpingostomy for unruptured ectopic pregnancy and subsequent fertility: 1980–1992

Study	Year	No. treated	No. of successful treatments	Tubal patency HSG[b]	Patent	Subsequent fertility No. included[c]	Pregnancy	Ectopic pregnancy
Bruhat et al.[1a]	1980	60	57	12	9	28	21	3
Daniell & Herbert[2]	1984	22	22	21	17	21	5	1
Pouly et al.[3]	1986	321	306			118	102	26
Johns & Hardie[4a]	1986	15	15	9	9			
DeCherney & Diamond[5]	1987	79	77			69	43	7
Bornstein et al.[6]	1987	16	16			4	3	2
Reich et al.[7]	1988	65	65	26	26	38	19	6
Brumsted et al.[8]	1988	10	9					
Silva[9]	1988	8	7			6	4	0
Vermesh et al.[10]	1989	30	26	20	16	18	10	1
Henderson[11]	1989	17	14					
Huber et al.[12]	1989	9	9	9	9			
Karsten & Seifert[13]	1990	12	12	6	6	12	3	1
Keckstein et al.[14]	1990	22	21	16	14			
Mecke et al.[15]	1991	251	236			143	83	23
Chapron et al.[16]	1991	63	55					
Verco[17]	1991	10	10					
Chapron et al.[18]	1992	26	25			11	8	1
Mottla et al.[19]	1992	5	5					
Total		1041	987 (94.7%)	98	88 (89.8%)	440	280 (63.6%)	68 (24.3%)

[a]Excluded from totals as included in a subsequent cumulative report.
[b]HSG denotes hysterosalpingography, a method of documenting tubal patency.
[c]Number of women seeking to become pregnant.

heal by "secondary intention" or is reapproximated. Salpingotomy implies opening a fallopian tube by an incision, whereas salpingostomy infers making a new opening (ostium). The term salpingostomy has also come to mean that the tubal incision is left open after evacuating its contents, with subsequent closure by secondary intention, whereas salpingotomy implies primary surgical closure of the tube.

After the 1980 report by Budowick et al.,[23] there was controversy regarding whether most tubal pregnancies develop inside the fallopian tube or in the extraluminal loose adventitial tissue between the tubal serosa and muscularis. An extraluminal location has rarely been reported by surgeons performing conservative procedures for tubal pregnancy, and it can be inferred that most tubal pregnancies develop in the limited space of the fallopian tube.

Historical Perspective

Reports of laparoscopic treatment using salpingectomy and salpingotomy are numerous. Manhes is generally recognized as the first to treat ectopic pregnancy using laparoscopy in 1970.[1] By 1975 Shapiro and Adler[24] and Soderstrom[25] had described laparoscopic partial salpingectomy using electrocoagulation.

The credit for pioneering the laparoscopic treatment of ectopic pregnancy belongs to Bruhat and his colleagues[1] in France, who were the first to perform laparoscopic salpingotomy and fimbrial expression. During the 10 year period 1974–1984 a total of 321 cases of tubal pregnancy in 295 women were treated endoscopically, and currently more than 90% of tubal gestations are managed in this manner.

11. Ectopic Pregnancy

THE AMERICAN FERTILITY SOCIETY CLASSIFICATION OF TUBAL PREGNANCIES

Patient's Name _____ Date _____ Chart # _____

Age _____ G _____ P _____ Sp Ab _____ VTP _____ Ectopic _____ Infertile Yes _____ No _____

Other Significant History (i.e. surgery, infection, etc.) _____

HSG _____ Sonography _____ Photography _____ Laparoscopy _____ Laparotomy _____

TUBAL PREGNANCY

	Right	Left	Contralateral Tube & Ovary
Infundibular	_____	_____	Normal _____ Absent _____
Ampullary	_____	_____	Abnormal _____
Isthmic	_____	_____	_____
Interstitial	_____	_____	_____
Size (cm)	_____	_____	_____

Treatment (Surgical Procedures):
Laparoscopy _____
  No Surgery _____
  Surgery _____
    Expression _____
    Linear Salpingostomy _____
      Sharp Dissection _____
      Laser _____
      Cautery _____
Laparotomy _____
  Linear Salpingostomy _____
    1° Closure _____
    2° Closure _____
  Segmental Resection _____
    1° Anastomosis _____
    2° Anastomosis Planned Yes _____ No _____

Other: _____

Additional Findings: _____

DRAWING

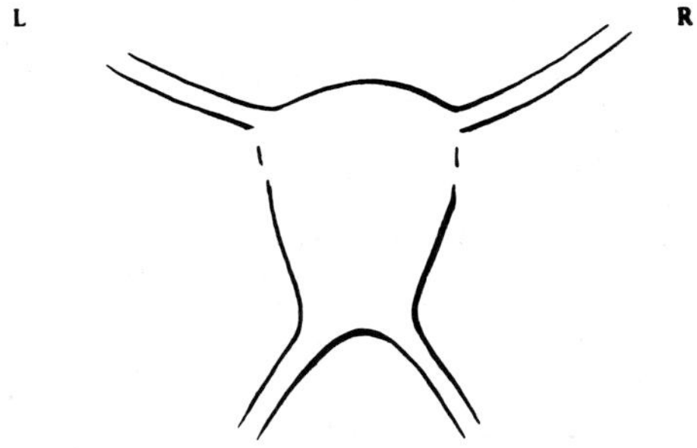

L   R

For additional supply write to:
The American Fertility Society
2140 11th Avenue, South
Suite 200
Birmingham, Alabama 35205

Prognosis for Conception & Subsequent Viable Infant*

_____ Excellent (> 75%)
_____ Good (50-75%)
_____ Fair (25%-50%)
_____ Poor (< 25%)

*Physician's judgment based upon adnexa with least amount of pathology.

Recommended Followup Treatment: _____

Property of
The American Fertility Society

Figure 11.1. American Society for Reproductive Medicine classification of tubal pregnancies. From Fertil Steril 1988;49:944–55. (Reproduced with permission of the publisher, The American Society for Reproductive Medicine (formerly the American Fertility Society))

There were 15 (5%) failures (i.e., incomplete removal of trophoblast); seven were treated with a second laparoscopic procedure and eight via laparotomy. Of 118 patients desiring pregnancy and followed for more than 12 months, 76 (64%) had an intrauterine gestation, 5 after laparoscopic treatment of a second ectopic gestation; and 26 (22%) had a subsequent ectopic pregnancy. More importantly, 53 of 62 women (85%) with no history of infertility and 23 of 56 women (41%) with a history of infertility achieved an intrauterine pregnancy. Eleven of twenty-four women (46%) had an intrauterine pregnancy after removal of an ectopic gestation from their sole remaining tube, but 7 (29%) in this group had a second ectopic pregnancy.[3]

Dubuisson et al. reported 100 cases of salpingectomy in 1987; they used thermocoagulation and transection of the isthmus, mesosalpinx, and tuboovarian ligament.[26] The reasons for treatment were hemoperitoneum of more than 100 ml ($n = 12$), tubal rupture ($n = 32$), and an ampullary pregnancy larger than 3 cm in diameter ($n = 42$). Two laparotomies, one for severe adhesions and the other for a large retrouterine hematocele, were necessary. The average operating time was 37 minutes, with more recent procedures requiring 15–40 minutes. The average postoperative stay was 2 days, and no immediate or delayed postoperative hemorrhage or fever occurred.[26]

One of the authors of this chapter (H.R.) managed 64 tubal pregnancies laparoscopically, including six with rupture, three located interstitially, and one in the ovary. Since 1983 laparoscopic procedures have been his primary method of managing tubal pregnancy (the last 61 cases).[7,22]

Diagnosis

There is no substitute for sound clinical judgment and an understanding of the pathophysiology involved. Although many protocols for the diagnosis of ectopic pregnancy have been devised, there are always exceptions to the rule. Ruptured ectopic gestations have occurred with hCG levels < 5 mIU/ml and > 50,000 mIU/ml. Likewise, many ectopic pregnancies do not present with the classic triad of amenorrhea, abnormal vaginal bleeding, and abdominal pain. An appreciation of the risk factors for ectopic pregnancy is important (although many patients have none). Cacciatore et al screened 225 asymptomatic pregnant women at risk (history of prior ectopic pregnancy, tubal or pelvic surgery, pelvic inflammatory disease, or current use of an intrauterine device) and found 55 ectopic pregnancies (24.4%) using a protocol that included β-hCG assays and early ultrasonography.[27] Asymptomatic women at risk with a positive pregnancy test and women presenting with any of the classic symptoms should have the diagnosis excluded.

The following discussion of a diagnostic protocol for suspected ectopic pregnancy should be considered only for those patients who are hemodynamically stable with a nonacute abdomen but with signs or symptoms suggesting possible ectopic pregnancy.

Waiting for quantitative β-hCG values or transvaginal ultrasonography results in the presence of orthostatic hypotension or a surgical abdomen is not ideal management. Such patients should be considered for immediate surgery as soon as basic laboratory results (CBC, hCG, blood type and screen) are available. In the nonemergent setting, the following guidelines may be applied.

Use of the hCG β-subunit assay to diagnose an ectopic pregnancy was first reported in the literature by Kosasa and colleagues in 1973.[28] Utilizing a discrimination zone, the hCG level during each ectopic pregnancy was found to be lower than that for intrauterine pregnancies of comparable gestational age. A subsequent publication by Kosasa and coworkers revealed that a small percentage of ectopic pregnancies could have hCG levels consistent with an intrauterine gestation, but that the rate of rise in each case was markedly slower than that of a normal pregnancy.[29] Subsequent investigations of asymptomatic women at risk for ectopic pregnancy have shown that some normal intrauterine pregnancies (ca. 2–3%) fail to exhibit normal doubling times for hCG, whereas approximately 30–40% of early asymptomatic

11. Ectopic Pregnancy

Figure 11.2. Diagnosis of ectopic pregnancy.

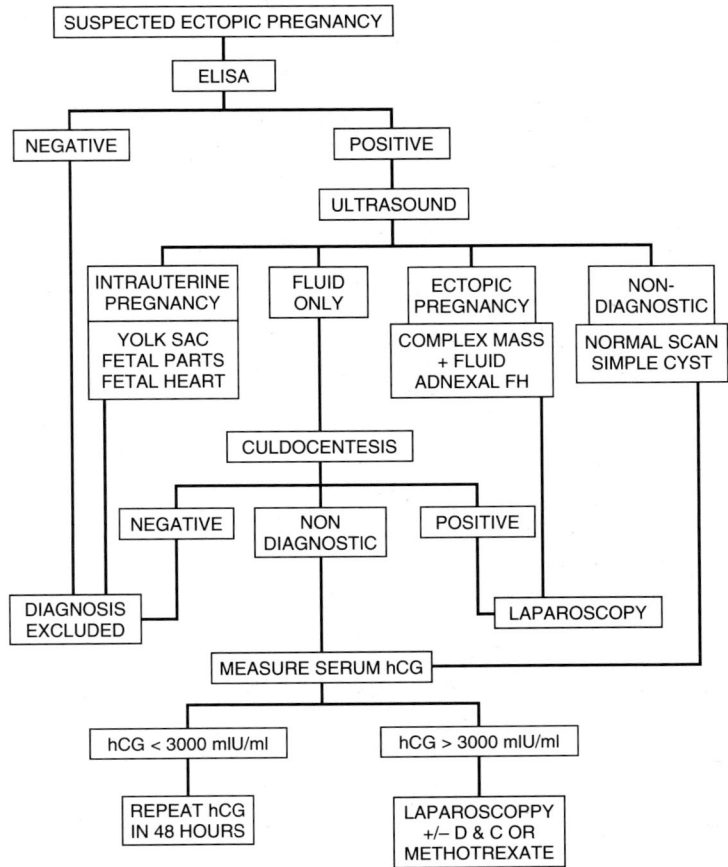

ectopic pregnancies show hCG doubling consistent with a normal pregnancy.[30] A combination of modalities is therefore optimal for accurate diagnosis.

A nonsurgical approach using serial β-hCG titers combined with ultrasonography for the diagnosis of ectopic pregnancy was first described by Kadar et al. in 1981.[31,32] Many minor variations of the original algorithm have been devised, but all involve the combined use of ultrasonography and a sensitive hCG assay, as well as serial hCG testing in some patients. The value of serial hCG testing as originally described, though questioned by some, has been repeatedly validated,[33–35] and its use has been extended to patients with falling hCG values.[36]

Valid estimates and fiducial limits for the discriminatory zone have also been established for vaginal sonography.[37] The discriminatory hCG zone, as described by Kadar et al, is the hCG value above which the gestational sac of an intrauterine pregnancy can *always* be imaged with ultrasonography (6500 mIU/ml for a transabdominal scan and 3000 mIU/ml for a vaginal one). This level should not be confused with the lowest level at which a sac *may* be visualized, which can be as low as 800 mIU/ml. The diagnostic evaluation that remains valid to this day is summarized in Figures 11.2 and 11.3.

The underlying concept was that in normal pregnancies there must be an hCG concentration below which the gestational sac can never be imaged sonographically, a concentration above which it can always be identified, and an intervening zone when it can be imaged in some patients but not in others. In other words, the serum hCG concentration is used to determine whether the gestational sac of an intrauterine pregnancy should be detectable sonographic-

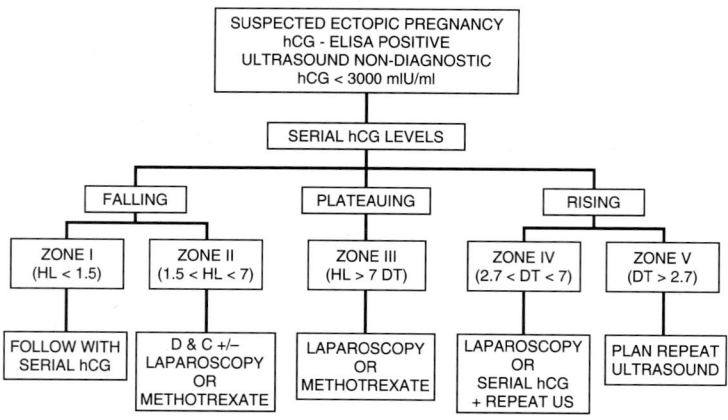

Figure 11.3. Serial hCG patterns in suspected ectopic pregnancy. (DT = Doubling Time; HL = Half Life)

ally. Because the date of the last menstrual period is frequently uncertain or unreliable, the serum hCG provides a more reliable yardstick by which to interpret the ultrasonographic findings than gestational age.

An hCG concentration above the discriminatory zone and a gestational sac that cannot be imaged provides presumptive evidence of an ectopic pregnancy. However, if the serum hCG level is below the discriminatory zone, failure to image a gestational sac is a nondiagnostic finding that may mean nothing more than that the intrauterine pregnancy is too early to be imaged sonographically. If an intrauterine pregnancy is imaged, however, it is taken to be evidence that an ectopic pregnancy does not exist because combined intrauterine and ectopic (heterotopic) pregnancies are uncommon.[31]

It should be emphasized that an appreciation of individual risk factors and adequate clinical suspicion are necessary for a timely diagnosis of ectopic pregnancy. In the situation of patients conceiving during fertility therapy, the incidences of ectopic pregnancy and multiple gestation are considerably higher than usual. During laparoscopy *both* fallopian tubes should be carefully examined even when an ectopic gestation in obviously present on one side.

Briefly, women of childbearing age who complain of abdominal pain, abnormal vaginal bleeding, or both must be examined and a urinary pregnancy test performed. For practical reasons, urinary enzyme-linked immunosorbent assay; (ELISA) pregnancy tests are now sensitive enough for a negative result to exclude the diagnosis. If the pregnancy test is positive, a vaginal ultrasound scan is performed that can provide a definitive diagnosis of ectopic or intrauterine pregnancy in 50–70% of cases. If the ultrasound findings are nondiagnostic and the patient is clinically stable, the serum hCG concentration is measured by radioimmunoassay (RIA). If the hCG concentration is > 3000 mIU/ml, a presumptive diagnosis of ectopic pregnancy is established. If the serum hCG concentration is < 3000 mIU/ml, the concentration is measured again 48 hours later and the doubling time (half-life) of hCG calculated.

Fortunately, there is now only one hCG standard available, and all hCG assays are standardized against it. The standard, formerly called the international reference preparation (IRP or 1st-IRP) has been renamed by the World Health Organization (WHO) as the 3rd international standard (3rd IS).

Some have advocated algorithms based on a serum progesterone measurement instead.[38] The use of serum progesterone measurements had its origins in the observation by Radwanska et al that the serum progesterone increased little during the first trimester of normal pregnancy, and that serum progesterone concentrations were lower in the presence of ectopic and aborting pregnancies than with normal intrauterine ones.[39] Thus it appeared that an age-independent measurement was available for first-trimester pregnancies that might be useful for differentiating normal and abnormal pregnancies. Rather implausibly, Mathews et al.[40] and Yeko et al.[41] subsequently suggested that ectopic and nonectopic gestations could be differentiated with 100% reliability on the basis of a single serum progesterone determination, an observation that has not withstood the test of time.[42-44] Although Stovall and colleagues[45] still favor a diagnostic algorithm centered on measuring the serum progesterone concentration, we have not found it to be useful in clinical practice.[39,44]

Color Doppler studies may eventually refine our ability to discriminate accurately between complete and incomplete intrauterine spontaneous abortions versus ectopic pregnancy.[46] Experience is currently still limited, as is the availability of the technology, making it impractical for widely utilized protocols.

Selection of Therapy

The optimal surgical management of tubal pregnancies has been a matter for debate since the turn of the twentieth century and remains so today. The debate originally centered on whether to save or remove the affected tube and subsequently on what type of operation to perform if the tube was to be removed or conserved. The advent of laparoscopic surgery did little to resolve these questions because each type of operation can be performed endoscopically just as well as via laparotomy; rather, controversy increased because additional questions were raised about the safety and efficacy of laparoscopic operations. Even before published data clearly established the advantages of laparoscopic surgery, however, the debate moved on to where it is today, focused on the place of nonsurgical therapy.

Compounding the problem of the many treatment options available has been an inability to interpret the results obtained with various operations. This lack of data is due to the fact that pregnancy rates after surgery (both tubal and intrauterine) have rarely been adjusted for the many factors other than the treatment itself that affect outcome following management of a tubal pregnancy. It is therefore not surprising that identical operations yielded statistics as disparate as live birth rates of 100% and 50%, for example, and recurrent ectopic pregnancy rates of 0% and 20%.[47,48]

A number of procedures have been virtually abandoned, such as resection of the ampulla, cornual resection at the time of salpingectomy, salpingo-oophorectomy, and under most circumstances "milking" of the tube. It also became apparent that salpingotomy incisions did not require closure, and that this operation yielded results comparable to those of segmental tubal resection, except perhaps in the case of isthmic pregnancies. Thus one was essentially left with a choice between salpingectomy and salpingotomy, which simply took one back to the original debate over the relative merits of conservative versus ablative operations.

Salpingotomy Versus Salpingectomy

Despite little conclusive support from published data, it is now widely accepted that a conservative operation is almost always preferred over an ablative one for women who are desirous of future child-bearing. It is not our intention to try to resolve this controversy because it is impossible to settle the dispute dispassionately with the evidence at hand. Suffice it to say that despite incontrovertible evidence that salpingotomy can restore the reproductive function of an oviduct after a tubal pregnancy and that repeat ectopic pregnancies are distributed with equal frequency between the conserved tubes and their contralateral counterparts, it does not follow that preservation of the affected tube, when the patient has another functional one, increases her chance of bearing a living child without increasing her risk of having another ectopic gestation.[49] In fact, most case series give no indication that tubal conservation increases subsequent live birth rates,[50-53] and in fact many show it to be associated with a trend toward higher rates of recurrent ectopic pregnancy. It is also incontestible that complications (hemorrhage, persistent trophoblast), however few, are more frequent after salpingotomy than after salpingectomy, which makes salpingotomy contraindicated in women who do not wish to bear more children. Despite these uncertainties, solid indications for salpingotomy can be identified, as discussed more fully elsewhere.[49]

Tubal conservation is clearly indicated if the pregnancy is located in a woman's only remaining tube or if the contralateral tube is occluded. The procedure is about three times more likely to result in a live birth than is in vitro fertilization; and if conception occurs, a term pregnancy is at least twice as likely as an ectopic pregnancy. Tubal conservation may be contraindicated if the contralateral tube and ovary appear to be normal and patent on intraoperative chromotubation but the gravid tube shows evidence of preexisting disease or has been operated on before for a previous ectopic pregnancy or blockage. When both tubes show evidence of prior disease, the decision to conserve the gravid tube when it has been operated on previously or when it appears to have been damaged much more than the opposite one is not easy and must be made on an individual basis, using as one's guide the extent to which the gravid fallopian tube has been damaged in absolute terms (amount of scarring, mobility, and length) and relative to the opposite side.

If the contralateral adnexa appears to be completely normal and patent at intraoperative chromotubation, the case for tubal conservation is not compelling. Those who favor salpingotomy argue that if a salpingectomy is performed and another ectopic pregnancy occurs, the opportunity to save what is then the only remaining tube may not present. This argument is the strongest one that justifies salpingotomy under these circumstances; but it is a weak one, as this eventuality is likely to occur in fewer than 5% of cases after salpingectomy. It has also been argued that intra-operative chromotubation is unreliable and that a normal-appearing tube may nonetheless be diseased. However, the problem with chromotubation is that a patent tube may appear blocked (usually because blood or decidua occlude the cornua), and patency on intraoperative chromotubation is clearly a valid finding. The case against salpingotomy is that when the contralateral tube and ovary are normal even the most favorable results obtained show no increase in the subsequent live birth rate. Tubal conservation probably does increase the recurrent tubal pregnancy rate, however, even if only by about 5%; and the risk of early and late postoperative hemorrhage is also greater.

Based on the available information, therefore, one can legitimately either perform a conservative or an extirpative operation in the presence of a normal contralateral adnexa. For example, if the pregnancy in the tube is small and unruptured and shells out easily at salpingotomy without bleeding, the tube should almost certainly be conserved. If there is a large ruptured tubal pregnancy present, however, or if after attempting a salpingotomy there is persistent bleeding from the tube, there is a much lower "threshold" for deciding to remove the gravid tube if the contralateral adnexa is normal than if the affected tube is the patient's only oviduct or if the contralateral adnexa is severely diseased.

Salpingotomy Versus Segmental Resection

Segmental tubal resection or partial salpingectomy is the procedure of choice whenever a gravid oviduct is to be conserved but its wall is ruptured or there is persistent or uncontrollable bleeding from the tube following salpingotomy. Although segmental resection with primary or delayed anastomosis has been advocated for the treatment of all tubal pregnancies on the grounds that salpingotomy conserves what is an abnormal implantation site, there is no evidence that better results are obtained by resecting the implantation site than by salpingotomy. Salpingotomy therefore remains the conservative operation of choice for tubal pregnancies.

There is persuasive evidence that the reproductive performance of women following conservative surgery for a tubal pregnancy is worse if the pregnancy is located in the isthmus than in the ampulla. Hallatt stated, without giving figures, that the intrauterine/ectopic pregnancy ratio after conservative surgery was about four times higher when the pregnancy was located in the ampulla than when it was in the isthmus.[54]

Ectopic pregnancy in the isthmic portion of the fallopian tube is uncommon. Whether the reproductive performance of women with isthmic pregnancies is any better after segmental tubal resection than after salpingotomy remains to be determined. DeCherney and Boyers have argued strongly that it is, but their argument is based on rather meager evidence. In a retrospective audit, they found that three of four women with unruptured isthmic pregnancies who were treated by salpingotomy had tubal occlusion on hysterosalpingography, and none conceived, whereas three of six women who were treated by segmental resection and delayed anastomosis delivered live infants, and one of six so treated had a recurrent tubal pregnancy.[55] However, Pouly et al[3] reported much better results with laparoscopic salpingotomy, as did Smith et al.[56] in a subsequent, randomized, prospective clinical study. Despite the small sample in the Smith et al.[56] study, all women who tried to become pregnant after salpingotomy conceived with an intrauterine pregnancy, results that provide a striking contrast to those reported by DeCherney and Boyers.[55]

In the series of 109 consecutive tubal pregnancies compiled by Reich et al;[7] there were nine isthmic tubal pregnancies; six were treated by partial salpingectomy and three by salpingotomy. No subsequent pregnancy occurred in either group. A future laparotomy for microsurgical tubal anastomosis is always necessary following laparoscopic partial tubal resection if a solitary tube is present.[7] This procedure can sometimes be avoided by a salpingotomy approach.

The optimal treatment of the unruptured isthmic pregnancy must therefore be considered subjective because the available data do not provide compelling evidence for treating women with isthmic and ampullary pregnancies differently. Because salpingotomy is much simpler, it should still be regarded as the operation of choice.

Laparoscopic Versus Abdominal Salpingotomy

Despite early skepticism, abundant data, including some from randomized trials, demonstrate that compared with the open operation laparoscopic salpingotomy is associated with a shorter hospital stay, shorter postoperative convalescence, reduced requirement for analgesia after surgery, and less postoperative adhesion formation.[8,10,57,58] Live birth rates are similar, but the recurrent ectopic pregnancy rate, surprisingly, tends to be lower for reasons that are unclear.[10,49]

An only absolute contraindication to laparoscopy is a hemodynamically unstable patient. Initially, the procedure was considered applicable to only a select group of patients (unruptured ampullary pregnancies < 3 cm with an otherwise normal pelvis and contralateral tube), but Reich et al.[7] were among the first to show that virtually all tubal pregnancies could be managed endoscopically unless the patient was hemodynamically unstable.

Laparoscopic Versus Nonsurgical Therapy

Since the mid 1980s increasing numbers of carefully selected patients with suspected or confirmed ectopic pregnancy have been managed nonsurgically. It is difficult to make direct comparisons between surgical and medical management, as patients qualifying for nonsurgical therapy are generally at early stages of pregnancy, stable, have low hCG levels, minimally impressive ultrasound findings, and no clinical evidence of rupture. Surgeons by default, inherit the difficult cases. Despite this scenario, medical therapy does have an important role in the management of ectopic pregnancy. As our diagnostic acumen continues to improve—hopefully resulting in earlier detection of ectopic gestations, often prior to tubal rupture—a greater proportion of patients will meet the criteria for nonsurgical therapy. Stovall and Ling reported that 41% of patients seen in their emergency department for possible ectopic pregnancy (all symptomatic) fit the criteria for medical management.[46] In the office setting, working with women at risk (as described above) or with infertility and careful monitoring of menses usually result in suspicion of ectopic gestation while the woman is still asymptomatic, allowing an even higher proportion of patients to choose nonsurgical care.

Diagnosis and Selection

Until nonsurgical diagnostic protocols had been proposed and evaluated, the use of methotrexate for treatment of ectopic pregnancy was somewhat illogical. Although it provides (in selected cases) results as good as conservative surgical therapy, it does not seem to be better in terms of resolution of the ectopic pregnancy, tubal patency, subsequent intrauterine pregnancy, or risk of repeat ectopic gestation. Time to complete resolution is roughly equivalent to conservative surgical management but can be psychologically more stressful to both patient and surgeon. Thus although diagnostic laparoscopy remained part of the standard evaluation prior to methotrexate therapy, no benefit accrued to the patient even though she might experience higher stress and cost.

Current nonsurgical diagnostic protocols allow consideration of medical therapy with potential savings in cost, pain, and hospital time. The diagnostic protocol prior to medical therapy need be no different than that prior to surgical therapy. Stovall et al. have advocated monitoring with serum progesterone levels, which generally add little to surgical decision making but may assist in the choice of nonsurgical protocols.[44,46] Progesterone levels < 5 ng/ml in untreated patients who are otherwise clinically stable are commonly observed, but these patients can be diagnosed by monitoring hCG levels and possibly vaginal ultrasonography. Those with levels > 25 ng/ml likely have an intrauterine pregnancy; but as previously discussed, the diagnosis is probably evident from the hCG level and ultrasound scans. (Any patient with a surgical abdomen still requires exploration.) Progesterone levels may also predict the outcome of methotrexate therapy. Ransom et al. examined a small number of patients receiving methotrexate for ectopic gestations (meeting the usual criteria). Of 11 patients with progesterone levels > 10 ng/ml, 6 eventually required surgical intervention, whereas all 10 patients with serum values < 10 ng/ml were successfully managed with medical measures alone.[59]

Dilatation and curettage has also been advocated[46] in the diagnostic protocol to distinguish an ectopic gestation from an intrauterine spontaneous abortion. Although this choice may make sense if curettage can be performed in the emergency room or office under local anesthesia, it could be argued that the cost and morbidity of dilatation and curettage meets or exceeds that of a single dose of methotrexate, which might simply be given in a presumptive fashion even without curettage results. This situation certainly exists when it is necessary to utilize a surgical suite for the procedure. Whereas a failing intrauterine pregnancy does not require the use of methotrexate, the presence of false-positive and false-negative results on curettage does obligate similar long-term follow up of hCG levels for either diagnosis, resulting in almost no cost savings if methotrexate is not given. Similarly, nearly all reported side effects from methotrexate administration occur if more than a single dose is given, which would not be necessary in the case of a spontaneous abortion treated mistakenly.

Observation

It has long been known that a number of tubal pregnancies resorb spontaneously without treatment, and observation alone with no active intervention is an appropriate way to manage a woman with a presumed ectopic pregnancy who has minimal symptoms, hCG concentrations < 1000 mIU/ml and falling (half-life < 1.5 days), and an adnexal mass (if visualized) of < 3.5 cm.[60] Perhaps one of three early ectopic gestations can be managed in this fashion, with 30% eventually requiring surgical management or methotrexate.[61] The type of patient who goes on to have a chronic ectopic pregnancy must be better defined.

Fernandez et al. conducted a long-term follow-up of a group of 49 patients treated conservatively, including 16 with expectant management.[61] Of these women, nine desired subsequent pregnancy, eight demonstrated tubal patency on the side of the ectopic pregnancy by hysterosalpingogram, and eight eventually achieved one or more normal pregnancies with the only recurrent ectopic gestation occurring in one of the three women who did not desire pregnancy. The average time to conception was 16.6 months.

Women who have a relatively small (< 3.5 cm), unruptured pregnancy, preferably with no fetal cardiac activity or maternal hepatic or renal insufficiency, and are comfortable with treatment can be managed with methotrexate therapy.

Local Injection of Methotrexate

Intratubal injection of methotrexate theoretically has the advantages of being a simple surgical technique producing fewer side effects than systemic injection. In an early randomized prospective trial, laparoscopic tubal injection of methotrexate was discontinued after only seven patients had been treated because of the high failure rates.[19] Subsequent analysis of this report suggested that the concentration and volume of methotrexate (25 mg/7 ml) might have been inappropriate, and the criteria defining failure may have been too broad.[62] A later prospective randomized trial with a larger number of patients (29 with intratubal methotrexate, 24 with laser salpingotomy) reported better results utilizing 20 mg/0.8 ml, with equal treatment failures in each group (10–12%) and similar tubal patency rates after therapy (65–75%).[63] In this study it was recognized that rising or plateaued hCG rates did not necessarily represent failure, as many of these cases resolved. The patients were highly selected in this study, as only patients with masses < 4 cm diameter were included.

One long-term follow-up study of 33 patients treated with ultrasound guided local injection of methotrexate reported a 70% success rate for therapy (10 required eventual laparoscopy).[61] Of the 17 women in this study desiring future pregnancy, 15 had patency demonstrated by hysterosalpingography on the side of the ectopic pregnancy. Four patients had only one tube at the time of treatment, and all four exhibited tubal patency after treatment; two conceived. Eight other patients became pregnant, with seven term deliveries. The average time to conception was 8.6 months.

Although these and similar studies may have demonstrated that in selected cases methotrexate injection could be as effective as salpingotomy, they did not demonstrate any real advantage except that it is a marginally easier technique. Patients still undergo the cost, pain, and risks of surgery. Several other investigations have demonstrated equivalent success with ultrasound guided percutaneous[64] and transvaginal[65,66] injection. A similar technique, transcervical fallopian tube cannulation with local delivery of methotrexate has also been described.[67] These initial studies had similar selection restrictions and were not controlled. Success rates were similar to those seen with systemic therapy, and in fact a pharmacokinetic study suggested little difference in peak serum levels after intratubal and intramuscular injection.[68] Because the local injection techniques require additional expertise and are more invasive, they seem to offer little advantage over systemic therapy.

Systemic Methotrexate

Early large trials of methotrexate therapy utilized multiple doses of methotrexate (1 mg/kg IM every other day for four doses) alternating with leucovorin (0.1 mg/kg IM every other day).[69,70] Therapeutic failures occurred in about 5% of cases; the figures for tubal patency, subsequent intrauterine pregnancy, and repeat ectopic pregnancy were all similar to those for surgical therapy. Criteria for this therapeutic choice are the same as those described above. More recently, successful therapy has been described utilizing a single intramuscular dose of methotrexate 50 mg/m^2.[60,71,72] This regimen has the advantage of producing fewer side effects and costing less. It is important to recognize that abdominal cramping is a common symptom (15–30% of patients) 3–7 days after methotrexate administration and does not call for surgical intervention if it is the only symptom. Likewise, reversal of hCG levels to zero is a slow process, averaging 4 weeks and occasionally taking up to 8–10 weeks.[71,72]

Cost

In an interesting retrospective analysis of records and billing statements of all patients treated for ectopic pregnancy at San Francisco General Hospital in 1991, Creinin and Washington[73] estimated that 15 of 50 patients (30%) would have been eligible for methotrexate therapy. When all direct and indirect surgical costs were compared to estimated costs of methotrexate therapy (including laboratory evaluation, long term follow up, and surgical management of failures), the use of medical management for appropriate patients was calculated to save 24%, or $161,000, for these 50 cases. On a national basis the saving would amount to $270 million annually. Although these amounts are substantial, all of the cases reported in this study were managed by laparotomy, adding substantially to the hospital costs and indirect costs (lost wages). Use of laparoscopy has been found to decrease direct costs by $1500–2000 when compared to laparotomy, with an additional decrease in indirect costs expected.[10] Thus similar cost savings would be expected nationally if most ectopic pregnancies were handled laparoscopically.

Equipment

Laparoscopic electrosurgical techniques are ideally suited for tubal pregnancy surgery. Bipolar forceps, which permit high-frequency low-voltage current (25–50 watts) to be passed through its jaws, are used for desiccation of the proximal tube, its mesosalpinx, and in rare cases the infundibulopelvic ligament with enclosed ovarian vessels and the uteroovarian ligament[74] (Fig. 11.4).

A knife electrode is an excellent instrument for correcting a tubal occlusion with a salpingotomy incision. The blades of the laparoscopic scissors can be used in a similar fashion, as can the CO_2 laser. The knife electrode is connected to a low-voltage electrosurgical generator, and unipolar cutting current (40–80 watts) is used (Table 11.2). Pure cutting current is critical for precision and to minimize the low-grade thermal coagulation zone in surrounding tissue. Coagulation current is used only for fulgurating specific blood vessels or hemorrhagic ovarian cysts.

Throughout most laparoscopic procedures a suction-irrigator-dissector is essential for evacuating smoke, removing clots, retracting tissues, atraumatically elevating the tube or ovary, irrigating the fallopian tube and cul-de-sac, and developing surgical planes (aquadissection). Viable products of conception, without surrounding organized blood clots, can often be evacuated completely from a fallopian tube using a suction-irrigator; trophoblastic tissue with surrounding blood clots can be irrigated from the tubal lumen using the hydraulic pressure of the fluid irrigant.

A laser beam can be used to incise the tube and perform a laparoscopic salpingostomy. The laser is usually not practical for unscheduled (emergency) surgery. The insurance policies of many hospitals mandate that a separate "laser

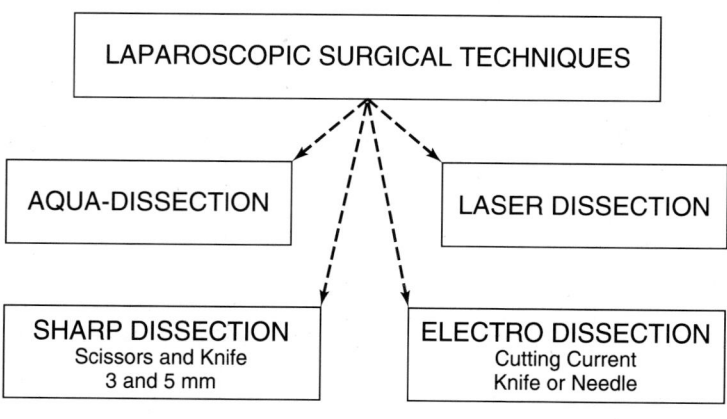

Figure 11.4. Laparoscopic surgical techniques.

Table 11.2. Wolf knife electrode

Setting	Valleylab SSE2 electrosurgical generator			SSE2 with low-power attenuator		
	Cut	Blend	Coag	Cut	Blend	Coag
0	0	0	0	0	0	0
1	0	0	0	0	0	0
2	70	35	20	0	0	0
3	150	85	30	5	0	0
4	195	115	40	15	2	0
5	220	145	55	25	5	2
6	250	160	65	30	8	3
7	280	175	75	40	10	5
8	310	190	90	50	12	7
9	340	220	100	60	15	9
10	370	260	120	70	20	10

Power is in watts. The apparatus is monopolar. Settings in boldface should be avoided.

nurse" be present for laser surgery in addition to the necessary scrub and circulating nurses, often an impossibility during the middle of the night.

Basic Techniques

All operations are performed under general anesthesia with endotracheal intubation. Steep Trendelenburg position (30°) is helpful, as is a high-flow CO_2 insufflator capable of delivering CO_2 at 10 L/min. This step is followed by insertion of a uterine manipulator for tubal lavage and uterine manipulation. A 10 mm laparoscope is inserted through a vertical intraumbilical incision, and lower quadrant 5 mm puncture sites are established just below the pubic hairline and lateral to the inferior epigastric vessels. The aquadissector, the "workhorse instrument," in most cases is placed on a sterile table behind the surgeon and connected to wall suction and to a pressurized source of irrigant (usually Ringer's lactate). The tubing of the aquadissector, which is manipulated by the surgeon's left hand, frequently kinks when stretched across the abdomen to a right-sided abdominal puncture site. It is important for the operator to be consistent with incisions, regardless of the pathology involved; such consistency results in a reproducible procedure with a resultant reduction in intraoperative decision-making. Devices or assistants can be used to stabilize the laparoscopic trocar sleeve, allowing the surgeon to operate with two hands, each holding a lower quadrant instrument.

Any adhesions on the contralateral tube are usually treated during the same laparoscopic procedure. At the close of each procedure excess CO_2 is expelled, and 2 L of Ringer's lactate is left in the peritoneal cavity to keep visceral surfaces separated during the early healing process. Postoperatively, Rh immunoglobulin (RhIg) is administered to unsensitized Rh-negative patients with an ectopic pregnancy (50 μg RhIg is usually adequate to prevent sensitization). Documentation of successful treatment includes weekly quantitative β-hCG titers until a negative test is attained.

Evacuation of Hemoperitoneum

Usually the suction-irrigator is sufficient to evacuate the hemoperitoneum, including large clots. In cases of tubal rupture the patient may be unstable, and the hemoperitoneum and clots may be excessive. For these cases it is best to insert an 11 mm left lower quadrant trocar (similar to the umbilical trocar) and thread the wall suction tubing directly through it (DAVOL Suction Tubing with a diameter of .25 inch; Cranston, RI.) Wells Johnson (Tucson, AZ) aspiration tubing, with an internal diameter of 0.281 inch, can also be attached just above the trumpet valve of an 11 mm trocar sleeve. By aspirating the larger clots directly, one can avoid obstructing the suction-irrigation device. Visualization of the site of rupture or active bleeding can thus be rapidly obtained and treatment initiated. If prompt control is impossible, immediate laparotomy should be considered.

Laparoscopic Salpingectomy

After following evacuation of any hemoperitoneum, Kleppinger bipolar forceps and laparoscopic hook scissors are introduced successively to desiccate and cut the tube and its mesosalpinx. Bipolar continuous sinusoidal wave current (cutting) at 25 watts should be used (Fig. 11.5). An endpoint monitor is essential to indicate the completion of desiccation and avoid char sticking to the forceps, as carbonization occurs thereafter. A loop ligature can also be used around the distended tube to perform salpingectomy safely (Fig. 11.6).

The segment of tube with its enclosed ectopic pregnancy is then removed from the peritoneal cavity through the 11 mm umbilical trocar sleeve, using forceps placed through the operating port of a right-angle operating laparoscope. The laparoscope, forceps, sleeve, and portion of the tube within the trocar sleeve are removed in one motion, resulting in either complete or partial removal of the tube, which can then be grasped with a hemostat and teased out through the umbilical incision. The laparoscope and sleeve are reinserted and final inspection performed. Removal of a fallopian tube in this manner may result in a "milking" process, leaving products of conception extruded from the

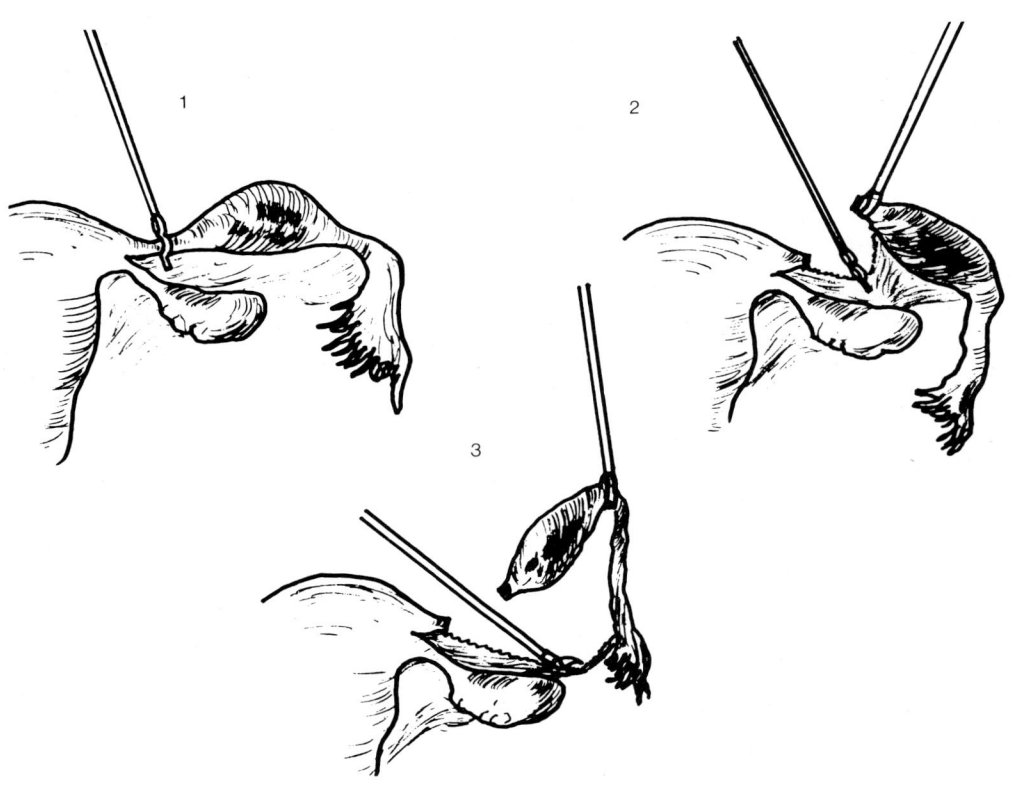

Figure 11.5. (1) Coagulation of the tube adjacent to a tubal pregnancy using bipolar forceps. (2) Coagulation of the mesosalpinx. (3) Division of the mesosalpinx using laparoscopic scissors. (Reprinted with permission from the American College of Obstetricians and Gynecologists (Obstet Gynecol 1986;67:301))

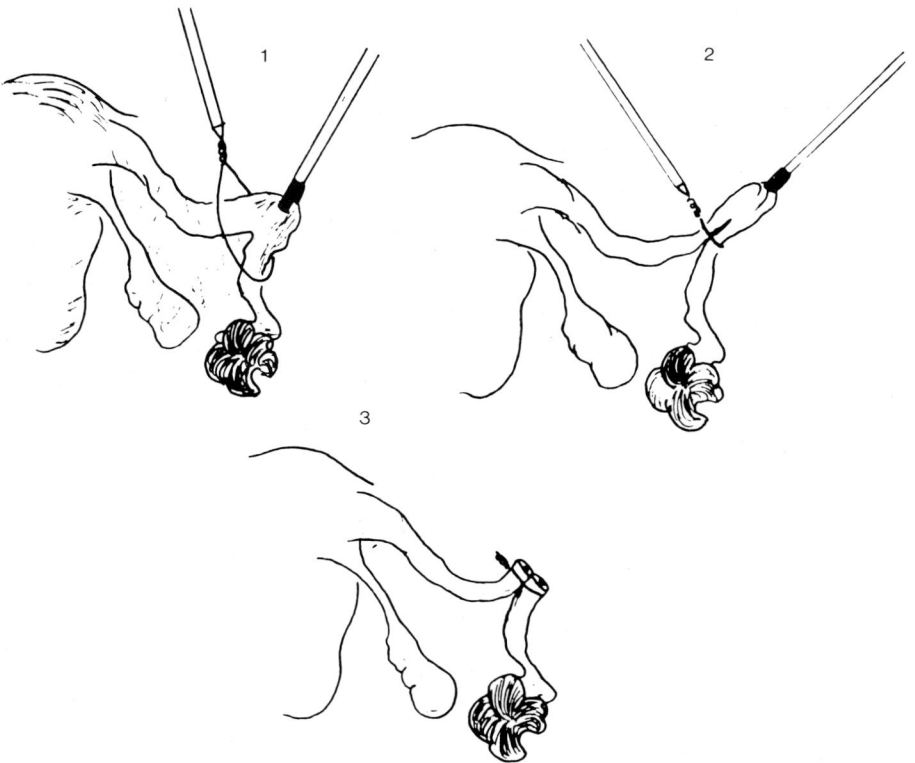

Figure 11.6. (1) Placement of the Endoloop around a tubal pregnancy. (2) Tightening of the Endoloop knot using a pusher. (3) End result after excision of the segment of the tube with its enclosed pregnancy. (Reprinted with permission from the American College of Obstetricians and Gynecologists (Obstet Gynecol 1986;67:301))

tube in the peritoneal cavity as it is being pulled through the trocar sleeve. They can then be removed with the aquadissector or biopsy forceps. Salpingotomy (ampullotomy) with aspiration of the products of conception may be considered for reducing its volume before extraction of the tube through the umbilical trocar sleeve, thereby preventing the "milking" effect.

The umbilical extension technique developed by one of the authors (H.R.) is a better method for removing of tubes containing products of conception from the peritoneal cavity. The umbilical incision is always made inside the umbilicus, overlying the area where skin, deep fascia, and parietal peritoneum of the anterior abdominal wall meet. This incision can be enlarged using the operating laparoscope with scissors in the operating channel. The tip of the laparoscope is placed 1 cm from the tip of the trocar sleeve, which is then gently removed from the peritoneal cavity. The peritoneum is first visualized and can then be incised downward in the midline with the scissors in the operating channel of the operating laparoscope. Next, the deep fascia is identified and incised to add another 1–2 cm to the incision. Finally, the skin incision inside the umbilicus can be extended upward to incorporate the superior wall of the umbilical fossa.[75]

The products of conception can also be removed through a lower quadrant 5- or 11-mm trocar sleeve. Alternatively, a culdotomy can be made using laparoscopic techniques: A sponge at the end of a ring forceps is placed just behind the cervix to identify the posterior cul-de-sac. A second sponge or probe is placed in the rectum and then removed; this step confirms the anatomic relation of the rectum to the posterior vagina and thus serves to identify any abnormal tenting of the rectum in this area. A 2- 3-mm spot size CO_2 laser beam with power set at 60–100 watts continuous is then directed through the laser laparoscope to make a transverse culdotomy incision directly over the posterior fornix sponge. Alternately, a spoon electrode at 150 watts cutting current can be employed. Thereafter the usually large tubal pregnancy can be pushed through the incision made from above or pulled through from below with laparoscopic biopsy forceps, ring forceps, or the surgeon's fingers, all under direct visualization.

Laparoscopic Partial Salpingectomy (Midtube Resection)

Kleppinger bipolar forceps are used to coagulate the tube on each side of the distention made by the tubal pregnancy. The resultant desiccated areas are then divided with laparoscopic hook scissors. The mesosalpinx supplying the involved tubal segment is next coagulated and divided, and the tube segment is removed from the peritoneal cavity through the 11 mm umbilical trocar sleeve or by laparoscopic culdotomy.

With another technique, a loop ligature (Endoloop) can be placed around the tube segment with its enclosed ectopic pregnancy. This loop is inserted into a special applicator and introduced into the pelvis through the 5 mm trocar sleeve. The tube and its mesosalpinx are divided with laparoscopic scissors. Should the loop ligature slip, the pedicle can always be regrasped and either another Endoloop ligature placed or complete hemostasis obtained using bipolar forceps (Fig. 11.6).

Laparoscopic Salpingotomy

After evacuation of the hemoperitoneum, the tuboovarian complex is mobilized usually with the aid of an aquadissector. In many cases a "phlegmon" of tube–ovary exists that should be separated using the aquadissector.

The knife electrode is used to make a 1- to 2-cm incision (Fig. 11.7) in the antimesenteric border over the point of maximal tubal dilatation using cutting current (50–80 watts). Alternatively, scissors or the CO_2 laser at 25–35 watts superpulse can be used. Tubal layers are often identified (i.e., serosa followed by stretched muscularis mucosa) prior to entering the tubal lumen. Occasionally a blood clot is expressed from the extraluminal space prior to separately opening the muscularis mucosa.

Often after placing the salpingotomy incision products of conception begin to extrude. At this point the aquadissector is used to suction loose, friable products of conception that may be present with viable ectopic pregnancies. In cases where a blood clot has formed firmly around the products of conception, irrigation from the aquadissector can be used to mobilize the clot with its enclosed gestational tissue. Occasionally it is necessary to insert atraumatic grasping forceps into the tube to mobilize the products of conception with a spreading motion prior to using the aquadissector to effect expulsion. These same forceps are also used to check the lumen of the tube after evacuation. Finally, toothed biopsy forceps are necessary in some cases to grasp and tease out products of conception closely adherent to the tubal wall.

Removal of the products of conception from the peritoneal cavity is accomplished as previously described using the 11 mm umbilical trocar sleeve and the operating laparoscope with enclosed biopsy forceps. Sometimes the products of conception can be reduced to small segments using biopsy forceps and the aquadissector.

The fallopian tube is then irrigated distally with the aquadissector and proximally through a cervical Cohen cannula. The salpingotomy incision is usually left open. If the defect is large or marked eversion of mucosa occurs, a 4–0 Vicryl or polydioxanone suture (PDS: Ethicon Z-420) can be placed.[76] Should bleeding from the tubal edge or implantation site be present after evacuating the products of conception, compression with grasping forceps should be attempted prior to resorting to electrosurgical coagulation, laser, or a suture. Frequently, 5 minutes of pressure at the salpingotomy edge results in complete hemostasis. In other instances, lifting the adnexa above the pelvic brim—in effect, kinking the mesosalpingeal vessels—yields a similar result.

If uncontrollable hemorrhage occurs during evacuation of the ampulla, the segment of the

11. Ectopic Pregnancy

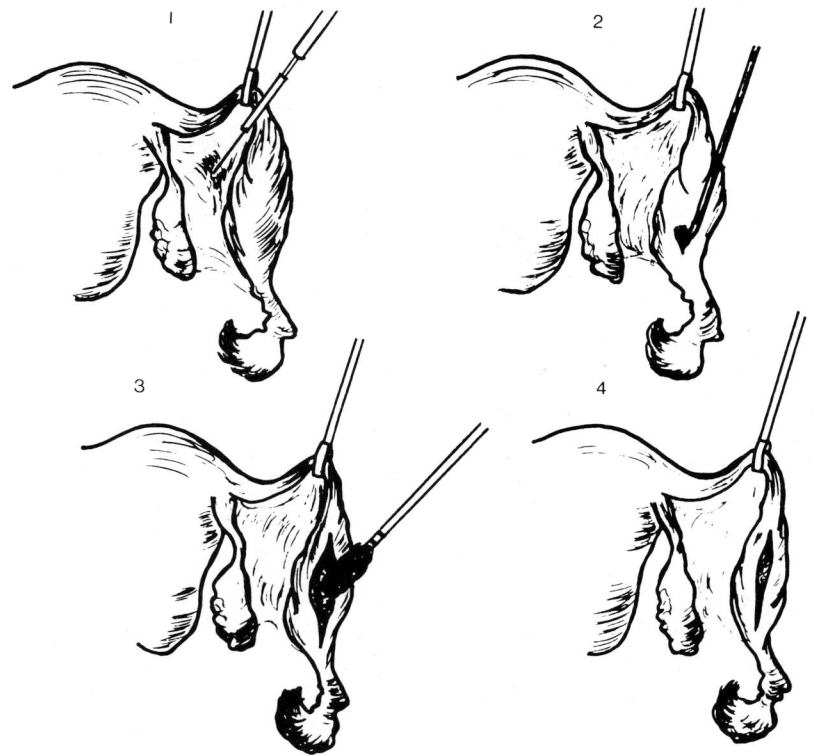

Figure 11.7. (1) Vasopressin injection into the mesosalpinx. (2) Salpingotomy incision with knife electrode electrosurgery. (3) Evaluation of products of conception from the tube. (4) Salpingotomy incision left open at the end of the procedure. (Reprinted with permission from the American College of Obstetricians and Gynecologists (Obstet Gynecol 1986;67:301))

tube can be loosely ligated with an Endoloop as described by Semm.[77] The cul-de-sac and subphrenic space are irrigated and evacuated. After 5–10 minutes the ligature is released. In most cases the bleeding subsides. If not, selected areas in the mesosalpinx can be suture ligated; or if the contralateral tube appears normal, salpingectomy or partial salpingectomy can be performed as previously described.

The mesosalpinx can be infiltrated with a dilute vasopressin solution (Fig. 11.7) before salpingotomy (Pitressin; Parke Davis, Morris Plains, NJ) as first described by Bruhat's group.[1] A mixture of 20 U (one ampul) in 50 ml of normal saline works well, though more dilute or more concentrated solutions may be used. A 5 mm injection and puncture cannula can be used through the lower quadrant trocar sleeves. Alternatively, a 22-gauge spinal needle can be inserted directly through the skin at the pubic hairline usually just lateral to the inferior epigastric vessels. Care must be taken at initial insertion into the mesosalpinx to avoid direct injection into the blood vessels by gently puncturing the serosa prior to infiltration of the solution. Thereafter 10–20 ml of the solution can be infiltrated, which should cause a grossly visible swelling in the mesosalpinx.

The pharmacologic effect of vasopressin persists for approximately 2 hours and is probably sufficient to allow physiologic hemostasis to occur. It cannot be overemphasized that great care is necessary during penetration of the mesosalpingeal peritoneum to avoid vessel laceration or intravascular injection, which can cause arterial hypertension. Extravascular injection itself can induce a moderate increase in the arterial blood pressure or moderate bradycardia. Complications from vasopressin administration have been reported, and both Bruhat's group and we no longer use it during laparoscopic procedures.

Fimbrial Evacuation of Tubal Pregnancy

Fimbrial evacuation, tubal aspiration without salpingotomy, and tubal abortion without salpingotomy refer to the technique of removing products of conception at or near the fimbrial end of the tube using either suction or grasping forceps and, on occasion, using grasping forceps to gently push the products of conception toward the fimbrial end (milking). In some cases tubal abortion is already in progress.

Concern regarding incomplete removal of trophoblast and increased tubal damage has resulted in the condemnation of fimbrial evacuation of a tubal pregnancy using either laparoscopic or laparotomy techniques, especially after the 1980 study by Budowick et al., which implied that most tubal pregnancies occur in the extraluminal space.[23] The findings of Sherman et al. may encourage the laparoscopic surgeon to reconsider this method. In a laparotomy series Sherman's group successfully expressed 31 unruptured tubal gestations through the fimbriated end of the tube. Of 27 women followed for more than 3 years, 25 later conceived, resulting in 23 term pregnancies, 2 spontaneous abortions, and no repeat ectopic pregnancies.[78]

If most ampullary tubal pregnancies rapidly invade the tubal wall and grow in the loose connective tissue between mucosa and serosa, milking the ectopic pregnancy out of the fimbria would cause further tubal destruction. We have not seen a high incidence of extraluminal tubal pregnancies and have treated 8 of the last 18 tubal pregnancies by "aqua-expression." With this technique, in selected cases of nonviable intraluminal ampullary ectopic pregnancy, the tip of the aquadissector is inserted through the open end of the affected tube into the ampulla, and fluid under pressure is used to dislodge and expel the intraluminal products of conception with surrounding blood clot (a tubal cast) without a salpingotomy incision. They can then be aspirated from the peritoneal cavity. There were no intraoperative or postoperative complications. β-hCG titers were in the nonpregnant range 2 weeks after surgery in all cases.[79]

hCG Monitoring After Conservative Therapy

Several tacit assumptions underlie the policy of screening for residual trophoblastic activity after conservative therapy for tubal pregnancy. The first assumption is that in the absence of residual functioning trophoblast the serum hCG level falls unabatedly and in a predictable manner. The second assumption is that a period of renewed trophoblastic growth is required for symptoms to develop. The third assumption is that during this preclinical stage renewed trophoblastic growth manifests first as a delayed rate of fall in the serum hCG levels and eventually by rising serum hCG values.

Vermesh et al. described the use of serial postoperative hCG and progesterone measurements following conservative operative treatment of tubal pregnancies. They found that even in patients with persistent trophoblastic activity hCG levels fell precipitously during the early postoperative period, reaching 13–25% of the baseline value by 3 days after surgery and 6–25% by 6 days. Thereafter the serum hCG in the "persistent ectopic" group and the "resolved ectopic" group diverged, there being no overlap at all between the groups by the 12th postoperative day. However, Vermesh et al. did not clarify the definition of persistent trophoblastic activity inasmuch as two of six patients with this diagnosis had continually decreasing hCG values and were managed by simple observation.[80]

Conversely, in a study of 32 women treated with laparoscopic laser salpingotomy ($n = 14$) or local injection of methotrexate ($n = 18$), Thompson et al. found that in 29 cases there was plateauing of hCG levels sometime during the first 17 days, most commonly during the first week after therapy.[81] Although this finding might seem understandable in the case of local methotrexate injection (because of additional trophoblast proliferation while the antimetabolic action of methotrexate is taking effect), it was also found in most of the salpingotomy cases. Reaction to plateaus or slight increases in hCG levels, especially during the first week after therapy, can lead to overtreatment with methotrexate or unnecessary repeat surgery, both modalities increasing the side effects.

"Normal" limits for the rate of hCG clearance are difficult to define because the dynamics of hCG clearance are complex, involving at least two half-lives (an initial half-life of 5–6 hours and a second, slower one of 11–38 hours). The between-patients variation in the rate of hCG clearance is also large. Part of the reason may be that unless a pregnancy is terminated by salpingectomy or hysterectomy some trophoblast is always disseminated into the circulation and continues to secrete hCG. With tubal pregnancies the presence or absence of trophoblastic tissue within the tubal wall is an added factor that complicates and increases the variability of hCG clearance rates. Consequently, no hCG pattern invariably presages continued trophoblastic growth or predicts resolution of the pregnancy.

Because the bulk of the trophoblast is removed during surgery (barring gross technical errors), hCG levels invariably fall precipitously during the first few days after surgery even in patients destined to develop symptoms from continued trophoblastic growth. There is therefore no merit in measuring the hCG concentration earlier than a week after surgery because hCG levels in women with persistent and resolving trophoblastic activity overlap before this time.[80] Therefore hCG measurements should commence 1 week after conservative surgery, but the optimal method for monitoring patients has not been defined, and few studies have been undertaken to identify those at particular risk for developing this problem. Those who have an hCG concentration > 1000 mIU/ml at 1 week after surgery are probably at greater risk,[82] and hCG titers should be monitored every 3 days. If the level is < 1000 mIU/ml at 1 week after surgery, the assay can be performed at weekly intervals until the levels become negative or at least < 100 mIU/ml.

In the absence of symptoms, intervention is not indicated so long as hCG levels continue to fall, however slowly. Rising values are more ominous but do not invariably presage continued trophoblastic growth. A reasonable compromise between overtreatment and undertreatment is to intervene if the rate of increase is "normal" (i.e., the doubling time is < 2.7 days) or to follow subnormally increasing levels for a few days with repeat measurements to ensure that the rising pattern persists (because it often does not) before intervening. We intervene with chemotherapy and have always used methotrexate 50 mg/m² IM, which is effective with uncomplicated trophoblastic disease.

Persistent Trophoblastic Tissue and Persistent Ectopic Pregnancy

Successful conservative treatment of tubal pregnancy is documented by declining quantitative β-hCG levels. Persistent trophoblastic tissue has been described and implies the continued presence or growth of trophoblastic tissue within the tube or peritoneal cavity after conservative surgery. It should be suspected if serum levels of β-hCG are detectable 2 weeks postoperatively. Thereafter titers should be followed and a tentative diagnosis made if titers plateau or rise. A second laparoscopy or a regimen of methotrexate may then be considered, with laparoscopy being the preference if clinical symptoms of tubal rupture or hemorrhage are present.

In at least 40% of tubal pregnancies the trophoblast penetrates the tubal wall, and some trophoblastic tissue is left behind if the implantation site is not removed, as is the case with a salpingotomy. This tissue usually degenerates; but in about 5% of cases, instead of resorbing, the residual trophoblastic tissue persists and resumes growing until the patient eventually develops symptoms due to intraperitoneal hemorrhage or a pelvic mass. The frequency of this complication is ill-defined. It is also slightly more common after laparoscopic salpingotomy than after abdominal salpingotomy. Stock attributed the problem to incomplete evacuation of the trophoblastic tissue.[83] Seifer et al.,[84] in a comparison of 11 patients with persistent trophoblastic tissue with those whose pathology resolved postoperatively, noted an association with small pregnancies (< 2 cm), early pregnancies (< 6 weeks from last menses), and persistence. They speculated that it may be caused by poorly defined planes between trophoblast and the implantation site due to less hemorrhage prior to surgery. They recommended careful follow-up of patients who have an early ectopic gestation.

Persistent ectopic pregnancy implies the presence of persistent trophoblastic tissue within the fallopian tube after salpingotomy or fimbrial aspiration. Persistent ectopic pregnancy presents with signs of intraperitoneal hemorrhage or pain referable to a pelvic mass usually 10 days or more after the original surgery and occasionally as early as 1 week later.[85]

Serial hCG monitoring after conservative operations has been instituted in the hope of forestalling this problem by identifying persistent trophoblastic activity at an asymptomatic stage. Serial ultrasound imaging of the adnexal mass (at least in patients managed with methotrexate therapy initially) has been shown to be of little value and is potentially misleading. Brown et al. followed 18 patients treated with methotrexate and found that resolution of the mass took up to 3 months, in some cases well beyond the point of negative hCG titers.[86] Enlarging masses did not predict treatment failure (this finding might logically be extrapolated to postsurgical management), and ultrasonography overall did not contribute to management decisions.

If laparoscopy is the chosen approach, a second salpingotomy procedure is usually effective. Alternatively, a partial salpingectomy procedure can be done using either the Endoloop ligature or bipolar coagulation.

In our series of 109 consecutive tubal pregnancies treated laparoscopically, one persistent ectopic pregnancy occurred and was treated with a second laparoscopic salpingotomy procedure 4 weeks later. Four other women had persistent β-hCG titers: Laparoscopy 4 weeks later revealed ectopic trophoblastic tissue on the pelvic side wall and cul-de-sac peritoneum. Treatment consisted of excision with laparoscopic biopsy forceps, laser vaporization, or both.[7,87]

Persistent trophoblastic tissue has been successfully treated with methotrexate without a laparoscopic procedure.[88] Criteria for utilization of methotrexate versus laparoscopy in this circumstance should be similar to the choice for the initial therapy. When more intense abdominal symptoms are present, if hCG levels are > 5000 mIU/ml, if hepatic function tests or hematologic values are abnormal, or if a patient does not take prescribed medication, laparoscopy is the preferred choice. In most other situations, especially asymptomatic serial increases in hCG levels, methotrexate may be most appropriate. Care must be taken in this situation to monitor the patient for signs of tubal rupture, which can occur at a considerable interval (2–4 weeks) after the initial therapy.

Reproductive outcome in 50 women treated for persistent ectopic therapy and followed for at least 1 year afterward has been reported by Seifer et al.[89] Treatment for persistent ectopic gestation was repeat salpingotomy in seven cases, partial or complete salpingectomy in 27 (half of the surgical interventions were laparoscopic), and methotrexate in 16; 32 of these 50 women attempted pregnancy after treatment (5 salpingotomy, 16 salpingectomy, and 11 methotrexate). Four of the women attempting a pregnancy had only one fallopian tube. Conceptions occurred in 3 of 5 women after salpingotomy (one miscarriage), 12 of 16 after salpingectomy, and 4 of 11 after methotrexate (two miscarriages). There was a significant correlation between having a normal contralateral tube (probably a higher percentage of women undergoing salpingectomy) and subsequent conception. Patients treated with methotrexate took longer to conceive but had been advised to use contraception for 4 months after therapy. The cumulative clinical pregnancy rate by life table analysis was 59% at 36 months. These rates are comparable to those seen after primary therapy of ectopic pregnancy.

Special Situations

Cornual (Interstitial) Ectopic Pregnancy

Cornual ectopic pregnancy is rare, and few reports exist regarding its treatment via laparoscopy. Both Johns et al.[7] and Reich et al.[90] have noted isthmic tubal pregnancies bordering on cornual pregnancies; that is, the proximal portion of the tubal dilatation caused by the ectopic pregnancy was in the uterine wall. These three cases were treated laparoscopically

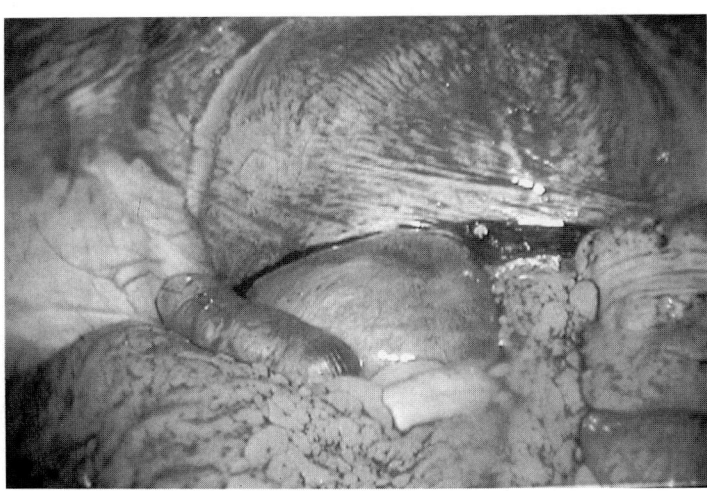

Figure 11.8. Left tubal pregnancy seen with surrounding hemoperitoneum.

by segmental resection resulting in preservation of most of the distal portion of the tube but destruction of much interstitium, making the success of a future anastomosis unlikely.[7,90] Tubal implantation would still be possible, however.

The diagnosis of interstitial ectopic pregnancy may be missed at laparoscopy. It may be suspected when the endometrial cavity is empty and both fallopian tubes look normal despite a β-hCG value indicating an existing pregnancy. Bulging or nodularity is usually present in the cornual area.

Methotrexate may be considered for treatment of cornual ectopic pregnancy, and there are two reports documenting its successful use.[91] Tanaka et al. in 1982 reported a case where an interstitial ectopic pregnancy was diagnosed at laparotomy, following which the abdomen was closed and the patient treated with methotrexate.[92]

Subsequently, three slightly larger series documented 12 cases of interstitial pregnancy treated with methotrexate (or KCl in two cases of heterotopic pregnancy), either systemically or locally injected.[93-95]

Extraluminal Tubal Pregnancy

In most cases of extraluminal ectopic pregnancy, when opening the tubal serosa over the most distended portion of the tube products of conception are evident and may extrude. If spontaneous extrusion does not occur, as there is no surrounding muscularis, trophoblastic tissue must be removed in pieces, with special care taken not to avulse the normal tube. Thereafter irrigation with the aquadissector produces distention of the tube without flow of irrigant out of the fimbrial end. The operator can err by trying to open the tube further if bleeding is present (Fig. 11.8–11.13).

In our experience with these cases, it is rarely necessary to enter the tubal lumen. Occasionally the blood clot or products of conception encircle the space between the serosa and the muscularis. After removing the bulk of the products of conception and obtaining hemostasis with pressure or electrosurgical fulguration with an electrode or an argon beam coagulator, the surgeon should end the procedure and follow the patient carefully with β-hCG titers. Adjuvant therapy with methotrexate may be considered.

Ruptured Tubal Pregnancy

In the series of 109 consecutive tubal pregnancies compiled by Reich et al.,[7] there were 16 cases of ruptured tubal pregnancy. Total or partial salpingectomy was performed in 13 of these patients and salpingotomy in 3. Subsequently, two women had intrauterine pregnancies. Another woman who underwent salpingectomy has since had two pregnancies in her remaining tube, both treated by laparoscopic salpingotomy.[7]

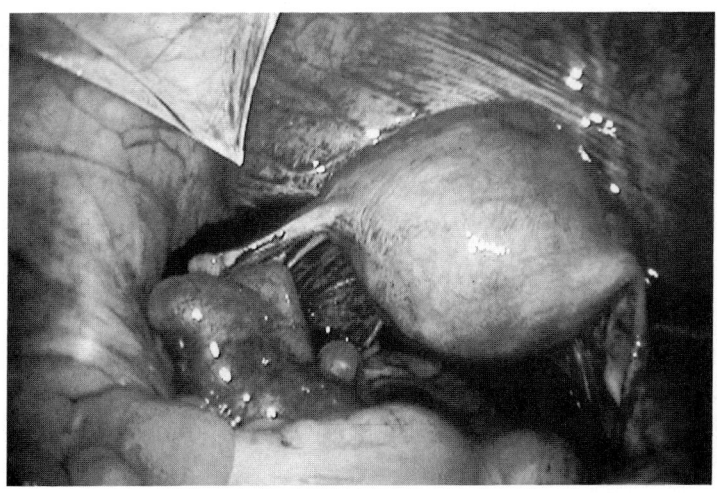

Figure 11.9. Trendelenburg position exposes the uterus, tubes, and ovaries. Left-sided 5 mm trocar is inserted lateral to the rectus muscle.

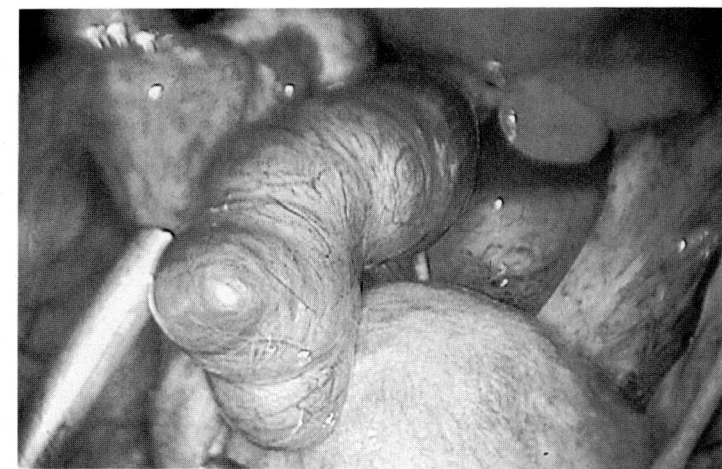

Figure 11.10. Ectopic pregnancy occupies the ampulla of the left fallopian tube and can be seen distending the tubal serosa, indicating a probable extraluminal location between the tubal serosa and muscularis.

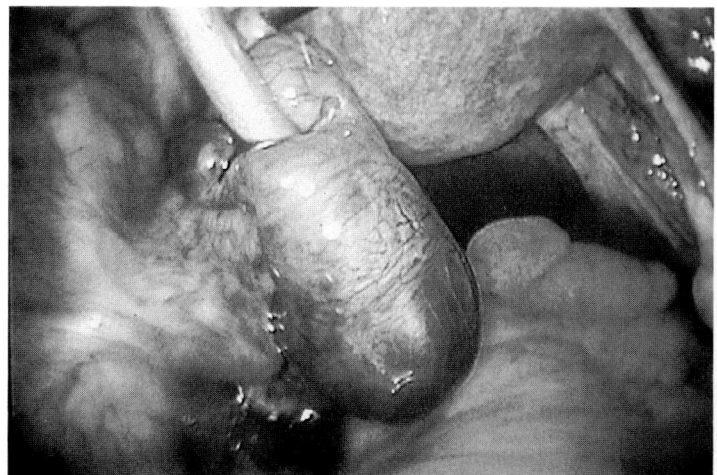

Figure 11.11. Aquadissector is inserted into the salpingotomy incision in the tubal serosa and is used to flush out the ectopic gestation.

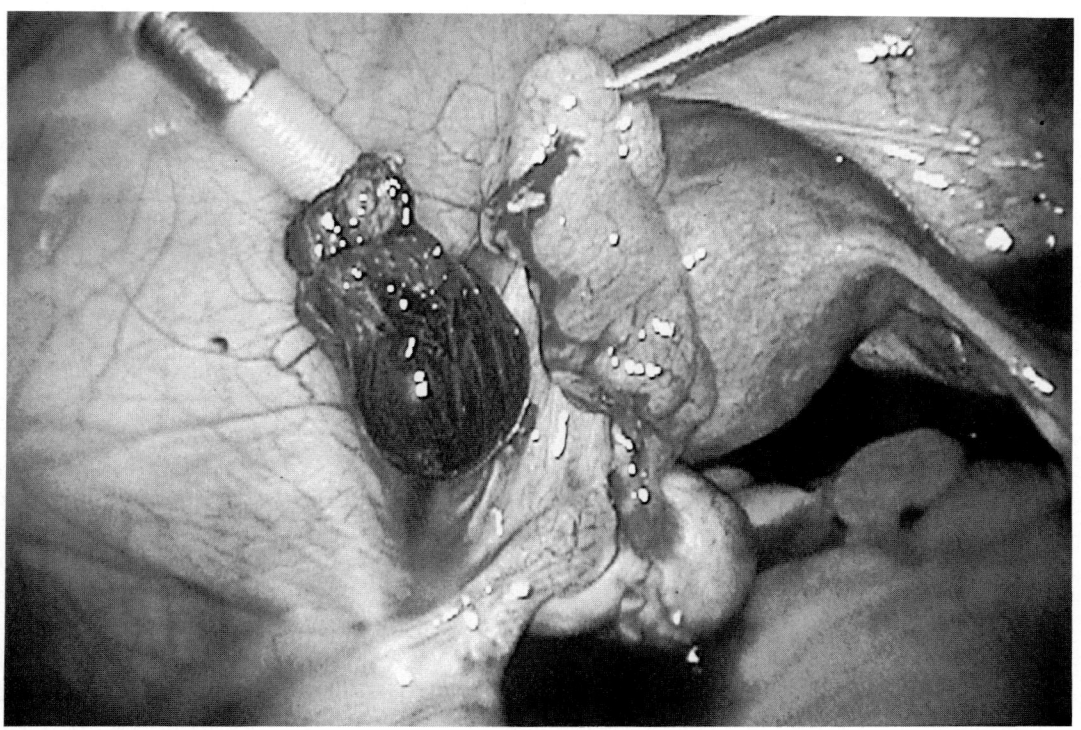

Figure 11.12. Intact products of conception noted after being flushed out of the fallopian tube.

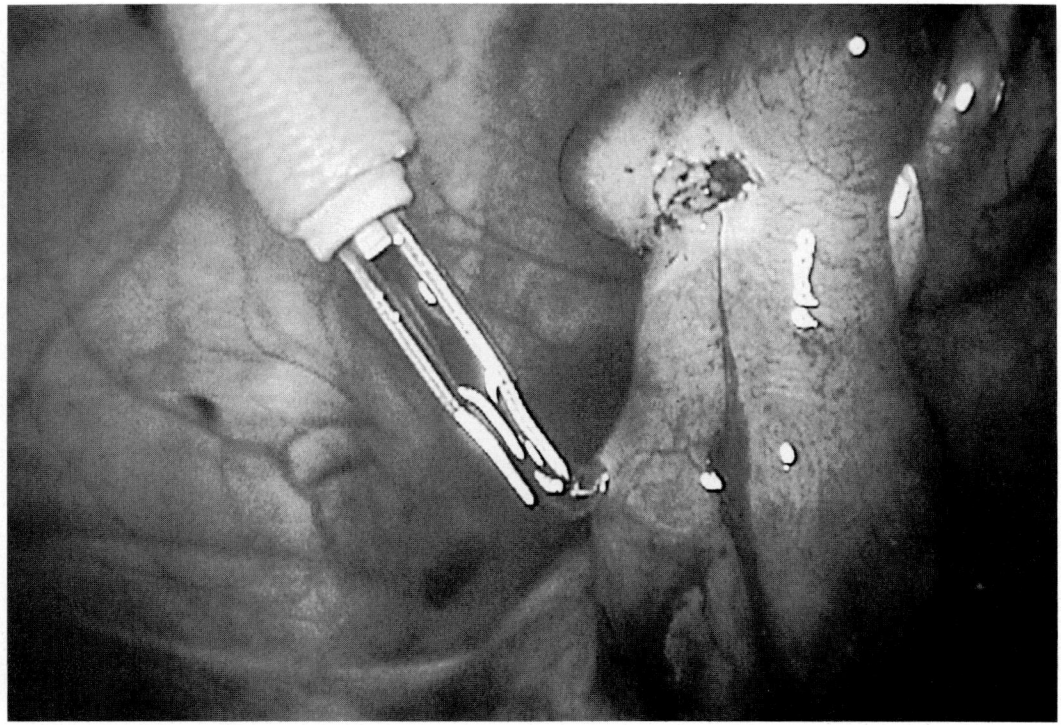

Figure 11.13. Microbipolar forceps are used to obtain hemostasis at the original salpingotomy incision.

In the series of Bruhat et al. of 118 women whose tubal pregnancies were treated by laparoscopic salpingotomy while still desiring fertility, a ruptured tube was present in 47.[1] Intrauterine pregnancies were later recorded in 27 of these women (57%) and recurrent ectopic pregnancy in 9 (19%). A ruptured tube was present in 32 of the 100 women who underwent laparoscopic salpingectomy reported by Dubuisson et al.[26]

Although many clinicians believe that laparoscopy may cause treatment delay in the patient with a ruptured tubal pregnancy who is in shock, the expert laparoscopist can control bleeding as quickly as most gynecologists with laparotomy regardless of the extent of hemoperitoneum. Although only one of four women with ruptured tubal pregnancy treated by one of the authors (H.R.) was in shock, all had at least 500 ml of hemoperitoneum. The woman in shock was admitted from the emergency room to the operating room. After induction of anesthesia, active bleeding was controlled within 5 minutes using Kleppinger bipolar forceps to coagulate the 13-week gestation tube and its mesosalpinx. After receiving 2 U of packed cells, the patient was discharged on the first postoperative day.

It should be emphasized that the Kleppinger bipolar forceps is a potent bipolar coagulator-desiccator that can effectively coagulate the tube and mesosalpinx despite active arterial or venous bleeding. We have used this instrument to coagulate the ovarian vessels in more than 300 laparoscopic salpingo-oophorectomy procedures.[96,97]

A ruptured tubal pregnancy is an almost absolute contraindication for a conservative approach. When the contralateral tube is absent, segmental resection or evacuation of products of conception after establishment of complete hemostasis may be considered—but only by the most expert laparoscopist. In most cases it is better to consider in vitro fertilization as the only hope for an intrauterine pregnancy in these women.

Cervical Pregnancy

Although not amenable to laparoscopic therapy, cervical ectopic pregnancy is a rare but potentially catastrophic event. Six reports document methotrexate therapy in 12 women, all with resolution.[98-103] This approach to this unusual clinical presentation remains highly experimental but with more experience may prove to be the therapy of choice.

Ovarian Pregnancy

Ovarian ectopic pregnancy, when recognized, can be treated much like any other ovarian cyst of unknown etiology (i.e., shelled out, often intact, through a superficial ovarian cortex incision). Ovarian pregnancy should be suspected in women with hCG titers above 3000 mIU/ml, an empty uterus as seen by ultrasonography, and no evidence of a tubal pregnancy at laparoscopy. The ovary is bivalved, perpendicular to its long axis starting at its most dependent part where cystic area meets solid tissue. Thereafter the cortex over the cystic area can be lifted with grasping forceps and the dissector inserted to gently aquadissect the gestational sac from surrounding ovarian tissue. Often an intact sac can be removed from inside the ovary with little ovarian bleeding. The ovary usually falls together without suturing.

There is at least one case report of treatment of ovarian pregnancy (thought to be a corpus luteum at laparoscopy but with biopsy of ovarian stroma showing villi) postoperatively with methotrexate, with subsequent resolution.[104] Recorded hCG levels in this case never exceeded 50 mIU/ml.

Chronic Ectopic Pregnancy

Fifty cases of chronic ectopic pregnancy among 882 ectopic pregnancies (5.7%) over a 3.5 year period were reported in 1982 by Cole and Corlett.[105] This condition is usually the direct result of a tubal abortion or ruptured ectopic pregnancy in which the hemodynamic insult is subclinical and self limiting and causes an inflammatory response to surrounding structures with resultant dense adhesions and occasional abscess formation involving the fallopian tube, ovary, small and large bowel, and omentum. The β-hCG level is frequently low owing to nonviable trophoblastic tissue. In the Cole and

Corlett series, 86% of the women had pain, 80% a mass, and 68% bleeding. Operative procedures included salpingectomy (20 cases), salpingo-oophorectomy (17 cases), and salpingo-oophorectomy with abdominal hysterectomy (13 cases). Twelve women had an infection as part of the chronic ectopic process, four with abscess formation.[105]

We have treated two chronic ectopic pregnancies laparoscopically, one by partial salpingectomy and the other by salpingectomy.[7] The surgical techniques involved are similar to those described for laparoscopic treatment of pelvic abscess.[106,107] It must be stressed that acute and subacute adhesions (i.e., adhesions of relatively recent onset) are amenable to laparoscopic lysis. The key is careful blunt dissection using the aquadissector until all structures are separated. Thereafter salpingectomy can be performed using bipolar forceps to coagulate the fallopian tube and its mesosalpinx. Intravenous antibiotics should be administered if any sign of purulent material is present; the patient is then discharged on an antibiotic effective against *Chlamydia*.

Conclusion

Ectopic pregnancy, a complex yet increasingly common condition that can occur in a variety of locations and under a diverse set of circumstances, can be appropriately managed using minimally invasive techniques with emphasis on tubal preservation. Advantages of laparoscopic treatment over conventional surgical management include minimal cosmetically placed incisions, short hospital stay, and a significant reduction in recuperation time. Laparoscopic advantages over medical management include accurate assessment of pregnancy status and location, the ability to lyse tuboovarian adhesions and evaluate the contralateral tube, confirmation by direct visualization of adequate treatment and complete hemostasis, and evacuation of all blood clots at the close of the procedure, usually "under water" after the replacement of CO_2 peritoneum by Ringer's lactate solution.

Considering the diversity and complexity of the problem, it is not surprising that controversy exists regarding whether primary laparoscopic surgical treatment of an early unruptured tubal pregnancy offers any advantages for tubal preservation over expectant management, medical treatment with methotrexate, or transvaginal injection of the ectopic pregnancy under sonographic guidance with hypertonic glucose, KCl, or methotrexate. The answer to this question awaits studies with long-term follow-up to determine tubal patency, fertility outcome, and subsequent recurrence of ectopic pregnancies following each of these treatment modalities. These studies must include documentation of the ectopic pregnancy location, including whether it has penetrated the muscularis mucosa, an accurate description of its viability, and if surrounding blood or clot is present. This documentation may not be obtainable using medical treatment, which is also unlikely to improve the underlying tubal compromise. Intensely sclerosing agents, such as methotrexate, may increase tubal adhesions when injected into the tubal lumen. Is there a place for adjuvant medical therapy following a surgical procedure? Viable extraluminal ectopic pregnancy, interstitial pregnancy, and cervical pregnancy may prove to be the ultimate testing ground for the use of methotrexate and transvaginal injection.

References

1. BRUHAT MA, MANHES H, MAGE G, POULY JL: Treatment of ectopic pregnancy by means of laparoscopy. Fertil Steril 1980;33:411.
2. DANIELL JF, HERBERT CM: Laparoscopic salpingostomy utilizing the CO_2 laser. Fertil Steril 1984;41:558.
3. POULY JL, MAHNES H, CANIS M, BRUHAT MA: Conservative laparoscopic treatment of 321 ectopic pregnancies. Fertil Steril 1986;46:1093.
4. JOHNS DA, HARDIE RP: Management of unruptured ectopic pregnancy with laparoscopic carbon dioxide laser. Fertil Steril 1986;46:703.
5. DECHERNEY AH, DIAMOND MP: Laparoscopic salpingostomy for ectopic pregnancy. Obstet Gynecol 1987;70:948.
6. BORNSTEIN S, KAHN J, FAUSONE V: Treatment of ectopic pregnancy with laparoscopic resection

in a community hospital. J Reprod Med 1987; 32:590.
7. REICH H, JOHNS DA, DECAPRIO J, ET AL: Laparoscopic treatment of 109 consecutive ectopic pregnancies. J Reprod Med 1988;33:885.
8. BRUMSTED J, KESSLER C, GIBSON C, ET AL: A comparison of laparoscopy and laparotomy for the treatment of ectopic pregnancy. Obstet Gynecol 1988;71:889.
9. SILVA PD: A laparoscopic approach can be applied to most cases of ectopic pregnancy. Obstet Gynecol 1988;72:944.
10. VERMESH M, SILVA PD, ROSEN GF, ET AL: Management of unruptured ectopic gestation by linear salpingostomy: a prospective, randomized clinical trial of laparoscopy versus laparotomy. Obstet Gynecol 1989;73:400.
11. HENDERSON SR: Ectopic tubal pregnancy treated by operative laparoscopy. Am J Obstet Gynecol 1989;160:1462.
12. HUBER J, HOSMANN J, VYTISKA-BINSTORFER E: Laparoscopic surgery for tubal pregnancies utilizing laser. Int J Gynaecol Obstet 1989;29:153.
13. KARSTEN U, SEIFERT B: Introduction and results in the endoscopic treatment of extrauterine pregnancy. Zentralbl Gynaekol 1990;112:467.
14. KECKSTEIN J, HEPP S, SCHNEIDER V, ET AL: The contact Nd:YAG laser: a new technique for conservation of the fallopian tube in unruptured ectopic pregnancy. Br J Obstet Gynaecol 1990; 97:352.
15. MECKE H, ARGIRIOU C, SEMM K: Treatment of tubal pregnancy by pelviscopy—complications, pregnancy and recurrence rates. Geburtsh Frauenheilkd 1991;51:549.
16. CHAPRON C, QUERLEU D, CREPIN G: Laparoscopic treatment of ectopic pregnancies: a one hundred cases study. Eur J Obstet Gynecol Reprod Biol 1991;41:187.
17. VERCO CJ: Nonlaser videolaparoscopic surgery for ectopic gestation. Aust NZ J Obstet Gynaecol 1991;31:168.
18. CHAPRON C, POULY JL, WATTIEZ A, ET AL: Results of conservative laparoscopic treatment of isthmic ectopic pregnancies: a 26 case study. Hum Reprod 1992;7:422.
19. MOTTLA GL, RULIN MC, GUZICK DS: Lack of resolution of ectopic pregnancy by intratubal injection of methotrexate. Fertil Steril 1992;57:685.
20. PAUERSTEIN CJ, CROXATTO HB, EDDY CA, ET AL: Anatomy and pathology of tubal pregnancy. Obstet Gynecol 1986;67:301.
21. STOCK RJ: Histopathologic changes in tubal pregnancy. J Reprod Med 1985;30:923.
22. REICH H, FREIFELD M, MCGLYNN F, REICH E: Laparoscopic treatment of tubal pregnancy. Obstet Gynecol 1987;69:275.
23. BUDOWICK M, JOHNSON TR, GENADRY R, ET AL: The histopathology of the developing tubal ectopic pregnancy. Fertil Steril 1980;34:169.
24. SHAPIRO HI, ADLER DH: Excision of an ectopic pregnancy through the laparoscope. Am J Obstet Gynecol 1973;117:290.
25. SODERSTROM RM: Unusual uses of laparoscopy. J Reprod Med 1975;15:77.
26. DUBUISSON JB, AUBRIOT FX, CARDONE V: Laparoscopic salpingectomy for tubal pregnancy. Fertil Steril 1987;47:225.
27. CACCIATORE B, STENMAN U-H, YLöSTALO P: Early screening for ectopic pregnancy in high-risk symptom-free women. Lancet 1994;343:517.
28. KOSASA TS, TAYMOR ML, GOLDSTEIN DP, LEVESQUE LA: Use of a radioimmunoassay specific for human chorionic gonadotropin in the diagnosis of early ectopic pregnancy. Obstet Gynecol 1973;42:868.
29. KOSASA TS, LEVESQUE LA, GOLDSTEIN DP, TAYMOR ML: Clinical use of a solid-phase radioimmunoassay specific for human chorionic gonadotropin. Am J Obstet Gynecol 1974;119:784.
30. KADAR N, FREEDMAN M, ZACHER M: Further observations on the doubling time of human chorionic gonadotropin in early asymptomatic pregnancies. Fertil Steril 1990;54:783.
31. KADAR N, DEVORE G, ROMERO R: Discriminatory hCG zone: its use in the sonographic evaluation for ectopic pregnancy. Obstet Gynecol 1981; 58:156.
32. KADAR N, CALDWELL BV, ROMERO R: A method of screening for ectopic pregnancy and its indications. Obstet Gynecol 1981;58:162.
33. KADAR N, ROMERO R: Further observations on serial hCG patterns in ectopic pregnancy and abortions. Fertil Steril 1988;50:367.
34. DAYA S: Human chorionic gonadotropin increase in normal early pregnancy. Am J Obstet Gynecol 1987;156:286.
35. FRITZ MA, GUO S: Doubling time of human chorionic gonadotropin (hCG) in early normal pregnancy: relationship to hCG concentration and gestational age. Fertil Steril 1987;47:584.
36. KADAR N, BOHRER M, KEMMAN E, SHELDON R: The hCG–time relationship in early gestation: a prospective randomized study. Fertil Steril 1993; 60:409.
37. KADAR N, BOHRER M, KEMMAN E, SHELDON R: The discriminatory hCG zone for endovaginal

sonography: a prospective, randomized study. Fertil Steril 1994;61:1016.
38. CARSON SA, BUSTER JE: Ectopic pregnancy. N Engl J Med 1993;329:1174.
39. RADWANSKA E, FRANKENBERG J, ALLEN E: Plasma progesterone levels in normal and abnormal early human pregnancy. Fertil Steril 1978;30:398.
40. MATHEWS CP, COULSON PB, WILD RA: Serum progesterone levels as an aid in the diagnosis of ectopic pregnancy. Obstet Gynecol 1986;68:390.
41. YEKO TR, GORRILL MJ, HUGHES LH, ET AL: Timely diagnosis of early ectopic pregnancy using a single blood progesterone measurement. Fertil Steril 1987;48:1048.
42. BUCK RH, JOUBERT SM, NORMAN RJ: Serum progesterone in the diagnosis of ectopic pregnancy: a valuable diagnostic test. Fertil Steril 1988; 50:752.
43. HUBINONT CJ, THOMAS C, SCHWERS JF: Luteal function in ectopic pregnancy. Am J Obstet Gynecol 1987;156:669.
44. KADAR N, BLUMENTHAL S: Serum progesterone levels in ectopic pregnancy. Infertility 1992; 15:7.
45. STOVALL TG, LING FW, COPE BJ, ET AL: Preventing ruptured ectopic pregnancy with a single serum progesterone. Am J Obstet Gynecol 1989; 160:1425.
46. STOVALL TG, LING FW: Ectopic pregnancy—diagnostic and therapeutic algorithms minimizing surgical intervention. J Reprod Med 1993; 38:807.
47. VALLE JA, LIFCHEZ AS: Reproductive outcome following conservative surgery for tubal pregnancy in women with a single fallopian tube. Fertil Steril 1983;39:316.
48. DECHERNEY AH, MAHEAUX R, NAFTOLIN F: Salpingostomy for ectopic pregnancy in the sole patent oviduct. Fertil Steril 1982;37:619.
49. KADAR N: Ablative versus conservative operations. In Diagnosis and Treatment of Extrauterine Pregnancies, Kadar N (ed). New York, Raven Press, 1990, pp 112–128.
50. DECHERNEY AH, KASE N: The conservative surgical management of unruptured ectopic pregnancy. Obstet Gynecol 1979;54:451.
51. TOUMIVARA L, KAUPPILA A: Radical or conservative surgery for ectopic pregnancy? A follow up study of fertility of 323 patients. Fertil Steril 1988;50:580.
52. THORBURN J, PHILIPSON M, LINDBLOM B: Fertility after ectopic pregnancy in relation to background factors and surgical treatment. Fertil Steril 1988;49:595.
53. SULTANA CJ, EASLEY K, COLLINS RL: Outcome of laparoscopic versus traditional surgery for ectopic pregnancies. Fertil Steril 1992;57:285.
54. HALLATT JG: Tubal conservatism in ectopic pregnancy: a study of 200 cases. Am J Obstet Gynecol 1986;154:1216.
55. DECHERNEY AH, BOYERS SP: Isthmic ectopic pregnancy: segmental resection as the treatment of choice. Fertil Steril 1985;44:307.
56. SMITH HO, TOLEDO AA, THOMPSON JD: Conservative surgical management of isthmic cornual pregnancies. Am J Obstet Gynecol 1987; 157:604.
57. MURPHY AA, NAGER CW, WUJEK JJ, ET AL: Operative laparoscopy versus laparotomy for the management of ectopic pregnancy: a prospective trial. Fertil Steril 1992;57:1180.
58. LUNDORFF P, HAHLIN M, KALLFELT B, ET AL: Adhesion formation after laparoscopic surgery in tubal pregnancy: a randomized trial versus laparotomy. Fertil Steril 1991;55:911.
59. RANSOM MX, GARCIA AJ, BOHRER M, ET AL: Serum progesterone as a predictor of methotrexate success in the treatment of ectopic pregnancy. Obstet Gynecol 1994;83:1033.
60. KADAR N: Treatment of ectopic pregnancy after pelvic inflammatory disease. In Pelvic Inflammatory Disease, Berger GS, LV Westrom (eds). New York, Raven Press, 1992, pp 139–162.
61. FERNANDEZ H, LELAIDIER C, BATON C, ET AL: Return of reproductive performance after expectant management and local treatment for ectopic pregnancy. Hum Reprod 1991;6:1474.
62. FERNANDEZ H, LELAIDIER C: Critical comparisons of alternative therapies for ectopic pregnancy. Fertil Steril 1993;59:246 [letter].
63. O'SHEA RT, THOMPSON GR, HARDING A: Intra-amniotic methotrexate versus CO_2 laser laparoscopic salpingotomy in the management of tubal ectopic pregnancy—a prospective randomized trial. Fertil Steril 1994;62:876.
64. PORRECO RP: Percutaneous, ultrasound-directed ablation of ectopic pregnancy with methotrexate: a report of three cases. J Reprod Med 1992;37:363.
65. FERNANDEZ H, BENIFLA J-L, LELAIDIER C, ET AL: Methotrexate treatment of ectopic pregnancy: 100 cases treated by primary transvaginal injection under sonographic control. Fertil Steril 1993; 59:773.
66. TULANDI T, ATRI M, BRET P, ET AL: Transvaginal intratubal methotrexate treatment of ectopic pregnancy. Fertil Steril 1992;58:98.

67. RISQUEZ F, FORMAN R, MALEIKA F, ET AL: Transcervical cannulation of the fallopian tube for the management of ectopic pregnancy: prospective multicenter study. Fertil Steril 1992; 58:1131.
68. SCHIFF E, SHALEV E, BUSTAN M, ET AL: Pharmacokinetics of methotrexate after local tubal injection for conservative treatment of ectopic pregnancy. Fertil Steril 1992;57:688.
69. SAUER MV, GORRILL MJ, RODI IA: Non-surgical management of unruptured ectopic pregnancy: an extended clinical trial. Fertil Steril 1987; 48:752.
70. STOVALL TG, LING FW, GRAY LA, ET AL: Methotrexate treatment of unruptured ectopic pregnancy: a report of 100 cases. Obstet Gynecol 1991; 77:749.
71. STOVALL TG, LING FW, GRAY LA: Single-dose methotrexate for treatment of ectopic pregnancy. Obstet Gynecol 1991;77:754.
72. GLOCK JL, JOHNSON JV, BRUMSTED JR: Efficacy and safety of single-dose systemic methotrexate in the treatment of ectopic pregnancy. Fertil Steril 1994;62:716.
73. CREININ MD, WASHINGTON AE: Cost of ectopic pregnancy management: surgery versus methotrexate. Fertil Steril 1993;60:963.
74. HULKA J, REICH H: Electrosurgical hemostasis. In Textbook of Laparoscopy (2nd ed). Philadelphia, Saunders, pp 196–199.
75. HULKA J, REICH H: Umbilical extension. In Textbook of Laparoscopy (2nd ed). Philadelphia, Saunders, p 182.
76. REICH H, CLARKE C, SEKEL L: A simple method for ligating with straight and curved needles in operative laparoscopy. Obstet Gynecol 1992;79:143.
77. SEMM K: Operative Manual Endoscopic Abdominal Surgery. Year Book, 1987.
78. SHERMAN D, LANGER R, HERMAN A, ET AL: Reproductive outcome after fimbrial evacuation of tubal pregnancy. Fertil Steril 1987;47:420.
79. REICH, H, DECAPRIO J, MCGLYNN F, KREDENTSER J: Aquaexpression for laparoscopic removal of distal tubal pregnancies. Gynaecol Endosc 1992;1:69.
80. VERMESH M, SILVA PD, SAUER MV, ET AL: Persistent tubal ectopic gestation: patterns of circulating beta-human chorionic gonadotropin and progesterone, and management options. Fertil Steril 1988;50:584.
81. THOMPSON GRStJ, O'SHEA RT, HARDING A: Beta hCG levels after conservative treatment of ectopic pregnancy: is a plateau normal? Aust NZ J Obstet Gynaecol 1994;34:96.
82. LUNDORRF P, HAHLIN M, SJOBLOM P, LINDBLOM B: Persistent trophoblast after conservative treatment of tubal pregnancy: prediction and detection. Obstet Gynecol 1991;77:129.
83. STOCK RJ: Persistent tubal pregnancy. Obstet Gynecol 1991;77:267.
84. SEIFER DB, GUTMANN JN, DOYLE MB, ET AL: Persistent ectopic pregnancy following laparoscopic linear salpingostomy. Obstet Gynecol 1990; 76:1121.
85. KADAR N: Conservative operations. In Diagnosis and Treatment of Extrauterine Pregnancies, Kadar N (ed). New York, Raven Press, 1990, pp 112–128.
86. BROWN DL, FELKER RE, STOVALL TG, ET AL: Serial endovaginal sonography of ectopic pregnancies treated with methotrexate. Obstet Gynecol 1991;77:406.
87. REICH, H, DECAPRIO J, MCGLYNN F, ET AL: Peritoneal trophoblastic tissue implants after laparoscopic treatment of tubal ectopic pregnancy. Fertil Steril 1989;52:337.
88. HOPPE DE, BEKKAR BE, NAGER CW: Single-dose systemic methotrexate for the treatment of persistent ectopic pregnancy after conservative surgery. Obstet Gynecol 1994;83:51.
89. SEIFER DB, SILVA PD, GRAINGER DA, ET AL: Reproductive potential after treatment for persistent ectopic pregnancy. Fertil Steril 1994;62:194.
90. REICH, H, MCGLYNN F, BUDIN R, ET AL: Laparoscopic treatment of ruptured interstitial pregnancy. J Gynecol Surg 1990;6:135.
91. BRANDES MC, YOUNGS DD, GOLDSTEIN DEP, ET AL: Treatment of cornual pregnancy with methotrexate: case report. Am J Obstet Gynecol 1986;155:655.
92. TANAKA T, HAYASHI H. KUTSUZAWA T, ET AL: Treatment of interstitial ectopic pregnancy with methotrexate. Fertil Steril 1982;37:851.
93. FERNANDEZ H, ZIEGLER DD, BOURGET P, ET AL: The place of methotrexate in the management of interstitial pregnancy. Hum Reprod 1991;6:302.
94. TIMOR-TRITSCH IE, MONTEAGUDO A, MATERA C, VEIT CR: Sonographic evolution of cornual pregnancies treated without surgery. Obstet Gynecol 1992;79:1044.
95. PEREZ JA, SADEK MM, SAVALE M, ET AL: Local medical treatment of interstitial pregnancy after in-vitro fertilization and embryo transfer (IVF-ET): two case reports. Hum Reprod 1993; 8:631.
96. MANN WJ, REICH H: Laparoscopic adnexectomy in postmenopausal women. J Reprod Med 1992;37:254.

97. REICH H, JOHNS DA, DAVIS G, DIAMOND MP: Laparoscopic oophorectomy. J Reprod Med 1993;38:497.
98. KAPLAN BR, BRANDT T, JAVAHERI G, SCOMMEGNA A: Nonsurgical treatment of a viable cervical pregnancy with intra-amniotic methotrexate. Fertil Steril 1990;53:941.
99. YANKOWITZ J, LEAKE J, HUGGINS G, ET AL: Cervical ectopic pregnancy: review of the literature and report of a case treated by single-dose methotrexate therapy. Obstet Gynecol Surv 1990;45:405.
100. THOMAS RL, GINGOLD BR, GALLAGHER MW: Cervical pregnancy. A report of two cases. J Reprod Med 1991;36:459.
101. TIMOR-TRITSCH IE, MONTEAGUDO A, MANDEVILLE EO, ET AL: Successful management of viable cervical pregnancy by local injection of methotrexate guided by transvaginal ultrasonography. Am J Obstet Gynecol 1994;170:737.
102. PELEG D, BAR-HAVA I, NEUMAN-LEVIN M, ET AL: Early diagnosis and successful nonsurgical treatment of viable combined intrauterine and cervical pregnancy. Fertil Steril 1994;62:405.
103. MARCOVICI I, ROSENWEIG BA, BRILL AI, ET AL: Cervical pregnancy: case reports and a current literature review. Obstet Gynecol Surv 1994;49:49.
104. CHELMOW D, GATES E, PENZIAS AS: Laparoscopic diagnosis and methotrexate treatment of an ovarian pregnancy: a case report. Fertil Steril 1994;62:879.
105. COLE T, CORLETT RC: Chronic ectopic pregnancy. Obstet Gynecol 1982;59:63.
106. REICH H, MCGLYNN F: Laparoscopic treatment of tuboovarian and pelvic abscess. J Reprod Med 1987;32:747.
107. REICH H: Endoscopic management of tuboovarian abscess and pelvic inflammatory disease. In Operative Gynecologic Endoscopy, Sanfilippo JS, Levine RL (eds). New York, Springer-Verlag, 1989, pp 118–132.

12
Distal Tubal Reconstructive Surgery

Lisa M. Peacock and John A. Rock

Obstruction of the distal fallopian tube is one of the most common causes of female infertility. Tubal reconstruction and adhesiolysis performed by an open abdominal approach utilizing microsurgical techniques have been the classic management for this cause of infertility. Today sophisticated laparoscopic instrumentation allows minimally invasive correction of certain pathologic conditions of the fallopian tube and ovary. Proximal obstruction may still be best corrected through traditional methods, but distal obstruction can, in select cases, be corrected through endoscopic techniques, which are associated with decreased perioperative morbidity, mortality, and expense.

Etiology

The most common cause of tubal damage is salpingitis, which is usually secondary to pelvic inflammatory disease (PID). Pathogens such as *Chlamydia trachomatis* can cause acute symptoms, or they may instead work silently, causing significant chronic damage with gross anatomic distortion of the tubes and progressive destruction of the mucosal surfaces. PID can cause fimbrial agglutination leading to phimosis or to complete obstruction with subsequent hydrosalpinx, destruction of the tubal cilia, loss of the normal mucosal folds (rugae), inflammation, and adhesion formation. All of these contributing factors markedly distort the normal relations between the fallopian tube and ovary, preventing ovum capture and migration.

Endometriosis can also cause adhesion formation with distortion of tubal anatomy; and as with PID, the severe, protracted disease with its resultant inflammatory response and adhesion formation can cause distal tubal agglutination or obstruction. Distal tubal disease also may be caused by previous abdominal or pelvic surgery with resultant trauma to serosal surfaces and by such inflammatory conditions of the abdomen or pelvis as appendicitis, diverticulitis, inflammatory bowel disease, and tuberculous salpingitis.

Diagnosis

The damaged distal tube is assessed after thorough medical and surgical histories, careful pelvic examination, routine infertility testing (i.e., semen analysis, confirmation of ovulatory status, and postcoital testing), and hysterosalpingography (HSG) prior to laparoscopic intervention to assess distal tubal architecture. Performed under fluoroscopic guidance, HSG can be used to ascertain the presence of distal obstruction or intraluminal adhesions, the extent of determining prognosis and stage of disease.[1] HSG provides only limited information regarding tubal thickness or rigidity, pelvic peritoneal disease, and other pelvic or adnexal adhesions. Assessment of these remaining factors must await laparoscopy, when complete visualization of pelvic structures and possible concurrent surgical correction of pelvic pathology can be undertaken.

Prognosis and Contraindications

To achieve the ultimate goal of the pelvic reconstructive surgeon—restoration of normal anatomy and reproductive function—it is mandatory that tissue trauma be avoided as much as possible by using precise surgical techniques. Meticulous excision of adhesions that alter important anatomic relations and interfere with ovum capture is critical. Restoration of tubal patency, liberation of the ovary, and reapproximation of the distal tube with the unencumbered ovarian surface are mandatory for normal reproductive function. The pelvic reconstructive surgeon must assess each patient with these goals in mind to determine the appropriateness of and the route for possible surgical intervention.

Studies utilizing traditional microsurgical techniques have identified a number of factors that affect the ultimate success of surgical tubal reconstruction and that also define those patients for whom surgical reconstruction may be contraindicated because of an extremely poor prognosis. The American Society for Reproductive Medicine (ASRM) classification committee on distal tubal occlusion noted that tubal function subsequent to surgical reconstruction depends on the status of the fallopian tube at the time of surgical intervention.[1] This committee formulated a scoring system based on several factors affecting postsurgical tubal function, including (1) the diameter of the distal ampullary segment, (2) the thickness of the tubal wall, (3) the presence of mucosal or rugal folds at the neostomy site, and (4) the extent and type of adhesions. Donnez and Casanas-Roux[2] reported an inverse association between ampullary diameter (evaluated by HSG) and pregnancy outcome: In particular, dilation of 3 cm is associated with a poor prognosis for pregnancy. Conversely, the presence of rugal folds on HSG is positively correlated with the chance of pregnancy.[3-5] Other investigators have found that rigid, thick tubal walls also are indicative of a poor prognosis,[4,5] as are dense, occlusive periadnexal and pelvic adhesions.[6-8] Thus multiple studies have confirmed the associations of degree of tubal distention, thickness of the (tubal) wall, the presence of rugal folds on HSG, and the severity of periadnexal adhesions with ultimate pregnancy outcomes.[3-9]

Based on a careful preoperative evaluation including HSG and diagnostic laparoscopy, an assessment can be made as to the appropriateness of surgical intervention for the purpose of tubal reconstruction. Conditions that may contraindicate reconstruction and hence could indicate referral for advanced assisted reproductive technologies such as in vitro fertilization (IVF) include intraluminal adhesions, the absence of fimbria, the presence of a large hydrosalpinx (> 3 cm in diameter), extremely thick-walled fallopian tubes, and dense obliterative adhesions fixing the adnexae and surrounding structures to the pelvic side walls or to other pelvic organs. Consideration must also be given to other factors pertinent to the patient's fertility, including age > 35 years, severe oligospermia,[10] previous tuberculous salpingitis,[1] a failed previous surgical tubal reconstruction, and the presence of anti-sperm antibodies. Cases that fall into the "moderate" category by classification[1] are, in contrast to those on either end of the spectrum, more difficult to assess for appropriateness of surgical correction. In these cases decisions must take into account numerous individual medical and socioeconomic factors in order to formulate a plan for the most appropriate method of treatment.

The prudent practitioner (after careful evaluation as to the best approach for tubal reconstruction) makes the decision to proceed with laparoscopic reconstruction based not only on the severity of pelvic pathology but also on one's own level of skill, experience, and previous training. Performed correctly in properly selected cases, laparoscopic distal tubal surgery is comparable with respect to outcome and has the distinct advantage of limiting length of hospital stay, expense, morbidity, and mortality.

General Technique

Because the patient's position during laparoscopic investigation must allow free range of motion of all operative ports and instrumentation, the Allen Universal Stirrups and the dorsal "ski" position are preferred. This stirrup rests the weight of the patient's leg on the heel and sole of the foot, with 0° of flexion between the thigh and the torso. After all operative ports are placed, the patient is put in steep Trendelenburg position to displace the bowel away from the pelvic basin.

To reduce the number and size of abdominal puncture sites, it is preferable to use the operative laparoscope introduced through an umbilical sheath together with an adjunctive 5 mm suprapubic port (usually only one, just lateral to the midline) for the use of graspers, irrigator-suction wand, and so on. The operative port of the laparoscope is used for passage of a fiberoptic or CO_2 laser, wave-guide scissors, aspirating needles, and blunt probes. With the ports placed in this manner, generally only two ports are required to accomplish the necessary dissection and excisions.

In general the CO_2 laser is preferred to other wavelengths or energy sources because of the precision of application possible, the minimal thermal spread from the delivery point, and its ready availability at most centers. Use of a wave guide in particular allows close approximation of the delivery tip to the tissue surface with subsequent reduction of carbon char formation. The tip of the wave guide also can be utilized for fine blunt dissection of loose areolar and peritoneal surfaces, obviating the need for additional instrumentation through additional ports and taking best advantage of the magnification properties of the laparoscope. Continuous or superpulse laser mode (20 watts) with close approximation of the laser tip to the desired target generally results in a clean, precise line of dissection. Laser backstopping can easily be achieved for the CO_2 laser via pooling of pelvic irrigant, hydrosufflation, or use of any of the nonreflective probes or cannulas.

When positioning and port placement are completed, the pelvic and abdominal structures are carefully inspected. A methodic routine should be established to ensure that the assessment is complete each time. Abdominal wall, omental, or bowel adhesions should be lysed during this assessment to expose the pelvic viscera and anterior abdominal wall. Only after the pelvic viscera are adequately visualized should adhesiolysis of the fallopian tube and ovary be undertaken to restore normal pelvic anatomy.

Delicate tubal and ovarian tissues should be handled with great care using fine atraumatic instrumentation. Manipulation of structures and avoidance of excessive countertraction, which can cause avulsion or laceration of contiguous structures, may be accomplished by grasping adhesions. Careful attention should be paid to the normal anatomic landmarks of the fallopian tube and ovary to avoid inadvertent injury to structures of vital function, including the fimbria ovarica and mesosalpingeal and ovarian vasculature. In addition to using existing adhesions, the uteroovarian ligament is useful for attaching atraumatic graspers to facilitate salpingoovariolysis. Adhesiolysis is achieved through a fine layer-by-layer approach using the laser, hook scissors, and blunt probe dissection. The line of cleavage between the structures being separated should be identified and followed to avoid dissection into critical structures. Hydrodissection can be useful when attempting to avoid critical vascular or anatomic structures (e.g., the ureter). The judicious use of countertraction in conjunction with transection of the adhesive fibers in a perpendicular or crosswise pattern greatly facilitates the ease of resection. Adhesions should be completely excised all the way to the base of the cul-de-sac to eliminate their interference with reproductive function.

Meticulous hemostasis should be maintained throughout dissection and adhesiolysis. Either a defocused CO_2 laser beam or microbipolar electrocautery can be safely used with limited thermal injury spread. We avoid unipolar cautery because of the inherent risks of the development of undesired conduction pathways and subsequent occult injury to abdominal structures such as the bowel or bladder. The adhesiolysis should proceed in a methodic fashion, moving from well identified anatomic landmarks caudad down to the base of the cul-de-sac. The cardinal rule during adhesiolysis (applicable to both open abdominal and laparoscopic dissection) is to identify all structures prior to division or coagulation to avoid blind destruction or entry into vital pelvic structures.

In addition to hemostasis, meticulous dissection, and gentle handling of tissues under laparoscopic magnification, the prevention of adhesion reformation is assisted by the use of warm Ringer's lactate to irrigate, hydrodissect, and remove all blood and carbonized debris from the pelvis. For deserosalized and denuded peritoneal or tuboovarian surfaces, oval patches of methylcellulose (absorbable membrane, Interceed; Johnson & Johnson) placed in strategic locations may prevent the reformation of postoperative adhesions. Attention should be directed in particular to the posterior broad ligament and ovarian fossa, the pelvic side wall, and the tuboovarian fossa. To maximize the efficiency of this artificial membrane, meticulous hemostasis must be achieved and gentle saturation of the product performed with low-flow Ringer's lactate irrigant. In addition to the above-mentioned adhesion prevention measures, prophylactic antibiotics are administered prior to initiation of the operative procedure and in some cases for several days postoperatively. Other possible antiadhesion measures described by investigators include terminal irrigation with heparinized (5000 U/L) irrigant, with intraperitoneal instillation of 1–2 L of Ringer's lactate. Such irrigation at the conclusion of the procedure facilitates hydroflotation and separation of contiguous peritoneal surfaces during the initial stages of healing. Care must be taken, however, to avoid fluid overload and electrolyte disturbances when instilling these osmotic fluids.

Fimbrioplasty

When complete adhesiolysis has been achieved, the distal portion of the fallopian tube can be mobilized for correction of phimosis or clubbing of the fimbriated end. Hydrodistention of the fallopian tube is first achieved by means of transcervical insufflation through a cannulated uterine manipulator with diluted indigo carmine dye. The distal tube is stabilized with an atraumatic grasper, and adhesion bands are released by laser, scissors, or micropoint electrocautery (Fig. 12.1) in order to identify the tubal dimple (i.e., the convergent cicatricial lines of closure). These landmarks frequently are not visible, and careful incision is necessary to minimize damage to the normal fimbrial tissues. One should note that the tubal aperture is generally located high on the antimesosalpingeal end of the hydrosalpinx and away from the fimbria ovarica.

If the aperture is readily identifiable after transection of phimosing bands, the fimbriated end can be progressively dilated using 3 mm alligator-type forceps or tongs (Fig. 12.2). The closed forceps is advanced distally through the constricted aperture without use of excessive force. Once the forceps is beyond the area of terminal constriction and is inside the tubal lumen, its jaws are opened and then gently withdrawn in the open position through the phimosed end of the fallopian tube. Satisfactory blunt dilation of distal agglutinations generally can be achieved with one or more passes of the forceps using the same technique. The axis of the instrument can be rotated with each pass.

Perifimbrial adhesion bands should be transected with shallow laser or micropoint cautery in the avascular planes. If necessary, radial incisions can be made to facilitate eversion of the fimbriated end, and even further eversion can be facilitated by brushing the tubal serosa proximal to the fimbria with a defocused CO_2 laser beam at low wattage to cause mild desiccation and constriction of the serosal surface.[11]

Results of laparoscopic fimbrioplasty compare favorably with traditional microsurgical technique. Crude intrauterine pregnancy rates after open abdominal microsurgical fimbriopla-

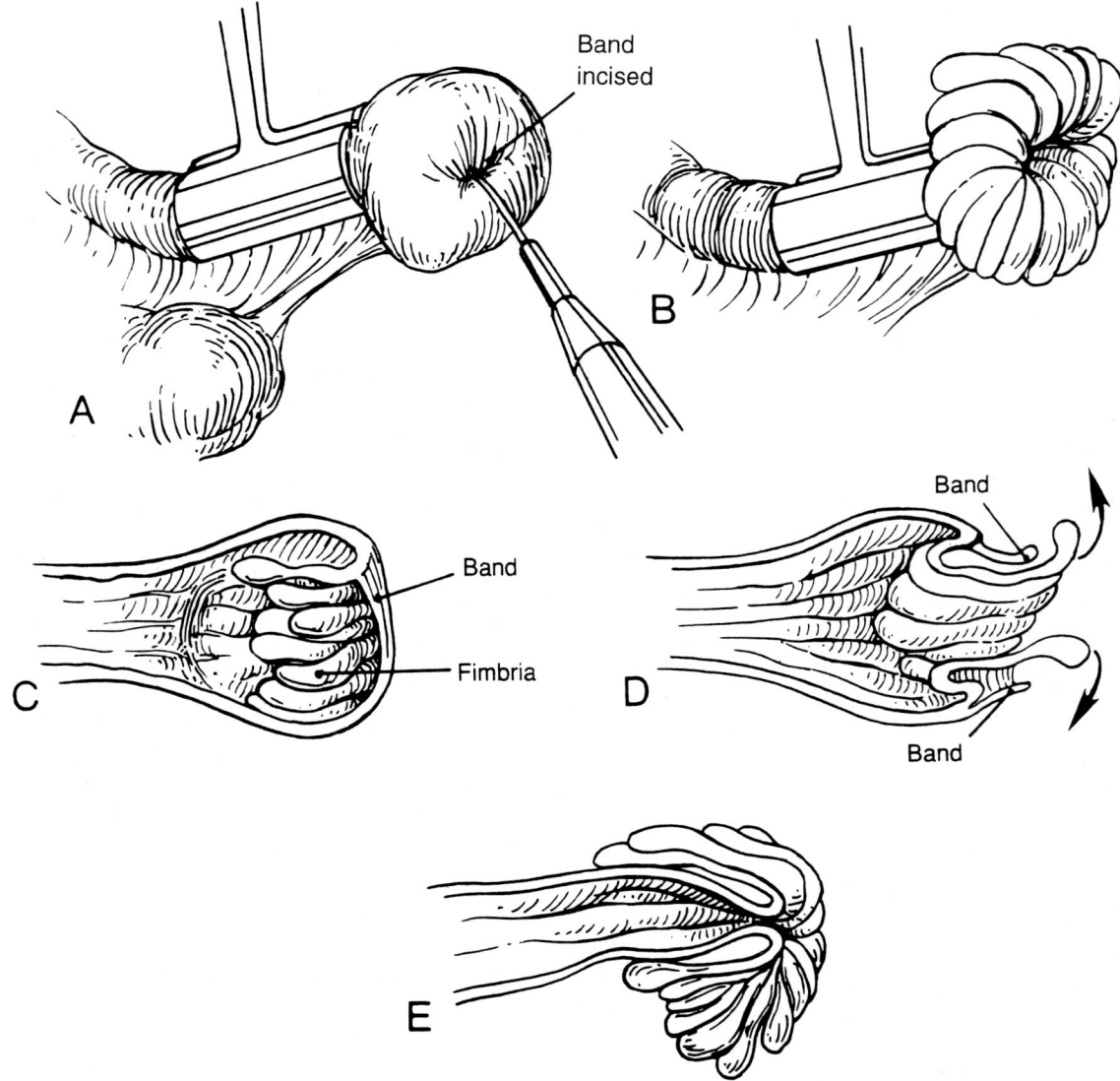

Figure 12.1. Complete distal fimbrial obstruction without significant hydrosalpinx or fimbrial destruction. (A) Whitish scar is incised. (B) Fimbrial strands are revealed. Some agglutination may be noted. Small forceps may be used to dilate the phimotic os. (C) Cross section reveals strands by peritoneal band. (D) When the band is incised the fimbriae are released. (E) Fimbriae assume their normal anatomic position. (From Murphy AA: Reconstructive surgery of the oviduct. In *Female Reproductive Surgery*, Rock JA, Murphy AA, Jones HW Jr (eds). Baltimore, Williams & Wilkins, 1992, reprinted with permission)

sty have been reported at 49%, 68%, and 70%, respectively.[8,10,12] Intrauterine pregnancy rates after laparoscopic fimbrioplasty are reported as 31%, 35%, and 50%, respectively.[13–15] Tubal patency at 6–8 weeks postoperatively has been reported at 64% in laparoscopic cases.[14] Ectopic pregnancies have been cited at a rate of 40% (two of five patients) for laparoscopic procedures[14] and 10% (one of eight patients) for abdominal procedures,[8] but these results must be interpreted cautiously owing to the small sample sizes of both studies.

Figure 12.2. Fimbrial agglutination. (A) Tongs, ampulla dilator, or small crile may be inserted into the phimotic tube in the closed position. (B) Instrument is opened and carefully withdrawn in that position. This maneuver may be repeated at various angles to allow symmetric dilatation. The fimbriae should then be examined for interfimbrial adhesions, which should be carefully lysed. (From Murphy AA: Reconstructive surgery of the oviduct. In *Female Reproductive Surgery,* Rock JA, Murphy AA, Jones HW Jr (eds). Baltimore, Williams & Wilkins, 1992, reprinted with permission)

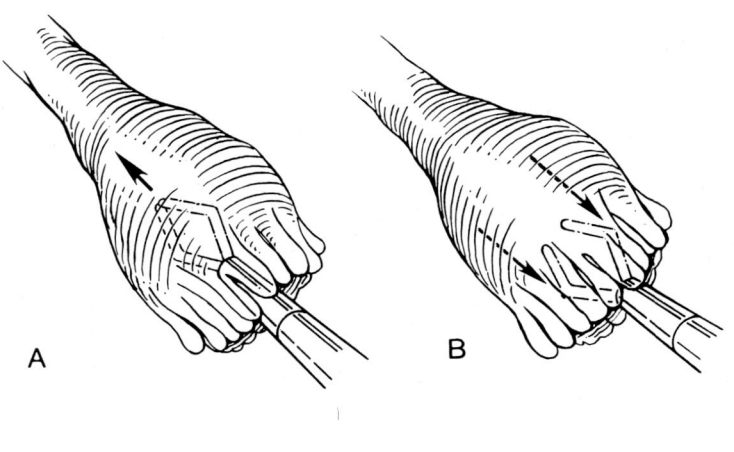

Salpingoneostomy

In 1980 an ad hoc committee of the International Federation of Fertility and Sterility (IFFS) defined fimbrioplasty to mean "the reconstruction of existent fimbria" and defined salpingoneostomy, in contrast, to be "the surgical creation of a new tubal ostium in a totally occluded fallopian tube."[16] The term salpingoneostomy is further defined by the site at which the new aperture is created (i.e., terminal, ampullary, isthmic, or a combination of types between the two tubes). Terminal salpingoneostomy has been (still is?) the procedure of choice because of its anatomic result and because success rates associated with ampullary and isthmic procedures are unacceptably poor.

Pregnancy rates are low whether the repair is completed laparoscopically or abdominally because of the advanced degree of tubal damage associated with complete distal tubal obstruction and the usual association of hydrosalpinx and loss of rugal folds with inherent damage to the ciliated mucosal lining. Given the lack of significant success regardless of methodology, laparoscopic salpingoneostomy still has the previously stated advantages of low cost, morbidity, and mortality compared to open abdominal microsurgical reconstruction. In addition, a laparoscopic repair can be completed at the time of the diagnostic laparoscopy, obviating the need for the second anesthetic and surgical procedure that usually are necessary if the traditional microsurgical approach is undertaken.

The principles for dissection, mobilization, and hemostasis apply, of course, to the fimbrioplasty (or any laparoscopic) procedure, as does the method of hydrodistention of the obstructed fallopian tube by transcervical retrograde insufflation of dilute indigo carmine dye until the distal ends of the fallopian tubes bulge under pressure of the fluid (Fig. 12.3A). The distal tube should by this time have been adequately mobilized and stabilized with an atraumatic grasper to allow precise incision of the obstructed tube. A variety of instruments may be used to score and then incise the obstructed end, including scissors, micropoint cautery, or high power density laser beam. Care should be taken to identify and incise at the already avascular scarred regions and to avoid, if possible, incising across healthy fimbrial tissue (Fig. 12.3B). After the surface of the hydrosalpinx has been scored along avascular lines of agglutination, the lumen is entered. There is a consequent efflux of the distending dye, and readjustment of the stabilizing grasper may be necessary. If a fine atraumatic grasper is being used, the scarred edge of the newly created ostium can be grasped. Hemostasis can be achieved with microbipolar or micropoint cautery as previously noted.

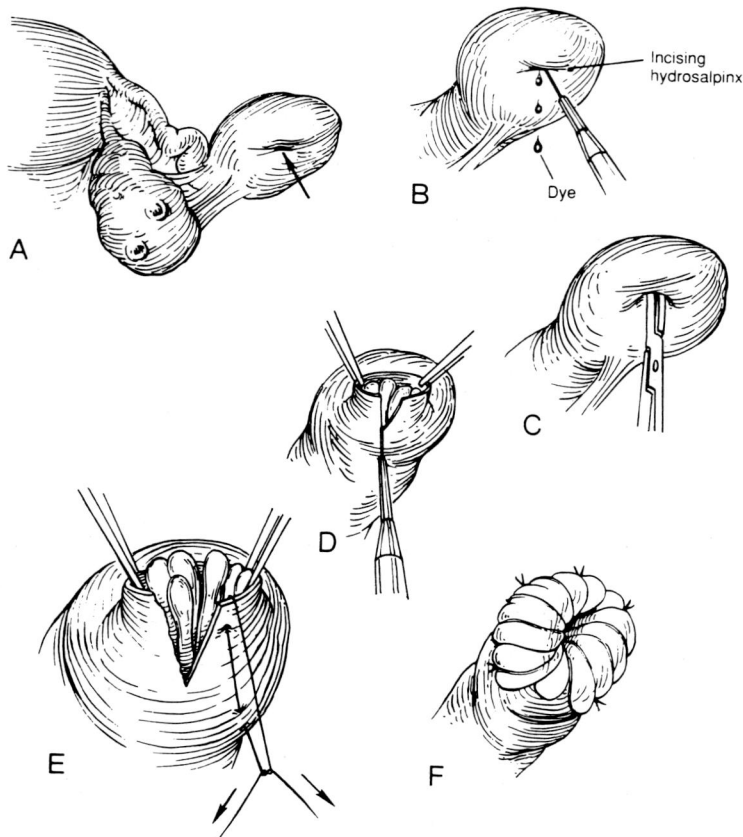

Figure 12.3. Distal fimbrial obstruction with moderate hydrosalpinx and complete fimbrial destruction. (A, B) Incision is made over the whitish scar on the distended hydrosalpinx. (C) Ostium is dilated with a fine forceps. (D) Incision is extended at 6 o'clock toward the fimbria ovarica. (E, F) Cuff salpingostomy is achieved after eversion of the mucosa using 7-0 polyglactic suture. (From Murphy AA: Reconstructive surgery of the oviduct. In *Female Reproductive Surgery*, Rock JA, Murphy AA, Jones HW Jr (eds). Baltimore, Williams & Wilkins, 1992, reprinted with permission)

After the tube is opened the edges must be everted to maintain patency. The number of additional radial incisions should be limited to as few as are necessary to allow adequate eversion of the fimbria. As has previously been shown to be possible in open abdominal cases, a single incision eversion procedure is possible with laparoscopy[17] and may help minimize tissue damage. Frequently, however, one or two additional radial incisions are required to adequately evert the fimbriated end (Fig. 12.3D–E). The simplest eversion technique utilizes the defocused laser at low wattage (3–5 watts) to brush the serosal surface 360° at 0.5–1.0 cm proximal to the fimbriated end, thereby desiccating and causing contraction of the serosa with subsequent eversion of the fimbriated end. Care must be taken to avoid overzealous application of any thermal source to the serosa because subsequent damage to the underlying mucosa can lead to later stenosis or obstruction.

Attempt, instead, to make a broad application, producing a generous degree of eversion to prevent postoperative reocclusion by reapproximation of the cut edges of the hydrosalpinx. A similar result can be achieved with other thermal sources, such as endocoagulation or electrocoagulation; however, the degree of thermal spread may then be more difficult to control than with the CO_2 laser.

In cases in which eversion cannot be satisfactorily achieved by thermal flowering techniques, fine sutures may be used to attach the cut edge to the ampullary serosa to create an ostial cuff (Fig. 12.3F). Typically 4-0 polydioxanone (PDS) suture is used to place one or more anchoring stitches in either an intracorporeal or extracorporeal fashion as described by Reich.[18] This technique can be especially useful in the presence of a thickened tubal wall refractory to thermal eversion. In addition to absorbable suture, endoscopic absorbable staples may be used to ensure that eversion is adequate.

The completed salpingoneostomy reconstruction is ideally recorded by videography or other recording method. Patency should be tested by transcervical retrograde insufflation with dilute indigo carmine dye. The previously described copious irrigation and antiadhesion adjuncts should be applied prior to terminating the procedure.

The success of distal tubal reconstructive procedures depends largely on the preoperative condition of the fallopian tube and the presence and degree of periadnexal adhesions. Intrauterine pregnancy rates after microsurgical salpingoneostomy for mild degrees of tubal disease have ranged from 58.8% to 86.0%, whereas rates for severe cases ranged only from 5% to 19%.[4,5,8] Overall pregnancy rates achieved by laparoscopic methods are comparable with crude pregnancy rates and range from 14.0% to 28.5%. Ectopic pregnancy rates range from 5% to 10%.[13,14,18–20] As is the case with abdominal salpingoneostomy, the pregnancy rates for laparoscopic reconstructions are inversely correlated with the severity of tubal disease. Cases with preserved fimbria and ciliated mucosa demonstrate the greatest success rates.[21]

One must keep in mind when interpreting the literature on this subject that most of the previously noted studies had small sample sizes, no controls, and inadequate descriptions of surgical technique, precluding direct comparison of results. In addition, experimental documentation of the degree of tubal disease was frequently lacking, classifications of the disease were ill-defined, or the definition was so highly subjective that comparisons could not be made from study to study.

Given that only 10% of cases of distal tubal occlusion are diagnosed early (when disease is mild) and that 60% are first diagnosed as severe disease, the overall prognosis is poor.[8] As with any surgical procedure, patient selection is critical for maximizing successful outcome. Some laparoscopic studies have demonstrated significantly lower pregnancy rates compared to salpingoneostomy performed by laparotomy.[14,20] In view of this finding the prudent practitioner not highly skilled in endoscopic techniques may use a microsurgical approach via laparotomy in the case of mild tubal disease to gain a two- to threefold greater chance of success. Cases of moderate to severe tubal disease that are associated with success rates nearly comparable for either the laparoscopic or the abdominal approach can be reconstructed at the time of diagnostic laparoscopy. Postoperative pregnancy rates are low, and such women ultimately may still require IVF to achieve pregnancy.

Success rates for IVF have been shown to be highest in cases for which the indication for treatment is tubal disease. In vitro teams across the country are demonstrating pregnancy rates of 19–33% per transfer and live birth rates of 15–20% per cycle.[22] Thus in situations in which the expected pregnancy rate is significantly higher with IVF than with surgical reconstruction, the surgeon should extensively counsel the patient in this regard. Because the final decision concerning the treatment approach ultimately may incorporate the several factors previously mentioned (e.g., religion, socioeconomic circumstances) a formulation of distinct and unchanging criteria for the abandonment of surgical reconstruction in favor of IVF is not feasible.

Second-Look Laparoscopy

In an effort to increase the effectiveness of tubal reconstructive procedures and theoretically to reduce the formation of dense permanent adhesions, second-look laparoscopy has been advocated in a number of preliminary reports in the literature.[23–26] However, studies comparing patients undergoing second-look laparoscopy with those expectantly managed after reproductive surgery report that no significant difference can be demonstrated in cumulative pregnancy rates over 1–3 years.[27,28] Although more than half of the adhesions that were lysed at first-look surgery did not recur when graded at the second-look procedure, success rates were not significantly different.[27] There may be a slight reduction in the time elapsed from initial surgery to pregnancy with second-look laparoscopy; but, once again, overall cumulative pregnancy rates were not found to be significantly increased.[28] In light of the added expense and morbidity associated with an additional surgical procedure that has not yet proved to have a clear-cut advantage, we cannot at this time advocate early second-look laparoscopy for the improvement of intrauterine pregnancy rates after reproductive surgical procedures.

Conclusion

The advent of sophisticated endoscopic instrumentation and techniques has established the laparoscopic method of reproductive surgery as an alternative to traditional microsurgical techniques performed by laparotomy. It is the responsibility of the reproductive surgeon always to appraise each patient individually and to select those who may best be served by the particular method of reconstruction. It is also imperative that each surgeon take into account his or her level of skill and experience. Surgical correction of a distal tubal obstruction must be undertaken only when a clear-cut advantage is present over the currently available advanced assisted reproductive technologies such as IVF.

Referenecs

1. AFS classifications of adnexal adhesions, distal tubal obstructions, tubal pregnancies, mullerian anomalies of 12 intrauterine adhesions. Fertil Steril 1988;49:944.
2. DONNEZ J, CASANAS-ROUX F: Prognostic factors of fimbrial microsurgery. Fertil Steril 1986;46:200.
3. YOUNG P, EGON J, BARLOW J, ET AL: Reconstructive surgery for infertility at the Boston Hospital for Women. Am J Obstet Gynecol 1970;108:1092.
4. MAZE G, PARLY J, JOLISSIERE J, ET AL: A preoperative classification to predict the intrauterine and ectopic pregnancy rates after distal tubal microsurgery. Fertil Steril 1986;46:807.
5. BOER-MEISEL M, VELDE E, HABBEMA J, ET AL: Predicting the pregnancy outcome in patients treated for hydrosalpinx: a prospective study. Fertil Steril 1986;45:23.
6. HULKA J: Adnexal adhesions: a prognostic staging and classification system based on a five year survey of distal surgery results at Chapel Hill, North Carolina. Am J Obstet Gynecol 1982;144:141.
7. ROCK JA, KATAGOMA KP, MARTIN ET, ET AL: Factors influencing the success of salpingostomy techniques for distal fimbrial obstructions. Obstet Gynecol 1978;52:591.
8. SCHLAFF W, HARSIAKOS D, DAMEWOOD M, ET AL: Neo-salpingostomy for distal tubal obstruction: prognostic factors and report of vaginal technique. Fertil Steril 1990;54:984.
9. SINGHAL V, LI TC, COOKE ID: An analysis of factors influencing the outcome of 232 consecutive tubal microsurgery cases. Br J Obstet Gynaecol 1991;98:628.
10. SCHOGSMAN R: Tubal microsurgery versus in vitro fertilization. Acta Eur Fertil 1984;15:5.
11. MAGE G, BRUHAT M: Pregnancy following salpingostomy: comparison between CO_2 laser and electrosurgery procedures. Fertil Steril 1983;40:472.
12. PATTON GW: Pregnancy outcome following microsurgical fimbrioplasty. Fertil Steril 1982;37:150.
13. METTLER L, GIESEL H, SENUN K: Treatment of female infertility due to tubal obstruction by operative laparoscopy. Fertil Steril 1979;32:384.
14. FAZIZ J: An assessment of the role of operative laparoscopy in tuboplasty. Fertil Steril 1983;39:476.
15. GOMEL V: Salpingo-ovariolysis by laparoscopy in infertility. Fertil Steril 1983;40:607.
16. GOMEL V: Classification of operations for tubal and peritoneal factors causing infertility. Clin Obstet Gynecol 1980;23:1259.
17. KOSASA T, HALE R: Treatment of hydrosalpinx using a single incision eversion procedure. Int J Fertil 1988;33:391.
18. REICH H: Laparoscopic treatment of extensive pelvic adhesions, including hydrosalpinx. J Reprod Med 1987;32:736.
19. DONNEZ J, NISOLLE M, CASARA-ROUX F: CO_2 laser laparoscopy in infertile women with adnexal adhesions and women with tubal occlusions. J Gynecol Surg 1989;5:47.
20. DANIELL J, HERBERT C: Laparoscopic salpingostomy utilizing the CO_2 laser. Fertil Steril 1984;41:558.
21. NEZHAT C, WINER WK, COOPER JD, ET AL: Endoscopic infertility surgery. J Reprod Med 1989;34:107.
22. In vitro fertilization-embryo transfer in the United States: 1988 results from the IVF-ET registry; Medical Research International and the Society for Assisted Reproductive Technology. Fertil Steril 1990;53:13.

23. DIAMOND M, DANIELL J, MARTIN D, ET AL: Tubal patency and pelvic adhesions at early second-look laparoscopy following intraabdominal use of the carbon dioxide laser: initial report of the intraabdominal laser study group. Fertil Steril 1984;42:717.
24. JANSEN R: Early laparoscopy after pelvic operations to prevent adhesion: safety and efficacy. Fertil Steril 1988;49:26.
25. RAJ S, HULKA J: Second-look laparoscopy in infertility surgery: therapeutic and prognostic value. Fertil Steril 1982;38:325.
26. DANIELL JP, HAWAG D: Short-interval second-look laparoscopy after infertility surgery. J Reprod Med 1983;28:281.
27. TRIMBOS-KEMPER T, TRIMBOS J, VAN HALL E: Adhesion formation after tubal surgery: results of the eighth-day laparoscopy in 188 patients. Fertil Steril 1985;43:395.
28. TULANDI T, FALIONE T, KAFKA I: Second-look operative laparoscopy 1 year following reproductive surgery. Fertil Steril 1989;52:401.

13
Laparoscopic Tubal Reanastomosis

D. Alan Johns

The reversal of female sterilization procedures has challenged gynecologists for years. The first descriptions of gynecologic microsurgery were directed toward treatment of pelvic adhesive disease and distal tubal occlusion. In 1974 Gomel adapted these techniques to accomplish reanastomosis of electively occluded fallopian tubes.[1] Microsurgical instrumentation, operating microscopes, and extremely small sutures were quickly incorporated into gynecologic microsurgery. The microsurgical principles and techniques described by Gomel during the 1970s have been widely accepted, resulting in (so far) two decades of excellent results.

Twenty years of data have confirmed the safety, efficacy, and outcome of conventional microsurgical tubal reanastomosis by laparotomy. Rates of patency, pregnancy, and ectopic gestation are accepted and reproducible among authors. Undoubtedly, the ability of the surgeon to apply microsurgical principles has been the key to this success.[2]

Coinciding with concerns over rising health care costs, the first reports of outpatient tubal reanastomosis came in 1991.[3] Principles and techniques developed during the 1970s were used through smaller skin incisions, permitting shorter hospital stays and quicker recovery. This quest for smaller "access" incisions continued into the 1990s.

The intrusion of laparoscopy in all areas of operative gynecology naturally led to attempts at endoscopic tubal reanastomosis. Although few reports of this new technique are available, widespread interest in endoscopic surgery continues to encourage its investigation. Despite the paucity of information available on endoscopic microtubal reanastomoses, the objective of this chapter is to review and compare available data on tubal reanastomosis at laparotomy, minilaparotomy, and laparoscopy.

Preoperative Evaluation (All Patients)

Prior to this rather expensive procedure, every patient should undergo thorough preoperative counseling and evaluation. Simple confirmation of ovulatory status is mandatory. In oligoovulatory patients, successful ovulation induction should be documented preoperatively.

Adequate semen parameters, determined by semen analysis, should be present, ideally with progressively motile sperm in ovulatory cervical mucus. Any factors potentially diminishing the chances of pregnancy should be evaluated, corrected, and carefully discussed with the patient.

Operative reports from the sterilization procedure should be reviewed to determine the type of procedure performed and the likelihood of adequate tubal segments being present. Patients who have undergone irreversible sterilization procedures (fimbriectomy) should be identified prior to surgery and referred for assisted reproductive technology. Evaluation of the proximal tubal segments by hysterosalpingography is occasionally helpful for preoperative assessment.

Expected tubal patency rates and ectopic and intrauterine pregnancy rates should be candidly discussed with the patients judged to be candidates for surgery. Alternatives to reanastomosis (in vitro fertilization; IVF) should also be discussed. Currently available success rates of each should be provided to the patient.

Tubal segments varying greatly in diameter are often encountered, including cornual-isthmic, isthmic-ampullary, and isthmic-infundibular segments. Successful reanastomosis of such tubal segments requires experience and skill. Gynecologists interested in performing these procedures must be familiar with microsurgical principles and techniques in order to afford patients the best chance of success.

Tubal Reanastomosis by Laparotomy

Technique

Conventional microsurgical tubal reanastomosis has been described in numerous textbooks and journals.[2] An operating microscope is recommended, although operating loupes (with maximum 6× magnification) are commonly used. Standard microsurgical instruments are required. Use of 8-0 to 10-0 sutures is advised. Adherence to traditional microsurgical principles is mandatory.

Prior to the skin incision, a method for tubal insufflation is established. A 10F pediatric Foley catheter introduced through the cervix into the uterine cavity provides a simple route for tubal insufflation. Packing the vagina with surgical gauze elevates the uterus, making the adnexal structures more accessible. Uterine manipulators are occasionally helpful but may interfere when positioning the uterus and adnexae for optimal exposure.

Depending on the method of sterilization, many surgeons perform a diagnostic laparoscopy as the initial step of the procedure. Tubal segments are assessed, any concomitant pathology evaluated, and the appropriate surgical approach planned. Optimally, the reanastomosed tube should measure at least 5 cm in length at the conclusion of the procedure. If the tubal segments are inadequate for reanastomosis or other pathology precluding the planned procedure is encountered, the patient has not been committed to laparotomy. Additionally, the surgeon may treat adnexal adhesive disease laparoscopically, allowing the reanastomosis to be accomplished through a minimal Pfannenstiel incision.

After access to the pelvis has been established via a Pfannenstiel incision and treatment of any associated adnexal adhesive disease has been completed, the length and condition of proximal and distal tubal segments is carefully noted. The fallopian tube to be approached initially is elevated and isolated with warm moistened laparotomy pads. "Packing" the bowel away from the operative field is rarely necessary and may contribute to diminished postoperative bowel function. A Kirshner retractor is helpful when small (4–6 cm) incisions are used.

The proximal tubal stump is identified and dilated with fluid via the transcervical catheter. The distal segment of the proximal stump is incised until normal tubal lumen is identified. Insufflation confirms the patency of this tubal segment. Whether the tube should be transected with laser, electrosurgery, or scissors is debatable, but there appears to be little difference when microsurgical principles (e.g., gentle tissue handling, careful hemostasis, continuous irrigation) are observed.

After identifying the distal tubal segment, the fimbria is closely inspected. Abnormalities (e.g., adhesions, phimosis) are noted and corrected as necessary. The proximal end of the distal tubal segment is incised and the patency of this segment confirmed. It is imperative that meticulous hemostasis be maintained during this portion of the procedure, and unipolar microneedle electrosurgery is particularly suited to this task. Excessive damage to the tubal lumen from heat, pressure,

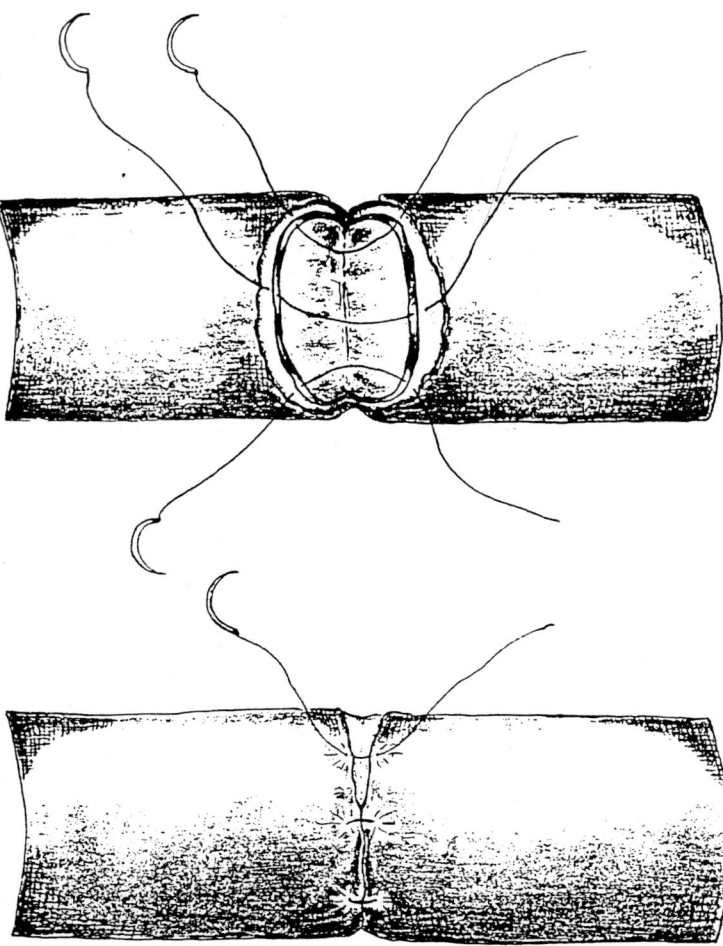

Figure 13.1. 2-layer closure of mid segment reanastomosis.

desiccation, or poor technique may ultimately lead to tubal scarring and should be avoided at all costs. Constant irrigation of the segments intraoperatively minimizes desiccation of the tubal serosa and subsequent adhesion formation.

If the tissue at the "newly opened" ends of the segment does not appear viable (i.e., fibrotic and does not bleed easily), another 0.5–1.0 cm portion should be removed until the remaining segments are healthy in appearance and bleed easily (demonstrating adequate vascularity).

After both tubal segments have been prepared, they are brought into alignment by approximating the mesosalpinx with 4-0 to 6-0 absorbable, non-reactive suture material (Fig. 13.1). This maneuver brings the prepared ends of the tubes into relatively close apposition, simplifying placement of 8-0 to 10-0 sutures for reapproximation of the lumen. The remainder of the mesosalpingeal defect is then closed.

The tubal lumen is reapproximated (usually in two layers) with fine, monofilament, nonreactive, absorbable suture. The first layer approximates the muscularis of the tube and the second layer the serosa. Some authors recommend against passing suture material through the tubal lumen, whereas others believe this practice has no effect on subsequent patency. Depending on the size of the lumen, three to eight interrupted sutures in each layer are required to appropriately reanastomose the tube. A stent of 0 to 2-0 nylon passed into the lumen of each tubal segment may aid the surgeon in avoiding placement of sutures into or through the lumen.

This technique, although conveyed here in an abbreviated manner, reflects generally accepted principles for microtubal reanastomosis. Virtually all published data on this topic recommend similar procedures, equipment, and techniques.[4-8] Reported success rates (patency, intrauterine pregnancy, extrauterine pregnancy) are based on these principles and must be the basis for comparison when discussing laparoscopic tubal reanastomosis.

Outcome

Microsurgical tubal reanastomosis via laparotomy is in general an uncomplicated surgical procedure. Infection, intraoperative and postoperative bleeding, and postoperative ileus may occur but are rare. Most authors report no major intraoperative or postoperative complications in their series.[3-9] Postoperative hospital stays of 2–4 days are common. Recovery is similar to that after most commonly performed gynecologic laparotomy procedures.

Numerous articles have been published examining pregnancy rates following microsurgical tubal reanastomosis at laparotomy. Utilizing microsurgical principles, pregnancy rates of 40–90% have been reported.[2-5,7-9] Tubal patency rates vary depending on the type of reanastomosis performed. Cornualisthmic anastomoses are associated with the lowest reported patency rates (20%) and ampullary–ampullary anastomoses with the highest (88.8%).[2,6]

Ectopic pregnancy rates of 1–23% have been reported after tubal reanastomosis, with most authors reporting an incidence of 4% or less. The higher ectopic rates have been associated with cases in which microsurgical techniques were not used.[6] After reanastomosis, spontaneous abortion rates as high as 17% have been reported,[6] although most authors do not believe reanastomosis adversely affects these rates.

In summary, the experienced, skilled surgeon using accepted microsurgical techniques at laparotomy can anticipate the following: tubal patency in up to 90%, pregnancy in up to 90%, ectopic gestation rate of 4% or less, and few operative complications. Unfortunately, there are no reported data examining costs related to this procedure.

Minilaparotomy (< 6 cm Incision)

The desire to reduce medical costs has spawned efforts to perform some gynecologic procedures through ever smaller incisions. If successful, these procedures performed via "minilaparotomy" offer the combination of shorter hospital stays and reduced patient recuperation time.

Data currently available on outpatient microsurgical tubal reanastomosis by minilaparotomy suggest that the technique offers tubal patency rates, intrauterine and ectopic pregnancy rates, operative time, and complications comparable to those achieved by the same procedure performed at laparotomy.[3] With a shorter hospital stay and quicker recovery, minilaparotomy offers significant economic advantages over traditional modes of access (laparotomy) for tubal reanastomosis. It should be noted that we are comparing virtually the same surgical procedure, only performed through different sized abdominal incisions. If all other factors are equal, reductions in cost and morbidity are important advantages in today's health care environment.

In my series of 26 patients undergoing outpatient microsurgical tubal reanastomosis via minilaparotomy, the operating time averaged 118 minutes, and all patients were discharged within 23 hours of their procedure. Furthermore, 85% of the reanastomosed tubes were subsequently found to be patent, and 70% of patients attained an intrauterine pregnancy. No complications occurred and all patients recovered within 2 weeks or less[10].

Laparoscopic Tubal Reanastomosis

The quest to perform gynecologic procedures endoscopically has evolved to include a laparoscopic approach to tubal reanastomosis. Laparoscopic video technology and improved equipment for laparoscopic suturing have allowed these attempts to proceed. If the laparoscopic surgeon expects to achieve the same pregnancy rates attainable at laparotomy, however, microsurgical principles and techniques must be observed.

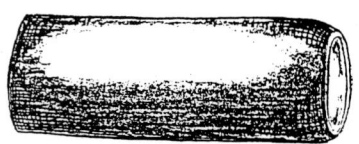
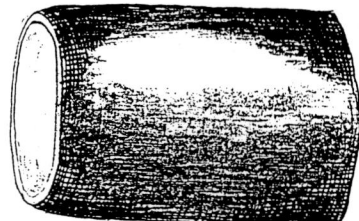

Figure 13.2. Reanastomosis of tubal segments of differing lumen diameter.

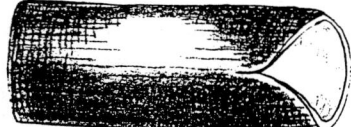

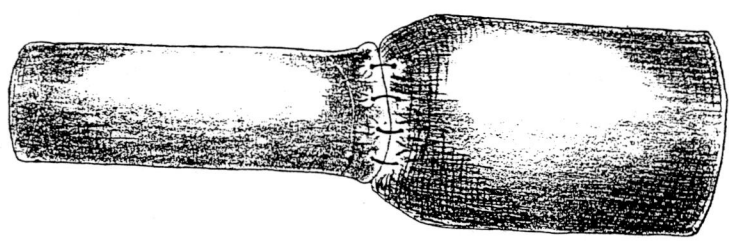

Reanastomosis via laparoscopy presents unique technical problems for the surgeon. Preparation of the tubal segments, hemostasis, and precise placement of fine suture material are comparatively simple procedures at laparotomy. The same procedures at laparoscopy can be frustrating and time-consuming. The result of frustration and extended operative time often is associated with poor technique and increased tissue damage, both of which decrease the probability of success.[11] Surgeons reporting on their attempts at laparoscopic reanastomosis have strictly adhered to microsurgical principles during these procedures, including the use of magnification (the laparoscope), fine suture material, precise hemostasis, and careful atraumatic technique.[11–14]

Preparation of the occluded end of the distal tubal segment has proved to be one of the more challenging steps in the procedure. Adhesions commonly obscure this area, making identification of the tubal lumen difficult. The distal tubal segment must be stabilized and the lumen precisely opened to create the appropriate diameter necessary to match that of the proximal segment. Transection of this segment at the proper angle for reanastomosis has proved to be an endoscopic challenge[11] (Fig. 13.2).

Reich et al. reported the use of stents to maintain the tubal segments in close apposition. Stabilizing the two segments close together facilitates precise laparoscopic placement of 6-0 to 8-0 sutures. Intracorporeal knot tying techniques, though difficult and tedious, are required for securing these sutures.

Koh has reported laparoscopic tubal reanastomosis using 7-0 and 8-0 sutures and standard microsurgical techniques. The difficulty of suture placement was partially overcome with newly designed laparoscopic needle holders. Even with instruments specifically designed for the procedure, however, Koh reported operative times from 2.5 to 6.0 hours.[14]

Results

Three groups have reported outcomes of outpatient microsurgical reversal of tubal sterilization by either laparoscopy or combined laparoscopy and minilaparotomy.[3,11,14] Their three papers represent 28 patients. The operative times for these patients ranged from 65 minutes to 5.5 hours. The patency rates were not calculable, as many of the patients did not have follow-up hysterosalpingography. The ectopic pregnancy rate was cited in only one paper (at 18%). The pregnancy rates in this small group of patients range from 35% to 50%. The authors reported no postoperative complications, and all patients were discharged on the day of their surgery.

By any parameter, laparoscopic tubal reanastomosis is currently inferior to the same procedure performed via laparotomy or minilaparotomy. The only advantage currently offered by the laparoscopic version of tubal reanastomosis is a recovery time shortened from 7–14 days (minilaparotomy) to 2–7 days (laparoscopy).

Conclusions

Tubal reanastomosis at laparotomy remains the "gold standard" to which other methods must be compared. Twenty years of microsurgical experience confirm its safety and efficacy. Fortunately, however, surgical expertise continuously advances and improves. Operative laparoscopy has proved to be one of the most influential innovations in gynecologic surgery, and attempts at laparoscopic tubal reanastomosis is an integral aspect of this trend.

In gynecologic surgery, small abdominal incisions usually result in short hospitalizations and quick recoveries. This trend toward small incisions led to a number of gynecologic procedures being performed via minilaparotomy. Microtubal reanastomosis requires a relatively small operative field and therefore is ideal for this approach. Because the same microsurgical techniques are possible with either laparotomy or minilaparotomy, outcomes are similar with either approach.

Operative laparoscopy offers the surgeon an opportunity to diagnose and treat adnexal pathology with minimally invasive techniques, permitting the reanastomosis to be completed through a small incision. Possibly, the role of the laparoscope in tubal reanastomosis lies in preparation of the tubal segments for reconstruction via minilaparotomy.

When all parameters have been evaluated, the procedure associated with the best outcome, fewest complications, and lowest cost will prevail. When currently available data are reviewed, microsurgical tubal reanastomosis performed via minilaparotomy with an outpatient (< 23 hours) hospitalization represents the most cost-effective method by which a previously sterilized patient may attain pregnancy (Table 13.1).

Laparoscopic tubal reanastomosis is certainly in its infancy. Improved laparoscopic skills coupled with new instrumentation and suture material may decrease the operative time. Experience should improve the pregnancy rates. In the past the laparoscopic approach to treatment of ectopic pregnancy moved from an anomaly to an accepted standard. Laparoscopy may ultimately prove to be the new "gold standard" for tubal reanastomosis.

Table 13.1. Data for three microsurgical techniques for tubal reanastomosis

Factor	Laparotomy	Minilaparotomy	Laparoscopy
Operative time (minutes)	97	100–179	150 (65–360)
Complications (%)	<1	<1	<1
Hospital stay (hours)	17–60	3–23	<6
Recovery (days)	14–42	7–14	1–3
Cost ($)	Unknown	5724	Unknown
Patency rate (%)	44–64	70–89	Unknown
Pregnancy rate (%)	50–96	71	35
Ectopic rate (%)	1–23	6	18

References

1. GOMEL V: Tubal reanastomosis by microsurgery. Fertil Steril 1977;28:59.
2. GOMEL V: Microsurgical reversal of female sterilization: a reappraisal. Fertil Steril 1980;88:587.
3. SILVA PD, SCHAPER AM, MEISCH JK, SCHAUBERGER CW: Outpatient microsurgical reveral of tubal sterilzation by a combined approach of laparoscopy and mini-laparotomy. Fertil Steril 1991; 55:696.
4. MCLAUGHLIN DS, BONAVENTURA LM, JARRETT JC: Tubal reanastomosis: a comparison between microsurgical and microlaser techniques. Microsurgery 1987;8:83.
5. MCDONELL CF, DAUGHTREY P, HOLLOMAN J, MILLER D: Microsurgical reversal of female sterilization. NC Med J 1992;53:142.
6. VERCHUYSSE PH, BOECKX W, BROSENS I: Microsurgical reversal of female mechanical sterilization techniques. Contraception 1988;38:99.
7. GOMEL V, YARALI H: Infertility surgery: microsurgery. Curr Opin Obstet Gynecol 1992;4:390.
8. GILLETT WR, MARTIN WL, ROMANS SE: Reversal of female sterilization: outcome of 210 referrals. NZ Med J 1993;106:173.
9. GALEN DI, JACOBSON A: A successful microsurgical reanastomosis program in a community hospital. J Reprod Med July 1996;7:595.
10. JOHNS DA: Outpatient tubal reanastomosis: a review of 26 patients. 1994; In press.
11. REICH H, MCGLYNN F, PARENTE C, ET AL: Laparoscopic tubal anastomosis. J Am Assoc Gynecol Laparosc 1993;1:16.
12. TSIN DS, MAHMOOD D: Laparoscopic and hysteroscopic approach for tubal anastomosis. J Laparoendosc Surg 1993;3:63.
13. KATZ E, DONESKY B: Laparoscopic tubal anastomosis: a pilot study. J Reprod Med 1994;39:497.
14. KOH CH: Laparoscopic tubal reanastomosis. MVP Video J Obstet Gynecol 1993;6.

14
Endometriosis

David B. Redwine

Since the classic description by Cullen in 1920,[1] endometriosis has attracted sustained and well deserved attention by clinicians, researchers, and patients. That such a common disease could remain so mystifying after so many decades suggests that fundamental concepts regarding the disease may be in error.

Definition

Endometriosis is a disease process of glandular elements and associated stroma. The tissue involved somewhat resembles native endometrium but exists in locations remote from the endometrium. Several generations of gynecologists have believed that endometriosis is simply ectopic native endometrium, but application of this concept has not resulted in conceptual or therapeutic breakthroughs, in part because endometriosis differs significantly from native endometrium (Table 14.1).

The important fundamental differences between endometriosis and native endometrium help explain the frustrations that accompany the understanding and treatment of the disease since the early part of this century. This frustration is compounded needlessly by confusion when a biopsy-proved absence of endometriosis is accepted as scientific proof of its presence[2] or when the visual opinion of the surgeon is substituted for histology. The presence of glands and stroma remains the gold standard for the histologic diagnosis of endometriosis (Fig. 14.1).

Etiology

The etiology of endometriosis remains debatable. If its etiology were known, rational and effective treatment might be developed. Some argue that knowing the etiology of endometriosis is unnecessary for understanding the disease and the development of therapy against it (M. Vernon, personal communication, 1993), whereas others disagree with this position.

Sampson's Theory

Although many theories of origin have been advanced and reviewed in the literature,[4,5] Sampson's theory of reflux menstruation historically has been the most popular theory advanced to explain the origin of endometriosis. This theory holds that menstrual blood is regurgitated through the fimbriated ends of the fallopian tubes each cycle during menses, carrying with it viable cells from the lining of the uterus that attach to peritoneal surfaces, implant, and develop into endometriosis.

Table 14.1. Differences between endometriosis and native endometrium

Characteristic	Endometriosis	Native endometrium
Visual appearance	Protean	Proliferative, secretory
Histology	Varying degrees of differentiation	Well differentiated, in cycle
Menstrual cycle histology	Unpredictable	Predictable
Hormone receptors	Low and varying levels	Normal levels
Hormone response	Varying	Predictable
Frequency of cyclic bleeding	Uncommon	Always in ovulatory cycles
Associated fibrosis	Occurs	Does not occur

A modification of this theory seeks to invoke a selective deficiency of the immune mechanism to explain attachment and implantation of viable endometrial cells in some, but not all women undergoing reflux menstruation.[5] With this scheme, a competent immune system is able to reject refluxed endometrial cells and so prevent the development of endometriosis, whereas the disease develops in women with defective immune systems. For example, natural killer (NK) cell activity is decreased in the peritoneal fluid of patients with endometriosis compared to that of normal controls,[6] apparently because of a depressive effect by a serum component.[7] Complete excision of pelvic endometriosis therefore does not improve NK function.[6] How-

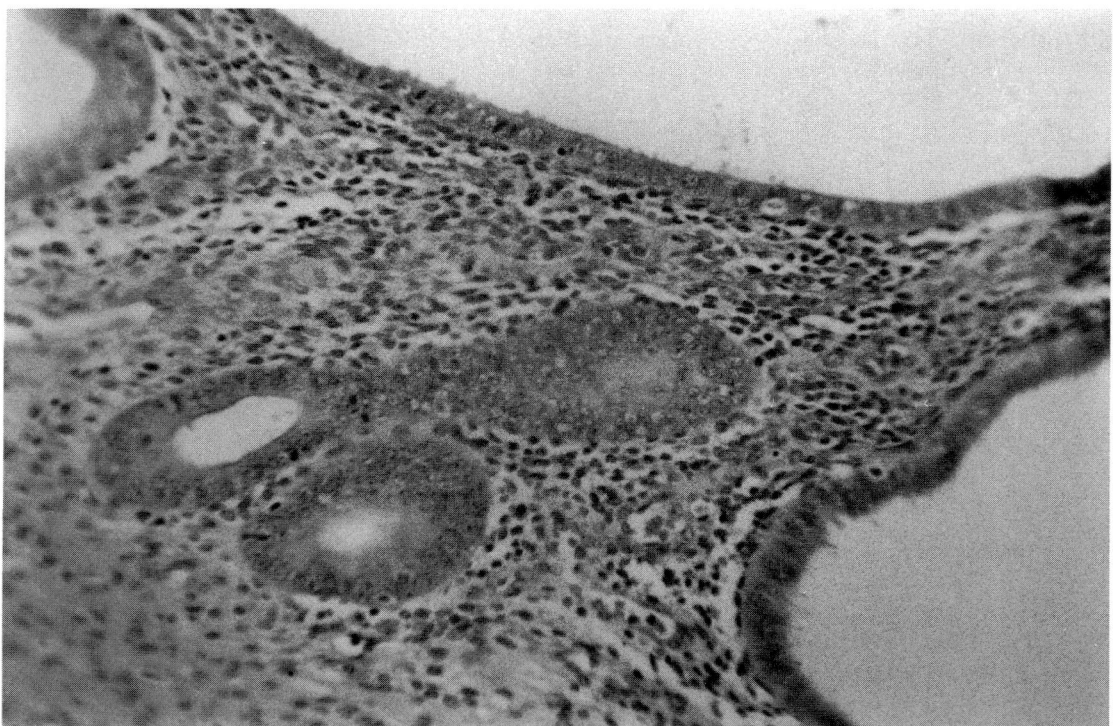

Figure 14.1. Histologic appearance of endometriosis. Glandular epithelium with surrounding stroma is the "gold standard" for the histologic diagnosis of endometriosis. This photomicrograph depicts well differentiated endometriosis. However, there is disparity in the size of glands, which indicates a possible asynchronous response to hormonal effects. In some patients, individual glands contain epithelium of varying levels of differentiation.

ever, the NK deficits that have been observed are variable and are present even in some normal adults.[8] Although glucocorticoid treatment may enhance fertility in patients with endometriosis,[9] there currently is no other immunologic therapy with application to endometriosis.

Although many of the putative steps involved in Sampson's theory have been demonstrated, the sine qua non of this theory is the demonstration of initial peritoneal attachment of refluxed endometrial cells or groups of cells. These attached groups of cells must be small enough to have traversed the smallest diameter of the isthmus of the fallopian tube, which measures at most 200 μm in diameter. The chronologically ordered sequence of (1) attachment to the peritoneum of single or multiple endometrial cells followed by (2) implantation and (3) proliferation should be easy to prove by light microscopy, but virtually all published photomicrographs of endometriosis depict established disease. Even studies on microscopic endometriosis have failed to find evidence of the initial peritoneal attachment of refluxed endometrium, and undetected "microscopic" endometriosis invariably seems to exist as subperitoneal disease in the few patients who have been found to harbor such subtle disease.[10–15] Abundant evidence for initial attachment should have been found by now, as it is assumed by supporters of the Sampson theory that reflux menstruation is common and is the main mode of origin of disease. Because confirmatory evidence has never been produced in more than 70 years of exhaustive study of the disease, the absence of microscopic evidence of initial attachment of endometrial cells effectively casts doubt on Sampson's theory about the etiology of endometriosis. Endometriosis has also been reported in many locations within the female body, which cannot be explained by reflux menstruation,[16–18] and has even been reported in elderly men undergoing estrogen therapy for advanced prostatic cancer, though a rare occurrence.[19,20] Recurrence after complete excision is much lower than would be predicted by this theory.[21,22]

Adherence to Sampson's theory of origin carries significant risks. The assumption that endometriosis is always a geographically spreading disease has led recent generations of gynecologists to abandon surgical therapy in favor of medical therapy, the hope being that medical therapy would retard the "dandelion spread" that is supposed to occur with this disease and that would make surgical therapy ultimately futile and associated with a high rate of recurrence. This assumption appears to have been accepted by a leap of faith rather than because it is supported by scientific evidence. Any failures of medical or surgical therapy can conveniently be explained by this theory of origin that predicts such failures, so clinicians do not have to question the scientific rationale or clinical efficacy of their treatments if they assume that "the disease always comes back."

Other Theories

Although the glandular and stromal complexes of endometriosis have received most of the attention over the years, it seems increasingly likely that there may be several related pathologic states in patients with the disease, including ovulation disorders and immune system changes. Although pain associated with pelvic pathology is what brings most patients to their physicians, a systemic, expanded view of endometriosis is needed in which the entire patient is considered, not just the pelvic endometriosis.[23] In the vacuum left by the continued lack of supporting evidence for Sampson's theory, metaplasia of embryologically patterned tracts of peritoneum emerges as a more rational etiology of endometriosis that would more likely explain the implant in the body. Such tracts, composed of surface peritoneum and sub peritoneal substrate, may be laid down in the embryo, perhaps enabled in utero by slight inborn defects of the fetal immune system that can persist and are identifiable in the adult.

Epidemiology

The prevalence of endometriosis has been estimated to range between 1% and 53% depending on the group of women under study,[24] although 10% is a commonly mentioned rate for the general population. The youngest patient reported with the disease was 10.5 years old[25] and the oldest more than 78 years old.[26] Five million American women are affected by the disease,[24] which makes endometriosis a common gynecologic condition. Because surgery is required for its definitive diagnosis, prevalence estimates of endometriosis are subject to Berkson's fallacy[27] and may not be representative of the total population of women. At surgery, incomplete identification of endometriosis can have a profound impact on our understanding of the disease.[28] A familial tendency has been described.[29]

Natural History

Conventional wisdom has long held that endometriosis is a progressive disease, owing in large part to adherence to Sampson's theory. Progression is thought to occur in several ways with advancing age: more widespread involvement of the pelvis, more invasiveness of individual lesions, and accompanying adhesions. Sampson's theory of reflux menstruation certainly suggests that patients should develop more widespread and extensive pelvic involvement with advancing age as repetitive monthly reflux menstruation seeds the pelvis. However, newly diagnosed older patients do not exhibit more pelvic areas of involvement,[30] nor is there an increase in surface pelvic involvement, although some lesions can become more invasive locally.[31-33] Most untreated patients do not exhibit progression of their disease,[34] and the seemingly "new" disease may simply be an illusion resulting from the age-related change in color of lesions from subtle to more obvious forms.[35] The natural history of the disease after excision at laparotomy and laparoscopy seems benign, with a 19% incidence of new, minimal endometriosis observed by 5 years after surgery, even with no intervening medical therapy.[21,22]

Other investigators have found that the stage of endometriosis, as measured by the revised American Fertility Society (rAFS) classification system,[36] does not increase with advancing age in populations of patients with endometriosis.[37] Moreover, even in a large referral practice spe-

Table 14.2. Distribution of rAFS stages[a]

rAFS stage	No. of patients	%
I	634	51.1
II	280	22.5
III	123	9.9
IV	205	16.5
Total	1242	100.0

[a]Excludes patients with previous hysterectomy or hysterectomy and bilateral oophorectomy.

cializing in the surgical treatment of endometriosis, lower rAFS stages of disease are more frequent than higher stages (Table 14.2). It should be noted, however, that the rAFS classification system of endometriosis has critical faults that render it incapable of determining disease extent accurately. The inability to account for intestinal disease, an emphasis on ovarian disease at the expense of more common peritoneal disease, an inability to distinguish increasingly widespread peritoneal involvement, and an inability to gauge disease accurately in women with previous hysterectomy and oophorectomy negatively affect the accuracy and precision of the system. For example, there are at least 78 ways to score 20 points. With more than 110,000 possible combinations of point totals, it is not consistently reproducible in clinical practice.[38]

Thus, the available evidence suggests that endometriosis is a positionally static disease that does not exhibit geographic spread with advancing age but may undergo varying degrees of local invasion. This natural history results in a low degree of persistence or recurrence after surgical destruction. If tracts of embryologically patterned subperitoneal substrate are not completely destroyed, the growth factors involved in the wound healing process may allow induction of new disease in a few patients. Such new disease is usually minimal and superficial.

Symptomatology

Patients with endometriosis present with pain, infertility, or an asymptomatic pelvic mass. Pain is almost three times more common than infertility as a symptom,[30] so the historical emphasis

Table 14.3. Distribution of endometriosis among women undergoing conservative excision (n = 953)

Area of endometriosis	No. of patients with disease in area	%
Pelvic areas		
Cul-de-sac	721	75.7
Left broad ligament	549	57.6
Right broad ligament	473	49.6
Left uterosacral ligament	417	43.8
Right uterosacral ligament	375	39.3
Bladder	340	35.7
Left ovary	153	16.0
Right ovary	144	15.1
Fundus	126	13.2
Left tube	85	8.9
Right tube	55	5.8
Intestinal areas		
Sigmoid	173	18.2
Rectal nodule	105	11.0
Ileum	36	3.8
Appendix	20	2.1

When nodularity (Plate 23) and tenderness are present, they are strongly suggestive of the presence of endometriosis,[39] although as many as 20% of patients may be asymptomatic.[30]

Symptoms associated with endometriosis are not always caused by the disease. The only way to determine if a symptom is caused by endometriosis is to apply a treatment that has been shown to eradicate the disease and observe whether the symptom is eliminated.

Diagnosis

The correct diagnosis of endometriosis begins in the office by identifying symptoms due to endometriosis. The cardinal symptom of endometriosis is pain. Thus clinicians should strongly consider endometriosis as the most likely diagnosis in women presenting with pelvic pain. If a patient with pelvic pain is presumed to have a sexually transmitted disease (STD) in the presence of a normal white blood cell (WBC) count and a normal erythrocyte sedimentation rate (ESR), is afebrile, and repeatedly fails to respond to multiple antibiotics, endometriosis should be considered. If the physician chooses empiric therapy with birth control pills or nonsteroidal antiinflammatory drugs, and if symptomatic improvement has not occurred after two or three menstrual cycles, endometriosis should be considered. Similarly, recurrent pain after initial improvement with conservative measures should prompt consideration of en-

on infertility seems misdirected. The geographic distribution of the disease parallels pathways of organogenesis across the dorsal coelomic cavity, with the cul-de-sac being most frequently involved (Table 14.3). Symptoms are frequently associated with the geographic location of the disease, although intestinal symptoms are nonspecific and may be caused by peritoneal or intestinal endometriosis (Table 14.4).

Table 14.4. Pain symptoms associated with location of endometriosis

Symptom	Cul-de-sac	Uterosacral ligaments	Ovary	Rectal nodule	Ileal nodule
Dyspareunia	+	+	−	+	−
Rectal pain	+	+	−	+	−
Rectal pain with sitting	−	−	−	+	−
Dyschezia	−	−	−	+	−
Dyschezia during menses	+	+	−	+	−
Flank pain	−	±	+	−	−
Pain radiating to flank	−	−	+	−	−
Pain radiating down leg	−	+	−	−	−
Right lower quadrant pain	−	+ (right)	+ (right)	−	+
Left lower quadrant pain	−	+ (left)	+ (left)	−	−
Nausea, constipation, diarrhea	+	+	+	+	+

dometriosis. Patients who require narcotic pain pills for analgesia should undergo a surgical diagnosis.

The cardinal sign of endometriosis is tenderness of the cul-de-sac or uterosacral ligaments, with or without nodularity. This sign can be detected with the internal examining hand without external palpation. It is fortunate that the cul-de-sac and uterosacral ligaments are among the most commonly involved areas, as they are easily reached on pelvic examination (Plate 23).

Imaging tests are not particularly helpful for the diagnosis or management of endometriosis. Intestinal endometriosis almost never penetrates the bowel lumen, so intestinal studies are commonly negative even in patients with severe intestinal endometriosis. Although there is a correlation between the tumor marker CA 125 level and the severity of endometriosis,[40] the CA 125 level can be elevated with other benign or malignant conditions.[41] Because production of CA 125 is not specific to endometriosis[42] it is not clinically useful for its management.

Surgery is usually necessary to establish a firm diagnosis, but the surgeon must be familiar with the appearance of endometriosis. Its visual manifestations are protean, often subtle,[43,44] and are often much different than the black powderburn lesion many clinicians were trained to identify. Endometriosis assumes many color manifestations and is sometimes even colorless in young patients.[35,45] An awareness of the wide range of visual appearances possible with endometriosis and the more common appearance of atypical, or "nonclassic" lesions indicates that a large degree of visual selection bias has been operative with this disease.[46] For this reason much of the literature before 1984, which may have focused on hemorrhagic forms of the disease, may not be applicable to a true understanding of the disease. Any visual abnormality of the pelvic peritoneum must be considered possible endometriosis unless proved otherwise by biopsy; and errors of visual identification have contributed directly to the confusion surrounding the disease.[46] Biopsy remains useful for clarifying the confusion about what is or is not endometriosis.

Parallel to the concept of subtle endometriosis is that of microscopic disease. Clinicians must be aware of the criteria of normal peritoneum in order to distinguish abnormal peritoneum that may harbor endometriosis.[47]

Treatment

Treatment options include observation, symptomatic treatment with medical therapy, or surgical therapy. Currently, no medical therapy is U.S. Food and Drug Administration (FDA)-approved specifically for treatment of infertility associated with endometriosis.[48]

Observation

Because endometriosis does not seem to spread geographically in the pelvis with advancing age and medical or surgical treatment of stage I or II endometriosis has not been clearly shown to be superior to no treatment in patients with no other cause of infertility,[49-51] observation may be appropriate for infertile endometriosis patients with a low level of painful symptoms, However, observation places some patients at risk of increasing local invasion and associated adhesions and is contrary to the clinical dictum that it is easier to treat a disease in its early stages than in later stages. Also, simply because a patient with significant pain is also infertile is not justification for continued observation.

Symptomatic Treatment

Ovarian suppression with birth control pills, danazol, or gonadotropin-releasing hormone (GnRH) agonist therapy may reduce or eliminate pain associated with endometriosis.[52] Modern therapy with GnRH agonists carries a high rate of side effects that cause many patients to abandon therapy before a typical 6-month course has been completed. Because all medical therapy is based on the still-unproven twin notions that pregnancy and the menopause physically eradicate endometriosis, it comes as no surprise that medical therapy results in a high rate of disease persistence: Minimal and mild endometriosis persist in at least 78% of patients at the conclusion of 6 months of medical therapy.[52] The persistence rate may be even higher if

Plate 1. Patient's position for laparoscopic hysterectomy.

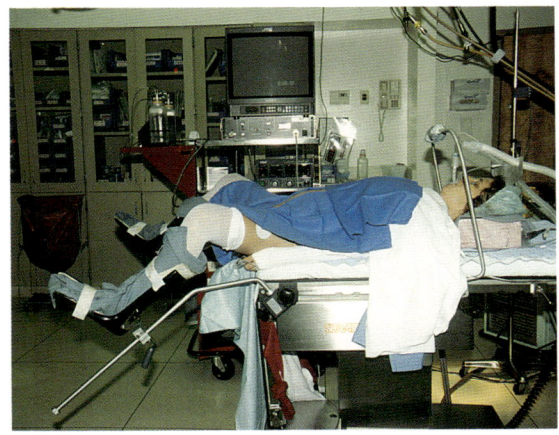

Plate 2. White line. Upper border of the vesico-uterine fold is identified as a white line when the assistant pushes the uterus upward. Above the white line, the peritoneum is firmly attached to the uterus. There is a distance of 2.0 to 2.5 cm between the white line and the dome of the bladder, and the peritoneum is loosely attached to the cervix.

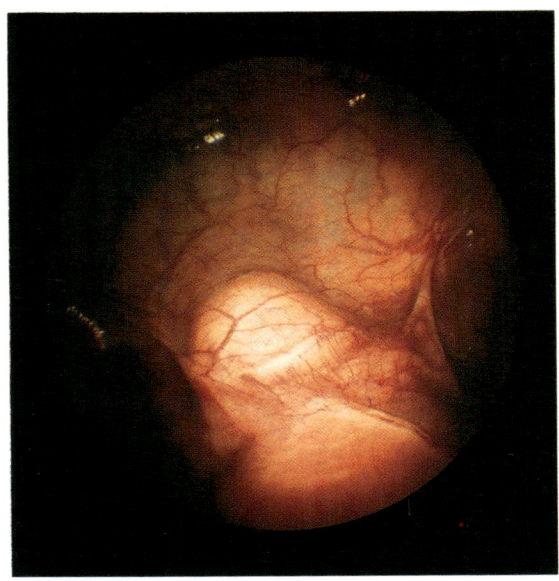

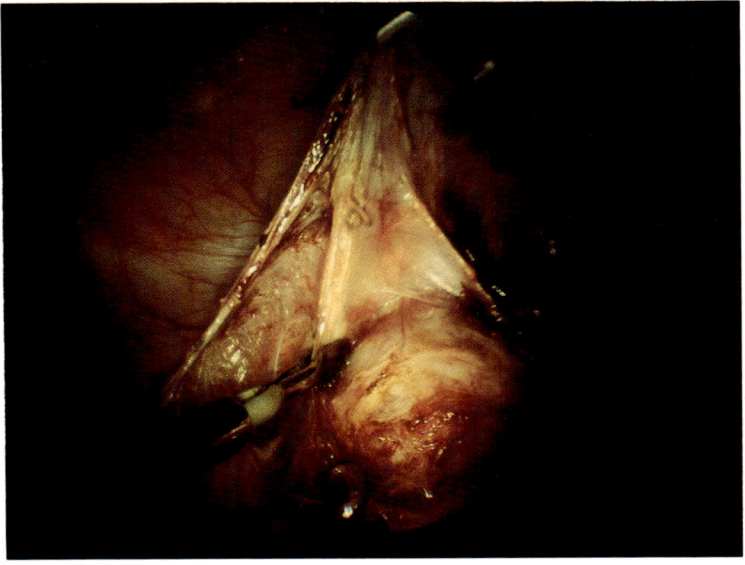

Plate 3. Bladder pillars must be coagulated before division.

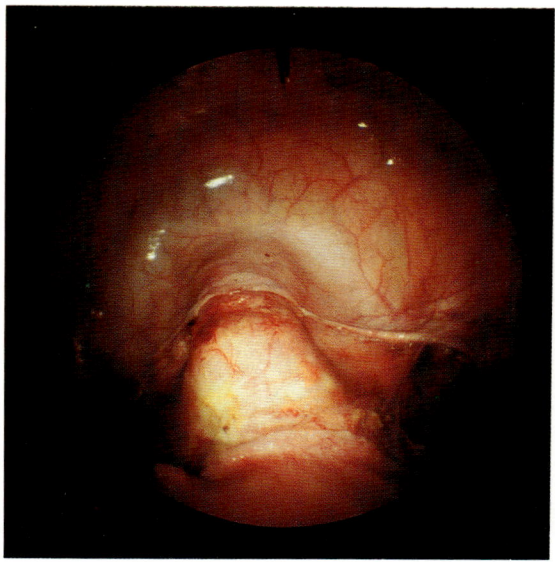

Plate 4. Bladder had been dissected down to the upper segment of the vagina. The pearly white appearance of the vesicocervical and vesicovaginal spaces can be identified.

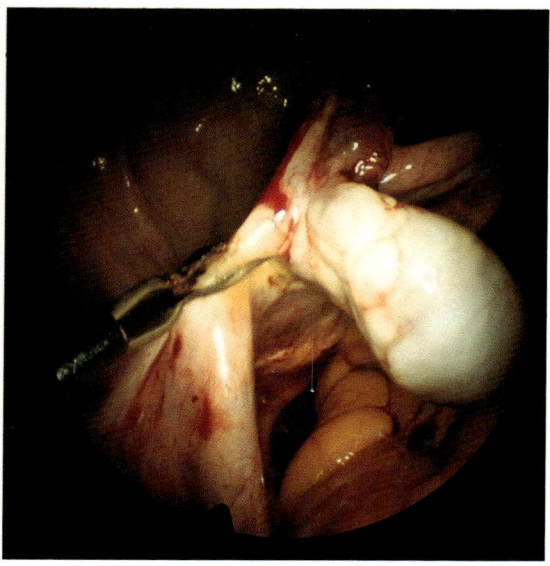

Plate 5. Infundibulopelvic ligament is desiccated with bipolar forceps.

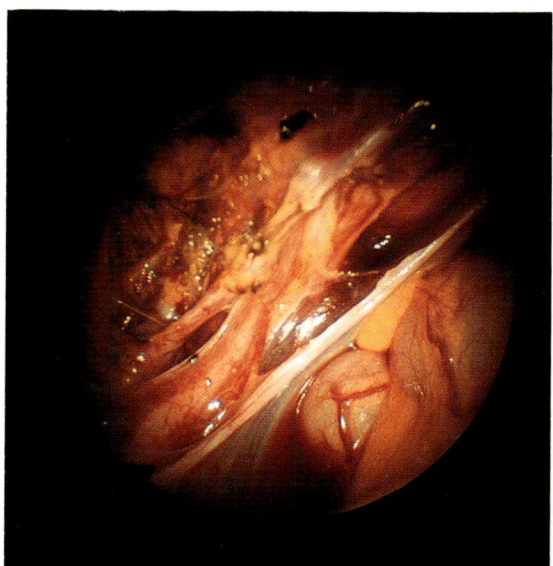

Plate 6. Ureter at the level of the ureteric canal. The roof of the ureteric canal is the uterine artery. The cardinal ligament lies below the ureter.

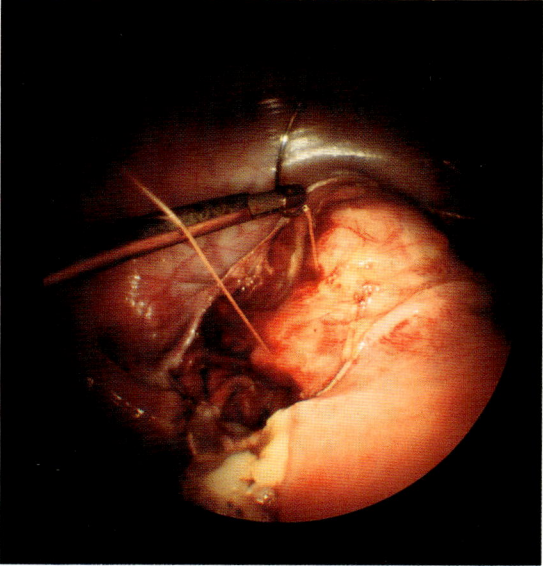

Plate 7. 0 Vicryl suture with CT-1 needle is used to suture-ligate both the uterine artery and the cardinal ligament.

Plate 8. Endo GIA-30 is used to staple and divide the uterine vessels and part of the cardinal ligament. The ureter must be identified before the automatic stapling device is fired.

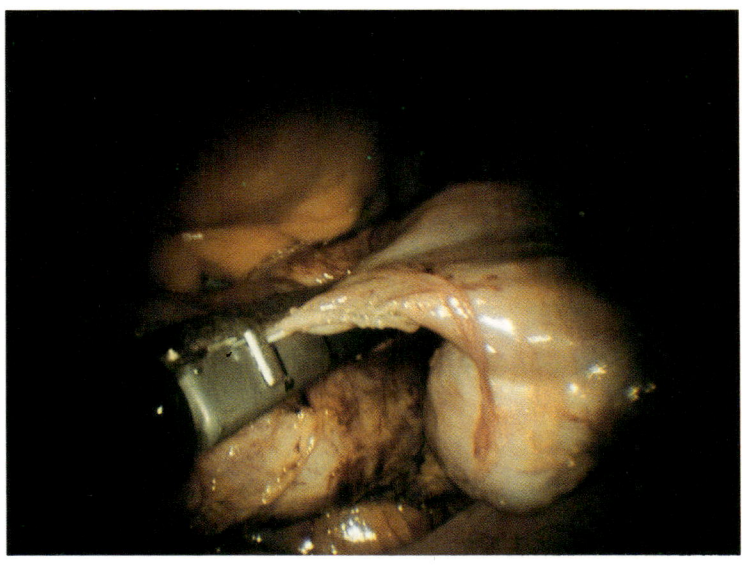

Plate 9. After circumferential culdotomy, the uterus is completely detached from the vagina, maintaining the pneumoperitoneum.

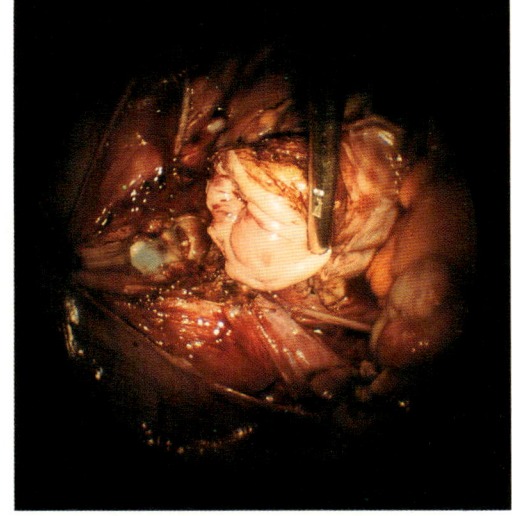

Plate 10. Vaginal cuff is closed with three interrupted figure-of-eight sutures. The uterosacrocardinal ligaments are sutured to the corner of the vaginal cuff to provide good suspension of the vagina.

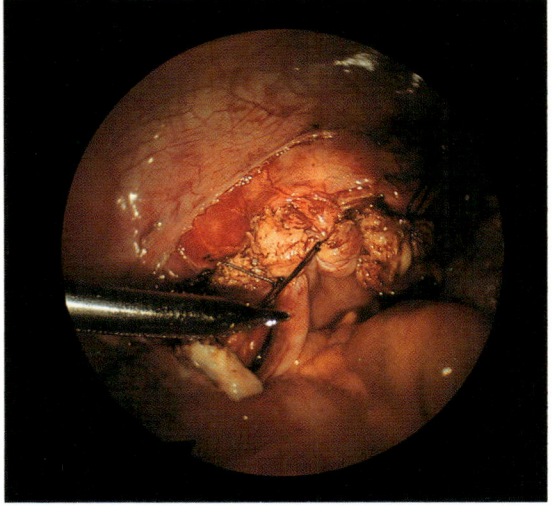

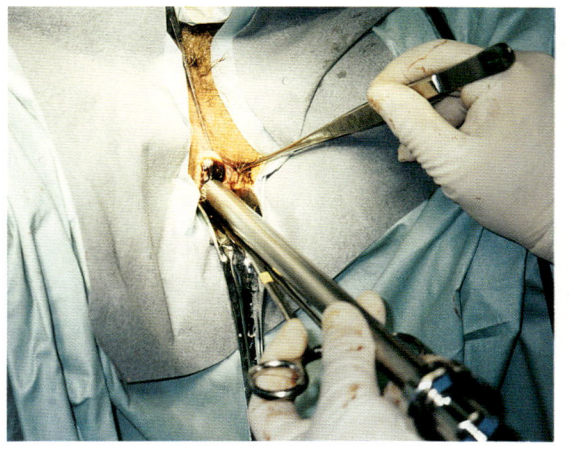

Plate 11. Coring of cervix with 15 mm CURT set.

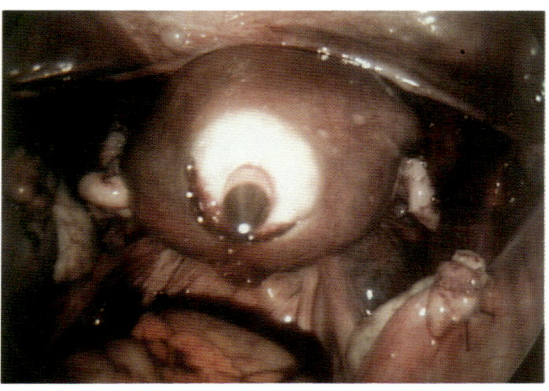

Plate 12. CURT perforates fundus. Intrafascial cervico-fundal tissue cylinder is removed.

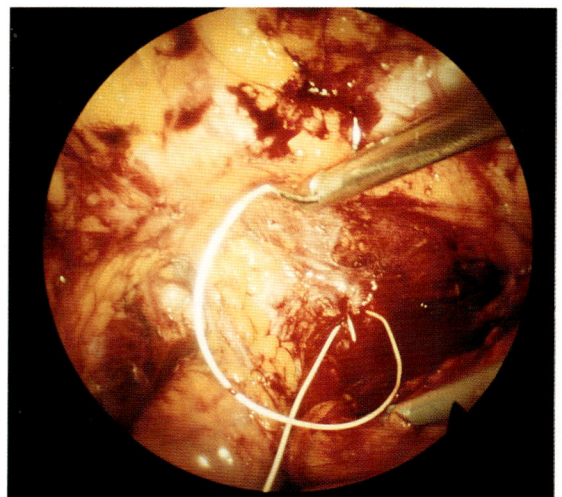

Plate 13. Double bite is taken of the whole thickness of the anterior vaginal wall but not penetrating the vaginal mucosa.

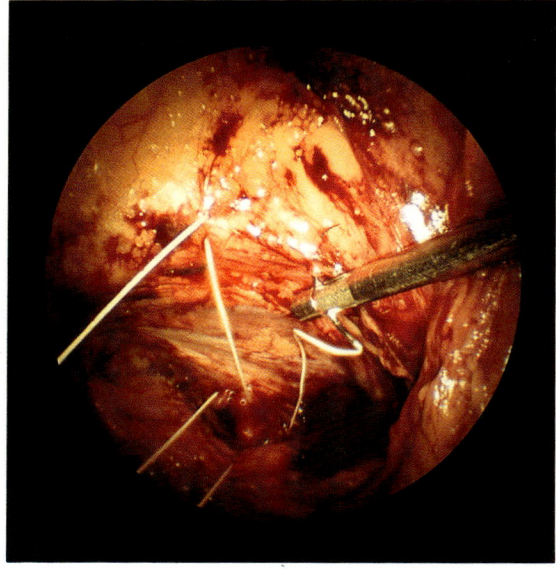

Plate 14. Deep bite of Cooper's ligament is critical to provide good suspension.

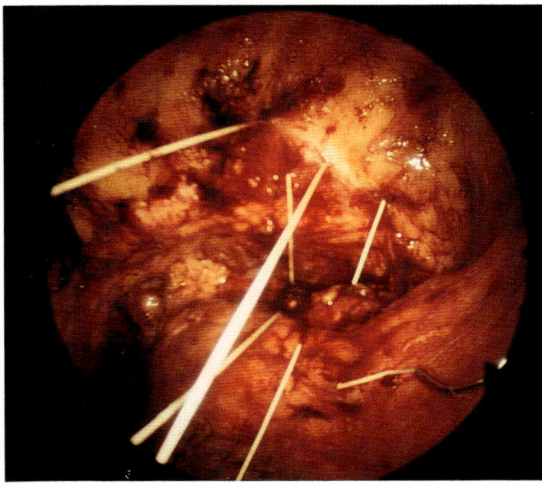

Plate 15. Two sutures are placed on each side of the urethra. The first suture is placed at the mid-urethral level and the second at about the U-V junction. Both sutures are placed at least 2 cm from the urethra and then through Cooper's ligament on the ipsilateral side.

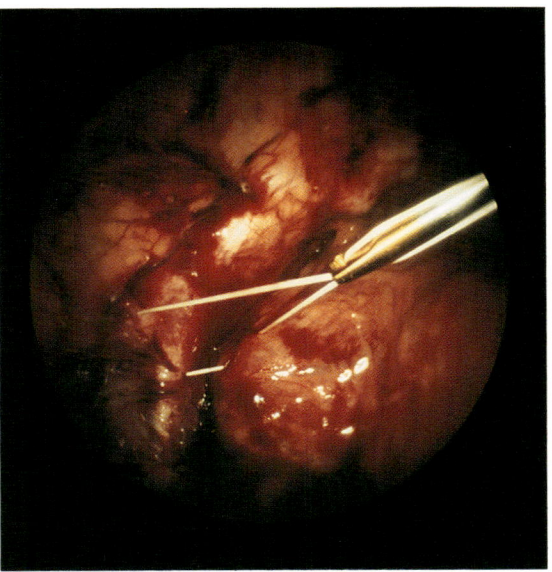

Plate 16. Extracorporeal knot-tying technique with a Clarke knot pusher. The knot is tied without undue tension.

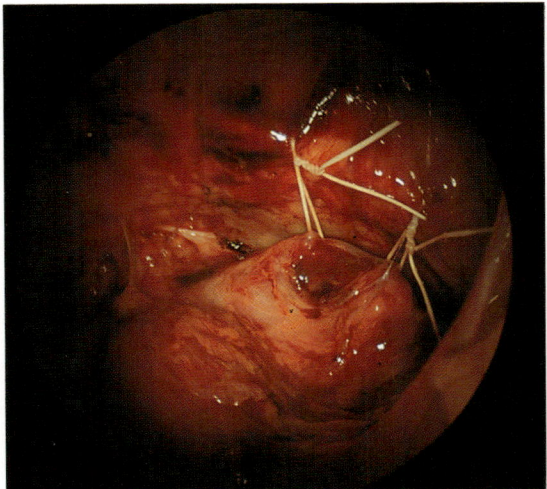

Plate 17. The knot should not be tied too tightly. It is not necessary to have the vaginal wall in direct contact with Cooper's ligament.

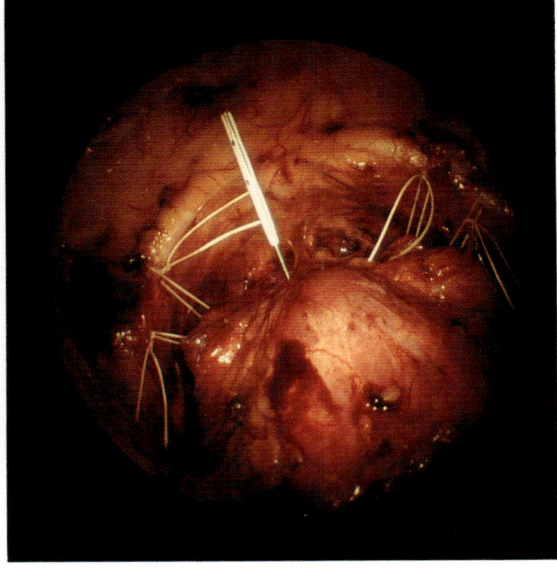

Plate 18. Banano suprapubic catheter is inserted into the bladder under direct visualization.

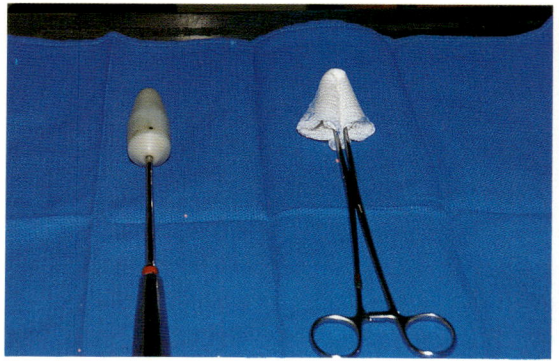

Plate 19. Rectal probe and vaginal manipulator are important instruments for rectocele and enterocele repairs.

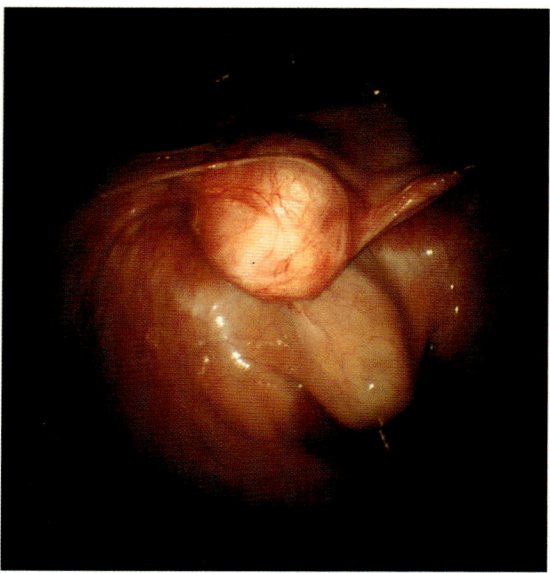

Plate 20. Laparoscopic view of the rectum and vagina with the rectal probe inside the rectum and the vaginal manipulator inside the vagina.

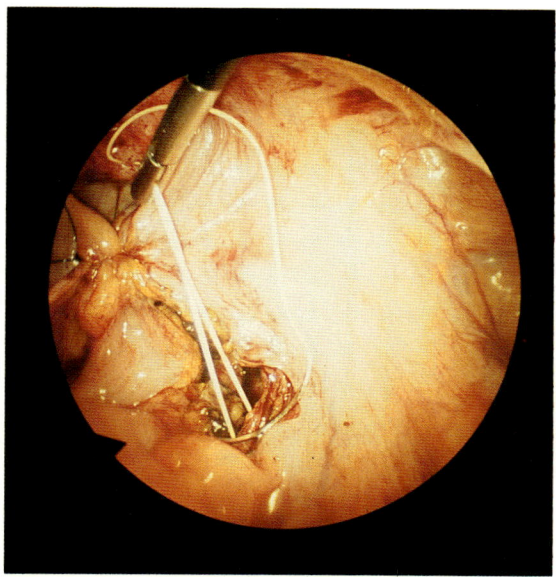

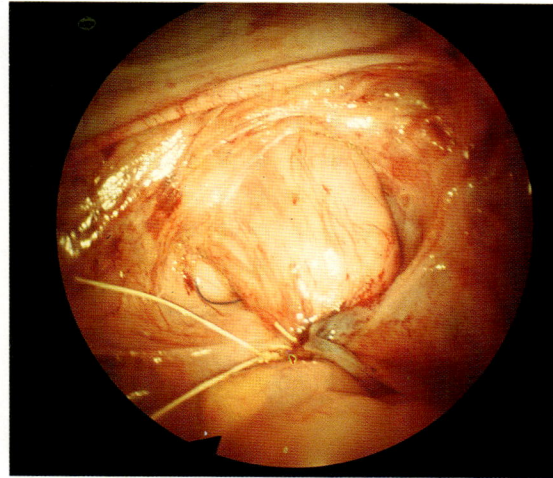

Plate 22. Completion of vaginal vault sacrospinous suspension.

Plate 21. Strength of the suture should be tested by forcefully pulling on it to make sure that the suture is placed deep in the sacrospinous ligament.

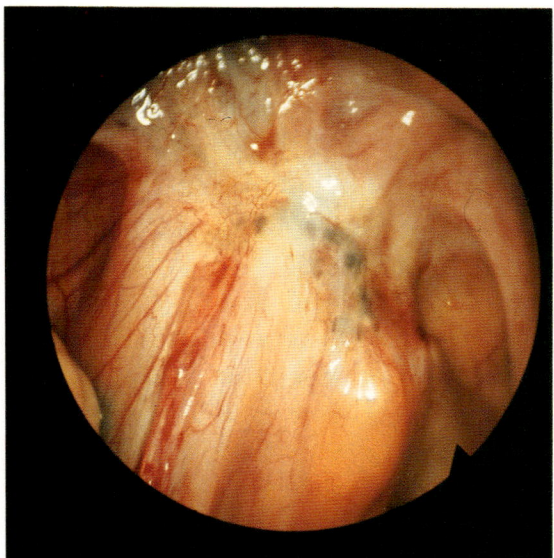

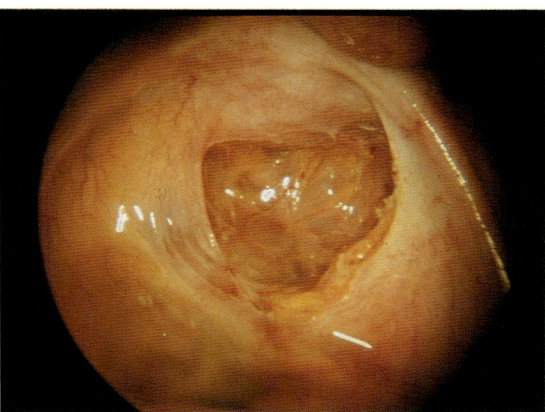

Plate 24. Right cul-de-sac after excision of endometriosis with the CO_2 laser. Note the lack of lateral thermal damage with the use of high power density. (Courtesy of Dan C. Martin, M.D.)

Plate 23. Invasive endometriosis of the left uterosacral ligament with partial obliteration of the cul-de-sac. This patient had a tender, palpable nodule in the left uterosacral ligament and symptoms including left-sided pelvic pain, deep dyspareunia, and painful defecation throughout the month. Note that the rectum is tented into the uterosacral ligament and is itself involved by invasive disease. Surgical therapy must address invasive disease of both the ligament and the bowel wall.

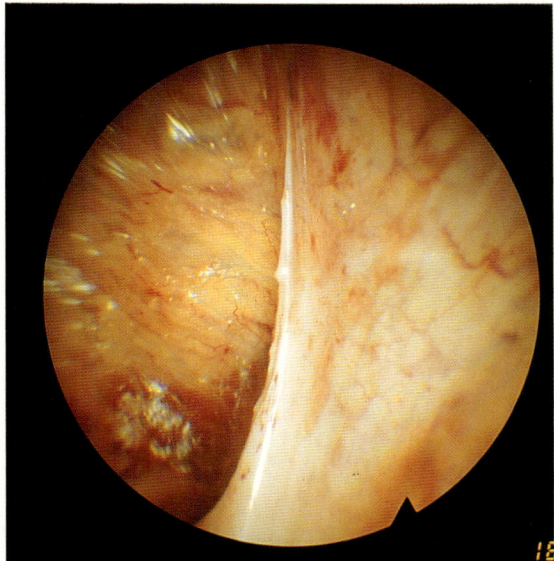

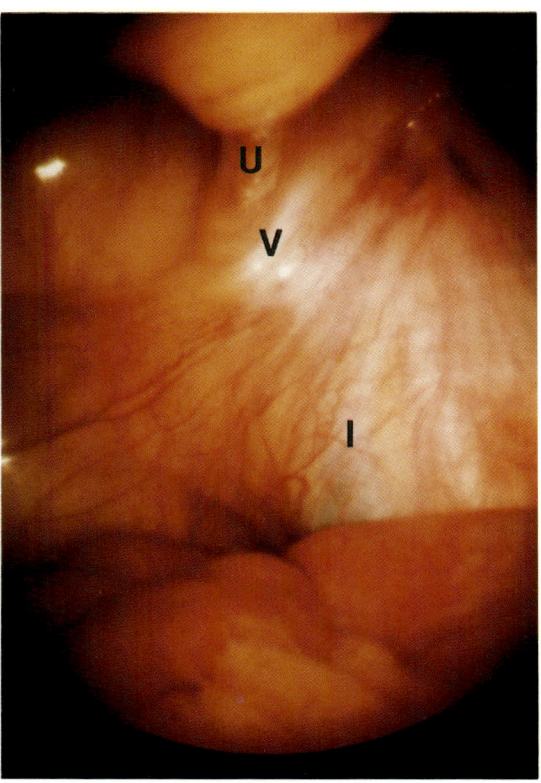

Plate 25. Close-up view of the left cul-de-sac after excision of endometriosis with 3 mm monopolar scissors. Note the lack of lateral thermal damage with the use of high power density.

Plate 26. Laparoscopic view of the iliac–obturator region. U, obliterated umbilical artery; V, vas deferens; I, iliac vessels. (From Gomella LG, et al: *Laparoscopic Urologic Surgery.* New York, Raven Press, 1994, with permission)

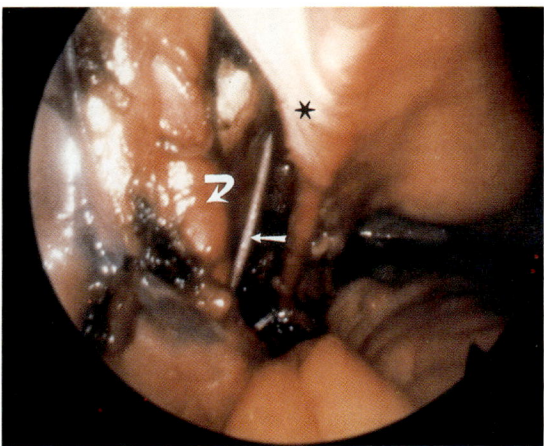

Plate 27. Complete left obturator lymph node dissection. Small arrow shows the obturator nerve; curved arrow indicates the external iliac vein; star is situated just lateral to the left obliterated umbilical artery. (From ref. 25, with permission)

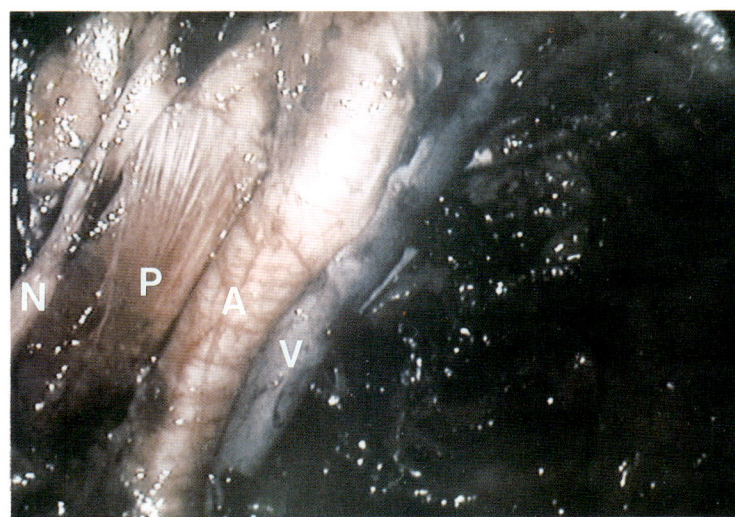

Plate 28. Left extended pelvic lymph node dissection for cancer of the bladder. V, external iliac vein; A, external iliac artery; P, psoas muscle; N, genitofemoral nerve.

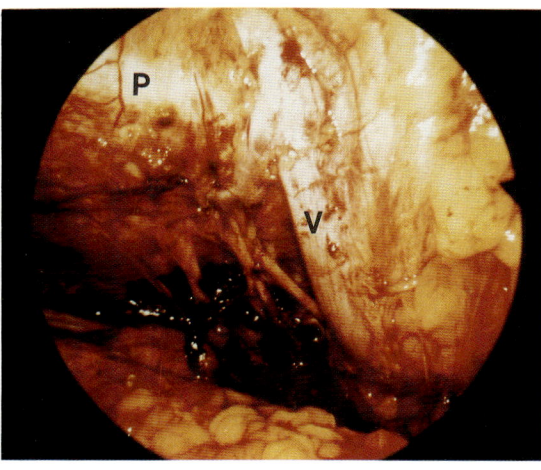

Plate 29. Balloon expansion of the extraperitoneal space of Retzius. P, pubic bone; V, external iliac vein.

subtle forms of the disease were overlooked at second-look laparoscopy performed during ovarian suppression.[53] Low-dose oral contraceptive steroids have been found in a randomized trial to produce pain relief equivalent to the GnRH agonist goserelin,[54] but early recurrence of pain is common[52,54,55] after medical therapy. It is generally accepted that medical therapy is far less effective than excision for eradicating the disease.[55] Medical therapy does not enhance fertility[56] and is not FDA-approved for treatment of infertility associated with endometriosis. The only clear indication for medical therapy in the treatment of endometriosis therefore is for temporary pain relief in patients who must delay surgery.

Because ovarian suppression may treat other estrogen-responsive sources of pain such as adenomyosis[57] leiomyomas,[58] pain at ovulation, or primary dysmenorrhea, medical therapy appears to be better than it really is for the treatment of endometriosis. Although it may be seen as an added benefit, the scientific process is confounded by measuring the response of symptoms rather than the response of the disease. Symptom recurrence following medical therapy is common. A pilot study of chronic GnRH therapy with estrogen add-back was shown to produce pain relief in six of eight patients treated for 24 months.[59] The medical effects of maintaining millions of women chronically on such experimental medical suppression is unknown, and the economic impact of such maintenance therapy would be far greater than effective surgery, which eradicates the disease.

Surgical Treatment

Successful surgical treatment of endometriosis depends on the following:

1. A technique, without intervening medical or surgical therapy that long-term follow-up confirms has eradicated or reduced the disease
2. A technique that can be used safely without limitations anywhere in the body
3. A technique that can be replicated widely by practicing clinicians
4. A technique that can eradicate deeply invasive disease

Confirmation of Therapeutic Efficacy of Surgical Treatment of Endometriosis

How well a surgical therapy eradicates endometriosis is an important question. The prognosis for symptom relief following a specific type of surgery depends heavily on published scientific validation of the completeness of eradication of the disease, particularly as endometriosis may invade from 1 cm to several centimeters underneath the visible peritoneal surface.[60–62] If pain or infertility are caused by endometriosis, complete eradication of the disease provides symptom relief of variable duration, depending on which theory of origin explains the etiology of the disease. Because not all symptoms are caused by endometriosis and because the response of symptoms does not necessarily reflect the response of the disease, surgical efficacy is best evaluated by data on second-look surgery to answer the following questions: (1) after a particular surgical therapy, what is the frequency of subsequent surgical interventions required to alleviate symptoms? (2) In reoperated patients, how often is endometriosis found? (3) When endometriosis is identified, how extensive is it? If medical therapy routinely follows surgical therapy, the long-term results may no longer be specific for the surgical effect.

Electrosurgery

Electrocoagulation is commonly used to treat endometriosis at laparotomy or laparoscopy. For effective performance of electrocoagulation, the clinician must have guidance regarding the electrosurgical generator used, the wattage setting, the active electrode, and the specific technique employed. None of the most influential articles on unipolar electrocoagulation[63–68] of endometriosis supplies all these details, so electrocoagulation of endometriosis remains relatively undescribed in the literature. All authors recommend caution and describe limitations on use over underlying vital structures such as the bowel, urinary tract, or large vessels. Because 61% of patients have lesions > 2 mm deep and 25% have lesions > 5 mm in depth[60] (Fig. 14.2) complete destruction of invasive endometriosis by electrocoagulation is difficult without en-

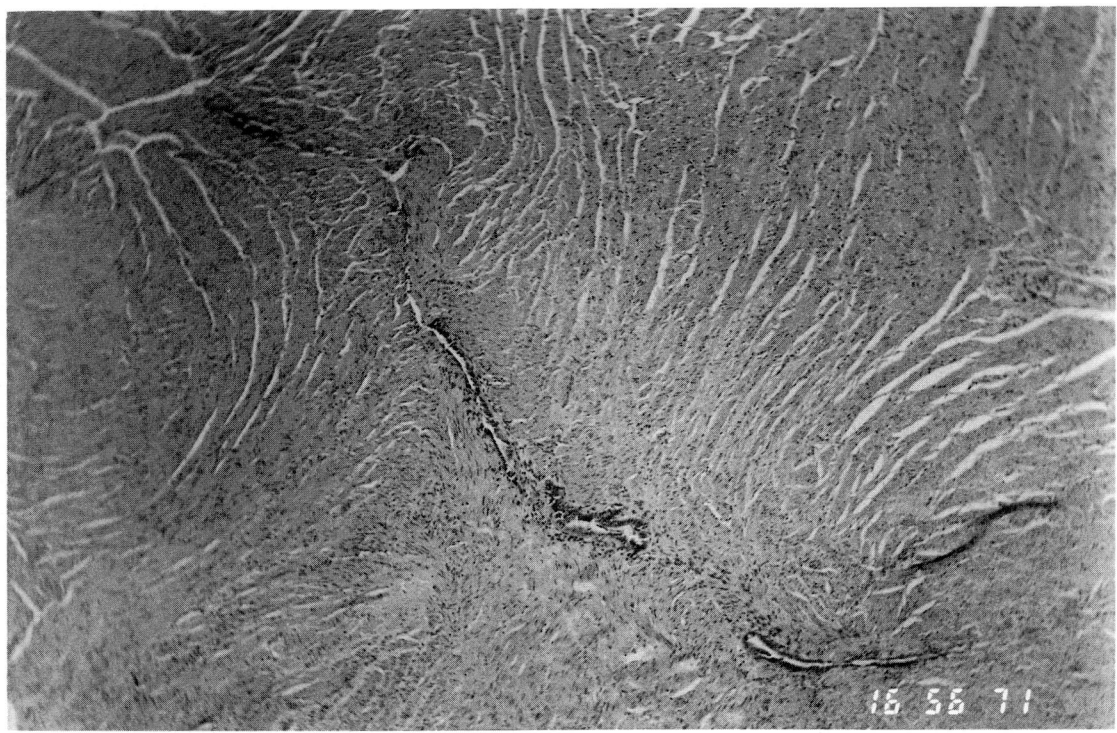

Figure 14.2. Glandular elements with sparse surrounding stroma located more than 10 mm deep within a fibrotic rectal nodule associated with complete obliteration of the cul-de-sac. To eradicate all disease detection of the presence or absence of such disease within a nodule is mandatory, and efforts to completely remove (and destroy) such structures is paramount.

dangering underlying structures. Superficial endometriosis could theoretically be destroyed by electrocoagulation, but the depth of invasion is not always predictable from the visible surface changes.[61] Because no pathology report is returned after electrocoagulation, all surgical findings and results are subject to the opinion of the surgeon. Finally, electrocoagulation has not been validated with respect to efficacy of physical destruction of endometriosis of any stage. It has been only loosely studied with respect to relief of the symptoms of pain and infertility. If significant uterosacral ligament disease is present, symptom recurrence was anecdotally noted to be more frequent,[63] probably as a direct result of the inability to completely destroy endometriosis by superficial electrocoagulation. Coupled with confusion over the terms "fulguration," "electrocautery," and "electrocoagulation," it is impossible to consistently duplicate the effects of electrocoagulation of endometriosis in clinical practice. Hence its use as front-line surgical therapy can be questioned.

Laser Vaporization

The CO_2 laser is the most commonly used laser for vaporization of endometriosis, although KTP[69] and Nd:YAG[70] lasers [71] have also been used. Compared to electrocoagulation, laser vaporization of endometriosis is well described with respect to hardware used, power settings, techniques, and tissue effects. Unwanted lateral thermal damage is limited when high power densities are used.[71] Laser vaporization has been studied primarily with respect to relief of symptoms of pain or infertility but has not been validated by follow-up studies as being effective for long-term eradication or reduction of endometriosis. Laser vaporization has limited use over vital structures, although aquadissection may provide protection against damage to underlying structures. Aquadissection, however, does not dissect the dense fibrosis that may accompany endometriosis. Laser vaporization does not produce a specimen for pathology, so therapeutic endpoints are defined at the discretion of the surgeon. Although superficial disease may be completely destroyed by laser vaporization, the result more frequently is debulking of endometriosis rather than complete surgical eradication, particularly when dealing with invasive disease with surrounding fibrosis.

Excision

Reproducible and understandable excisional techniques exist that allow treatment of invasive endometriosis anywhere in the pelvis or intestinal tract. Excision of endometriosis, whether at laparotomy[21] or laparoscopy,[23] has been shown by life-table analysis to result in a persistence or recurrence rate of 19% at 5 years after surgery. Excision can be performed with sharp dissection,[72] electrosurgery,[73] or laser.[74–76] Electroexcision is significantly faster than sharp dissection.[73]

Excision results in a pathology report that validates the scientific process and removes the bias introduced by a surgeon's visual opinion of tissue histology. Histologically confirmed absence of endometriosis, however, should not be accepted as scientific proof of the presence of disease.[2] Acceptance of benign pathology as malignant would be unacceptable in oncology, and no less discipline should be allowed for the study of endometriosis.

Excision of peritoneal endometriosis may require superficial or deep excision depending on the pathology. One of the principles of safe surgery is separation of diseased tissue from healthy tissue before dealing with the diseased tissue, and only excision allows strict adherence to this principle.

Monopolar electroexcision is performed with high current density. A 3- or 5-mm scissors is passed down the operating channel of a 10 mm laparoscope inserted through an all-metal cannula in the umbilicus. A Valleylab Force 2 or Force 4 generator is used, set at 90 watts of pure cutting current and 50 watts of coagulation current. The active electrode is activated before touching the tissue; otherwise pillowing of tissue can occur around the electrode tip with a decrease of current density and a resulting coagulation effect rather than a clean cut. The cutting current is used primarily on the peritoneum and for fine incisions. If 90 watts produces a coagulation effect rather than a clean cut, the wattage setting can be increased to 110 (watts) as needed. The footprint of the 3 mm scissors may be as small as 0.2 mm^2, resulting in a current density applied to the tissue of approximately 45,000–55,000 watts/cm^2. This current results in a surgical energy equivalent to that available with many lasers. As has been found with lasers (Fig. 14.2), high current density in monopolar electrosurgery results in a clean cut (Plates 24, 25) and "what you see is what you get." In a porcine model, such high current density produced little or no lateral thermal burn (E. Bieber, R. Tucker, and D.B. Redwine, unpublished data).

The coagulation waveform carries a voltage several times higher than the cutting waveform,[77] so this waveform is useful for retroperitoneal and parenchymal cutting, as through the insertion of the uterosacral ligament into the posterior cervix. Either waveform can be used for cutting or coagulation, as the surgeon's experience dictates. The speed of the electrode as it is drawn or pushed across the tissue is an important determinant of the surgical effect, as a slow speed results in a longer dwell time and increased coagulation effects.

It is important to understand that during monopolar electrosurgery for endometriosis the electrode is activated only for short intervals and for a fraction of the total time of surgery. Most of the surgical effect is accomplished by blunt dissection to isolate tendrils or columns of tissue, which can then be transected with electrosurgery.

Superficial peritoneal endometriosis can be resected by grasping and tenting up normal peritoneum adjacent to the endometriotic lesion, and then cutting across the pleat of tissue

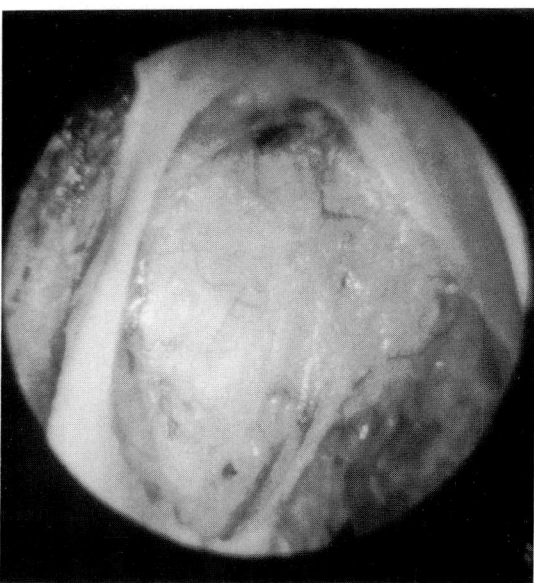 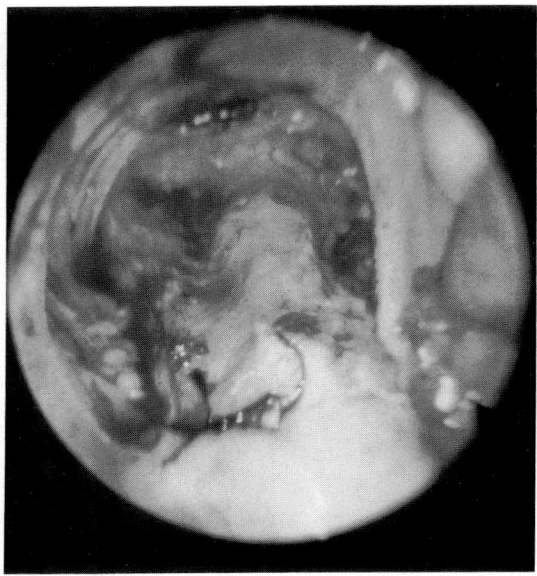

Figure 14.3. Superficial endometriosis studding the cul-de-sac has been removed by excision. Note the wall of the rectum lying just medial to the left uterosacral ligament. The rectum is invested within fatty tissue underneath the cul-de-sac and may lie relatively hidden, thus increasing the potential for trauma to the area.

Figure 14.4. Partial thickness bowel resection has been performed on the lower rectosigmoid colon and closed with 3-0 silk suture. Note that the left uterosacral ligament has been resected for treatment of an invasive nodule seen in Plate 23. The right uterosacral ligament remains intact to the right of the rectum. The right ovary and fimbriated end of the right tube are seen on the edge of the frame to the right. The rectovaginal septum has been developed bluntly distally, and the muscularis of the rectum contrasts with the shiny serosa of the proximal sigmoid.

created. The peritoneum can then be bluntly separated from the underlying structures using blunt dissection and excised. This technique allows safe treatment of endometriosis over the bowel (Fig. 14.3), urinary tract, or large vessels.

Resection of the uterosacral ligament is frequently necessary to treat endometriosis completely. A releasing incision is created in normal peritoneum lateral to the involved ligament, and a blunt probe is used to separate the ligament from the adjacent ureter and vessels. Occasionally, dense retroperitoneal fibrosis requires mechanical or electrosurgical ureterolysis or angiolysis. Once the ligament has been separated from the lateral vital structures, a peritoneal incision is made medially. Partial obliteration of the cul-de-sac sometimes requires this second peritoneal incision to be made on the contralateral side of the adherent rectum. The uterosacral ligament can then be transected at its insertion into the posterior cervix and dissected off the pelvic floor. With partial obliteration of the cul-de-sac (Plate 23) the incision is carried across the posterior cervix above the point of adherent attachment of the colon, and an intrafascial dissection is carried down the posterior cervix, removing a plane of tissue perhaps 2 mm thick. This intrafascial dissection is carried posteriorly until the rectovaginal septum is encountered distal to the involved bowel. The lateral attachments of the rectum can be severed to mobilize the bowel, and a partial-thickness (Fig. 14.4), full-thickness, or segmental bowel resection[78–80] is performed as needed. Endometriosis of the bowel rarely penetrates the mucosa (Fig. 14.5). Most frequently, endometriosis involving the colon can be removed by the technique of mucosal skinning, whereby the involved layers of muscularis are dissected off the

14. Endometriosis

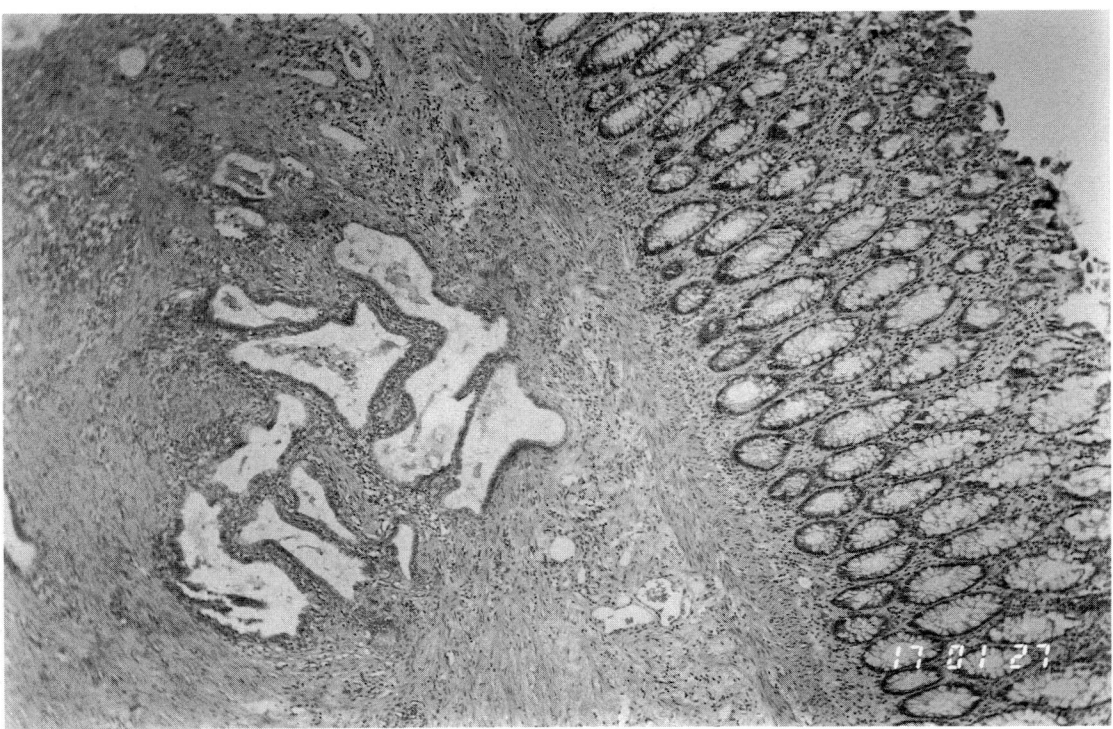

Figure 14.5. Histologic appearance of colonic endometriosis. Note the nest of endometriosis in the submucosa of the colonic wall without penetration of the mucosal layer.

mucosa without entry into the bowel lumen. In experienced hands this procedure can sometimes be accomplished without a bowel preparation. If a full-thickness bowel resection is performed, the mucosa is closed with running 3-0 chromic suture. The seromuscularis is closed with interrupted 3-0 silk suture applied longitudinally so as not to constrict the diameter of the bowel. If bowel surgery is anticipated, 4 L of oral colonic lavage (Abbott, Chicago, IL) can be given the afternoon before surgery and two enemas the evening before surgery. For patients unable to tolerate this type of bowel preparation, enemas until clear the morning of surgery usually cleanse the colon sufficiently to allow bowel surgery. A 4-day clear liquid diet may also be helpful in such patients.

Peritoneal regeneration occurs after excision (Fig. 14.6), although if surgery occurs on or around the ovaries, adhesions may result.[22]

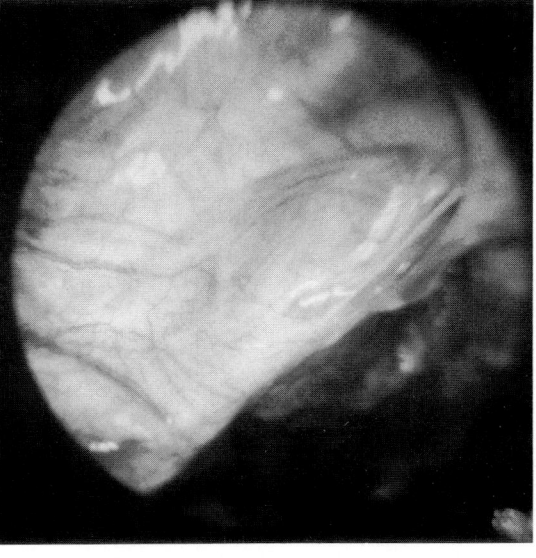

Figure 14.6. Regenerated peritoneum of the left broad ligament. Note the relative lack of retroperitoneal fat.

Hysterectomy and Bilateral Salpingo-oophorectomy

Although total abdominal hysterectomy and bilateral salpingo-oophorectomy (TAH/BSO) is commonly referred to as "definitive" treatment of endometriosis and is offered to patients as a cure for their disease, there is no scientific evidence that either the absence of the ovaries[81–86] or a menopausal level of estradiol is cytotoxic or cytocidal to endometriosis. Removal of the uterus, tubes, and ovaries eliminate endometriosis in fewer than 5% of patients[87]; therefore 95% of patients with such treatment could still harbor disease. Although removal of the uterus, tubes, and ovaries may relieve pain, the pain that is relieved could be from uterine, ovarian, or tubal origin rather than due to endometriosis. Symptomatic patients with previous TAH/BSO have an increased incidence of intestinal disease and an increased incidence of obliteration of the cul de sac. Therefore surgeons must be prepared to treat intestinal endometriosis in such patients. In those with previous TAH/BSO and continuing pain, excision of endometriosis results in pain relief in most patients.[87]

Complications

The best means of dealing with complications is to prevent their occurrence. To this end, adherence to the principles of safe surgery are paramount: extensive knowledge of anatomy, separation of healthy tissue from diseased tissue before destruction of the diseased tissue, and good visualization of the surgical target. Surgeons apply their expertise mainly with the sense of touch and the sense of sight. Anything hindering these senses can lead to unsafe surgery.

Endometriosis may be accompanied by invasion and fibrosis that involves adjacent structures, such as the ureter. When normal anatomy is distorted, blunt separation of the fibrotic area with ureterolysis is necessary in order not to traumatize the ureter. During ureterolysis considerable traction can be applied to the ureter by grasping it with atraumatic graspers, a technique that is occasionally helpful for obtaining the proper angle of surgical attack and may spell success or failure of the surgical effort. When the ureter is injured, it may be repaired over a stent. Blunt, sharp, or precise laser or electrosurgical dissection is frequently necessary to separate the fibrotic area from other pelvic structures and vessels. Such safe separation of healthy tissue from diseased tissue is routine during excision of endometriosis. Such separation is not always accomplished before application of laser vaporization or electrocoagulation; and surgeons using these modalities must always be aware of possible violation of this principle of safe surgery.

When bleeding occurs, an attempt should be made to isolate the vessel, particularly if it is buried in fat, otherwise electrocoagulation of the bleeder may be inefficient or unsafe. During resection of the uterosacral ligaments, the surgeon must anticipate the presence of rather large vessels lateral and deep to the uterosacral ligaments. Avoidance of these vessels is usually possible, and they can be safely controlled with bipolar or monopolar coagulation, as the ureter is usually placed well laterally.

If the bowel is lacerated during surgery, it should be repaired primarily with 3-0 chromic

Table 14.5. Complications among 825 conservative laparoscopies for excision of endometriosis

Complication	No. of patients		
	Occurrences	Reoperation	Transfusion
Fever, possible infection	4	0	0
Bleeding	5	2	1
Bladder perforation	1	0	0
Peroneal nerve paresis	1	0	0
Clinical deep vein thrombosis	1	0	0

on the mucosa and interrupted 3-0 silk on the seromuscular layer. Copious irrigation and prophylactic antibiotics should be used.

Among 825 laparoscopies for conservative excision of endometriosis performed by this author, 12 patients (1.4%) had notable complications (unpublished data). (Table 14.5).

Outcome

Symptom response after conservative excision of endometriosis has been measured by pain scales administered preoperatively and postoperatively, with a score of 1 representing no problem and a score of 5 representing the presence of a symptom(s) to a debilitating degree. Excision of endometriosis results in significant reduction of symptoms that appears to be lasting in most of the patients in my series. This response of symptoms parallels the surprisingly low rate of recurrence of new disease after aggressive excision at laparotomy[21] or laparoscopy.[22] Aggressive laparoscopic treatment of endometriosis with laser has been shown to be equivalent to treatment at laparotomy[88,89] with respect to fertility outcomes, particularly for advanced disease.

There are no reported studies that detail long-term rates of reoperation, recurrence, or pain relief following laser vaporization or electrocoagulation. Clinicians must therefore be guided by their own experience when recommending these treatment modalities to their patients.

References

1. CULLEN TS: The distribution of adenomyomas containing uterine mucosa. Arch Surg 1920; 1:215.
2. FAYEZ JA, VOGEL MF: Comparison of different treatment methods of endometriomas by laparoscopy. Obstet Gynecol 1991;78:660.
3. HANEY AF: The pathogenesis and aetiology of endometriosis. In Modern Approaches to Endometriosis, Thomas E, Rock J (eds). Dordrecht, Kluwer Academic Publisher, 1991, pp 3–19.
4. SAMPSON JA: Peritoneal endometriosis due to the menstrual dissemination of endometrial tissue into the peritoneal cavity. Am J Obstet Gynecol 1927;14:422.
5. GLEICHER N, EL-ROEIY A, CONFINO E, ET AL: Is endometriosis an autoimmune disease? Obstet Gynecol 1987;70:115.
6. OOSTERLYNK DJ, MEULEMAN C, WAER M, ET AL: The natural killer activity of peritoneal fluid lymphocytes is decreased in women with endometriosis. Fertil Steril 1992;58:290.
7. KANZAKI H, WANG H-S, KARIYA M, ET AL: Suppression of natural killer cell activity by sera from patients with endometriosis. Am J Obstet Gynecol 1992;167:257.
8. PROSS HF, BAINES MG: Studies of human natural killer cells: in vivo parameters affecting normal cytotoxic function. Int J Cancer 1976; 18:593.
9. SIMON C, GOMIZ E, MIR A, ET AL: Glucocorticoid treatment decreases sera embryotoxicity in endometriosis patients. Fertil Steril 1992;58:284.
10. VASQUEZ G, CORNILLIE F, BROSENS IA: Peritoneal endometriosis: scanning electron microscopy and histology of minimal pelvic endometriotic lesions. Fertil Steril 1984;42:696.
11. MURPHY AA, GREEN WR, BOBBIE D, ET AL: Unsuspected endometriosis documented by scanning electron microscopy in visually normal peritoneum. Fertil Steril 1986;46:522.
12. REDWINE DB: Is "microscopic" peritoneal endometriosis invisible? Fertil Steril 1988;50:665.
13. REDWINE DB, YOCOM L: A serial section study of visually normal peritoneum in patients with endometriosis. Fertil Steril 1990;54:648.
14. NEZHAT F, ALLAN CJ, NEZHAT C, ET AL: Non-visualized endometriosis at laparoscopy. Int J Fertil 1991;36:340.
15. HAYATA T, MATSU T, KAWANO Y, ET AL: Scanning electron microscopy of endometriotic lesions in the pelvic peritoneum and the histogenesis of endometriosis. Int J Gynecol Obstet 1992;39:311.
16. ROCK JA, MARKHAM SM: Extra pelvic endometriosis. In Endometriosis, Wilson EA (ed). New York, Alan R. Liss, 1987, pp 185–206.
17. MITCHELL GW: Extrapelvic endometriosis. In Endometriosis: Contemporary Concepts in Clinical Management, Schenken RS (ed). Philadelphia, Lippincott, 1989, pp 307–328.
18. MARKHAM SM: Extrapelvic endometriosis. In Modern Approaches to Endometriosis, Thomas E, Rock J (eds). Dordrecht, Kluwer Academic, 1991, pp 151–182.
19. OLIKER AJ, HARRIS AE: Endometriosis of the bladder in a male patient. J Urol 1971;106:858.

20. BECKMAN EN, LEONARD GL, PINTADO SO, ET AL: Endometriosis of the prostate. Am J Surg Pathol 1985;9:374.
21. WHEELER JM, MALINAK LR: Recurrent endometriosis. Contemp Gynecol Obstet 1987;16:13.
22. REDWINE DB: Conservative laparoscopic excision of endometriosis by sharp dissection: life table analysis of reoperation and persistent or recurrent disease. Fertil Steril 1991; 56:628.
23. REDWINE DB: Mulleriosis: the single best fit model of origin of endometriosis. J Reprod Med 1988; 33:915.
24. BERGER GS: How many women are affected by endometriosis? Contemp Obstet Gynecol 1993; October:47.
25. GOLDSTEIN DP, DECHOLNOKY C, EMANS J: Adolescent endometriosis. J Adolesc Health Care 1980; 1:37.
26. HAYDON GB: A study of 569 cases of endometriosis. Am J Obstet Gynecol 1942;43:704.
27. BERKSON J: Limitations of the application of four-fold table analysis to hospital data. Biometrics 1946;2:47.
28. REDWINE DB: The visual appearance of endometriosis and its impact on our concepts of the disease. Prog Clin Biol Res 1990;323:393.
29. SIMPSON JL, ELIAS S, MALINAK LR, ET AL: Heritable aspects of endometriosis. I. Genetic studies. Am J Obstet Gynecol 1980;137:327.
30. REDWINE DB: The distribution of endometriosis in the pelvis by age groups and fertility. Fertil Steril 1987;47:173.
31. KONINCKX PR, CORNILLIE FJ: Deeply infiltrating pelvic endometriosis: a new entity. In Endometriosis, Shaw RW (ed). Carnforth, UK; Parthenon, 1990, pp 31–43.
32. KONINCKX PR, MEULEMAN C, DEMEYERE S, ET AL: Suggestive evidence that pelvic endometriosis is a progressive disease, whereas deeply infiltrating endometriosis is associated with pelvic pain. Fertil Steril 1991;55:759.
33. CORNILLIE FJ, OOSTERLYNCK D, LAUWERYNS JM, ET AL: Deeply infiltrating pelvic endometriosis: histology and clinical significance. Fertil Steril 1990; 53:978.
34. THOMAS E, COOKE ID: Successful treatment of asymptomatic endometriosis: does it benefit infertile women? BMJ 1987;294:1117.
35. REDWINE DB: Age related evolution in color appearance of endometriosis. Fertil Steril 1987; 48:1062.
36. THE AMERICAN FERTILITY SOCIETY: Revised American Fertility Society classification of endometriosis: 1985. Fertil Steril 1985;43:351.
37. MARANA R, MUZII L, CARUANA P, ET AL: Evaluation of the correlation between endometriosis extent, age of the patients and associated symptomatology. Acta Eur Fertil 1991;22:209.
38. HORNSTEIN MD, GLEASON RE, ORAV J, ET AL: The reproducibility of the revised American Fertility Society classification of endometriosis. Fertil Steril 1993;59:1015.
39. RIPPS BA, MARTIN DC: Focal pelvic tenderness, pelvic pain and dysmenorrhea in endometriosis. J Reprod Med 1991;36:470.
40. PITTAWAY DE, DOUGLAS JW: Serum CA-125 in women with endometriosis and chronic pelvic pain. Fertil Steril 1989;51:68.
41. FRANSSEN AMHW, VAN DER HEIJDEN PFM, THOMAS CMG, ET AL: On the origin and significance of serum CA-125 concentrations in 97 patients with endometriosis before, during, and after buserelin acetate, nafarelin, or danazol. Fertil Steril 1992; 57:974.
42. MCBEAN JH, BRUMSTED JR: In vitro CA-125 secretion by endometrium from women with advanced endometriosis. Fertil Steril 1993;59:89.
43. STRIPLING MC, MARTIN DC, CHATMAN DL, ET AL: Subtle appearance of pelvic endometriosis. Fertil Steril 1988;49:427.
44. MARTIN DC, HUBERT GD, VANDERZWAAG R, ET AL: Laparoscopic appearances of peritoneal endometriosis. Fertil Steril 1989;51:63.
45. FALLON J, BROSNAN JT, MANNING JJ, ET AL: Endometriosis: a report of 400 cases. RI Med J 1950;33:15.
46. REDWINE DB: The visual appearance of endometriosis and its impact on our concepts of the disease. Prog Clin Biol Res 1990;323:393.
47. REDWINE DB: Is "microscopic" peritoneal endometriosis invisible? Fertil Steril 1988;50:665.
48. The evaluation and treatment of endometriosis. American Fertility Society guideline for practice. Birmingham, AL, The American Fertility Society, 1992.
49. SEIBEL MM, BERGER MJ, WEINSTEIN FG, ET AL: The effectiveness of danazol on subsequent fertility in minimal endometriosis. Fertil Steril 1982;38:534.
50. BAYER SR, SEIBEL MM, SAFFAN DS, ET AL: Efficacy of danazol treatment on minimal endometriosis in infertile women: a prospective, randomized study. J Reprod Med 1988;33:179.
51. COLLINS JA, WRIXON W, JANES LB, ET AL: Treatment-independent pregnancy among infertile couples. N Engl J Med 1983;309:1201.
52. REDWINE DB: Treatment of endometriosis-associated pain. Infertil Reprod Med Clin North Am 1992;3:697.

53. EVERS JLH: The second-look laparoscopy for evaluation of the result of medical treatment of endometriosis should not be performed during ovarian suppression. Fertil Steril 1987;47:502.
54. VERCELLINI P, TRESPIDI L, COLOMBO A, ET AL: A gonadotropin-releasing hormone agonist versus a low-dose oral contraceptive for pelvic pain associated with endometriosis. Fertil Steril 1993; 60:75.
55. WALLER KG, SHAW RW: Gonadotropin-releasing hormone analogues for the treatment of endometriosis: long-term followup. Fertil Steril 1993; 59:511.
56. HUGHES EG, FEDORKOW DM, COLLINS JA: A quantitative overview of controlled trials in endometriosis-associated infertility. Fertil Steril 1993; 59:963.
57. GROW D, FILER RB: Treatment of adenomyosis with long-term GnRH analogues: a case report. Obstet Gynecol 1991;78:538.
58. FRIEDMAN AJ, REIN MS, HARRISON-ATLAS D, ET AL: A randomized placebo-controlled, double-blind study evaluating leuprolide acetate depot treatment before myomectomy. Fertil Steril 1989; 52:728.
59. FRIEDMAN AJ, HORNSTEIN MD: Gonadotropin-releasing hormone agonist plus estrogen-progestin "add-back" therapy for endometriosis-related pelvic pain. Fertil Steril 1993;60:236.
60. MARTIN DC, HUBERT GD, LEVY BS: Depth of infiltration of endometriosis. J Gynecol Surg 1989; 5:55.
61. KONINKCX PR, MARTIN DC: Deep endometriosis: a consequence of infiltration or retraction or possibly adenomyosis externa? Fertil Steril 1992; 58:924.
62. REDWINE DB: Laparoscopic en bloc resection for treatment of the obliterated cul de sac in endometriosis. J Reprod Med 1992;37:695.
63. HASSON HM: Electrocoagulation of pelvic endometriotic lesions with laparoscopic control. Am J Obstet Gynecol 1979;135:115.
64. DANIELL JF, CHRISTIANSON C: Combined laparoscopic surgery and danazol therapy for pelvic endometriosis. Fertil Steril 1981;35:521.
65. SEILER JC, GIDWANI G, BALLARD L: Laparoscopic cauterization of endometriosis for fertility: a controlled study. Fertil Steril 1986;46:1098.
66. MURPHY AA, SCHLAFF WD, HASSIAKOS D, ET AL: Laparoscopic cautery in the treatment of endometriosis-related infertility. Fertil Steril 1991; 55:246.
67. ARUMUGAM K, URQUHART R: Efficacy of laparoscopic electrocoagulation in infertile patients with minimal or mild endometriosis. Acta Obstet Gynecol Scand 1991;70:125.
68. SULEWSKI JM, CURCIO FD, BRONITSKY C, STENGER VG: The treatment of endometriosis at laparoscopy for infertility. Am J Obstet Gynecol 1980; 138:128.
69. DANIELL JF, MILLER W, TOSH R: Initial evaluation of the use of the potassium-titanyl-phosphate (KTP/532) laser in gynecologic laparoscopy. Fertil Steril 1986;46:373.
70. CORSON SL, UNGER M, KWA D, ET AL: Laparoscopic laser treatment of endometriosis with the Nd:YAG sapphire probe. Am J Obstet Gynecol 1989;160:718.
71. MARTIN DC: Tissue effects of lasers. Semin Reprod Endocrinol 1991;9:127.
72. REDWINE DB: Laparoscopic excision of endometriosis by sharp dissection. In Laparoscopic Appearance of Endometriosis, Martin DC (ed). Memphis: Resurge Press, 1990, pp 9–19.
73. REDWINE DB: Laparoscopic excision of endometriosis with 3 mm scissors: comparison of operating times between sharp excision and electro-excision. AAGL 1993;1:24.
74. MARTIN DC: Laparoscopic and vaginal colpotomy for the excision of infiltrating cul-de-sac endometriosis. J Reprod Med 1988;33:806.
75. MARTIN DC, VANDER ZWAAG R: Excisional techniques for endometriosis with the CO_2 laser laparoscope. J Reprod Med 1987;32:753.
76. DAVIS GD, BROOKS RA: Excision of pelvic endometriosis with the carbon dioxide laser laparoscope. Obstet Gynecol 1988;72:816.
77. HULKA JF: Power: electricity and laser. In Textbook of Laparoscopy, Hulka JF, Reich H (eds). Philadelphia, Saunders, 1994, pp 23–46.
78. REDWINE DB, SHARPE DR: Laparoscopic segmental resection of the sigmoid colon. J Laparoendosc Surg 1991;1:217.
79. SHARPE DR, REDWINE DB: Laparoscopic segmental resection of the sigmoid and rectosigmoid colon for endometriosis. Surg Laparosc Endosc 1992; 2:120.
80. NEZHAT F, NEZHAT C, PENNINGTON E: Laparoscopic proctectomy for infiltrating endometriosis of the rectum. Fertil Steril 1992;57:1129.
81. KEMPERS RD, DOCKERTY MB, HUNT AB, ET AL: Significant postmenopausal endometriosis. Surg Gynecol Obstet 1960;3:348.
82. VENTER PF, ANDERSON JD, VAN VELDEN DJ: Postmenopausal endometriosis: a case report. S Afr Med J 1979;56:1136.
83. METZGER DA, LESSEY BA, SOPER JT, ET AL: Hormone-resistant endometriosis following total ab-

dominal hysterectomy and bilateral salpingo-oophorectomy: correlation with histology and steroid receptor content. Obstet Gynecol 1991; 78:946.
84. SPENCE MR: Endometriosis occurring eight years after total abdominal hysterectomy and bilateral salpingo-oophorectomy. Am J Gynecol Health 1992;6:22.
85. SCHRAM JD: Endometriosis after pelvic cleanout. South Med J 1978;71:1414.
86. O'CONNOR DT: Endometriosis. In Current Review in Obstetrics and Gynaecology, Singer A, Jordan J (eds). Melbourne, Churchill Livingstone, 1987, pp 11–12.
87. REDWINE DB: Endometriosis persisting after castration: clinical characteristics and results of surgical management. Obstet Gynecol 1994;83:405.
88. ADAMASON GD, SUBAK LL, PASTA DJ, ET AL: Comparison of CO_2 laser laparoscopy with laparotomy for treatment of endometriomata. Fertil Steril 1992;57:965.
89. ADAMSON GD, HURD SJ, PASTA DJ, ET AL: Laparoscopic endometriosis treatment: is it better? Fertil Steril 1993;59:35.

15
Laparoscopic Treatment of Tuboovarian and Pelvic Abscess

Harry Reich and F. Michael Shaw

Approximately one million women in the United States are diagnosed with acute pelvic inflammatory disease (PID) annually.[1] By the year 2000 the projected direct and indirect costs of PID and its sequelae will approach $9 billion.[2] Risk factors include a sexually active adolescence, multiple sexual partners (especially a new partner within the last 2 months), failure to use a barrier contraceptive method, use of an intrauterine contraceptive device (increased risk the first months after insertion), intrauterine manipulative procedures, immunosuppression, and frequent douching. Bacterial vaginosis has now also been implicated as a risk factor.

In recent years, therapy for the spectrum of PID, from early salpingitis to unruptured tuboovarian abscess, has been antibiotics, with surgical intervention reserved for those who do not respond to medical therapy.[3] Although this approach avoids surgical intervention when medication is considered successful, prolonged contact between necrotic and inflamed tissue often results in dense fibrous adhesions that diminish reproductive potential and cause chronic pelvic pain.

The accepted antibiotic therapy for acute PID is administered on an outpatient basis, with hospitalization for parenteral antibiotics reserved for situations when the diagnosis is uncertain, surgical emergencies cannot be excluded, pelvic abscess is suspected, the patient is pregnant or an adolescent, the patient is unable to follow or fails to respond to outpatient management, or clinical follow-up cannot be otherwise obtained.[4] Guidelines for treatment of sexually transmitted diseases are listed in Table 15.1.[5] An unruptured adnexal abscess is managed with intravenous antibiotics; surgical intervention is considered only when the patient does not respond to antibiotics.

Antibiotic success implies the resolution of symptoms and the pelvic mass as judged by clinical or ultrasound examination, often at a significantly later date; it does not imply the resolution of pelvic adhesions that could result in future infertility. The literature confirms that when long-term resolution of symptoms and infertility is considered, medical treatment is usually doomed to failure even with current-generation antibiotics.

In reality, it is much easier to operate on acute PID than it is to deal with dense adhesions subsequently developed that obliterate normal anatomic relations and develop neovascularization by their chronicity. For example, second-look laparoscopic adhesiolysis soon after infertility surgical procedures is much easier than the original procedure for dense adhesion formation.[6] Electrosurgery, laser surgery, and sharp scissors dissection are all useful for chronic adhesive PID but play a small role in the

Table 15.1. Regimens for the treatment of pelvic inflammatory disease recommended by the CDC

Treatment	Comment
Inpatients	
Regimen 1	
Cefoxitin 2 g IV q6h *or* cefotetan 2 g IV q12h	The regimen is continued for at least 48 hours after the occurrence of substantial clinical improvement, after which doxycycline, 100 mg po bid, should be given until day 14 of treatment.
Doxycycline 100 mg IV or PO q12h,	
Regimen 2	
Clindamycin 900 mg IV q8h	The regimen is continued for at least 48 hours after the occurrence of substantial clinical improvement, after which doxycycline, 100 mg PO bid, *or* clindamycin, 450 mg PO qid, is given until day 14 of treatment.
Gentamicin 2 mg/kg body weight IV or IM (loading dose) followed by 1.5 mg/kg IV or IM q8h (maintenance dose)	
Outpatients	
Regimen 1	
Cefoxitin 2 g IM in a single dose plus concomitant probenecid 1 g PO *or* ceftriaxone 250 mg IM *or* another third-generation cephalosporin (e.g., ceftizoxime or cefotaxmine),	
Doxycycline 100 mg PO bid for 14 days,	
Regimen 2	
Ofloxacin 400 mg PO bid for 14 days,	
Clindamycin 450 mg PO qid for 14 days *or* metronidazole 500 mg PO bid for 14 days	

Adapted from ref. 5.

treatment of acute adhesion formation. Simply stated, the laparoscopic treatment of acute adhesions with or without abscess does not require the high level of technical skill prerequisite to excising an endometrioma, performing a salpingostomy, or even removing an ectopic pregnancy laparoscopically.[6–8] It is essentially an exercise in meticulous blunt dissection using a probe or aquadissector and can be performed by gynecologists experienced in operative laparoscopy using equipment available in most hospitals.[9–11]

Definition

Pelvic inflammatory disease is defined as an infection of the uterus, fallopian tubes, and pelvic peritoneum. *Pelvic abscess*, the most severe manifestation of this disease, is a localized collection of microorganisms (often both aerobic and anaerobic), inflammatory exudate, and necrotic debris separated from surrounding tissue by a fibrous capsule. An adnexal abscess that lacks a classic abscess wall and contains agglutinated uterine tube and ovary adherent to the adjacent pelvic and abdominal structures is termed a *tuboovarian complex*. True pelvic abscess with a classic abscess wall can occur in the ovary and following rupture of a diverticulum. Regardless of the terminology, purulent material exists in a collection within the pelvis. The terms adnexal abscess, tuboovarian abscess (TOA), tuboovarian complex, and pelvic abscess are used virtually interchangeably, with *pelvic abscess* implying extension of the adnexal abscess to involve most of the true pelvis.

Pathophysiology

Acute PID is usually an ascending infection. It is estimated that *Chlamydia trachomatis* and *Neisseria gonorrhoeae* are the most frequent causative organisms (i.e., more than half of all cases). It is of particular note that these organisms have been isolated from apparently normal-appearing fallopian tubes during laparoscopy.[12] Other bacterial organisms isolated from the upper genital tract in patients with acute PID include enteric pathogens, respiratory pathogens such as *Hemophilus influenzae*, and endogenous vaginal microorganisms.[13] Bacterial vaginosis is a common concurrent disorder of women with acute salpingitis, and bacterial vaginosis microorganisms are commonly isolated from the upper genital tract of affected women.[14] The role of bacterial vaginosis appears to be permissive: It alters the cervical mucus and allows ascent of microbiologic pathogens.

Hillis et al. described the early pathogenicity of PID.[15] They reported that animal studies of *Chlamydia* infection revealed marked inflammation and subsequent intraluminal fibrin deposition, accounting for the associated tubal damage. The peak effect was at 7–14 days. The pathogenicity of *N. gonorrhoeae* appears to be related to endotoxin and may initiate earlier destruction of tubal mucosa.[15]

Abscess is the end result of an acute or subacute infection beginning with an initial peritonitis stage where aerobic bacteria predominate, followed by the development of an intraabdominal abscess with emergence of anaerobic bacteria as the predominant flora. Abscesses contain a large number of organisms in high concentration but not in a rapid growth phase, making them less susceptible to responding to antimicrobial agents that require actively growing organisms for efficacy. The fibrinous capsule may inhibit adequate levels of antimicrobial agents from entering the abscess.[16] The anaerobic milieu may hinder host defense mechanisms, reducing the ability of neutrophils to phagocytize and kill bacteria. Thus therapy for abscesses must include some technique of adequate drainage along with appropriate antimicrobial agents.

Diagnosis

The diagnosis of an adnexal infection or abscess is suspected in women who have persistent pain and lower abdominal, adnexal, or cervical motion tenderness on examination. Because of the potential for serious long-term sequelae, even from mild disease, clinicians should have a high index of suspicion and a low threshold for making the diagnosis and initiating treatment.

Women with acute or subacute onset of lower abdominal pain and a palpable mass or sonographic evidence suggestive of a pelvic mass require early laparoscopy for diagnosis and treatment in association with antibiotic therapy: Even an "obvious TOA" may prove to be an endometrioma, hemorrhagic corpus luteum cyst, or an abscess surrounding a ruptured appendix (Figs. 15.1, 15.2). The routine use of laparoscopy to diagnose acute PID has become widespread in Europe and is accepted by virtually every gynecology department in Sweden.[17,18] The worldwide average rate of misdiagnosis of PID is 35% when laparoscopy has been used for confirmation. Conversely, PID can be an unanticipated finding at laparoscopy for pelvic pain. Laparoscopy can provide objective findings in all patients without PID, including ectopic pregnancy, appendicitis, endometriosis, adnexal torsion, ruptured or unruptured ovarian cyst, gastroenteritis, and other problems.[19]

Although laparoscopy provides information relating to the serosal surface of the fallopian tubes, it fails to exclude intraluminal infection.[20] Even the morphologically normal fallopian tube can demonstrate *C. trachomatis* or *N. gonorrhoeae* within the lumen of the tube.[13,21] In women with acute PID who delay treatment there may be devastating effects on future fertility; a delay of 3 days or more has been reported to produce a threefold increased risk of ectopic pregnancy, infertility, or both.[15]

Temperature, leukocyte count, C-reactive protein, CA 125, or erythrocyte sedimentation rate (ESR) may be elevated.[22] Endocervical cultures for *N. gonorrhoeae* and *Chlamydia* may be positive. One study indicated that endometrial biopsy has a diagnostic sensitivity of 89% and a specificity of 67% with laparoscopically confirmed disease.[23] The serum or urine human chorionic gonadotropin (hCG) level must be obtained and a negative result documented. Ultrasonography may demonstrate a large hydrosalpinx filled with dense fluid or an adherent

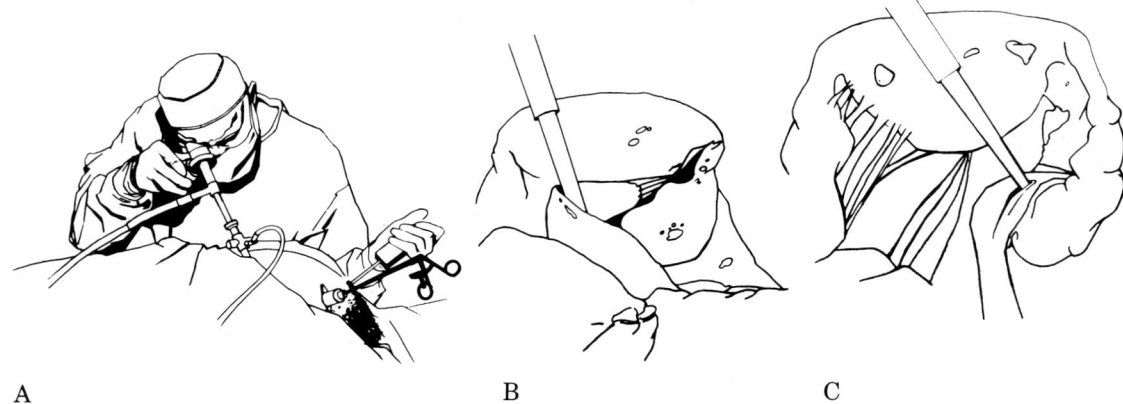

Figure 15.1. (A) Operative technique using laparoscope with beam splitter and two pubic hairline lower abdominal puncture sites, one with grasping forceps and the other with the Aquapurator. (B) Small bowel is separated from a right tuboovarian abscess using the Aquapurator. (C) Purulent material is drained and aspirated from a right tuboovarian abscess cavity.

adnexal mass; septations, air-fluid levels, internal echoes, and abscess cavity may be identified. Human immunodeficiency virus (HIV) testing should be considered especially in women with a pelvic abscess.[24]

More sophisticated diagnostic testing—including gallium 67 and indium 111-labeled or technetium 99m-hexamethylpropylenamineoxime- labeled white blood cell (WBC) scans and computed tomographic (CT) scans—is rarely necessary, as laparoscopy can determine the appropriate diagnosis.[25] After a presumptive diagnosis of PID/TOA is established, endoscopic diagnosis and management should be initiated within 24–48 hours. The procedure is explained to the patient and family including the risk/benefit ratio and other treatment alternatives. Informed consent is obtained and appropriately documented.

Historical Perspective

The commonly accepted belief that surgical intervention during acute pelvic infection would result in greater injury than waiting for the infection to subside dates back 85 years to a New York City report suggesting that early surgical intervention was associated with increased technical difficulty.[26] This opinion prevailed until relatively recently, even though the risks associated with surgical intervention have changed drastically since the early part of the twentieth century.

In 1973 Franklin and colleagues reported a series of 137 consecutive cases of acute pelvic abscess.[27] Of these women, 120 underwent conservative management including 35 posterior colpotomies (9 days average hospital stay), and

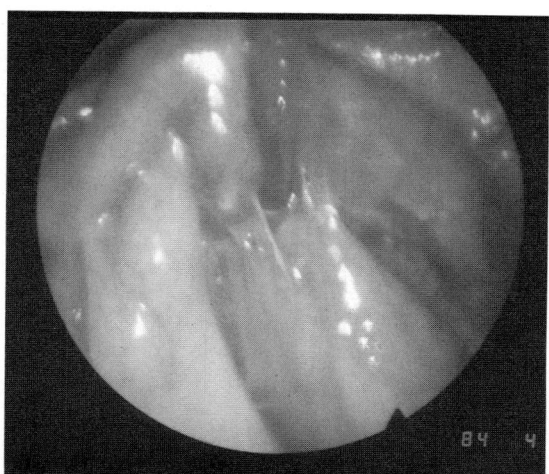

Figure 15.2. Using aquadissection, the small bowel is separated from the posterior uterus.

17 had immediate laparotomy, 10 for definitive diagnosis and 7 because of a presumed ruptured pelvic abscess. Of the 120 patients treated conservatively, 103 were followed for 2.5–8.0 years. The total failure rate was 26%. Twelve women (10%) required definitive surgery, usually hysterectomy and adnexectomy for "early failure" to respond to conservative management during their initial hospitalization; 19 (16%) required subsequent definitive surgery for persistent mass, pain, or hypermenorrhea. Among the 120 women, 10 subsequently conceived (8%).[27]

Ginsburg and colleagues reviewed 160 patients with TOA (1969–1979).[28] Of these women, 76 responded to medical therapy with no subsequent surgical intervention, and 84 (53%) required subsequent surgery. Intervention during the acute phase was accomplished in 50 patients because of failure to respond to the medical regimen (40 TAH/BSO, 4 unilateral adnexectomies, and 6 abscess drainage procedures), and 34 required subsequent surgery for persistent symptoms related to the abscess. Eighty percent of the women who responded to medical therapy or had no subsequent abscess-related surgery continued to experience persistent or recurrent disease. Of 120 women in whom reproductive function was preserved, 9 conceived (7.5%); no woman with a bilateral TOA conceived.[28]

Hager (1970–1974) documented poor success with medical therapy alone. Of 50 women with the original diagnosis of TOA, only five had successful medical treatment. Hager reported that response to antimicrobial therapy may be the most reliable way to distinguish women with salpingitis from those with salpingitis and TOA, as the latter group did not respond well to antibiotic treatment regimens.[29]

In 1983 Landers and Sweet reported their results of 175 of 232 women with TOAs treated with antibiotics alone.[30] Laparoscopic confirmation was obtained in 15 of these women. Twenty-five percent required surgical intervention as part of their original therapy, including 8 of 71 women initially treated with regimens including clindamycin. Long-term follow-up information was available for 58 women treated with antibiotics alone: 31% required subsequent surgery.[3,30]

Of these 71 patients with salpingitis treated with single-agent β-lactam, 17 also demonstrated *Chlamydia trachomatis* on endometrial tissue biopsy. In most of the women (16 of 17) the symptoms resolved. Twelve continued to have positive *Chlamydia* cultures, a well recognized risk factor for future episodes of PID and its sequelae.[31]

Hemsell and associates reported 41 women with pelvic abscesses treated with cefotaxime during 1980–1981.[32] Chronic pelvic pain and recurrent infection were infrequent during a 31- to 43-month follow-up period, but five women (12%) subsequently required TAH/BSO for a persistent adnexal mass, and a sixth underwent unilateral salpingo-oophorectomy for an asymptomatic adnexal mass (hydrosalpinx). A pregnancy rate of 20% (6 of 30) was reported.[32]

Diagnosis in the above and other studies was based on clinical and sonographic findings without laparoscopic assessment for subsequent evaluation.[33] The studies document that antimicrobial treatment of a formed TOA rarely results in complete resolution without adhesion formation. In addition, medical treatment resulted in prolonged initial hospitalization in most cases with a high rate of readmission. Medical treatment has not proved beneficial in ensuring fertility and can be justified only because ovarian preservation maintains the possibility of future in vitro fertilization (IVF).

Alternative Surgical Treatment

Primary surgical treatment (laparotomy) for an unruptured TOA within a few days of admission has always been controversial. Early TAH/BSO was advocated by Kaplan and associates who, during 1964–1966, treated 71 women with a presumptive diagnosis of pelvic abscess. Five patients required transfusion. Postoperatively, there were seven superficial and one subfascial wound infections and one evisceration. Cuff abscess occurred in three women.[34]

Colpotomy drainage can be performed for pelvic abscesses that dissect into the upper portion of the rectovaginal septum. Rubenstein and colleagues reported the results of 38 colpotomy procedures for pelvic abscess: 14 (37%) required additional surgery. The mean duration of hospitalization was 12.4 days (7.7 days after drainage).[35]

Rivlin reviewed the results of 59 colpotomy drainage procedures. Additional surgery during the same admission was performed in 13 cases and even more surgery at a later admission in 11 patients. Five of forty potentially fertile women (12.5%) had one or more successful pregnancies.[36] Rivlin and colleagues also reviewed the results of 348 colpotomy drainage procedures at two medical centers. There were 23 instances of diffuse peritoneal sepsis (6.5%) with six deaths attributable to this condition.[37]

Percutaneous Drainage

Van Sonnenberg and colleagues reported a 78% success rate with percutaneous drainage of 50 patients with pelvic abscesses.[38] Gerzof and colleagues successfully treated six of nine pelvic abscesses (67%) via percutaneous drainage.[39]

Worthen and Gunning reported percutaneous drainage of 35 pelvic abscesses secondary to pelvic inflammatory salpingitis. Nine patients with a total of eleven abscesses were treated by percutaneous catheter placement, with a success rate of 77%; two patients required surgical procedures. Nineteen women underwent percutaneous aspiration. Among them, there were 23 abscess cavities, 18 (78%) of which were successfully aspirated; one required surgical drainage. Seven women had abscess cavities that could not technically be drained or aspirated. Four of the seven responded to antibiotic therapy alone, and three required surgical drainage.[40] Long-term follow-up was not determined in any of these studies.

Laparoscopic Treatment

Historical Perspective

Laparoscopic treatment of pelvic abscess was first proposed in 1972.[41] Its successful use was documented in the 1984 report by Henry-Suchet et al.,[10] who treated 50 women with TOA using laparoscopic surgery and parenteral antibiotics. Their report was based on a continuous series of 569 women treated for laparoscopically verified acute PID during 1974–1983. Laparoscopy was performed within 24 hours of admission. After diagnosis of a recent TOA in 32 cases, the friable adhesions between the pelvic organs were lysed with a blunt probe and the purulent fluid drained. After the adnexae and bowel were freed, the peritoneal cavity was irrigated with a mixture of physiologic saline, antibiotics (doxycycline or minocycline), and an antiseptic (noxythiolin). In 18 patients with chronic dense adhesions, the bowel was mobilized from the pelvic organs, but the adnexa constituted a dense mass in which it was difficult to distinguish between pyosalpinx and ovary. In these instances the mass was aspirated with a needle, the abundant purulent fluid removed with suction, and the saline-antibiotic-antiseptic mixture instilled into the abscess cavity; that is, the adhesions between tube and ovary were not lysed. None had a drain placed. Parenteral antibiotics were initiated during laparoscopy immediately after bacteriologic samples were obtained and included combination therapy: a cephalosporin and an aminoglycoside initially and, more recently, cefotaxime or cefoperazone, tetracycline, and metronidazole. No complications occurred during or after laparoscopic treatment.

A rapid recovery was recorded in 45 of 50 patients (90%) with complete disappearance of the adnexal mass within 3–4 days and with reduction in hospitalization from an average of 15–20 days to 6–8 days. Early laparotomy was necessary in five cases: one TAH/BSO, two bilateral salpingectomies, and two patients underwent unilateral salpingo-oophorectomy. No abscess was identified in the two women who underwent unilateral salpingo-oophorectomy. The procedures were performed on the basis of ultrasound data despite clinical improvement [the ultrasound detected mass proved to be functional ovarian cyst(s) covered with adhesions in both cases]. Thus there were only three early failures of treatment.

Long-term follow-up was possible in 44 of these women: Six (13%) experienced persistent pelvic pain. Twenty-five underwent a second-look laparoscopy, which documented the absence of tuboovarian adhesions in 12, unilateral adhesions in 5, and bilateral adhesions with tubal obstruction in 8. The last group underwent laparotomy for pain ($n = 3$) or infertility ($n = 5$).

The series included 24 patients with bilateral abscesses: 12 recent and 12 chronic. Of the 12 women with recent bilateral TOA, seven subsequently underwent laparoscopy, with normal adnexae reported in five and mild adhesions in two. Three of these women had a subsequent intrauterine pregnancy. In addition, there were three intrauterine pregnancies following treatment of unilateral abscess. No pregnancies were recorded in the chronic abscess group.

The American experience with laparoscopic treatment of tuboovarian abscess is limited. In 1981 Adducci[42] described seven patients treated by laparoscopic lysis of pelvic abscess-loculations followed by colpotomy drainage under direct vision. Two other patients with loops of bowel adherent to the cul-de-sac underwent laparoscopic drainage of purulent fluid followed by lysis of adhesions; Penrose drains were then placed without laparotomy (laparoscopically). Average hospitalization was 4 days, with the longest stay 7 days. There were no intraoperative or subsequent complications, and follow-up examination revealed good resolution in all cases.

Freistadt[43] in 1985 reported the use of laparoscopy following colpotomy incision to direct the end of the Penrose drain into the abscess cavity. The drain was left in situ for 2–3 days with the aid of a vaginal suture. Three of the four women subsequently conceived.

In our experience from 1976 until 1993, 46 of 48 women with tuboovarian and pelvic abscess were treated with intravenous antibiotics and laparoscopic surgical procedure. One patient, a 37-year-old gravida 4, para 4, underwent laparoscopy for diagnosis alone early in the study followed by total abdominal hysterectomy after no response to antibiotic therapy. One 29-year-old gravida 1, para 1 underwent laparotomy for presumed ruptured appendix and was treated for bilateral TOA with preservation of all reproductive organs when we were consulted during the operative procedure. (She had two subsequent intrauterine pregnancies.) Of 46 laparoscopically managed cases, there were 25 unilateral TOAs, 14 bilateral TOAs, 4 diverticular abscesses, 1 vaginal cuff abscess, 1 postappendectomy abscess, and 1 rectal abscess secondary to a delayed bowel perforation. The average age was 28 years (range 10–61 years; median 25 years).

Of 46 women treated for abscess, 45 (98%) had complete clinical resolution. No laparoscopic complications occurred during the 10 year study period. Average operating time was 90 minutes, and average length of hospital stay (postlaparoscopy) was 3 days. Minimal adhesions were noted in the eight women who later underwent second-look laparoscopy.

All cases were performed under general anesthesia with endotracheal intubation. Since 1983, complete lysis of pelvic adhesions was performed in all patients including chronic abscesses with dense walls. Extensive debridement of necrotic exudate was also accomplished.

A 10-year-old girl with postappendiceal abscess was treated via laparoscopy 21 days after appendectomy and 5 days after development of a peritoneovaginal fistula. She had failed to respond to parenteral antibiotics and a surgical drainage procedure. She was discharged home on the third day after laparoscopy afebrile and pain-free; she returned to full activity by the fifth postoperative day.[9]

Pathophysiology

Important peritoneal defense mechanisms protecting the host from invading bacteria include absorption of the microbes from the peritoneal cavity via translymphatic absorption through specialized structures of the diaphragm for distribution to systemic defense systems, phagocytosis by macrophages and polymorphonuclear leukocytes, complement effects, and fibrin trapping.[44] Fibrin trapping and sequestration of the bacterial inoculum by the omentum and intestinal distention and the tuboovarian complex act to contain the infection initially, although abscesses eventually may form. Fibrin traps bacteria, thereby decreasing the incidence of septicemic death; unfortunately, thick fibrin deposits represent a barrier to in situ destruction by neutrophils, with resultant abscess formation. Once formed, the abscess walls inhibit the effectiveness of antibiotics and the ability of the host to resolve the infection.

Ahrenholz and Simmons studied the role of purified fibrin in the pathogenesis of intraperitoneal infection.[16] Implantation of 0.5% bovine fibrin clots containing 2×10^8 *Escherichia coli* into the rat peritoneal cavity compared to implantation of the same amount of *E. coli* in a similar volume of saline solution reduced the 24-hour mortality rate from 100% to 0%. However, the 10-day mortality rate with fibrin was 90%; and all of the rats developed intraperitoneal abscesses. A control group of animals receiving sterile clots lysed them over 1–2 weeks without abscess formation. As few as 10^2 *E. coli* per fibrin clot produced abscesses, but 10^7 or more were required to result in death; without fibrin, fewer than 10^7 *E. coli* neither killed nor produced intraperitoneal infection. Both late death and abscess size with 2×10^8 *E. coli* were directly proportional to the fibrin clot size but not to the concentration of fibrin in the clot. Operative debridement of the fibrin at 4 or 24 hours completely eliminated abscess formation in surviving animals. Ahrenholz and Simmons concluded that fibrin delays systemic sepsis, but the entrapped bacteria cannot be eliminated easily by normal intraperitoneal bactericidal mechanisms. As a result, abscess formation occurs. They also concluded that radical peritoneal debridement or anticoagulation may reduce the septic complications of peritonitis; that is, procedures that decrease fibrin deposition or facilitate fibrin removal, enzymatically or surgically, probably further decrease the incidence of intraperitoneal abscess formation and peritonitis.

Hudspeth successfully treated 92 patients with advanced generalized bacterial peritonitis by radical surgical debridement after the source of contamination had been eliminated.[45] The ages of these patients ranged from 3 to 69 years. All were critically ill, and more than 90% had mechanical intestinal obstruction. Although the operations were tedious and often prolonged (average operating time 3 hours), all patients survived, and postoperative complications were minimal. Hudspeth believed that treatment success resulted from preventing further contamination and restoring the peritoneum to a state that allows normal host defense mechanisms to clear any residual infection. He further emphasized that the obvious way to prevent residual abscess formation and allow the peritoneum to clear intraabdominal infection is to break down all inflammatory adhesions, remove all necrotic tissue, eliminate any possible anaerobic condition, and reduce the bacterial count to a practical minimum.

Success with laparoscopic treatment further substantiates the laboratory findings of Ahrenholz and Simmons.[16] Laparoscopic drainage of a pelvic abscess followed by lysis of all peritoneal cavity adhesions and excision of necrotic inflammatory exudate allows host defenses to control the infection. In addition, extensive direct peritoneal cavity irrigation facilitates débridement of peritoneal surfaces, debulks the peritoneal cavity of bacteria, and facilitates bacterial absorption into the bloodstream where antibiotics are more effective. Meticulous dissection and attention to detail when separating adhesions and debriding necrotic purulent exudate produce results that are efficacious.[9,45,46]

Surgical Technique

Laparoscopic treatment of pelvic abscess was first proposed by Dellenbach et al. in 1972.[41] The largest series of laparoscopic treatment of TOA (50 cases) was reported by Henry-Suchet et al. in 1984, using a technique of lysing recent friable adhesions with a rod despite the presence of acute infection.[10] Success with laparoscopic and laparotomy treatment of TOA by Henry-Suchet et al., Reich,[6] Hudspeth,[45] and Rivlin and Hunt[47] substantiated the laboratory work of Ahrenholz and Simmons.[16] Laparoscopic drainage of a pelvic abscess followed by lysis of peritoneal cavity adhesions and excision of necrotic inflammatory exudate allows host defenses to control the infection.

Preoperative Care

Parenteral antibiotics are initiated on admission to the hospital, usually 2–24 hours prior to

15. Laparoscopic Treatment of Tubo-Ovarian and Pelvic Abscess

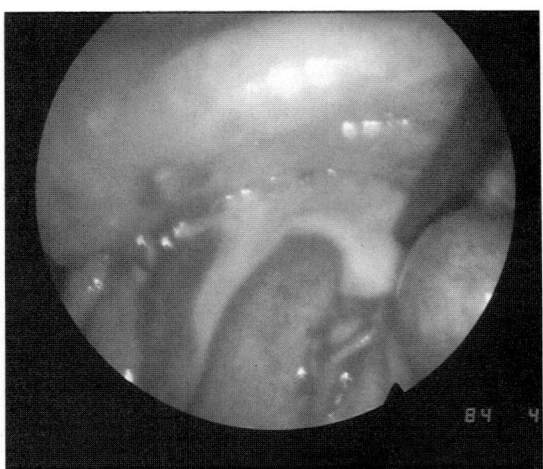

Figure 15.3. Purulent fluid in the abscess cavity is drained with minimal contamination of the pelvic cavity.

laparoscopy. Adequate and sustained blood levels of antibiotics are required to combat transperitoneal absorption of aerobic and anaerobic organisms during the operative procedure, which occurs mainly through the subdiaphragmatic lymphatics. We prefer cefoxitin 2 gm IV q 4 h from admission until discharge, usually on postoperative day 2 or 3. Oral doxycycline is initiated on the first postoperative day and continued for 10 days. Although clindamycin and metronidazole both have demonstrated the ability to enter abscess cavities and reduce bacterial counts therein, cefoxitin is used to simplify therapy to a single intravenous agent and assess further the efficacy of the laparoscopic surgical procedure; that is, the intravenous antibiotic alone cannot be considered the reason for the success of the therapy.

We advocate simultaneous hysteroscopy to inspect the endometrial cavity. Tissue is obtained for histology and *Chlamydia, N. gonorrhoeae,* and anaerobic and aerobic bacterial cultures. A uterine manipulator is then inserted. A 10 mm laparoscope is used through a vertical intraumbilical incision. Lower quadrant puncture sites are made above the pubic hairline and lateral to the rectus abdominis muscles (and thus the deep epigastric vessels) (Fig. 15.3).

The upper abdomen is examined, and the patient is placed in 20° Trendelenburg position before focusing attention on the pelvis. Attention to the upper abdomen may confirm the diagnosis of "old infection" if Fitz-Hugh-Curtis perihepatic adhesions are present.[48] A Foley catheter is inserted if the bladder is distended. Through the right-sided trocar sleeve, a blunt probe or a grasping forceps is inserted for traction and retraction. Through the left-sided trocar sleeve, a suction-irrigator-dissector (aquadissector) or a suction probe attached to a 50 cc syringe is inserted and used to mobilize omentum, small bowel, rectosigmoid, and tuboovarian adhesions until the abscess cavity is entered. Purulent fluid is aspirated as the operating table is returned to a 10° Trendelenburg position. Cultures should be obtained from the aspirated fluid and inflammatory exudate excised with biopsy forceps, especially exudate near the tubal ostium.

After the abscess cavity is aspirated, the aquadissector is used to separate the bowel and omentum from the reproductive organs and to lyse tuboovarian adhesions (aquadissection).[49] Aquadissection is performed by placing the tip of the aquadissector against the adhesive interface between bowel-adnexa, tube-ovary, or adnexa-pelvic side wall and by using both the tip and the pressurized fluid to develop a dissection plane that is extended bluntly or with additional fluid pressure. The grasping forceps place the tissue to be dissected on tension so the surgeon can identify the distorted tissue plane accurately prior to aquadissection. When the dissection is completed, the abscess cavity (necrotic inflammatory exudate) is excised in segments using a 5 mm biopsy forceps (Fig. 15.4).

It is important to remember that after ovulation purulent material from acute salpingitis may gain entrance into the ovary by inoculation of the corpus luteum, which may then become part of the abscess wall. Thus after draining the abscess cavity and mobilizing the entire ovary, a gaping hole of varying size may be noted in the ovary that had been intimately involved in the abscess cavity. This area should be well irrigated; it heals spontaneously. Significant bleeding is rarely encountered.

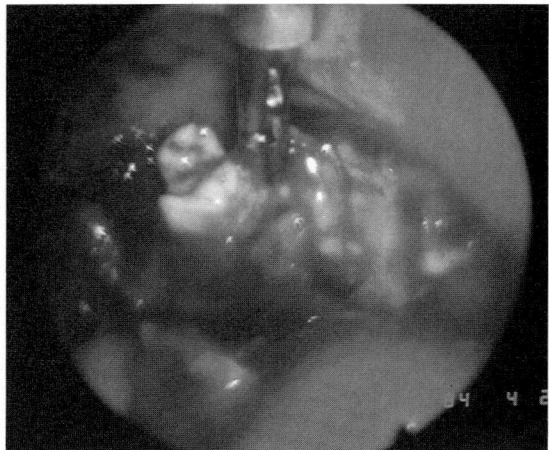 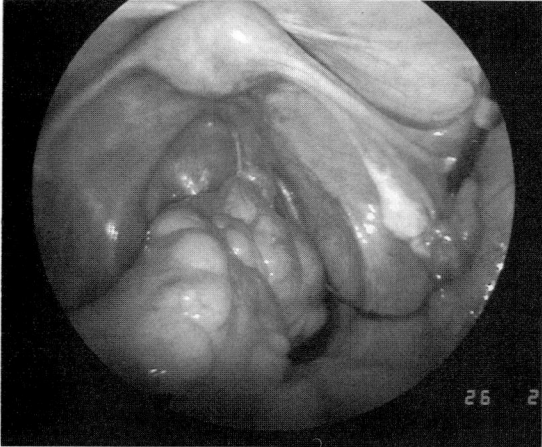

Figure 15.4. Fibrinous exudate, making up the abscess cavity, is excised from the peritoneal cavity.

Figure 15.5. This woman underwent a second laparoscopic procedure 1 year after the first. Minimal adhesions formed following laparoscopic treatment of the abscess.

The next step is to insert grasping forceps into the fimbrial ostia and spread them in order to free agglutinating fimbriae. Retrograde irrigation of the tube is performed with the aquadissector to remove infected debris and diminish the chance of recurrence. The fimbrial endosalpinx is assessed for future prognosis.

Tubal lavage with indigo carmine dye through a Cohen cannula is attempted. With early acute abscess, the tubes are rarely patent owing to interstitial edema. However, when the abscess process has been present for more than 1 week or the patient was previously treated with an antibiotic, lavage frequently documents tubal patency, and inspissated necrotic material may exit the tube.

The peritoneal cavity is irrigated thoroughly with Ringer's lactate solution until the effluent is clear. The total volume of irrigant may exceed 20 L. As part of this procedure, 2 L of Ringer's lactate solution is flushed into the upper abdomen (1 L on each side of the falciform ligament) to dilute any purulent material that may have gained access to these areas during the 20° Trendelenburg positioning. Reverse Trendelenburg position is then used for the "underwater" examination. The laparoscope and aquadissector are manipulated into the deep cul-de-sac underneath floating bowel and omentum, and this area is alternately irrigated and suctioned until the effluent is clear. An underwater examination is then performed to observe the completely separated uterine tubes and ovaries and to document complete hemostasis. At the close of each procedure, at least 3 L of Ringer's lactate is left in the peritoneal cavity to prevent fibrin adherence from forming between surgical surfaces during the early healing phase and to dilute the bacteria present.[49]

Blood loss is rarely more than 100 ml. Drains, antibiotic solutions, and heparin are not used. Second-look laparoscopy is encouraged (Fig. 15.5).

Postoperative Care

Postoperatively, the patient is ambulatory and on "diet as tolerated" after recovery from anesthesia. Leukocytosis and fever rarely persist past the first postoperative day. Discharge home is determined by resolution of pain and fever. Intravenous cefoxitin is continued until discharge, which usually occurs on the second postoperative day. Oral doxycycline is continued for 10 outpatient days. The patient is examined 1 week after discharge, and all restrictions are removed.

It is critically important to have the sexual partner undergo medical evaluation and be screened for sexually transmitted diseases. Although frequently asymptomatic, the partner is treated according to the U.S. Centers for Disease Control and Prevention (CDC) outpatient antibiotic regimen for PID.[50]

Complications

After treatment of acute PID and abscess, the most serious complications are inaccurate or delayed diagnosis and inadequate management. The result is often a lifetime of the sequelae of pelvic adhesive disease. Tubal factor infertility occurs in 8% of women after one episode of PID, in 20% after two episodes, and in 40% after three or more episodes.[51]

Complications of laparotomy treatment of pelvic abscess include superficial wound infection, wound dehiscence, bowel injury including delayed perforation of bowel secondary to unrecognized injury, bowel obstruction, persistent undrained collections, thrombophlebitis, pulmonary embolism, septic shock, and subdiaphragmatic collections with pleural effusion.

At laparoscopy the subphrenic region can be well visualized and irrigated directly. Delayed bowel perforation secondary to an unrecognized injury is a rare complication of laparoscopy, especially as laser and electrosurgery are used infrequently. Bowel injury, the most common serious operative complication of abscess surgery via laparotomy, occurs only when the bowel is the primary source for abscess formation.

Conclusion

"Treatment of infertility is glamorous gynecology. Treatment of pelvic inflammatory disease (PID), the most important preventable cause of infertility, afflicting an estimated 1 million American women yearly, is not glamorous gynecology . . . [and] must be one of the most neglected areas of American medicine."[52]

The goals of management for acute TOA are prevention of the chronic sequelae of infection, including infertility and pelvic pain, either of which often leads to further surgical intervention. Laparoscopic treatment in addition to intravenous antibiotics is effective and economical. It offers the gynecologist 100% accuracy in diagnosis while simultaneously accomplishing definitive treatment with a low complication rate.

It is encouraging that at least one health care plan emphasizes the importance of expedient management of acute PID. The Oregon health care plan, based on the concept of care-by-priority, created 17 ranked categories of health care services. The first nine were deemed "essential," the next four are classed as "very important," and the last four "valuable to certain individuals." The first category, "acute fatal; treatment prevents death and allows full recovery" recognizes that medical and surgical treatment of PID (and ectopic pregnancy) is critical. We salute the 11 members of the Health Services Commission for their difficult task and specifically for recognizing that early treatment of PID can prevent significant morbidity and mortality.[53]

Presently, many physicians are reluctant to advocate the routine use of laparoscopy for diagnosis and treatment of acute pelvic adhesions and pelvic abscess. However, it is well recognized that definitive diagnosis is essential, as even "obvious TOAs" may prove to be endometriomas, hemorrhagic corpus luteum cysts, or an abscess surrounding a ruptured appendix. The worldwide average rate of misdiagnosis of PID is 35% when laparoscopy has been used for confirmation.[17] Continued experience with laparoscopic treatment of pelvic abscess combined with intravenous antibiotic therapy indicates better results than early surgery or medical treatment alone with less risk to the patient.

Antibiotic success implies symptom resolution and, perhaps at a much later date, resolution of the pelvic mass, determined by clinical or ultrasound examination. It in no way ensures fertility and can be justified only because ovarian preservation affords the possibility of future candidacy for assisted reproductive technology. To be accurate, efficacy of antibiotic therapy must include long-term complications (ectopic pregnancy, infertility, pelvic pain) in addition to microbiologic response and symptomatic relief.[54]

Laparoscopy allows conservation of the uterine tube and ovary with subsequent fertility potential. Additionally, laparoscopy has a high degree of patient acceptance due to minimal incision size, short hospital stay, and early return to full activity. The combination of laparoscopic treatment and effective intravenous antibiotics is a reasonable approach to the spectrum of PID from acute salpingitis to ruptured TOA.

References

1. MCCORMACK WM: Pelvic inflammatory disease. N Engl J Med 1994;330:115.
2. WASHINGTON AE, KATZ P: Cost of and payment source for pelvic inflammatory disease. JAMA 1991;266:2565.
3. LANDERS D, SWEET R: Current trends in the diagnosis and treatment of tuboovarian abscess. Am J Obstet Gynecol 1985;151:1098.
4. Pelvic inflammatory disease: guidelines for prevention and management. MMWR Morb Mortal Wkly Rep 1991;40(RR-5):1–25.
5. Sexually transmitted diseases treatment guidelines. MMWR Morb Mortal Wkly Rep 1993;42:75.
6. REICH H: Laparoscopic treatment of extensive pelvic adhesions, including hydrosalpinx. J Reprod Med 1987;32:736.
7. REICH H, MCGLYNN F: Treatment of ovarian endometriomas using laparoscopic surgical techniques. J Reprod Med 1986;577.
8. REICH H, MCGLYNN F, REICH E: Laparoscopic treatment of tubal pregnancy. Obstet Gynecol 1987;69:275.
9. REICH H, MCGLYNN F: Laparoscopic treatment of tuboovarian and pelvic abscess. J Reprod Med 1987;32:747.
10. HENRY-SUCHET J, SOLER A, LOFFREDO V: Laparoscopic treatment of tuboovarian abscesses. J Reprod Med 1984;29:579.
11. REICH H: Endoscopic management of tuboovarian abscess and pelvic inflammatory disease. In Operative Gynecologic Endoscopy, Sanfilippo J, Levine R (eds), New York, Springer-Verlag, 1988, p. 118.
12. THJLS H, GNARPE J, LUNDKVIST O, ET AL: Diagnosis and prevalence of persistent Chlamydia infection in infertile women: tissue culture, direct antigen detection, and serology. Fertil Steril 1991;55:304.
13. SOPER D, BROCKWELL N, DALTON H, JOHNSON D: Observations concerning the microbial etiology of acute salpingitis. Am J Obstet Gynecol 1994;170:1008.
14. ESCHENBACH DA, HILLIER S, CRITCHLOW C, ET AL: Diagnosis and clinical manifestations of bacterial vaginosis. Am J Obstet Gynecol 1988;155:819.
15. HILLIS S, JOESOEF R, MARCHBANKS P, ET AL: Delayed care of pelvic inflammatory disease as a risk factor for impaired fertility. Obstet Gynecol 1993;168:1503.
16. AHRENHOLZ DH, SIMMONS RL: Fibrin in peritonitis. I. Beneficial and adverse effects of fibrin in experimental $E.\ coli$ peritonitis. Surgery 1980;88:41.
17. JACOBSON L, WESTROM L: Objectivized diagnosis of acute pelvic inflammatory disease. Am J Obstet Gynecol 1969;105:1088.
18. WESTROM L: Clinical manifestations and diagnosis of pelvic inflammatory disease. J Reprod Med 1983;28:703.
19. SCOTT H, ROSIN R: The influence of diagnostic and therapeutic laparoscopy on patients presenting with an acute abdomen. J R Soc Med 1993;86:699.
20. ABBOTT M: New directions in the diagnosis and treatment of pelvic inflammatory disease. J Antimicrob Chemotherap 1994;33:352.
21. STACEY C, MUNDAY P, THOMAS B, ET AL: *Chlamydia trachomatis* in the fallopian tubes of women without laparoscopic evidence of PID. Lancet 1990;336:960.
22. MOZAS J, JIMENA C, GILL T, ET AL: Serum CA-125 in the diagnosis of acute pelvic inflammatory disease. Int J Gynecol Obstet 1994;44:53.
23. PAAVONEN J, AINE R, TEISALA K, ET AL: Comparison of endometrial biopsy and peritoneal fluid cytologic testing with laparoscopy in the diagnosis of acute pelvic inflammatory disease. Am J Obstet Gynecol 1985;151:645.
24. HOEGSBERG B, ABULAFIA O, SEDLIS A, ET AL: Sexually transmitted diseases and human immunodeficiency virus infection among women with pelvic inflammatory disease. Am J Obstet Gynecol 1990;163:1135.
25. MOZAS J, CASTILLA A, ALARCON JL, ET AL: Diagnosis of pelvic inflammatory disease with 99m technetium-hexamethylpropylenamine-oxime-labeled autologous leukocytes and pelvic radionuclide scintigraphy. Obstet Gynecol 1993;81:797.
26. SIMPSON FF: The choice of time for operation for pelvic inflammation of tubal origin. Surg Gynecol Obstet 1909;9:45.

27. FRANKLIN E, HEVRON J, THOMPSON J: Management of the pelvic abscess. Clin Obstet Gynecol 1973;16:66.
28. GINSBURG D, STERN J, HAMOND R, ET AL: Tubo-ovarian abscess: a retrospective review. Am J Obstet Gynecol 1980;138:1055.
29. HAGER WD: Follow-up of patients with tubo-ovarian abscess(es) in association with salpingitis. Obstet Gynecol 1983;61:680.
30. LANDERS DV, SWEET RL: Tubo-ovarian abscess: contemporary approach to management. Rev Infect Dis 1983;5:876.
31. SWEET RL, SCHACTER J, ROBBIE MO: Failure of β-lactam antibiotics to eradicate Chlamydia trachomatis in the endometrium despite apparent clinical cure of acute salpingitis. JAMA 1983;250:2641.
32. HEMSELL D, SANTOS-RAMOS R, CUNNINGHAM G, ET AL: Cefotaxime treatment for women with community-acquired pelvic abscesses. Am J Obstet Gynecol 1985;151:771.
33. ROBERTS W, DOCKERY JL: Operative and conservative treatment of tubo-ovarian abscess due to pelvic inflammatory disease. South Med J 1984; 77:860.
34. KAPLAN A, JACOBS WM, EHRESMAN JB: Aggressive management of pelvic abscess. Am J Obstet Gynecol 1967;98:482.
35. RUBENSTEIN P, MISHELL D, LEDGER W: Colpotomy drainage of pelvic abscess. Obstet Gynecol 1976; 48:142.
36. RIVLIN M: Clinical outcome following vaginal drainage of pelvic abscess. Obstet Gynecol 1983; 61:169.
37. RIVLIN M, GOLAN A, DARLING M: Diffuse peritoneal sepsis associated with colpotomy drainage of pelvic abscesses. J Reprod Med 1982;27:406.
38. VAN SONNENBERG E, WITTICH GR, CASOLA G: Percutaneous drainage of 50 pelvic abscesses; pitfalls and refinements. In ARRS Scientific Program, 1985.
39. GERZOF S, JOHNSON W, ROBBINS A, NABSETH D: Expanded criteria for percutaneous abscess drainage. Arch Surg 1985;120:227.
40. WORTHEN N, GUNNING J: Percutaneous drainage of pelvic abscesses: management of the tubo-ovarian abscess. J Ultrasound Med 1986;5:551.
41. DELLENBACH P, MULLER P, PHILIPPE E: Infections utero annexielles aigues. Encycl Med Chir Paris Gynecol 1972;470:1410.
42. ADDUCCI JE: Laparoscopy in the diagnosis and treatment of pelvic inflammatory disease with abscess formation. Int Surg 1981;66:359.
43. FREISTADT H: The management of pelvic abscess by combined laparoscopy and colpotomy. Presented at the 14th Annual Meeting of the American Association of Gynecologic Laparoscopists, Anaheim, 1985.
44. SKAU T, NYSTROM P, OHMAN L, STENDAHL O: The kinetics of peritoneal clearance of *Escherichia coli* and *Bacteroides fragilis* and participating defense mechanisms. Arch Surg 1986;121: 1033.
45. HUDSPETH AS: Radical surgical debridement in the treatment of advanced generalized bacterial peritonitis. Arch Surg 1975;110:1233.
46. HULKA J, REICH H: Textbook of Laparoscopy (2nd ed). Philadelphia, Saunders, 1984.
47. RIVLIN M, HUNT J: Surgical management of diffuse peritonitis complicating obstetric/gynecologic infections. Obstet Gynecol 1986;67:652.
48. OWENS S, YEKO T, BLOY R, MAROULIS G: Laparoscopic treatment of painful perihepatic adhesions in Fitz-Hugh-Curtis syndrome. Obset Gynecol 1991;78:542.
49. REICH H: Aquadissection. In Endoscopic Laser Surgery, Baggish M (ed). Clinical Practice of Gynecology Series, Vol 2. New York, Elsevier, 1990, pp. 159–185.
50. GILSTRAP LC III, HERBERT WNP, CUNNINGHAM FG, ET AL: Gonorrhea screening in male consorts of women with pelvic infection. JAMA 1977; 238:965.
51. WESTROM L, JOESOEF R, REYNOLDS G, ET AL: Pelvic inflammatory disease and fertility: a cohort study of 1,844 women with laparoscopically verified disease and 657 control women with normal laparoscopic results. Sex Transm Dis 1992; 19:185.
52. WOLNER-HANSSEN P, ESCHENBACH D, PAAVONEN J, HOLMES K: Treatment of pelvic inflammatory disease: use doxycycline with an appropriate β-lactam while we wait for better data. JAMA 1986;256:3262.
53. HUSTON P: The Oregon plan: a rational way to "ration" care? OBG Management 1991;9:34.
54. BLACK JR: Antibiotic therapy for serious female pelvic infections. Infect Med 1987;10:435.

16
Laparoscopic Pelvic Lymph Node Dissection for Urologic Malignancies

J. Matthew Glascock and Howard N. Winfield

Of the major advancements in clinical surgery during the last half of the twentieth century, the development of laparoscopic intervention must be considered among the most important. Embraced by many surgeons today, the employment of laparoscopic surgical technique affords the patient numerous benefits. The postoperative morbidity often associated with an open surgical incision, the profound postoperative pain, a protracted inpatient stay, and a prolonged convalescence are greatly reduced by the utilization of laparoscopic surgery. For these reasons, laparoscopy is widely recognized as an excellent means of staging urologic pelvic malignancy. This chapter outlines the indications, contraindications, principles of patient selection, techniques, and complications associated with laparoscopic pelvic lymph node dissection (LPLND) for staging urogenital malignancy related to the urinary bladder and urethra and in men the prostate and penis.

Patient Selection

For patients with pelvic malignancy, especially urologic lesions, the status of the pelvic lymph nodes has a major impact on prognosis and subsequent therapeutic decisions.[1,2] Systematic dissemination of neoplastic disease, as evidenced by lymphatic metastasis, is generally understood to be a harbinger of incurable cancer. To forge ahead with aggressive therapeutic intervention without a thorough assessment of the lymph node status is unacceptable empiricism and, in the event that lymphatic dissemination has occurred, would consequently subject the patient to unwarranted morbidity.

In the past, attempts at assessing the pelvic lymph nodes utilizing noninvasive diagnostic modalities such as abdominopelvic computed tomography (CT), magnetic resonance imaging (MRI), and lymphangiography have been unsatisfactory owing to unacceptably low sensitivity and specificity.[3-9] Ultrasound- and CT-guided transcutaneous fine needle aspiration biopsy (FNAB) has been shown to be effective in the evaluation of enlarged pelvic nodes, but it is an operator-dependent technique that has no efficacy in detecting microscopic metastases in nonenlarged nodes. It is for this reason that pathologic evaluation of lymphatic tissue is required for accurate staging of urologic pelvic malignancy. Therefore pelvic lymph node dissection remains the "gold standard" for accurate assessment of lymph node status.[10]

Because of the minimally invasive nature of laparoscopy, LPLND presents an ideal means of obtaining lymphatic material for the accurate staging of urologic pelvic malignancy. It should be appreciated, however, that procedures intended to sample pelvic lymphatic tissues are indicated only in patients for whom knowledge of the lymph node status can direct further therapeutic decisions. Specifically, if some facet of the overall health of a patient precludes the possibility of surgery or the administration of radiation therapy with curative intent, the benefit of evaluating the lymph node status is negligible.

Special Indications

As with any evolving medical or surgical intervention, the indications for LPLND continue to be the subject for debate among practitioners of the art. Although LPLND is performed primarily for the surgical pathologic staging of patients with carcinoma of the prostate, the urologic applications of this technique are presently expanding to encompass the staging of cancers involving the urinary bladder, urethra, and penis.[11-20] These three primary malignancies, as well as the broad spectrum of gynecologic pelvic malignancies, should provide much future opportunity for redefining the role of LPLND in the evaluation of genitourinary cancer. Because lymph node metastasis from primary malignancy involving any one of the following sites has major prognostic and therapeutic implications, the use of laparoscopic lymph node staging to detect disseminated (and probably incurable) disease could potentially obviate the unnecessary morbidity associated with unsuccessful radical therapy.

Cancer of the Urinary Bladder

Extirpative surgery with curative potential is exceedingly unlikely in a patient with lymphatic dissemination of squamous cell carcinoma or adenocarcinoma of the urinary bladder. Similarly, during radical cystectomy the intraoperative detection of lymphatic metastasis from primary transitional cell carcinoma of the bladder suggests abortion of the procedure in favor of offering neoadjuvant chemotherapy. Likewise, the morbidity involved when proceeding with definitive radiotherapy for the treatment of bladder cancer would not be warranted in a patient with lymphatic metastasis. For these reasons, the lymph node status of patients with primary cancer of the urinary bladder plays a major role in determining the optimal therapeutic approach for each individual.[11,12,21-23]

The urinary bladder has a more proximal primary lymphatic drainage route. The extended pelvic lymph node dissection appropriate for the pathologic staging of bladder cancer is described later in this chapter.[24] It should be noted that before undergoing LPLND for staging bladder cancer, the patient is admitted to the hospital, and full bowel preparation is administered on the night prior to surgery in case urinary diversion is indicated.

We offer LPLND to patients with primary malignancy of the urinary bladder under the following conditions.[9]

1. Radiologic evidence of pelvic lymphadenopathy that is inaccessible by CT- or ultrasound-guided FNAB.
2. Patients who refuse radical cystectomy and desire definitive radiotherapy.
3. Patients being considered as candidates for partial cystectomy. The extirpation can then be approached through an extraperitoneal route following laparoscopic lymphadenectomy if histopathologic evaluation of the nodal tissue demonstrates the absence of malignancy.
4. Patients with squamous cell carcinoma or adenocarcinoma of the bladder. In the presence of lymph node positivity, curative radical cystectomy would be highly unlikely. In this situation, laparoscopic urinary diversion could be considered for palliation.
5. Clinical evidence of pelvic lymphadenopathy that cannot be visualized radiologically.

Cancer of the Urethra

Although rare, isolated carcinoma of the urethra is the only urologic cancer that is more common in the female than the male population.[19] Unfortunately, because of the insidious onset of symptoms, patients generally present with advanced disease. Tumors involving the distal urethra generally metastasize to the superficial and deep inguinal nodes. More proximal lesions involve primarily the external and internal iliac as well as the obturator lymph node chains, although some overlapping of the respective drainage fields is not unusual. In several reported series, lymphatic involvement at initial presentation can be as high as 35–50%, foreshadowing a grim prognosis for patients with this disease.[17] In 80–96% of cases palpable inguinal lymphadenopathy represents the metastatic spread of disease.

Because of the rarity of this disease, the possible approaches to its management comprise a subject of contention among the urologists. As with other genitourinary malignancies, radical exenterative surgery is contraindicated in patients with evidence of metastatic disease. We recommend extended laparoscopic pelvic lymph node dissection for patients with cancer of the urethra in the clinical situations listed below.[9]

1. Radiologic evidence of pelvic lymphadenopathy inaccessible through CT- or ultrasound-guided FNAB.
2. Prior to performing exenterative surgery for the treatment of tumors of the posterior urethra. Lymph node positivity would likely negate the curative potential of radical surgery.
3. In patients with locally invasive distal lesions.

Contraindications

Absolute contraindications to the performance of LPLND are in general the same as for any other laparoscopic procedure. Patients with generalized peritonitis, abdominal wall infection, coagulopathy not correctable by administration of blood products, and significant intestinal obstruction should be managed by alternative approaches. Relative contraindications to laparoscopy include obesity, previous major intraperitoneal surgery, abdominal aortic aneurysm, abdominal wall hernias, severe diverticular disease, and previous radiotherapy (Table 16.1). The relative importance of each contraindication evolves as the surgeon's confidence with the technique progresses. As always, the absolute and relative contraindications for general surgery with regard to anesthetic risk apply.

Table 16.1. Contraindications to laparoscopic surgery

Absolute contraindications
Generalized peritonitis
Abdominal wall infection
Nonreversible coagulopathy
Intestinal obstruction (significant)
Relative contraindications
Obesity
Previous major abdominal surgery
Abdominal aortic aneurysm
Abdominal wall hernia
Severe diverticular disease
Previous abdominopelvic radiotherapy

Preoperative Preparation

After a patient is selected for laparoscopic surgery, informed consent must be obtained. Because of the nature of the technique(s) involved specific potential complications rarely seen with the standard open procedure must be appreciated by the patient.[9,25,26] Potential major complications that should be discussed include vascular injury causing severe hemorrhage that may be voluminous enough to require transfusion, visceral injury including bowel or bladder perforation (which may require open repair), and the possibility of ureteral damage. It is also mandatory that the surgical candidate be informed of the possibility that intraoperative circumstances may necessitate conversion to an open procedure. Such circumstances include the aforementioned major complications as well as unsatisfactory dissection with poor lymphatic tissue yield and inadequate exposure due to anatomic aberrancy secondary to obesity, extensive adhesions from prior surgery, or previous radiation therapy. In addition, lymphedema and lymphocele formation, occasionally requiring percutaneous drainage, are potential complications that should be mentioned. The possibility of hematoma formation which, if infected, may subsequently require drainage is also discussed. Referred pain to the shoulder area as a result of diaphragmatic irritation brought on by CO_2 pneumoperitoneum is a postoperative side effect worthy of mention; and as with all surgical operations requiring general anesthesia, the attendant risks of pneumonia, myocardial infarction, stroke, and death are discussed. Other less common complications encountered during LPLND include infection, wound dehiscence, lower extremity deep venous thrombosis, and obturator nerve palsy.

Once informed consent is obtained and the surgery is scheduled, the surgical candidate receives specific instructions regarding the preoperative routine indicated by her individual circumstances. A healthy patient with no history of intraabdominal surgery or intraperitoneal pathology who is scheduled for LPLND only is directed to self-administer either an oral laxative such as Golytely or an enema on the night prior to surgery as a means of decompressing the colon and rectum. She is then instructed to report to the hospital for admission on the morning of surgery. For the patient with a medical history significant for previous abdominal surgery, peritonitis, chemotherapy, or radiation therapy, the greater likelihood of encountering extensive adhesions requiring lysis increases the risk of inadvertent enterotomy. In this situation the patient is ideally admitted to the hospital the night before surgery is planned so mechanical and antibiotic bowel preparation can be implemented. Also, with a patient for whom further surgery is planned should intraoperative evaluation of the lymphatic tissue specimen prove benign, the same formal bowel preparation is mandated the night prior to surgery.

After admission, and as part of the preoperative preparation, a blood type and antibody screen is indicated for all LPLND candidates should profound hemorrhage necessitate the administration of blood products. All patients receive three doses of a parenteral broad-spectrum antibiotic; one dose on call to the operating room and one dose every 8 hours postoperatively.

Operative Procedure

Upon arrival in the operating room, antiembolic pneumatic compression boots are placed on the patient. General anesthesia is preferred for LPLND because of analgesia, improved positioning, muscle relaxation and exposure. It is advisable that the anesthetic technique utilized not include the use of nitrous oxide as this inhalational agent is associated with distention of the intestines, which may interfere with proper exposure of the operative field during dissection.

After adequate general anesthesia is obtained, a Foley catheter for straight drainage and a nasogastric tube on low, constant suction are placed into the patient's bladder and stomach, respectively. Decompression of the bladder and stomach reduces the risk of iatrogenic injury during the procedure. The patient's arms are padded and placed at her sides, and wide adhesive tape across the chest and thighs is used to secure the patient to the operating table. The abdomen is then prepared and draped as for a traditional laparotomy. As a precaution, should the need for emergency laparotomy develop, it is advisable that a laparotomy setup be immediately available to the surgeon. Again, the surgeon's experience and confidence with laparoscopic surgical techniques replace this precaution in due time. The video monitoring equipment is arranged with an unobstructed view by the surgical team. If possible, dual video monitors allow the surgeons to view the monitors while squarely facing the patient.

Transperitoneal Laparoscopic Pelvic Lymph Node Dissection

After adequate pneumoperitoneum has been obtained and placement of a 10- or 11-mm subumbilical port has been accomplished, a 0° telescope is introduced into the intraperitoneal space through the port and a thorough and systematic survey of the abdominal contents to rule out injury or gross metastatic disease is performed.[27] Extensive adhesions or fatty tissue deposits in the vicinity of the umbilical ligaments are noted, as these findings may indicate the need for a modification of the standard "diamond" configuration for working port placement.

For most patients, the four-port "diamond" configuration is well suited to an intraperitoneal LPLND (Fig. 16.1). This arrangement features two lateral 5 mm working ports placed midway between the umbilicus and antero-

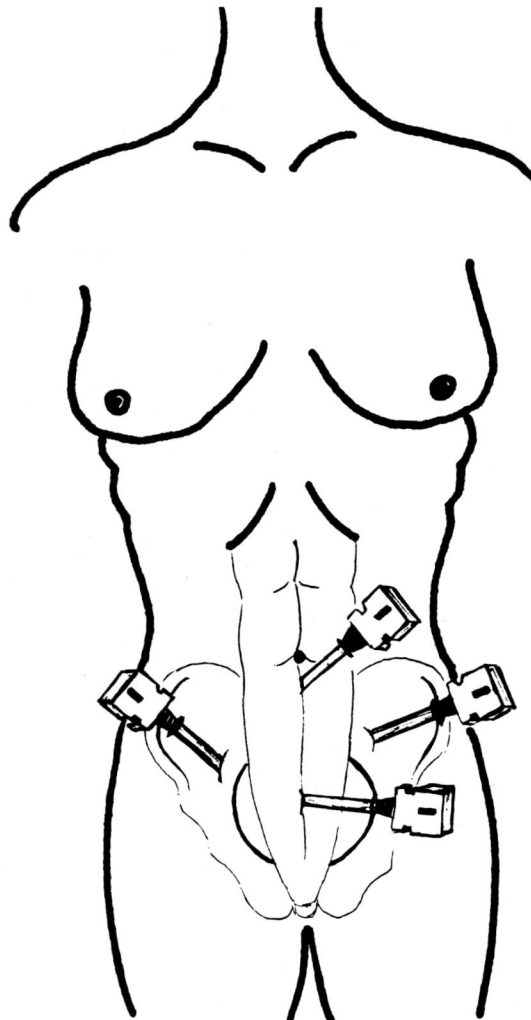

Figure 16.1. Diamond configuration of four laparoscopic ports for pelvic lymph node dissection.

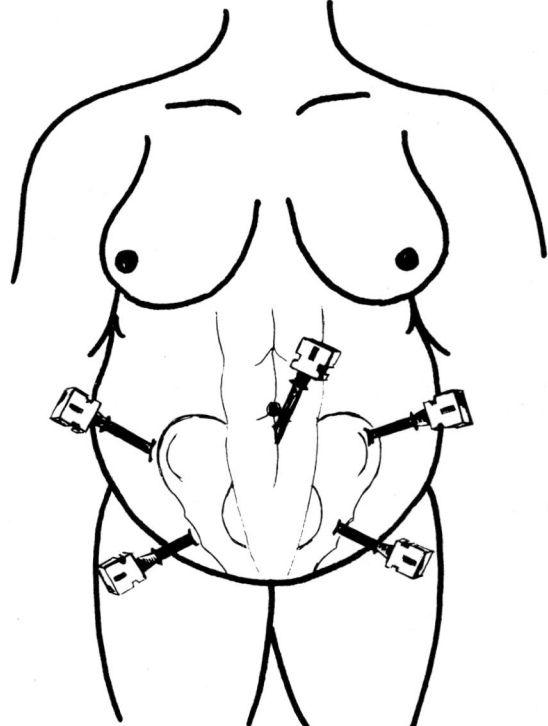

Figure 16.2. Horseshoe configurations of five laparoscopic ports for pelvic lymph node dissection in obese patients.

superior iliac spines along the lateral edge of the rectus muscle, and a 10- or 11-mm suprapubic midline port placed 3–5 cm above the pubic symphysis. All working ports are placed under direct laparoscopic visualization, and transillumination of the abdominal wall during the selection of puncture sites should decrease the risk of transecting the inferior epigastric vessels during port placement. An alternative arrangement for port placement in obese patients with an abundance of urachal fatty tissue is the inverted-U, or horseshoe, configuration (Fig. 16.2). The disadvantage of this alternative placement is the need for an additional laparoscopic port. The ports are secured to the abdominal wall by skin sutures. The Trendelenburg position is increased to 30°, and, in addition, 15°–30° of lateral rotation is obtained to further elevate the side of dissection, thereby mobilizing loops of bowel away from the operative field. At this point, adhesions interfering with proper exposure of the operative field may require lysis, particularly with dissection on the left side, as diverticular inflammation may create adhesions of the sigmoid colon to the pelvic side wall. By incising along the white line of Toldt, the sigmoid colon should be easily mobilized to allow a clear view of the iliac–obturator region. It is crucial to identify several important landmarks before beginning dissection of the pelvic lymph nodes. In the female patient, the round ligament should be seen coursing cephalad from the deep inguinal ring to its attachment point near the ovarian ligament on the uterine wall. The umbilical ligament should be seen extending from the anterior abdominal wall to its terminus off the internal iliac artery near the bifurcation of the common iliac artery. In nonobese patients, pulsations of the external iliac artery may be appreciated, suggesting its position underneath the posterior peritoneal membrane (Plate 26).

Obturator Lymph Node Dissection

The initial incision through the posterior peritoneal membrane begins at a point approximately midway between the obliterated umbilical artery and the internal inguinal ring high over the pubic bone; it is extended cephalad, medial to the external iliac artery, toward a point near the bifurcation of the common iliac artery. It is of the utmost importance to appreciate the proximity of the ureter to the bifurcation of the common iliac artery so as to avoid accidental injury of this structure. The external iliac vein is then exposed by careful dissection of all lymph node bearing fibrofatty tissue medial to the external iliac artery. The lateral extent of the dissection is thus formed by clearing all of the fibrolymphatic tissue off the anterior and medial surfaces of the external iliac vein using blunt and sharp dissection.

Gentle medial traction placed on the obliterated umbilical artery forms a plane delineating the medial boundary of the obturator node packet. Blunt dissection lateral to the obliterated umbilical artery is continued inferiorly to develop this plane to the level of the pubic bone and Cooper's ligament. This maneuver completes the inferior apex of the dissection. Venous anomalies are frequently noted in this area. For example, an accessory obturator vein may be encountered branching off the external iliac vein just as it exits the femoral canal. With careful manipulation, the distal lymphatic tissue may be passed underneath this vessel; but as is often the case, the accessory vein requires hemoclip ligation and division.

The distal extent of the lymph node packet is freed with cautious use of electrocautery. The free, distal aspect of the node packet is then grasped; and with proximal traction and blunt dissection at the base of the node packet, the underlying obturator nerve and vessels should come into view. During dissection of the lymph node packet toward the bifurcation of the common iliac artery, any small vessels or lymphatics encountered should be sealed with electrocautery. It must be remembered that as the dissection nears the bifurcation of the common iliac artery the proximity of the ureter puts it in jeopardy for unintentional injury. Once at the level of the common iliac bifurcation, the proximal lymphatic vessels are cauterized, with subsequent division resulting in a free lymph node packet.

With spoon-shaped or Russian laparoscopic forceps, the free lymph node packet is delivered through the 10- or 11-mm suprapubic port using a gentle twisting motion. The flap valve at the entrance to the port must be manually opened during extraction of the lymph node packet so as to avoid shearing and loss of lymphatic tissue within the barrel of the sheath. If immediate radical surgery is planned pending a negative histopathologic evaluation of the lymphatic tissue specimen, the lymph node packet is sent for immediate frozen (pathological) section, and attention is turned to the opposite side. The table is rotated in the opposite direction, the surgeons switch either sides or roles, and a similar dissection commences (Plate 27).

Extended LPLND

There are certain instances that indicate the need for a more extensive lymph node dissection.[9,24,28] The extended LPLND includes the excision of all lymphatic tissues found within an area bounded by the genitofemoral nerve laterally, the common iliac artery proximally, and the urinary bladder wall medially. To gain access to this broader region of dissection, more extensive mobilization of the sigmoid colon and cecoappendiceal regions is required. Greater exposure of the iliac region may be obtained through the use of an inverted V peritoneotomy,[29] which includes a second incision that originates at the same point over the pubic bone and continues posteromedially and equidistant to the initial incision. This incision forms a peritoneal free flap that, when elevated, allows more thorough exposure of the underlying obturator–iliac region. By gentle medial retraction of the external iliac artery and vein, full access to the lymphatic tissue deep to these vessels is achieved (Plate 28).

Extraperitoneal Laparoscopic Pelvic Lymph Node Dissection

As the technique for any newly proposed surgical procedure evolves from a "first-time" status to an accepted, routine operation, the developmental progression often suggests possible alternative approaches by which the same clinical end result can be obtained. Such is the case with LPLND. Over an 18 month period LPLND has been performed in selected cases by the authors via an extraperitoneal approach. Although the scope of the potential advantages and disadvantages of this novel approach are only now being fully characterized, it is evident that by maintaining the integrity of the peritoneum the risks of visceral injury, intraabdominal spillage of potentially tumor-laden lymphatic tissue, and postoperative development of intraabdominal adhesions associated with direct instrumentation of the intraabdominal contents may be avoided.

Creation of the Extraperitoneal Space

A 3 cm incision, beginning at the inferior crease of the umbilicus, is carried down to the level of the rectus abdominis fascia. The properitoneal space is then entered by splitting the rectus abdominis and transversus abdominis fasciae. By insinuating the finger, a properitoneal space is developed to the extent that a balloon dilation device can be introduced. Several dilation devices have been proposed. One approach involves use of a modified Gaur device consisting of a 16F red rubber (Robinson) catheter onto which the middle finger of a size 8½ Triflex surgeon's glove has been secured by silk-free ties.[30] Unfortunately, the 800–1000 ml of saline required to dilate the properitoneal space often ruptures the latex, necessitating a thorough search of the properitoneal space for glove fragments. Hence the finger cot of a transurethral resection drape in a similar configuration has been substituted, as the thicker polyethylene natural rubber material reduces the risk of rupture during the dilation process (Fig. 16.3).

With successful dilation, the space of Retzius is expanded to the extent that the pubic bone and external iliac vessels may be directly visualized (Plate 29). At this point, a Hasson type

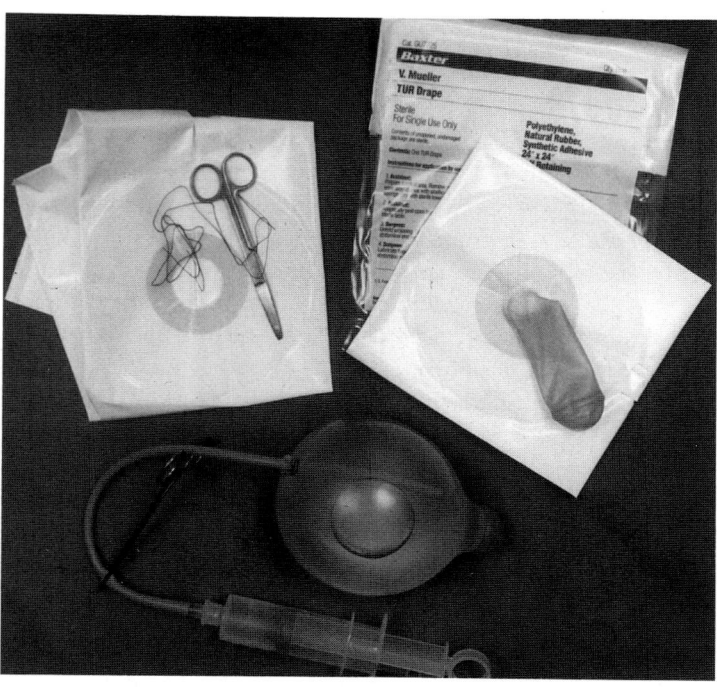

Figure 16.3. Polyethylene rubber material (TUR drape) used as a baloon-dilation device for creation of extraperitoneal space.

cannula is secured into the subumbilical incision and CO_2 insufflation proceeds up to 12–15 mm Hg through the cannula. In the standard "diamond" configuration, the working ports are then placed carefully in the properitoneal space so as to avoid traversing the peritoneal membrane. If the peritoneum is inadvertently entered, obliteration of the properitoneal space is likely. This eventuality necessitates converting the port placement from an extraperitoneal to an intraperitoneal position.

Once the ports are in place, LPLND proceeds in the same sequence as was described for the intraperitoneal approach. Some major intraoperative advantages of this approach are that it avoids the need to mobilize the sigmoid colon, it does not require extensive adhesiolysis, and it eliminates the need for retraction of loops of small bowel, which tend to interfere with exposure of the operative field. These advantages make the extraperitoneal approach ideal in situations where there is a high likelihood of encountering major intraabdominal adhesions from previous surgery, although a medical history significant for inguinal herniorrhaphy may prove to be a relative contraindication to this approach.

The potential disadvantages of the extraperitoneal approach include decreased working space and a distortion in the orientation of the anatomic landmarks. Fibrosis and scarring as a result of previous inguinal herniorrhaphy or any other extraperitoneal surgery may render the development of the properitoneal working space a formidable task indeed. Likewise, any subsequent surgery involving this area becomes much more difficult. Furthermore, the development of lymphoceles following extraperitoneal LPLND may occur more frequently. Presently, an ongoing randomized prospective study investigating the differences in (CO_2) metabolism (as well as many other intra- and postoperative characteristics) in patients undergoing either intraperitoneal or extraperitoneal LPLND is being evaluated. It is possible that the extraperitoneal approach allows greater subcutaneous emphysema development and CO_2 absorption resulting in iatrogenic hypercapnia.

At the conclusion of the laparoscopic procedure, the abdomen is thoroughly, systematically evaluated. Particular attention is directed to the operative sites to ensure that meticulous hemostasis has been achieved. The intraabdominal pressure is then lowered to approximately 5 mm Hg, and any venous bleeding that had been tamponaded during the higher intraabdominal pressures maintained throughout the procedure should become apparent. Because the physical presence of the ports may tamponade any potential bleeding from a lacerated abdominal wall vessel, the secondary ports are removed under direct laparoscopic visualization. The final port is removed over the laparoscope, with the laparoscope being the last instrument to exit the intraabdominal space. This technique guards against herniation of abdominal contents and allows final inspection for any hemorrhage that had been tamponaded by the camera port. In addition, digital exploration of the 10- or 11-mm port incisions may be used to rule out herniation before closure. Any residual CO_2 is expressed from the abdominal cavity, and all puncture sites that are 10 mm or larger are closed separately with a single 2-0 polydioxanone (PDS) suture on the fascia. All skin incisions are approximated with Steri-Strip closures and are covered with Tegaderm dressings. The nasogastric tube is removed before the patient is awakened, and she is then taken to the postanesthesia care unit for routine postoperative monitoring.

All patients are admitted to the hospital after laparoscopic surgery. They receive two postoperative doses of a parenteral, broad spectrum antibiotic, and their diet is advanced as tolerated. The Foley catheter should be removed as soon as the patient is alert. Ambulation should be tolerable on the evening of surgery and any postoperative pain manageable with oral analgesics. Narcotics are rarely indicated. Most patients are discharged on the first postoperative day and should be able to resume normal activity within 1 week.

Results

Since May 1990, LPLND has been performed on 195 patients for the operative staging of patients with urologic pelvic malignancy at the University of Iowa. Most ($n = 192$) of these

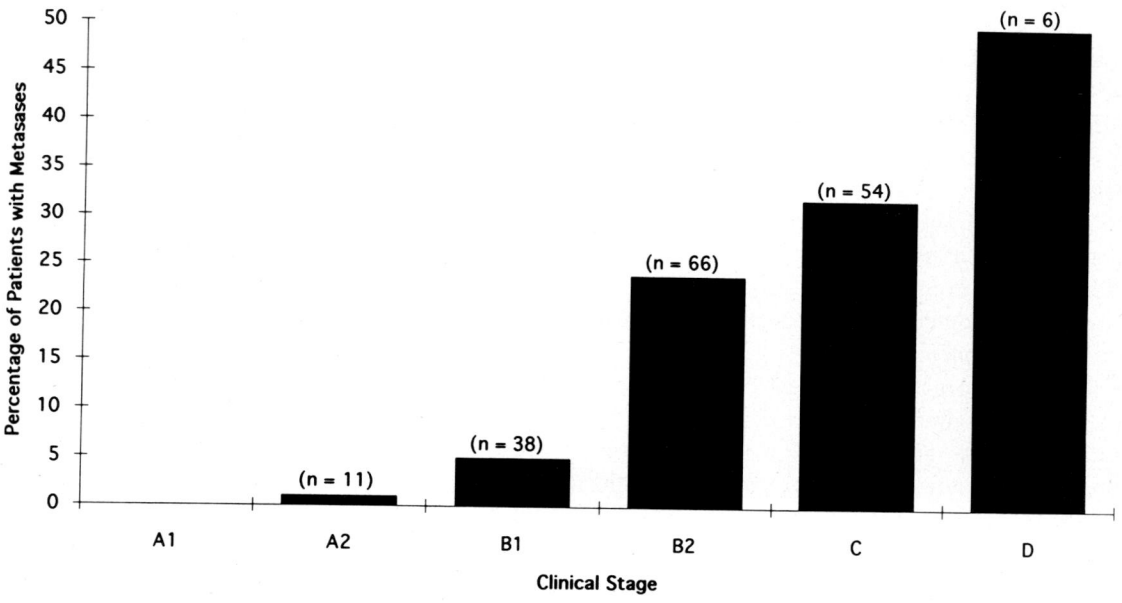

Figure 16.4. Increase in stage correlates with increased lymph node metastatic disease.

operations have been performed to stage cancer of the prostate. During the early experience, 26 of the initial 66 laparoscopic operations performed for cancer of the prostate were immediately followed by open exploration, which provided an opportunity to assess objectively the thoroughness of the laparoscopic procedure. Of these 26 patients, 15 underwent open surgery for radical retropubic prostatectomy, 10 were believed to have had an incomplete laparoscopic obturator lymphadenectomy, and one patient had laparoscopically induced hemorrhage from the most proximal portion of the obliterated umbilical artery and required open repair. The most proximal portion of the obliterated umbilical artery near its branch point off the internal iliac artery is widely patent. Of the patients who underwent laparoscopy followed by open lymphadenectomy, the mean number of lymph nodes laparoscopically obtained from the right and left sides was 2.5 and 2.3, respectively. The follow-up open lymphadenectomy yielded a mean of 0.96 and 1.3 additional lymph nodes from the right and left sides, respectively. Evaluation of these data suggests that more lymphatic tissue is missed laparoscopically on the left side. This finding is most likely due to the more difficult left-sided dissection resulting from dense adhesion of the sigmoid colon to the pelvic side wall in association with diverticular bowel disease. It is important to note that in 1 of the 26 patients undergoing immediate open exploration following LPLND a small amount of residual lymphatic tissue recovered near the bifurcation of the iliac vessels revealed a microscopic focus of metastatic adenocarcinoma. This finding occurred after the laparoscopically procured specimen was determined to be free of metastatic disease following frozen section histopathologic evaluation—corresponding to a roughly 4% false-negative rate in this series. However, in all patients with this type of cancer there exists the possibility of metastatic "skip lesions" involving the more proximal iliac lymphatics. In addition, patients who did not undergo open exploration following LPLND may have had foci of metastatic adenocarcinoma that were not detected laparoscopically. Figure 16.4 depicts the increasing percentages of ages of patients with lymphatic metastases within each clinical stage.

The mean duration for the performance of intraperitoneal LPLND for all patients in the series was 163 minutes (range 75–312 minutes).

Table 16.2. Comparison of intraperitoneal and extraperitoneal approaches to LPLND

Parameter	Intraperitoneal approach	Extraperitoneal approach
Age (years)	67	65
Gleason score	6.15	7.06
PSA	33.09	28.66
PAP (IU/L)	1.30	1.01
Operative duration (minutes)	163	162
Number of nodes obtained		
Left	4.54	3.00
Right	4.60	3.81
Postoperative inpatient duration (days)	1.30	1.12
Morphine (mg)	5.59	11.14
Tylenol 3 (tablets)	1.67	3.10
No analgesia required (% patients)	52	35

Results are averages.
PSA, Prostate-specific antigen; PAP, prostatic acid phosphatase.

It is of interest that, when considering the operative times for patients in the most recent half of the series, the mean duration of the procedure decreased from 163 to 147 minutes. This finding calls attention to the considerable learning curve associated with mastering this complex technique. It is also important to note that patient obesity is an important factor influencing operative duration. It was found that, on average, the procedure took an additional 25 minutes to perform in obese patients.

Because of its minimally invasive nature, patients tend to tolerate LPLND well, evidenced by the shorter inpatient duration and lower analgesic requirements seen in patients following this procedure. The mean postoperative inpatient duration following LPLND was 1.3 days, with 60% of patients being discharged from hospital early in the morning of the day after surgery. This timing compares well with the mean postoperative inpatient duration of 6.5 days for patients undergoing open pelvic lymphadenectomy.[9] In addition, 52% of patients required no analgesics following LPLND. Only 34% of patients required morphine for pain control (mean 5.59 mg per patient). Most of the patients taking morphine required only a single dose during the immediate postoperative period. In addition, 22% of patients took acetaminophen with codeine (30 mg codeine, Tylenol 3) at a mean dosage of 1.67 tablets per patient (Table 16.2).

As was previously mentioned, over the 18 months studied, LPLND was performed via an extraperitoneal approach in selected cases. Table 16.2 summarizes the basic patient characteristics and selected perioperative considerations between the two groups of patients. Interestingly, the average operative times for each approach are similar. Although the difference in sample size between these two groups of patients makes it difficult to draw statistically significant conclusions when comparing the data, a preliminary evaluation yields some interesting suggestions. It appears that the extraperitoneal approach produces a lower total number of lymph nodes than does the traditional intraperitoneal approach. This comparison is difficult to make; and as the sample size of patients in whom the extraperitoneal approach is used increases, this discrepancy will likely diminish. It is well known that there is a true disparity in the total number of lymph nodes in a given region between any two individuals. Hence it is the completeness of the individual dissection that is the important consideration when assessing the success of the procedure. It is also noted that the patients undergoing LPLND via the extraperitoneal approach have a slightly higher analgesic requirement. The pain associated with balloon dissection of the properitoneal space would reasonably account for this apparent discrepancy in analgesic requirements. However, more expe-

Table 16.3. Complications of laparoscopic pelvic lymph node dissection (University of Iowa experience, 195 cases)

Complication	No.
Hemorrhage	9
Controlled laparoscopically	8
Requiring open repair	1
Injury to external iliac artery	1
Injury to inferior epigastric vessels	6
Bleeding from obliterated umbilical artery	2
Bowel perforation/injury	4
Deep venous thrombosis/pulmonary embolism (S/P prostatectomy/ radiotherapy)	2
Wound infection/dehiscence	2
Abscess formation	1
Scrotal/suprapubic ecchymosis	3
Unsatisfactory dissection	1
Postoperative ileus	4
Urinary retention	4
Bowel obstruction	1
Obturator nerve neuropraxia, transient	1
Hypercarbia (extraperitoneal approach)	1
Postoperative sedation (anesthesia)	1
Intraoperative ST segment depression	1
Total	44

Table 16.4. Etiology of nine LPLND conversions to laparotomy[a] (University of Iowa experience, 195 cases)

Contributing factor	No.
Obesity	4
Previous abdominopelvic surgery/ radiotherapy	4
Bowel injury/enterotomy	2
Vascular injury	1
Unsatisfactory pathologic specimen	1
Equipment failure	1

[a]More than one contributing factor may apply in each case.

rience with the extraperitoneal approach is needed to determine whether a significant difference exists.

As was stated earlier, the presence of metastatic disease has major prognostic and therapeutic implications. The presence of disseminated disease is usually considered to be a contraindication to further radical surgical or radiotherapy. Likewise, hormonal manipulation is rarely, if ever, indicated for patients with local disease.

Although LPLND is a well tolerated procedure based on a review of our series, it is not an operation without a potential for significant complications.[9,325,26] Table 16.3 outlines the complications that occurred during our experience with LPLND. All vascular and bowel injuries became apparent intraoperatively and were subsequently corrected at the time of the initial surgery. For the nine procedures during which intraoperative complications necessitated conversion from laparoscopic to open surgery, Table 16.4 outlines the contributing factors. It is important to note the fact that obesity was a contributor in nearly one half of the cases that required the intraoperative conversion. In addition, nearly all of the cases in which major complications necessitated conversion from laparoscopic to open surgery occurred early in the series. More recently, however, the implementation of advanced laparoscopic techniques, such as laparoscopic suturing, facilitated the successful repair of several intraoperative complications that would have required open repair had they occurred earlier in the series. Again, the temporal distribution of surgical complications within the series attests to the significant learning curve associated with mastering the complex techniques required to perform LPLND.

With the current public and governmental interest in seeking an agreeable reorganization of the health care delivery system in the United States, the burden of objectively assessing the cost/benefit facet of surgical intervention now frequently falls primarily on the shoulder of the physician. Table 16.5 provides the findings of a retrospective financial analysis undertaken at our institution in which the pre-, intra-, and postoperative costs of LPLND were compared to those of open pelvic lymph node dissection. Because of the retrospective nature of the study (which encompassed the years 1988–1992), all dollar charges were corrected upward or downward to the base fiscal year of 1990–1991. As shown in Table 16.5, the intraoperative costs were approximately $2700 more expensive in the laparoscopic group. Postoperatively, however, there was a savings of close to $1400 for

Table 16.5. Cost analysis of laparoscopic versus open pelvic lymph node dissection for men with cancer of the prostate

Period	Cost[a] (average and range)	
	LPLND	Open PLND
Preoperative	$532 ($164–1452)	$693 ($171–1528)
Operative	$8075 ($6267–11,436)	$5332 ($4040–6377)
Postoperative	$842 ($399–2089)	$2161 ($1519–3331)
Pathology	$619 ($170–1153)	$538 ($181–1358)
Total	$10,068 ($7332–12,869)	$8724 ($6231–10,290)

Reprinted from ref. 31, with permission.
[a]Dollar amounts represent the 1990–1991 fiscal base year.

the laparoscopic group. The conclusion was that it is approximately $1300 more expensive to perform LPLND than open pelvic lymph node dissection for staging carcinoma of the prostate. Furthermore, it is the intraoperative expenses associated with longer operating room and anesthesia requirements, as well as the additional expense of disposable instrumentation, that combine to account for this cost discrepancy. However, it is indeed difficult to assign a monetary value to convalescence. It has been shown that the convalescent period following open pelvic lymph node dissection is at least 10 days longer than the mean post-LPLND convalescence. With more surgical experience and the judicious use of disposable instrumentation, the relative cost discrepancy between the two procedures will certainly diminish.

Conclusions

Since May 1990, LPLND has been performed more than 195 times at our institution; and to date it has been repeatedly shown to be an excellent, minimally invasive means to obtain lymphatic tissue for the pathologic staging of urologic pelvic malignancy. The standardization of LPLND as a staging procedure for gynecologic and other urologic pelvic malignancies should be a challenge accepted by all present and future practitioners. The temporal arrangement of complications within the series of LPLNDs at this institution betrays the short, steep nature of the learning curve. The likelihood of severe complications developing during laparoscopic surgery is greatly reduced by arming one's self with a thorough understanding and respect for the regional anatomy. Likewise, strict adherence to the basic principles of laparoscopic surgery is paramount to the elimination of many potential surgical misadventures.

The newly developed extraperitoneal approach to LPLND may further define the role of LPLND for staging urologic pelvic malignancy. Visceral injury and the development of postoperative bowel adhesions are just two complications that theoretically may be averted through the utilization of this technique. In addition, the confounding intraabdominal barriers seen in obese individuals are held in check through their retention by the intact peritoneal membrane. An ongoing study evaluating CO_2 metabolism, operative time, hospitalization, complications, analgesic use, and convalescence is currently under way at our institution.

Finally, although a previous study demonstrated a $1300 difference in the cost of performing an LPLND compared to the open lymph node dissection, there are numerous ways in which this discrepancy can be eliminated. Additional surgical experience and the development of dependable, reusable laparoscopic instruments present two immediate avenues of remediation.

Acknowledgments. We wish to acknowledge the work of our colleagues who were involved in the care of many of these patients: Drs. James F. Donovan, William A. See, Stefan A. Loening, and Richard D. Williams.

References

1. CLINE WA JR, KRAMER SA, FARNHAM R, ET AL: Impact of pelvic lymphadenectomy in patients with prostatic adenocarcinoma. Urology 1981; 27:129.
2. BEREK JS, HACKER NF, YAO-SHI F, ET AL: Adenocarcinoma of the uterine cervix: histologic variables associated with lymph node metastasis and survival. Obstet Gynecol 1985; 65:46.
3. MUKAMEL E, HANNA J, BARBARIC Z, ET AL: The value of computerized tomography scan and magnetic resonance imaging in staging prostatic carcinoma: comparison with the clinical and histologic staging. J Urol 1986;135:1231.
4. BENSON KH, WATSON RA, SPRING DB, ET AL: The value of computerized tomography in the evaluation of pelvic lymph nodes. J Urol 1981;126:63.
5. LOENING SA, SCHMIDT JD, BROWN RC, ET AL: A comparison between lymphangiography and pelvic node dissection in the staging of prostatic cancer. J Urol 1977;117:752.
6. PAULSON DF, PISERCHIA PV, GARDENER W: Predictors of lymphatic spread in prostatic adenocarcinoma: uro-oncology research group study. J Urol 1980;123:697.
7. RIFKIN MD, ZERHOUNI EA, GATSONIS CA, ET AL: Comparison of magnetic resonance imaging and ultrasonography in staging early prostate cancer. N Engl J Med 1990;323:621.
8. HAGANO T, NAKAI Y, TANIGUCHI F, ET AL: Diagnosis of paraaortic and pelvic lymph node metastasis of gynecologic malignant tumors by ultrasound-guided percutaneous fine-needle aspiration biopsy. Cancer 1991;68:2571.
9. WINFIELD HN, DONOVAN JF, SEE WA, ET AL: Laparoscopic pelvic lymph node dissection for genitourinary malignancies: indications, techniques, and results. J Endourol 1992;6:103.
10. PAULSON DF: The prognostic role of lymphadenectomy in adenocarcinoma of the prostate. Urol Clin North Am 1980;7:615.
11. DRETLER SP, RAGSDALE BD, LEADBETTER WF: The value of pelvic lymphadenectomy in the surgical treatment of bladder cancer. J Urol 1973; 109:414.
12. SKINNER DG: Management of invasive bladder cancer: a meticulous pelvic node dissection can make a difference. J Urol 1982;128:34.
13. SCHELLHAMMER PF, GRABSTALD H: Tumors of the penis. In Campbell's Urology (5th ed), Walsh PC, Gittes RF, Perlmutter AD, et al (eds). Philadelphia, Saunders, 1986, pp 1583–1606.
14. MCDOUGAL WS, KIRCHNER FJ JR, EDWARDS, RH, ET AL: Treatment of carcinoma of the penis: the case for primary lymphadenectomy. J Urol 1986; 136:38.
15. MUKAMEL E, DEKERNION JB: Early Versus Delayed Lymph Node Dissection Versus No Lymph Node Dissection for Carcinoma of the Penis. AUA Update Series, 1990, lesson 9.
16. HOPKINS SC, GRABSTALD H: Benign and malignant tumors of the male and female urethra. In Campbell's Urology (5th ed), Walsh PC, Gittes RF, Perlmutter AD, et al (eds). Philadelphia, Saunders, 1986, pp 1441–1462.
17. GRABSTALD H, HILARIS B, HENSCHKE U, ET AL: Cancer of the female urethra. JAMA 1966;197:835.
18. GRABSTALD H: Tumors of the urethra in men and women. Cancer 1973;32:1236.
19. LEVINE RL: Urethral cancer. Cancer 1980;45:1965.
20. SAROSDY MF: Urethral Carcinoma. AUA Update Series, 1987, lesson 6.
21. LEADBETTER WF, COOPER JF: Regional gland dissection for carcinoma of the bladder: a technique for one-stage cystectomy, gland dissection, and bilateral uretero-enterostomy. J Urol 1950;63:242.
22. WHITMORE WF, JR, MARSHALL VF: Radical total cystectomy for cancer of the bladder: 230 consecutive cases five years later. J Urol 1962;87:853.
23. LIESKOVSKY G, SKINNER DG: Role of lymphadenectomy in the treatment of bladder cancer. Urol Clin North Am 1984;11:709.
24. GOLIMBU M, MORALES P, AL-ASKARI S, ET AL: Extended pelvic lymphadenectomy for prostatic cancer. J Urol 1979;121:617.
25. WINFIELD HN, DONOVAN JF, SEE WA, ET AL: Urological laparoscopic surgery. J Urol 1991;146:941.
26. KAVOUSSI LR, SOSA E, CHANDHOKE P, ET AL: Complications of pelvic lymph node dissection. J Urol 1993;149:322.
27. KERBEL K, CLAYMAN RV: Basic techniques of laparoscopic surgery. Urol Clin North Am 1993; 20:361.
28. WINFIELD HN: Laparoscopic pelvic lymph node dissection for urologic pelvic malignancies. Urol Clin North Am 1993;1:33.
29. SEE WA, COHEN MB, WINFIELD HN: Inverted V peritoneotomy significantly improves nodal yield in laparoscopic pelvic lymphadenectomy. J Urol 1993;149:772.
30. GAUR DD, AGARWAL DK, PUROHIT KC: Retroperitoneal laparoscopic nephrectomy: initial case report. J Urol 1993;149:103.
31. TROXEL SA, WINFIELD HN: Comparative financial analysis of laparoscopic versus open pelvic lymph node dissection for men with cancer of the prostate. J Urol 1994;151:675.

17
Endoscopic Surgical Procedures During Pregnancy

Marcello Pietrantoni and Joseph S. Sanfilippo

Pregnant women and the puerperal patient are vulnerable to the same surgical ailments as nonpregnant women. Although there are similarities, there are also differences in the alterations of anatomy and physiology. Understanding these alterations during pregnancy is essential for the correct diagnosis and management of abdominal pain. Because of medical and legal concerns of the relative unknown effects of intervention during organogenesis, surgery is often delayed. A diagnosis of acute appendicitis or cholecystitis during pregnancy, however, requires prompt determination because of the associated increased morbidity.

Normal pregnancy often is accompanied by a number of symptoms that may also mimic "acute abdominal" surgical disorders. The incidence of acute surgical emergencies during pregnancy is between 0.5% and 1.0%.[1] Right upper quadrant abdominal pain during pregnancy or the puerperium usually presents a challenge for the obstetrician and surgical consultant. The laparoscopic surgeon must consider both the mother and the fetus when complaints of acute abdominal pain are elicited. Acute appendicitis is at times difficult to differentiate from acute cholecystitis. Subtle diagnostic differences relate to the continuous pain often seen with inflammation, as in appendicitis, whereas intermittent or colicky pain is more characteristic of an obstruction of a viscus.

Nonobstetric problems heralded by abdominal pain commonly involve acute appendicitis or acute cholecystitis. Other surgical considerations during pregnancy include torsion of an adnexa, an adnexal mass, rupture of a hemorrhagic corpus luteum (secondary to ovulation induction with, for example, human menopausal gonadotropin), and a perforated viscus (e.g., peptic ulcer or colonic diverticulum).

Vital medical complications are observed in approximately 15–20% of pregnancies, but surgical problems are relatively infrequent (1–2%).[2] Nonsurgical complications may include acute mesenteric adenitis, regional enteritis, acute gastroenteritis, urinary tract infection, pancreatitis, pneumonia, myocardial infarction, (early) herpes zoster, hepatitis, sickle cell crisis, acute intermittent porphyria, peptic ulcerative disease, diabetic neuropathy, and drug abuse. Operative endoscopy, as a diagnostic and a therapeutic technique, is now considered by many general surgeons the therapy of choice for several intraabdominal pathologic conditions. In fact, it is considered the new "gold standard" by many general surgeons.[3] Operative endoscopy can preclude unnecessary abdominal surgery, and in equivocal cases it can affect other diseases that require alternative therapy in 20–

40% of patients with abdominal pain.[4] The overall diagnostic accuracy of endoscopic evaluation of acute abdominal pain is better than 80%.[5] Laparoscopic cholecystectomy and appendectomy have been considered by some to be "minimally invasive" surgical procedures.[6] This approach has several conceivable advantages over the traditional laparotomy. A laparoscopic approach allows better visualization and a smaller scar, specifically in the obese patient in whom exposure is a problem. Total operative time is significantly less, and postoperative convalescence is undoubtedly reduced.[7] De novo adhesion formation is less probable, and brief hospital stays may translate into considerable economic gains.[8–10]

Thus awareness of the germane maternal physiologic and anatomic changes associated with these clinical problems is paramount. Medical and surgical evaluation calls for precise conclusions and appropriate operative intervention, as delay in treatment may lead to an increase in maternal and fetal morbidity.

Antenatal Considerations

The pregnant woman is unique for a number of reasons, particularly owing to the changes in maternal pathophysiology. Furthermore, medical complications may be encountered that are unique to pregnancy (e.g., pregnancy-induced hypertension and amniotic fluid embolism).

Of paramount relevance is a thorough history and physical evaluation as the pregnant patient presents with what appears to be a nonobstetric surgical problem.[11] Particular attention should be focused on the antenatal history, emphasizing any medical complications (e.g., cardiac disease, diabetes mellitus, chronic hypertension,

Table 17.1. Hematologic alterations during pregnancy

Laboratory test	Normal values	
	Nonpregnant	Pregnant
Total protein (g/dl)	6.5–8.6	85% of normal
Total bilirubin (mg/dl)	0.1–1.2	Unchanged
Serum albumin (g/dl)	3.5–5.0	2.5–4.5
Blood urea nitrogen (mg/dl)	10–25	5–15
Glucose (mg/dl)	70–110	65–100
Serum calcium (mEq/L)	4.6–5.5	4.2–5.2
Serum phosphate (mg/dl)	2.5–4.8	2.3–4.6
Alkaline phosphatase (IU/L)	35–48	35–150
Cholesterol (mg/dl)	120–290	177–345
Triglycerides (mg/dl)	33–166	130–400
Red blood cell count (cells/L)	$4.0 \times 5.2 \times 10^{12}$ to	$3.8 \times 4.4 \times 10^{12}$ to
White blood cell count (cells/L)	$5 \times 10 \times 10^9$ to	$5 \times 14 \times 10^9$ to
Hemoglobin (g/dl)	14 ± 2.0	> 11
Hematocrit (%)	36–41	33
Hemoglobin electrophoresis (%)		
Hb A	> 98.0	Unchanged
Hb A_2	< 3.5	Unchanged
Hb F	< 2.0	Unchanged
Platelets (cells/L)	$140 \times 440 \times 10^9$	Unchanged
Reticulocyte count (%)	0.5–1.0	1.0–2.0
Fibrinogen (mg/dl)	150–300	250–600
Bleeding time (Ivy) (minutes)	1–5	Unchanged
Serum creatinine (mg/dl)	0.8	0.6
Serum iron	50–110 g/dl	30–100 mg/dl

Modified from Sanfilippo J, Pietrantoni M: In *Operative Obstetrics*, Hankins G, Clark S, Gilstrap L, Cunningham FG (eds). Norwalk, CT, Appleton & Lange, 1995, with permission.

Rh status, asthma, sickle cell disease, chronic pelvic pain, maternal and fetal anomalies, and prior surgery). If there is vaginal bleeding, the placental location (central previa) is of major significance.

Second, pertinent laboratory analyses must be performed, with the definition of normal altered for a number of maternal factors (Table 17.1). If one is considering an operative procedure, accurate assessment of fetal viability and the presence of lethal anomalies by means of ultrasonography is suggested. Concern for anatomic alterations caused by encroachment of the gravid uterus up to the mid and upper abdominal quadrants must be noted. Contraindications for pursuing a laparoscopic approach for removal of either the appendix or gallbladder during pregnancy are dictated by the patient's clinical status and the gestational age. The gestational age at which the uterus would limit closed laparoscopic access to the abdominal cavity is of concern and remains a point of controversy. Advanced disease, abdominal sepsis, a retrocecal or walled-off perforated appendix, ileus, severe bleeding disorders, and late second or third trimester pregnancies are currently considered contraindications to endoscopic surgery.

The optimal time for elective nonobstetric surgery is during the second trimester, as there is a higher incidence of spontaneous abortion during the first trimester. Tocolysis should be a consideration for either elective or emergency cases starting at 24 weeks' gestation despite an intact survival of approximately 10%. Fetal heart rate monitoring with tocodynamometry may provide objective data not only preoperatively but intra- and postoperatively as well. The tocodynamometer enables the surgical team to detect the onset of premature labor. Fetal monitoring should be continued if uterine contractions or a nonreassuring fetal heart rate pattern is persistent. In pregnant women the supine position may cause significant uterine compression of the inferior vena cava and aorta; the former affects the venous circulation by diverting venous blood, potentially causing hypotension, fetal distress, or both. This situation may result in a decrease in the amount of regional anesthetic required. Therefore these patients should be positioned in the left lateral decubitus position with their right hip elevated. During endoscopy electronic control of the pneumoperitoneum must be carefully observed because excessive intraabdominal pressure may increase the resistance to blood flow in the vena cava.

A fundamental objective during the course of any surgical procedure is adequate oxygenation, as failure of such may result in substantial cell injury or cellular death, particularly in the pregnant patient. Oxygen demand and consumption are the same as in the healthy nonpregnant individual. However, in the critically ill patient oxygen transport may be impaired by three processes: lowered hemoglobin concentration (anemic hypoxia), decreased hemoglobin oxygen saturation (hypoxic hypoxia), and reduced cardiac output (stagnant hypoxia).[12] Demand is minimized by eliminating factors that increase the metabolic work of the cell (e.g., fever, pain, labored breathing, malnutrition, infection).

Visualization of the airway is also more difficult during pregnancy. Engorgement of the mucosal surface due to increased capillary blood flow may cause edema of the pharynx and larynx. Preoperative airway assessment by a modified Mallanpadanti test, which evaluates the oropharyngeal structures visible upon maximal mouth opening, is therefore recommended.[13] Other potential risk factors associated with difficult intubation include obesity; short neck; missing, protruding, or single maxillary incisors; receding mandible; facial edema; prior cervical orthopedic surgery; and swollen tongue.

Counseling patients for the potential perioperative increase in fetal morbidity and mortality is best done with institutional information. Prognosis for survival and outcome is best assessed knowing the gestational age and weight of the fetus.[14] In cases where preterm delivery may occur, the use of corticosteroids antenatally should be given due consideration. Antenatal steroid use in preterm infants have been demonstrated to decrease the incidence of respiratory distress syndrome.[15,16]

Maternal Physiology

During the initial maternal perioperative assessment, documenting vital signs (lateral decubitus position gives the lowest blood pressure reading), consideration for placement of an intravenous line, pulmonary artery catheterization, transcutaneous oximeter, complete blood count, blood type and screen, and cross-match if blood transfusion is a distinct possibility are recommended (Table 17.1). In addition, serum electrolytes, liver enzymes, electrocardiogram, urinalysis and culture, clotting profile, and plasma amylase and lipase assays may be obtained. The plasma lipase level is more sensitive than serum amylase during pregnancy. Autologous blood donation may be considered depending on the circumstances.[17] It should be remembered that the alkaline phosphatase level may be normally elevated during pregnancy and therefore is a less specific laboratory test; hepatic transaminase levels remain within the normal range.

Fundamental operative maternal–fetal considerations regarding surgery are related to the altered maternal anatomy and physiology: The circulatory system shows a 45–50% increase in plasma volume and 33% increase in erythrocytes, 10–20% increase in heart volume, 30–50% increase in resting stroke volume and cardiac output (4.5–6.0 L/min), 15–20% increase in heart rate, a decrease in systemic vascular resistance (mean 1210 ± 266 dynes/cm^{-5} per second), a decrease in pulmonary vascular resistance (mean 78 ± 22 dynes/cm^{-5} per second), and a reduced colloid oncotic pressure.[18,19] The respiratory system exhibits an increase in tidal volume, minute ventilatory volume, and minute oxygen uptake and a decreased functional residual volume.[20,21] The gastrointestinal system must also be considered, the most important concerns being delayed gastric emptying time, decreased esophageal tone, and incompetence of the esophageal-gastric sphincter.[22]

Preoperative prophylactic broad spectrum antibiotics should be administered to those patients at risk for infection (e.g., insulin-dependent diabetics, those with heart disease).[23] Although rare, rheumatic heart disease remains the most common cause of "heart disease" throughout the world. This patient population should receive prophylaxis in an effort to prevent bacterial endocarditis: ampicillin 2 g IV plus gentamicin 1.5 mg/kg IV at 30–60 minutes prior to surgery, with the dose repeated twice thereafter at 8 hour intervals. If the patient is allergic to penicillin, vancomycin is recommended. In patients with peritonitis or a viscus perforation, gentamicin 1.0–1.5 mg/kg, clindamycin 1.6–2.5 g IV, and metronidazole 2.0 g IV should be instituted.

Prophylactic low-dose heparin 8,000 U SC bid for the morbidly obese patient is recommended. Full heparinization is appropriate for patients with prior documented pulmonary embolism or deep venous thrombophlebitis.[24] Serial determination of the activated partial thromboplastin time (aPTT) is used to guide the heparin dose. Of note, although rare, the prothrombin time and the aPTT may be increased in the presence of preeclampsia.

A Kleihauer-Bethke test is recommended even in cases of minor trauma in order to evaluate fetomaternal bleeding.[25] It is important that 300 μg of Rh immune globulin be administered after any invasive procedures, such as abdomi-

Table 17.2. Evaluation of fetomaternal bleed

1. Size of hemorrhage: determine percent fetal RBCs present
   $$\frac{\text{Total no. fetal cells in 2000 total maternal RBCs}}{20}$$
   Average maternal blood volume = 5800 ml
   Average maternal hematocrit = 0.35%
   Average fetal hematocrit = 0.45%
2. Amount of transplacental hemorrhage
   $$\text{Transplacental hemorrhage} = 5800 \times (\% \text{ fetal cells in maternal circulation}) \times \frac{35}{45}$$

nal surgery by either laparoscopy or laparotomy, in the unsensitized Rh negative mother. The volume of blood required to produce sensitization is a point of concern, with as little as 0.1 ml of Rh-positive erythrocytes being sufficient to result in sensitization.[26] The size of the hemorrhage is calculated based on the percent of fetal red cells present (Table 17.2).

Fundamental Considerations

As with any surgical technique, a qualified surgical assistant is paramount. The purpose of such staff is essential in order to prevent complications due to malfunctioning instruments, to facilitate exposure, and to properly prepare the patient and equipment before surgery. Ideally, the first assistant should understand advanced endoscopic procedures.

Again there are many advantages to the laparoscopic technique. The patient's postoperative course is shortened with minimal use of analgesia; there is a reduced risk of atelectasis from postoperative hypoventilation. Patients are able to ingest a regular diet on the day of surgery and are usually discharged within 24 hours. The early ambulation afforded by the laparoscopic method decreases the risk of thromboembolic disease, particularly during pregnancy.[27] Definitively, diagnostic laparoscopy facilitates rapid exploration of any suspicious intraabdominal signs or symptoms of an illness (Table 17.3). This situation has arisen particularly in cases of questionable diagnosis of appendicitis, with a resultant reduction in unnecessary appendectomies of up to 50%.[28]

Albeit the surgical principles that apply to laparotomy also apply to operative laparoscopy, it is technically different. These technical limitations of laparoscopy include loss of depth perception, inability to directly palpate tissue, limitation of the number of instruments that can be used simultaneously, restriction of the angles available for approaching the surgical field, and increased distance from the surgical field to the surgeons' hands, which intensifies motion, making fine movements more arduous. Laparoscopy has a complication rate of less than 3%

Table 17.3. Emergent assessment of abdominal pain during pregnancy

History of abdominal pain
  Peptic ulcer disease
  Irritable bowel syndrome
  Hiatal hernia
  Pelvic inflammatory disease
  Tuboovarian abscess

Prior abdominal/pelvic surgery
  Exploratory laparotomy
  Cesarean section
  Ectopic pregnancy
  Cholecystectomy
  Appendectomy
  Adhesions

Pain characteristics
  Sharp or dull
  Manner of onset
  Location
  Persistent
  Intermittent

Secondary signs and symptoms
  Increased temperature
  Lightheadedness
  Acute loss of appetite
  Nausea/vomiting
  Abdominal soreness

From Vitale G, Sanfilippo J, Perissat J, (eds): *Laparoscopic Surgery: An Atlas for General Surgeons.* Philadelphia, Lippincott, 1995, with permission.

and a mortality rate of 0.1 per 1000 procedures.[29] The traditional approach (i.e., laparotomy) also has excellent results with a mortality of less than 0.1%.[30]

In most cases not associated with pregnancy the traditional approach to diagnostic endoscopy is to proceed with an umbilical port for placement of the endoscope and one or two suprapubic ports for the ancillary 5 mm trocar sleeves. During pregnancy these ancillary trocar sleeves are placed above the umbilicus and away from the uterus. For good intraabdominal visualization, a 10.5 mm cold light optic laparoscope with a 0° or 30° angle is recommended. Patients are placed in the Trendelenburg position to establish a pneumoperitoneum, for which the Veress needle is most commonly used for insufflation.[31] This needle is spring-loaded with a blunt probe surrounded by a sharp, beveled outer sleeve. Proper placement may be checked by the manometer reading. The filling procedure is performed up to a maximum intraabdominal pressure of 15–18 mm Hg. Excessive intraabdominal pressures of > 20 mm Hg when creating a pneumoperitoneum have been associated with gas embolism.[32] The use of a sharp trocar for laparoscopic insertion is imperative. The insertion should be controlled using appropriate force; it should be done slowly with a slight twisting motion. The endoscope is introduced into the abdomen through the hollow sheath created by the trocar containing a side port for continuous gas insufflation, as well as valves and gaskets that allow repeated insertion and removal of the laparoscope with minimal loss of CO_2. Consistency of technique may minimize bowel and vascular injuries. Vascular gas embolism, though rare, has been reported.[33] Although these complications are relatively uncommon, delay in identification may result in significant morbidity and mortality. Although endoscopy effectively allows excellent visualization of the intraperitoneal viscera, it does not provide such a picture of the retroperitoneum.

Patients at high risk for adhesion formation (i.e., those with previous bowel surgery or pelvic inflammatory disease) may be more appropriately managed with the open laparoscopic technique.[34] With this procedure the skin, subcutaneous tissue, fascia, and peritoneum are incised under direct observation, permitting insertion of the sleeve (with blunt trocar) for insufflation and laparoscope placement. Ancillary trocars of ≥ 5 mm are placed under direct visualization.

Laparoscopic appendectomy during pregnancy is certainly feasible, but perhaps the most important point is that of appropriate diagnosis. As noted subsequently, the position of the appendix changes throughout gestation, and the clinician must understand the varied location of signs and symptoms of acute appendicitis (Fig. 17.1).

Laparoscopic cholecystectomy is a relatively new operation that was first performed in France in 1987[35] and in the United States in 1988.[36] As of 1993 more than 85% of all chole-

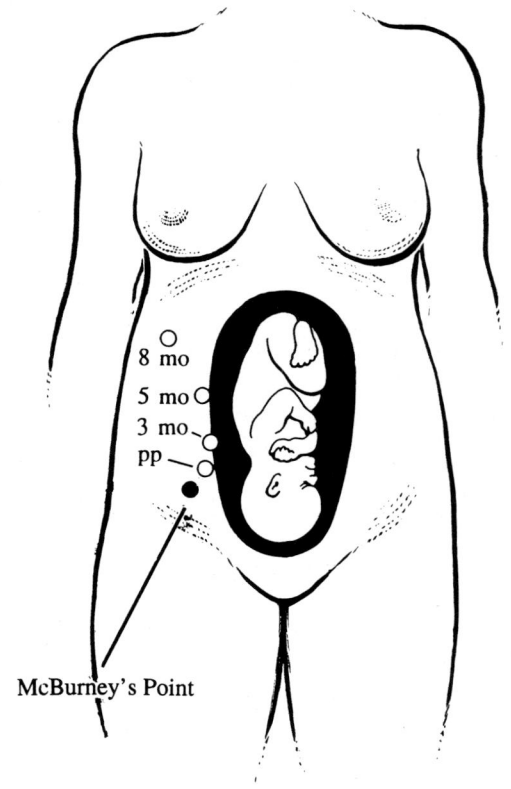

Figure 17.1. Migration of the appendix during pregnancy at various gestational ages. PP, postpartum. From Vitale G, Sanfilippo J, Perissat J, (eds): *Laparoscopic Surgery: An Atlas for General Surgeons*. Philadelphia, Lippincott, 1995, with permission.

cystectomies in the United States are performed by laparoscopy (Table 17.4). Most patients with symptomatic gallstones are candidates for laparoscopic cholecystectomy if they are able to tolerate general anesthesia and have no serious cardiopulmonary disease. As a rule, the indications for laparoscopic cholecystectomy are similar to those for open cholecystectomy. The death rate is relatively low for laparoscopic cholecystectomy (< 1%), although deaths have occurred owing to iatrogenic injuries to the bile duct or small bowel.[37]

Lastly the inability to tolerate general anesthesia, the presence of disseminated intravascular coagulation, or concurrent diseases that require exploratory laparotomy are absolute contraindications for any endoscopic procedure.

Table 17.4. Literature on cholecystectomy during pregnancy

Author	Study design	No. of pts.	Comments
Weber et al.[81]	First reported laparoscopic cholecystectomy during pregnancy	1	—
McKellar et al.[80]	Evaluated high incidence of fetal loss during first trimester and premature labor during third trimester in association with cholecystectomy	22	Elective abortion not recommended even when intraoperative cholangiogram was obtained. Tocolytic agents most efficacious
Bloch & Kelly[83]	Acute pancreatitis during pregnancy or postpartum	21	Acute pancreatitis associated with pregnancy, "gallstone pancreatitis"
Baillie et al.[77]	Extrahepatic biliary obstruction by gallstones	5	Four acute cholangitis, one gallstone pancreatitis. Treatment by endoscopic sphincterotomy
Van Beek et al.[82]	Gallstone disease evaluated in women < 30 years of age; correlation between age, pregnancy, obesity, and oral contraceptive use (retrospective study)	885	All underwent cholecystectomy. Relative risk 1:6 for pregnancy-related gallstone disease requiring cholecystectomy
Basso et al.[89]	Prospective antenatal study	512	Early gestation; age at menarche and oral contraceptives had no significant effect. Higher incidence of cholelithiasis in older women and patients with dysmenorrhea. Positive trend of cholelithiasis in patients with history of symptomatic gallstones
Schreiber[88]	Laparoscopic appendectomy	6	Complication rate 0.75, none of which occurred in the pregnant population

From Vitale G, Sanfilippo J, Perissat J (eds): *Laparoscopic Surgery: An Atlas for General Surgeons.* Philadelphia, Lippincott, 1995, with permission.

Anesthesia

Managing obstetric anesthesia is challenging and fraught with hazards. Anesthetic complications have the potential to result in significant maternal morbidity and mortality.[38] Each anesthetic option has different maternal and fetal risks. The mortality rate due to anesthetic complications is approximately 0.6 per 100,000 live births.

General anesthesia is the preferred method for most surgical emergencies during pregnancy. Adverse effects, though rarely serious, provide a good argument for preferential administration of a regional anesthetic such as an epidural or spinal application when surgery is indicated in women with early to mid second trimester pregnancies.[39] General anesthesia has the potential to induce fetal/neonatal depression (3% incidence) spontaneous abortion during the first trimester.[40] General anesthesia is usually produced with a rapid sequence induction (sodium pentothal; or Propofol-Diprivan, Stuart Pharmaceuticals) followed by nitrous oxide. Although rare, spinal and epidural blockades are not without complications. Paraplegia, arachnoiditis, postepidural puncture headache, and maternal hypotension (pharmacologic sympathectomy; systolic blood pressure < 100 mm Hg) have been reported to occur with an incidence ranging from 1.4% to 10.0%.[41,42]

Endotracheal intubation is the ventilatory method of choice, as mask ventilation alone increases the risk of hypoventilation, gastric distention, and aspiration of gastric contents. Difficulty with tracheal intubation appears to be the most common contributory factor to anesthesia-related maternal deaths.[43]

When general anesthesia is indicated, agents that produce maternal tachycardia should be avoided, specifically in patients with heart disease. Enflurane, isoflurane, and halothane may

Table 17.5. Obstetric anesthesia for endoscopic surgery

Give antacids for prophylaxis against pulmonary aspiration
Conduct rapid sequence induction
Secure a tenuous airway
Continuously monitoring PO$_2$ and end-tidal CO$_2$

be used to supplement nitrous oxide during maintenance of general anesthesia, but they are not without risk.[44,45]

Sedatives and anesthetics administered to the mother can have a profound effect on the neonate. Specifically, two areas on the venterolateral surface of the medulla are the respiratory center of the fetus and are highly vulnerable to both sedatives and anesthetics since they rapidly traverse the placenta and result in respiratory depression in the newborn.

Carbon dioxide gas is most often selected to establish a pneumoperitoneum for endoscopic procedures. There are few studies on the possible effects of excessive exposure. Cardiac anomalies have been associated when pregnant rats were exposed to 3% CO$_2$ and dental defects when levels as high as 30% were administered.[46,47] Vertebral anomalies in the offspring of rabbits exposed to 8% CO$_2$ for a few days have also been reported.[48] CO$_2$ rapidly forms carbonic acid on the parietal peritoneum, which can result in discomfort or pain. CO$_2$ pneumoperitoneum used during endoscopy also rarely causes other adverse local and systemic effects, such as gas emboli, hypercapnia, acidosis, and arrhythmias.[49]

Alternatively using nitrous oxide for peritoneal insufflation causes less irritation of the diaphragm. Nitrous oxide when administered over a long period (1–2 days) at 50% concentration, has been associated with increased spontaneous abortions, skeletal deformities, and small-for-gestational-age babies.[50] Nitrous oxide is preferred with local anesthesia, whereas CO$_2$ is the gas of choice with general anesthesia.

Another cause of fatality that may follow general anesthesia is pulmonary aspiration of gastric contents. Gastric emptying after the induction of anesthesia not only reduces postoperative nausea and vomiting but decreases the likelihood of gastric aspiration. Administering antacids shortly before induction of anesthesia has dramatically decreased mortality due to obstetric anesthesia, more so than any other practice[27] (Table 17.5).

Preterm Labor Management

Continuous electronic fetal heart rate (FHR) monitoring is advocated postoperatively. It may be accomplished by monitoring for suspected preterm labor via use of an external tocodynamometer and cervical examinations. Attempts to arrest premature labor may be accomplished with intravenous magnesium sulfate (6 g load and $\geq$ 2 g/hr maintenance). Indomethacin may be used (loading dose 50–100 mg rectal suppository and 25 mg PO maintenance q6h for 48 hours) provided the fetus is $\leq$ 32 weeks' gestation with normal amniotic fluid volume.[51] Indomethacin, however, has been associated with an increased incidence of necrotizing enterocolitis, prolonged fetal renal insufficiency, and oligohydramnios.[52] Long-term use of β-mimetics such as terbutaline (Brethine, Geigy Pharmaceuticals, Summit, NJ) or ritodrine hydrochloride (Yutopar, Astra Pharmaceuticals, Westborough, MA) is not recommended because of the significant metabolic and cardiovascular side effects (i.e., hyperglycemia, hypokalemia, fetomaternal tachycardia, chest pain, pulmonary edema, shortness of breath, cardiac dysrhythmia, and electrocardiogram "ischemic" changes, i.e., ST wave inversions). However, short-term use of β-mimetics such as terbutaline in doses of 0.25 mg q20min for not more than three doses can be prescribed. Notwithstanding, β-sympathomimetic agents should not be used in women with pyelonephritis or multiple gestation because of the increased risk for pulmonary edema.

Emesis during pregnancy may be treated medically with droperidol (a-butyrophenone, class C), prochlorperazine, or metoclopramide.[53-55] If vomiting is excessive or relentless, intravenous fluids and liberal use of antiemetic medications should be administered. This approach is in an effort to offset possible hypotension caused by the fluid loss. Narcotics should not be withheld, as pain per se may cause nausea and vomiting. Nonmedical treatments consist of positive reassurance, slow deliberate movements, warm blankets, and minimal pharyngeal suction.

Acute Appendicitis

Appendicitis is defined as an acute inflammation of the vermiform appendix. Most of the patients are between 5 and 30 years of age, with the incidence declining after age 40. Acute appendicitis, with an incidence of 1 per 2000 pregnancies, is the most common surgical condition during pregnancy. There is equal distribution with respect to incidence during each of the three trimesters and during the puerperium.[56,57] Unfortunately, the diagnosis is frequently delayed with obvious adverse sequelae. The delay is perhaps due in part to the confusing picture of nausea, vomiting, and abdominal discomfort observed with pregnancy, complemented by the normal "physiologic leukocytosis" (approximately 10,000–12,000/mm^3). A high index of suspicion for appendicitis is important for making the diagnosis. It is essential that the surgeon understand the change in location of the appendix during the progressive enlargement of the uterus with gestation (Fig. 17.1). Differential diagnoses include round ligament pain (spasm), adnexal torsion, and other gastrointestinal and genitourinary abnormalities (pyelonephritis). Dysuria occurs in up to 25% of pregnant women who have appendicitis during the third trimester.[58]

Diagnostic Evaluation

The initial visceral pain is typically gradual in onset, with an associated colicky pattern (secondary to smooth muscle contractions) that may reflect obstruction (fecalith or calculus). Classically, the pain is often referred to the epigastrium or periumbilical area, and it is often dull and diffuse in nature. The midepigastric pain is due to stretching of the appendix. During pregnancy, the enlarged uterus causes displacement of the appendix. The upward dislocation of the appendix by the uterus is accompanied by a shift of the inflamed appendix from the abdominal wall. Such displacement tends to minimize the signs of peritoneal irritation. Fewer than half of the pregnant patients with acute appendicitis have peritoneal signs.[59]

With respect to specifics for each trimester, during the first trimester the pain is primarily in the area of McBurney's point (65–90% of the time), and in 30% of patients it is noted in the pelvic area.[60,61] During the second trimester, the pain is associated with the lateral upward displacement of the appendix; frequently the point of maximal tenderness is above the iliac crest (75%). During the third trimester, pain and tenderness may be localized to the right costal margin (37%). These changes occur during pregnancy because of the progressive increase in the size of the gravid uterus, which displaces the base of the appendix.[61] The latter findings may be absent with a retrocecal appendix. Anorexia, accompanied by nausea and vomiting, often precedes the onset of pain by several hours.

Independent of the trimester, right lateral rectal tenderness is commonly noted; approximately 50% of patients have abdominal muscle spasm or guarding.[62] The uterus, because of its size and encroachment on the appendix, often intensifies pain. The pain is localized primarily to the area around the appendix (Fig. 17.1). It is essential that pain associated with uterine origin be differentiated from that of appendicitis. Uterine pain can frequently be alleviated by placing the patient in the left lateral (decubitus) position and providing hydration. Alder's sign (fixed tenderness) and Bryan's sign (tenderness in the right lateral position) may be used to differentiate uterine pain from signs that are indicative of appendicitis.[63] Temperature elevation (low grade, > 100.5°F) may also be associated with acute appendicitis. Sterile pyuria or hematuria may occur when the inflamed appendix lies in the vicinity of the ureter. Typically, leukocytosis associated with appendicitis increases only modestly (to 12,000–14,000/ml), with higher values suggesting perforation. Gangrene and perforation are more common in appendices with calculi. Patients may experience temporary relief at the time of perforation; but if the inflammation is not walled off, the pain usually becomes generalized.

Appendectomy Technique

Laparoscopy is done using general anesthesia, with a nasogastric tube and indwelling urinary catheter. The laparoscope is inserted at the level of the umbilicus. Working ports are placed in the right hypochondrium at the midclavicular line. Placement of additional ports varies depending on the patient's anatomy and intraoperative findings. After inspection of the peritoneal cavity, all fluid collections are aspirated for culture if perforation has occurred, and thorough lavage is performed in all four quadrants of the abdomen. The technique utilized for a laparoscopic appendectomy, as in the nonpregnant state, requires, first, for the appendix to be placed on traction with a guiding suture located at the distal end of the appendix. Second, blunt dissection into the avascular spaces of the mesoappendix with separate ligation or cauterization of the mesoappendiceal vessels is accomplished with bipolar forceps. The base of the vermiform appendix is doubly ligated with pretied sutures or hemoclips. The mucosa of the appendiceal stump is then coagulated with the bipolar forceps. The appendix is then removed through the 10- or 12-mm trocar sleeve. A purse-string suture may be placed with two needle holders prior to evaginating the appendiceal stump into the cecum. Some surgeons use a Z-suture or second closing procedure to secure the purse-string. It is not necessary to invert the stump in most cases. The suture area is inspected for complete hemostasis, and the operation is terminated by removing the trocar sleeves under direct vision with the endoscope. After deflation the incision is closed.

If the appendix ruptures, peritonitis often ensues; and the uterus attempts to wall off the abscess. Assertive, proper drainage minimizes the fetomaternal complications. Unfortunately, in many cases premature labor results, again underscoring the importance of early, appropriate diagnosis. Fetal morbidity and mortality significantly increase after appendiceal perforation.[64] The diagnostic error in pregnant women is approximately 25–40%.[65] The mortality rate associated with nonperforated appendicitis in the general population is 0.1%.[33] In comparison, mortality rates approach 7% for women during the third trimester.[33] Appendiceal perforation occurs with an incidence of up to 60% in pregnant women, in contrast to an incidence of 29% in the general population.[32] Therefore early, "aggressive" use of laparoscopy has repeatedly proved helpful for managing suspected appendicitis in the pregnant patient.

A series of 150 patients undergoing laparoscopic appendectomy was reported by Schreiber.[66] This series included six pregnant patients in all stages of gestation. The overall complication rate for the 150 patients was 0.75%, and there were no complications among the pregnant patients, thus attesting to the efficacy of a laparoscopic approach to acute appendicitis.

Cholecystitis

The incidence of acute cholecystitis during pregnancy is 0.03%; that is, it is more common during pregnancy due in part to the marked alteration in gallbladder physiology.[67] Gallstones are more common in women than in men, and estrogen receptors are known to be present in the gallbladder. Everson et al.[67] observed an increased risk of cholecystectomy in men treated with diethylstilbestrol, but at autopsy no increase in stone formation was noted. Possibly estrogens heighten the symptoms associated with gallbladder disease or magnify symptoms due to already existing stones. Physiologic evidence indicates that the elevated estrogen and progesterone levels during pregnancy promote the potential for the development of gallbladder disease.[68,69] Estrogen has a positive role in the regulation of progesterone biosynthesis; it increases low density lipoprotein (LDL) receptor uptake and promotes cytochrome P-450_{scc} enzymatic activity. Simply stated, estrogens cause an increase in cholesterol and a decrease in the secretion of bile acids.[70,71] Progesterone increases esterification but not cholesterol synthesis. It also produces smooth muscle relaxation, resulting in decreased gallbladder contractility and emptying, which is complicated by bile duct hypotonia. In addition, progesterone has been shown to inhibit the gallbladder's contractile response to cholecystokinin. These endocrine changes foster an effect on the composition of the bile acids and the kinetics of the gallbladder. Generally, the incidence of gallbladder disease during pregnancy increases progressively with each trimester. Pregnancy augments the saturation of cholesterol in bile and the circulating bile salt pool is decreased, resulting in production of more lithogenic bile.

Acute cholecystitis is the second most common nonobstetric cause of an acute abdomen during pregnancy (the most common cause is appendicitis).[72] There appears to be an association with advanced maternal age, obesity, diet, diabetes mellitus, ethnicity, familial hyperlipoproteinemia, hypertriglyceridemia (type IV), rapid weight loss, clofibrate therapy, cystic fibrosis, pancreatic insufficiency, Crohn's disease, and a history of cholecystitis episodes. Additionally, biliary tract disease tends to be more common in multiparous patients than in primiparas. Preexisting gallstones are not often a cause of cholecystitis in pregnant women, in part because the capability of the gallbladder to contract is inhibited by the increased circulating levels of progesterone.

It is estimated that up to 15% of the U.S. population has gallstones, but because approximately 50% of gallstones are asymptomatic, the actual prevalence is difficult to estimate.[73] Only 1–4% of asymptomatic patients with stones per year develop symptoms or a complication of gallstone disease. Cholecystitis, acute or chronic, is associated with stones in 90% of patients. During the second and third trimesters, fasting and residual volumes are twice as large as in the nonpregnant state, and the rate and percentage of bile expelled after stimulation diminishes. Gallbladder emptying is significantly slowed.[74] Cholecystectomy is performed in 3–8 per 10,000 pregnancies, accounting for more nonobstetric surgery during pregnancy than any other procedure except appendectomy.[75]

The obstetrician should be well versed in the various symptoms of clinical presentation among pregnant patients. Many times acute cholecystitis or cholelithiasis presents initially with biliary colic (misnamed "colic") manifested by nausea and associated vomiting and lasting up to 4–6 hours. Pain persists if the common bile duct is obstructed by a stone, and there is often radiation to the subscapular area, right flank, or shoulder. Right subcostal tenderness associated with temperature elevation is characteristic. The presence of persistent obstruction in the cystic duct causes distention, ischemia, and eventually bacterial infection. Ultrasonography appears to be efficacious (90% of cases) in diagnosing the presence of stones (echodense) or dilatation of the common bile duct. Approximately 85% of gallbladder stones are composed of cholesterol. Murphy's sign, which is severe pain under the right costal margin elicited by deep inspiration, is often positive; however, a positive sign and a palpable gallbladder occur in only 5% of pregnancies.[34] Laboratory tests sometimes show mild leukocytosis with a shift to the left and mild hyperbilirubinemia. The finding of minimally elevated alkaline phosphatase or amylase is not helpful during pregnancy, as the normal changes of pregnancy may confuse the issue.

Oral cholecystogram and intravenous cholangiography are contraindicated during pregnancy. Technetium 99m-iminodiacetic acid (Tc-IDA) scans of the gallbladder have been used during pregnancy with minimal risk of radiation exposure.[76] A chest radiograph may be helpful for preoperative evaluation because right lower lobar pneumonia or pleurisy can mimic cholecystitis.

As with acute appendicitis, there is a higher incidence of premature labor with fetal loss following the operative procedure.[77] Ideally, first trimester patients are treated conservatively until the second trimester at which time a cholecystectomy may be performed electively. The use of laparoscopic cholecystectomy, as for other laparoscopic procedures in general, during the first trimester of pregnancy is controversial for a number of reasons including the unknown effects of CO_2 pneumoperitoneum on the developing fetus.[78] CO_2 may cause hypercarbia and acidosis. During the second trimester patients are treated surgically as soon as the cholecystitis subsides; third trimester patients are managed medically until the postpartum period. Any patient who does not improve with medical management should undergo surgical intervention regardless of gestational age. There is 0.05% mortality among low risk individuals.[41] The efficacy of cholecystectomy during pregnancy without fetal loss, in part because of advances with respect to early diagnosis and anesthesia management, along with the use of tocolytic agents, have improved the prognosis.[79]

In a small series of 22 patients reported, the incidence of biliary stone disease during pregnancy was 0.05%.[80] Nine required cholecystectomy during pregnancy with no specific preponderance in surgical intervention during any one trimester. Common bile duct exploration was required in three of the nine patients. In addition, three had intraoperative cholangiography. Delay of appropriate surgical intervention does not appear to be warranted.

Weber and coworkers[81] reported the first laparoscopic cholecystectomy during pregnancy. The recovery time was significantly shortened compared with that required for laparotomy. Little has been reported with respect to gallstone management during the postpartum period.[82] However, Bloch and Kelly[83] reported a 22 year study in which acute pancreatitis developed in 21 women during pregnancy, 10 of which appeared within 6 weeks postpartum. Gallstones were the cause of pancreatitis in each patient. These authors recommended surgical treatment that included cholecystectomy and exploration of the common bile duct without operative cholangiography. Transcystic exploration of the common bile duct following laparoscopic cholecystectomy eliminates the need for a second procedure.

Laparoscopic Cholecystectomy Technique

Laparoscopic cholecystectomy requires sound knowledge of the relation between the hepatoduodenal ligament, triangle of Calot, porta hepatis, cystic artery and duct, hepatic and common bile duct, and gallbladder. Use of a 30° angled operative endoscope, rather than a 0° instrument, provides optimal circumferential visualization of the gallbladder and cystic duct. First, lysing of any omental, colonic, and duodenal adhesions not only aids in visualization but provides adequate exposure. Second, the visceral peritoneal veil should be dissected running from the ampulla to the hepatoduodenal ligament. The gallbladder is then grasped at its fundus (Hartman's pouch) and retracted anteriorly, cephalad, and laterally. This maneuver exposes the hilar structures. Once identified and freely dissected, the cystic artery and cystic duct may be clipped and transected. It is important to identify the cystic artery in order to avoid ligating the right hepatic artery. For similar reasons attention to the junction between the cystic duct and the common bile duct is equally important. Dissection is continued as the surgeon begins a surgical plane directly on the gallbladder wall in order to minimize bleeding. Electrosurgical vascular injuries tend to result in catastrophic hemorrhage that necessitates conversion to a laparotomy.

Sphincterotomy

It is estimated that up to 15% of patients undergoing cholecystectomy have common duct stones.[84] The best test for the diagnosis of gallstones during pregnancy is undoubtedly ultrasonography. These stones are a major source of morbidity, so their detection prior to a planned laparoscopic cholecystectomy is mandatory, especially if there is evidence of jaundice, recent pancreatitis, or a dilated common duct.

The endoscopic sphincterotomy procedure has been reported by Baillie et al.[77] They reported that extrahepatic biliary obstruction occurred in association with gallstones during pregnancy. Five patients, four of whom had acute cholangitis and one with gallstone pancreatitis, were treated by endoscopic sphincterotomy. It is of interest that all patients proceeded to deliver at term. Most gallstones can be extracted through the cystic duct with a stone basket or by dilating the cystic duct to allow insertion of a 10F (3 mm) choledochoscope through the common bile duct. The efficacy of endoscopic retrograde cholangiopancreatography (ERCP) and sphincterotomy must be considered. The success rate of endoscopic common duct stone extraction approaches 90–95% in expert hands.[45,85] To date only a few laparoscopic choledochostomies have been done, and they should be performed only by experienced laparoscopic surgeons.

Conclusion

The literature pertaining to the ever expanding indications for operative laparoscopy consists predominantly of descriptive studies. Few randomized controlled trials have been performed. In 1988 the American Association of Gynecologic Laparoscopists reported a serious complication rate of 15 per 1000 procedures, and a mortality of 5.4 per 100,000.[86] The rate of conversion from endoscopy to laparotomy ranges from 1.8% to 8.5% and tends to be highest early in a surgeon's experience. Therefore obstetrician-gynecologists must recognize their own limitations. Experience is increasing with the laparoscopic approach in the pregnant patient who requires surgical intervention for acute appendicitis or cholecystectomy. This technique avoids increased morbidity, prolonged hospital stay, and recovery complications associated with the more traditional approach (laparotomy). Additionally, there is no consensus as to the gestational age at which the uterus would limit laparoscopic access to the abdominal cavity. If the laparoscopic procedure is the more traditional type (closed-scope), 18–20 weeks' gestation is the upper age limit for this technique. The uterine fundus must be carefully assessed in relation to the umbilicus. As gestational age advances, there is greater risk for injury. Consideration of an "open laparoscopic technique" may be appropriate to minimize trauma to the viscera. This technique may be useful when adhesions are highly suspected, as they increase the possibility of visceral injury.[87] Laparoscopy with appendectomy has reportedly been performed as late as 25 weeks' gestation.[66]

Significant technical advances in the field of endoscopic surgery have paved the way to new horizons for the obstetrician-gynecologist and general surgeon worldwide.[89,90]

References

1. BARBER HRK, GRABER EA: Surgical Diseases in Pregnancy. Philadelphia, Saunders, 1974.
2. BARRON WM: The pregnant surgical patient: medical evaluation and management. Ann Intern Med 1984;101:683.
3. LEGORRETA AP, SILBER JH, CONSTANTINO GN, ET AL: Increased cholecystectomy rate after the introduction of laparoscopic cholecystectomy. JAMA 1993;270:1429.
4. REIERTSEN O, ROSSELAND AR, HOIVIK B, SOLHEIM K: Laparoscopy in patients admitted for acute abdominal pain. Acta Chir Scand 1985;151:521.
5. SUGERBAKER PH, SANDERS JH, BLOOM BS, WILSON RE: Preoperative laparoscopy in diagnosis of acute abdominal pain. Lancet 1975;1:442.
6. WOLF BM, GARDINER B, FREY CF: Laparoscopic cholecystectomy: a remarkable development. JAMA 1991;265:1573.
7. AZZIZ R, STEINKAMPF MP, MURPHY A: Postoperative recuperation: relation to the extent of endoscopic surgery. Fertil Steril 1989;51:1061.
8. LUNDORFF P, HAHLIN M, KALLFELT B, ET AL: Adhesion formation after laparoscopic surgery in tubal pregnancy: a randomized trial versus laparotomy. Fertil Steril 1991;55:911.
9. LEVINE RL: Economic impact of pelviscopic surgery. J Reprod Med 1985;30:655.
10. CHUNG RS, BROUGHAN TA: The phenomenal growth of laparoscopy cholecystectomy: a review. Cleve Clin J Med 1992;59:186.
11. HAMPTON JR, HARRISON MJG, MITCHELL JRA, ET AL: Relative contributions of history-taking, physical examination, and laboratory investigation to diagnosis and management of medical outpatients. BMJ 1975;2:486.
12. BARCROFT J: On anoxaemia. Lancet 1920;2:485.
13. MALLAMPATI SR: Clinical signs to predict difficult tracheal intubations (hypothesis). Can Anaesth Soc J 1983;30:316.
14. PHELAN JP: Fetal considerations in the critically ill obstetric patient. In Critical Care Obstetrics (2nd ed). Clark SL, Cotton DB, Hankins GDV, Phelan JP (eds). Boston, Blackwell Scientific, 1990, p 634.
15. LIGGINS GC, HOWIE RN: A controlled trial of antepartum glucocorticoid treatment for the preven-

tion of respiratory distress syndrome in premature infants. Pediatrics 1972;50:515.
16. COLLABORATIVE GROUP ON ANTENATAL STEROID THERAPY: Effect of antenatal dexamethasone administration on the prevention of respiratory distress syndrome. Am J Obstet Gynecol 1981;141:246.
17. ANDRES RL, PIACQUADIO KM, RESNICK R: A reappraisal of the need for autologous blood donation in the obstetric patient. Am J Obstet Gynecol 1990;163:1551.
18. UELAND K: Maternal cardiovascular dynamics. VII. Intrapartum blood volume changes. Am J Obstet Gynecol 1976;126:671.
19. SCHRIER RW, DUR JA: Pregnancy: an overfill or underfill state. Am J Kidney Dis 1987;9:284.
20. GILROY RJ, MANGURA BT, LAVIETS MH: Rib cage and abdominal volume displacements during breathing in pregnancy. Am Rev Respir Dis 1988;137:668.
21. CLARK SL, COTTON DB, LEE W, ET AL: Central hemodynamic assessment of normal term pregnancy. Am J Obstet Gynecol 1989;161:1439.
22. O'SULLIVAN GM, SUTTON AJ, THOMPSON SA, ET AL: Noninvasive measurement of gastric emptying in obstetric patients. Anesth Analg 1987;66:505.
23. HEMSELL D: Prophylactic antibiotics in gynecologic and obstetric surgery. Rev Infect Dis 1991; Suppl 10:S821.
24. HYERS TM, HULL RD, WEG JG: Antithrombotic therapy for venous thromboembolic disease. Chest 1986;89:26s.
25. VIRGILIO LA, SIMON NV: Measurement of fetal cells in the maternal circulation. Obstet Gynecol 1977;50:364.
26. BOWMAN JM: Hemolytic disease (erythroblastosis fetalis): maternal blood group immunization. In Maternal-Fetal Medicine: Principle and Practice, (3rd ed), Creasy RK, Resnick R (eds). Philadelphia, Saunders, 1989.
27. TALBERT LM, LANGDELL RD: Normal values of certain factors in the blood clotting mechanism in pregnancy. Am J Obstet Gynecol 1964;90:44.
28. ANTEBY SO, SHENKER JG, POLISHUK WZ: The value of laparoscopy in acute pelvic pain. Ann Surg 1875;181:484.
29. CHAMBERLAIN G: Gynaecological laparoscopy. Ann R Coll Surg Engl 1980;62:113.
30. PERISSAT J, COLLET D, BELLIARD R: Gallstones: laparoscopic treatment—cholecystectomy, cholecystotomy and lithotripsy. Surg Endosc 1990;4:1.
31. LUKACS D, VEREES E JR: Szaz eve szuletett Verees Elemer. Orv Hetil 1976;117:483.
32. SHULMAN D, ARONSON HB: Capnography in the early diagnosis of carbon dioxide embolism during laparoscopy. Can Anaesth Soc J 1984; 31:455.
33. YACOUB OF, CARDONA I JR, COVERLER LA, DODSON MG: Carbon dioxide embolism during laparoscopy. Anesthesiology 1982;57:533.
34. HASSON HM: Open laparoscopy. In Operative Gynecological Endoscopy, Sanfilippo J, Levine R (eds). New York, Springer-Verlay, 1989, pp 57.
35. DUBOIS F, ICARD P, BERTHELOT G, LEVARD H: Coelioscopic cholecystectomy: preliminary report of 36 cases. Ann Surg 1990;211:60.
36. NIH CONSENSUS CONFERENCE: Gallstones and laparoscopic cholecystectomy; NIH consensus development panel on gallstones and laparoscopic cholecystectomy. JAMA 1993;269(8).
37. WOLFE BM, GARDINER BN, LEARY BF, FREY CF: Endoscopic cholecystectomy: an analysis of complications. Arch Surg 1991;126:1192.
38. ENDLER GC, MARIONA FG, SOKOL RJ, STEVENSON LB: Anesthesia-related maternal mortality in Michigan. Am J Obstet Gynecol 1988;159:187.
39. HOOD DD: Anesthesia for cesarean section: minimizing risk and complications. Obstet Gynecol Clin North Am 1988;15:639.
40. KNILL-JONES RP, NEWMAN BJ, SPENCE AA: Anesthetic practice and pregnancy. Lancet 1975; 2:807.
41. JOUPPILA R, JOUPPILA P, KARINEN JM, HOLLMEN A: Segmental epidural analgesia in labor: related to the progress of labor, fetal malposition and instrumental delivery. Acta Obstet Gynecol Scand 1979;58:1350.
42. PARNASS SM, SCHMIDT KJ: Adverse effects of spinal and epidural anaesthesia. Drug Safety 1990; 5:179.
43. ROCKE DA, MURRAY WB, ROUT CC, GOUWS E: Relative risk analysis of factors associated with difficult intubation in obstetric anesthesia. Anesthesiology 1992;77:67.
44. FARRELL G, PRENDERGAST D, MURRAY M: Halothane hepatitis: detection of a constitutional susceptibility factor. N Engl J Med 1985;313:1310.
45. ANDREWS WW, RAMIN SM, MABERRY MC, ET AL: Effect of type of anesthesia on blood loss at elective repeat cesarean section. Am J Perinatol 1992;9:197.
46. HARING OM: Cardiac malformations in rats induced by exposure of the mother to carbon dioxide during pregnancy. Circ Res 1960;8:1218.
47. KING CTG, WILK A, MCCLURE FJ: Carbon dioxide induced acidosis in pregnant rats and cares sus-

17. Endoscopic Surgical Procedures During Pregnancy

ceptibility of their progeny. Proc Soc Exp Biol Med 1962;11:486.
48. SHEPARD TH: Catalog of Teratogenic Agent. Baltimore, Johns Hopkins University Press, 1986, p 262.
49. FITZGERALD SD, ANDRUS CH, BAUDENDISTEL LJ, ET AL: Hypercarbia during carbon dioxide pneumoperitoneum. Am J Surg 1992;163:186.
50. PEDERSON H, FINSTER M: Anesthetic risk in the pregnant surgical patient. Anesthesiology 1979: 51:439.
51. MOISE KJ: Effect of advancing gestational age on the frequency of fetal ductal constriction in association with maternal indomethacin use. Am J Obstet Gynecol 1993;168:1350.
52. GLOOR JM, MUCHANT DG, NORLING LL: Prenatal maternal indomethacin use resulting in prolonged neonatal renal insufficiency. J Perinatol 1993;8:425.
53. BAILEY PL, STREISAND JB, PACE NL, BUBBERS SJ: Transdermal scopolamine reduces nausea and vomiting after out-patient laparoscopy. Anesthesiology 1990;72:977.
54. TORNETTA FJ: Studies with the new antiemetic metoclopramide. Anesth Analg 1969;48:198.
55. PETTIT GP, SMITH GA, MCILROY WL: Droperidol in obstetrics: a double-blind study. Milit Med 1976;141:316.
56. BRANT HA: Acute appendicitis in pregnancy. Obstet Gynecol 1967;29:130.
57. BLACK WP: Acute appendicitis in pregnancy. BMJ 1960;1:1938.
58. MASTERS K, LEVINE BA, GASKILL HV, SIRINEK KR: Diagnosing appendicitis during pregnancy. Am J Surg 1984;148:768.
59. SARASON EL, BAUMAN S: Acute appendicitis in pregnancy: difficulties in diagnosis. Obstet Gynecol 1963;22:382.
60. BAER JL, REIS RA, ARENS RA: Appendicitis in pregnancy with changes in position and axis of the normal appendix in pregnancy. JAMA 1932; 98:1359.
61. HIBBARD LT: Cesarean section and other surgical procedures. In Obstetrics: Normal and Problem Pregnancies, Gabbe SG, Niebyl JR, Simpson JL (eds). New York, Churchill Livingstone, 1986.
62. ALDER SN: A sign for differentiating uterine from extrauterine complications of pregnancy and puerperium. BMJ 1951;2:1194.
63. SPITZER M, KAISER IH: Perforative appendicitis in the third trimester of pregnancy. NY State J Med 1984;84:132.
64. WEINGOLD AB: Appendicitis in pregnancy. Clin Obstet Gynecol 1983;26:801.
65. AUFSES AH JR: Biliary tract disease. In Pregnancy (2nd ed), Rovinsky JJ, Guttmacher A (eds). Baltimore, Williams & Wilkins, 1965, pp 251–253.
66. SCHREIBER JH: Laparoscopic appendectomy in pregnancy. Surg Endosc 1990;4:100.
67. EVERSON RB, BYAR DP, BISHOFF AJ: Estrogen predisposes to cholecystectomy but not to stones. Gastroenterology 1982;82:4.
68. DOWN RHL, WHITTING MJ, WATTS JM, JONES W: Effect of synthetic oestrogens and progestagens in oral contraceptives on bile lipid composition. Gut 1983;24:253.
69. LYNN J, WILLIAMS L, J. O'BRIEN, ET AL: Efects of estrogen upon bile: implications with respect to gallstone formation. Ann Surg 1973;178:514.
70. TRITAPEPE R, CESANA A, GANDINI R, TRIVELLINI G: Experimental research into the aetiopathogenesis of biliary calculosis. Panminerva Med 1969; 11: 410.
71. WOODHOUSE DR, HAYLEN B: Gallbladder disease complicating pregnancy. Aust NZ J Obstet Gynaecol 1985,25:233.
72. SIMON, JA: Biliary tract disease and related surgical disorders during pregnancy. Clin Obstet Gynecol l983;26:810.
73. BRAVERMAN DZ, JOHNSON ML, KERN F: Effects of pregnancy and contraceptive steroids on gall bladder function. N Engl J Med 1980;302:362.
74. HILL LM, JOHNSON CE, LEE RA: Cholecystectomy in pregnancy. Obstet Gynecol l975;46:291.
75. STAUFFER RA, ADAMS A, WYGAL J, LABERY JP: Gallbladder disease in pregnancy. Am J Obstet Gynecol 1982;144:661.
76. MARCUS CS, MASON GR, KUPERUS JW, MENA I: Pulmonary imaging in pregnancy: maternal risk and fetal dosimetry. Clin Nucl Med 1985;10:1.
77. BAILLIE J, CAIRNS SR, PUTMAN WS, COTTON PB: Endoscopic management of choledocholithiasis during pregnancy. Surg Obstet Gynecol 1990;171:1.
78. OSTMAN Pl, PANTLE-FISHER FM, FAURE EA, GLOSTEN B: Vasculatory collapse during laparoscopy. J Clin Anesth 1990;2:129.
79. PEOPLES JB: Cholecystectomy during pregnancy without fetal loss. Surg Gynecol Obstet 1992; 174:465.
80. MCKELLAR DP, ANDERSON CT, BOYNTON CJ, PEOPLES JB: Cholecystectomy during pregnancy without fetal loss. Surg Gynecol Obstet 1992; 174:465.
81. WEBER AM, BLOOM GP, ALLAN TR, CURRY SL: Laparoscopic cholecystectomy during pregnancy. Obstet Gynecol 1991;78:958.
82. VAN BEEK EJ, FARMER KC, MILLER DM, BRUMMELKAMP WH: Gallstone disease in women younger than 30 years. Neth J Surg 1992;43(3):60.

83. BLOCH P, KELLY TR: Management of gallstone pancreatitis during pregnancy in the postpartum period. Surg Gynecol Obstet 1989;168:426.
84. HUNTER JG, SOPER NJ: Laparoscopic management of common bile duct stones. Surg Clin North Am 1992;72:1077.
85. PHILLIPS EH, CARROLL BJ, PEARLSTEIN AR, ET AL: Laparoscopic choledochoscopy and extraction of common bile duct stones. World J Surg 1993; 17:22.
86. PETERSON HB, HULKA JF, PHILLIPS JM: American Association of Gynecologic Laparoscopists' 1988 membership survey on operative laparoscopy. J Reprod Med 1990;35:587.
87. HASSON, HM: Open laparoscopy: a report of 150 cases. J Reprod Med 1974;12:234.
88. BASSO L, MCCOLLUM PT, DARLING MR, ET AL: A study of cholelithiasis during pregnancy and its relationship with age, parity, menarche, breast-feeding, dysmenorrhea, oral contraception and a maternal history of cholelithiasis. Sur Obstet Gynecol 1992;175:41.
89. SOPER NJ, BRUNT LM, KERBL K: Laparoscopic general surgery. N Engl J Med 1993;330:409.

18
Principles of Pediatric Laparoscopy

Joseph S. Sanfilippo and Thom E. Lobe

Perhaps of all of the advances within the arena of laparoscopic surgery, the true "neophyte" is its application to the pediatric patient. Operative laparoscopy has now been performed successfully in preterm infants as well as neonates and young children.

The first report of endoscopic surgery was in the Babylonian Talmud (Niddah Treatise, Section 65b). It involved a lead funnel with a bent mouthpiece equipped with a wooden drain pipe introduced into the vagina, enabling direct visualization of the uterine cervix. Light reflected from a mirror placed in front of the exposed vulva enabled illumination of internal body structures, recorded by the Arabian physician Albukassim (912–1013 AD). We then move to the first endoscopic light source, which was attributed to the pioneering effort of Guilio Cesare Aranzi (1587). The subsequent application of the *camera obscura* was invented by the Benedictine monk Don Panuce. This work was followed by that of Bozzani in 1805, who used a tube and candle light to examine the urethra. Further innovative efforts were ascribed to Ott in 1901, who was the first to inspect abdominal viscera by focusing a head mirror into a speculum introduced through a small incision, perhaps the first truly laparoscopic procedure. Introduction of the pneumoperitoneum is attributed to Kelling and Jacobaeus, followed by introduction of the cystoscope (Nitze). The use of CO_2 insufflation is attributed to Zollikofer, and the insufflation needle we use daily is ascribed to the work of Veress.[1] As we continue on the historical perspective, Hope and subsequently Riddock were the first to diagnose an ectopic pregnancy through the laparoscope, as reported by Semm.[2]

From the pediatric perspective, the work of Gans provided the major impetus. He has encouraged pediatric surgeons to incorporate laparoscopy in the management of diseases in children.[3-5]

Perhaps the most pertinent issues regarding endoscopic surgery in the pediatric patient includes those of a procedural nature. First, which procedures can be performed, and how does one perform them? Second, what can be accomplished more efficaciously by laparoscopy than by the conventional operative approach to the extent that it should be performed preferentially because of its significant advantages? Accordingly, the risks and benefits of each proposed procedure must be carefully discussed with the parents and, when appropriate, the patient.

Instrumentation

The technologic advances with respect to instrumentation have enabled pediatric endoscopy, under certain circumstances, to become a frequent surgical procedure. Specifically, instru-

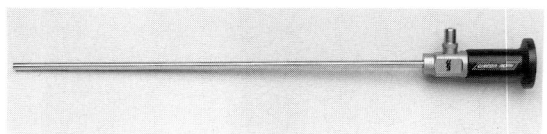

Figure 18.1. Pediatric 4.8 mm laparoscope. (Courtesy of Karl Storz Endoscopy-America, Culver City, CA)

ments ranging from 2 to 10 mm in diameter are used primarily, most often with a 0° or 30° lens configuration. Generally, the 0° scopes are the most practical and provide less disorientation, although 30° lenses are useful in specific instances: when it is necessary to "see around a corner" or at an angle and a second trocar is not desired. The right angle or operating laparoscopes have little use in most of our current operative endoscopic procedures and are probably not worth the additional expense if one is purchasing a new system. Another essential instrument is the lightweight videocamera system. There is currently significant discussion regarding the advantages of three-chip cameras versus the single-chip system.

Laparoscopy in infants and children requires small trocars and cannulas and delicate instrumentation (Fig. 18.1). The ideal trocar for the infant or small child is approximately 2.5 cm in length and remains fixed in the peritoneal cavity until it is no longer required. Currently, disposable and nondisposable instrumentation is available for the pediatric patient. Care must be exerted in that the screw-type fixation devices may tear the skin of the child or slip out easily because of their thin abdominal wall. Adhesive rings that secure the cannula in place are now available and are promising. It may be necessary to use Steri-Strips (3M, St. Paul, MN) or sutures to secure the cannulas in place after insertion.

Usually, general anesthesia is used with endotracheal intubation in this age group. Prophylactic (preoperative) antibiotics are recommended primarily to prevent trocar site infections.

For all infants and children the stomach and bladder should be emptied immediately prior to initiating the procedure. The stomach can be emptied with a suction catheter (nasogastric or orogastric tube). The bladder can be emptied using a Credé maneuver. A Verres needle can be used to establish a pneumoperitoneum even in the smallest infant. First, a stab incision is made in the skin at the inferior rim of the umbilicus, the length of which equals the diameter of the cannula to be used. The next step is to elevate the abdominal wall by grasping it on either side of the umbilicus as the Verres needle is introduced. It is easiest to introduce the needle perpendicular to the long axis of the patient, thereby avoiding insertion of the needle into the loose areolar subcutaneous tissue. The needle is best held at its shaft, like a dart; and the maneuver is a quick, shallow thrust into the peritoneal cavity until the retractable blunt end is heard to "pop" free into the abdomen. When the insufflation tubing is connected, the gas should flow at 0.5 L/min or faster. A slower rate of flow suggests that the needle is not in the proper location.

The exact volume of gas to be placed intraabdominally depends in part on the size of the patient. It is preferable to set the pressure limits with automatic insufflators at 6–8 mm Hg in the infant. For children, most procedures can be accomplished at pressures of 8–10 mm Hg; older children (adolescents) can better tolerate pressures of 10–12 mm Hg.

After the abdomen is insufflated, the umbilical trocar is introduced with a 5 mm cannula. Despite abdominal insufflation, the abdominal wall is elevated as the trocar is introduced. A twisting motion provides good control when inserting the trocar and sleeve.

Direct visualization of the trocar as it enters the abdomen is of the utmost importance when establishing secondary puncture sites. The trocar sites should be sutured closed in children, as the thin abdominal wall predisposes them to hernia formation at the trocar site.

It is advisable to administer metoclopramide (Reglan; A. H. Robins, Richmond, VA) to decrease the probability of nausea postoperatively. In children older than 8–10 years of age, a patch of Transderm-Scope (Ciba Pharmaceuticals, Edison, NJ) placed behind the ear is effective.

Children have less shoulder pain discomfort, in general, than do adults. Postoperative analgesic requirements are varied and best prescribed

Table 18.1. Laparoscopically Performed Procedures in Infants and Children

Appendectomy
Cholecystectomy
Trauma evaluation
Undescended testes
Varicocele
Small bowel obstruction
Abscess
Gallbladder shunts
Ventriculoperitoneal/Tenkoff catheters
Inguinal hernias
Pyloromyotomy
Nissen fundoplication
Tumor staging
Brachytherapy
Liver biopsy
Nephrectomy
Splenectomy
Bowel resection
Vagotomy
Pull-through for Hirschsprung's disease
Lymphadenectomy
Staging laparotomy
Vesicourethral reflux
Neonatal jaundice
Rectal prolapse
Acute pelvic inflammatory disease
Chronic pelvic pain correlation
Lysis of adhesions
Ovarian cyst
Adnexal torsion
Creation of neovagina

From: Sanfilippo JS, Lobe TE. Operative laparoscopy in the pediatric patient. In: *Laparoscopic Surgery: An Atlas for General Surgeons.* Vitale G, Sanfilippo JS, Perissat J (eds.). Philadelphia, Lippincott, 1995, p. 77

as necessary. A number of laparoscopic procedures can be accomplished in infants and children (Table 18.1).[6]

Acute Appendicitis

It is apparent that one of the most efficacious applications of laparoscopic surgery in the pediatric and adolescent patient is the treatment of appendicitis.[7,8] Most of the arguments against approaching this disease laparoscopically are by those unfamiliar with endoscopic surgery. There are several advantages of a laparoscopic approach, including a better cosmetic result (particularly important to young girls) and an early return to extracurricular activities after a brief recovery time (hours to days).

The complication rate of laparoscopic appendectomy is the same as for the open procedure.[9] Complications include minor local wound infections and an occasional intraabdominal abscess requiring drainage in association with a ruptured appendix. The latter complication can occur in the presence of a fecalith.

Following a laparoscopic appendectomy for acute uncomplicated appendicitis, patients are discharged 6–36 hours postoperatively and return to unrestricted activity as soon as they are comfortable (i.e., within 72 hours). With respect to a ruptured appendix, the advantages of laparoscopic appendectomy are not as obvious. The laparoscopic technique does offer an opportunity to treat the disease, however, and once antibiotic therapy is completed the patient quickly returns to a normal level of activity.

We have observed that approximately 40% of the appendices are ruptured at the time of laparoscopy. One approach suggested is to perform laparoscopy in patients who appear to have appendicitis uncomplicated by rupture or abscess formation. If laparoscopic appendectomy is undertaken and a ruptured appendix is discovered, it is often feasible to complete the appendectomy without laparotomy.

In cases of abdominal pain when the diagnosis is unclear, a laparoscopic approach proves advantageous. One must search for other possible causes of the acute abdominal signs and symptoms. It is easier to explore the abdomen via the laparoscope than through the conventional right lower quadrant incision. In the pediatric patient the ovaries and tubes can be atraumatically manipulated and inspected. The bowel can be inspected in its entirety, looking for a Meckel's diverticulum or other pathology, and the upper abdomen can be assessed for cholecystitis or abscess formation.

Technique

There are many laparoscopic approaches to appendectomy. The procedure can be performed using the laser, surgical clips, linear stapling

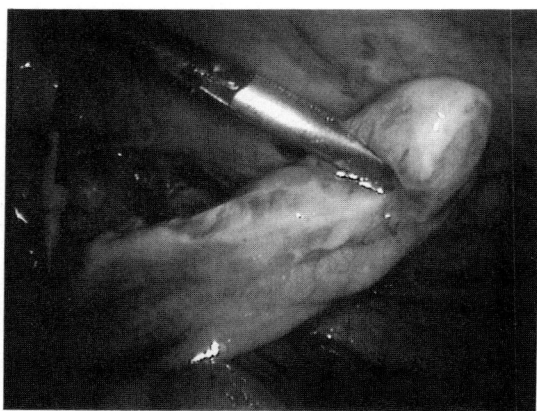

Figure 18.2. Appendix is held by an endoscopic grasper.

devices, endoscopic loops, or sutures. The initial approach to laparoscopic appendectomy requires placement of a nasogastric tube and a bladder catheter. The patient is placed supine in the Trendelenburg position. A pneumoperitoneum is established as described previously; and, depending on the size of the patient, a 5- or 10-mm laparoscope is introduced by way of the umbilicus into the peritoneal cavity. In general, a 5 mm laparoscope is used for patients under 10 years of age and a 10 mm laparoscope for older children.

On inspection of the peritoneal cavity, it is usually immediately obvious that there is inflammation in the right lower quadrant; a collection of peritoneal fluid is occasionally observed. Two additional cannulas are introduced to complete the operation, their size and location depending on the technique. Symmetric placement of the cannulas (ports) in the right and left lower quadrants below the "bikini line," lateral to the epigastric vessels on either side, is preferable. One 5 mm and one 12 mm port appear to be adequate. If a GIA stapler is used, a 12 mm port must be inserted to ensure ample room for proper instrument placement and function. To mobilize the appendix, a 5 mm reducing cap must be placed when 5 mm instruments are used with the larger ports so the pneumoperitoneum is not lost.

Two tissue graspers, at least one of which has a ratcheted handle, are used to mobilize the appendix so the tip (of the appendix) is secured in one of the graspers (Fig. 18.2). A closed grasper is helpful, serving as a blunt dissector in a manner similar to the blunt dissection performed during open cases. It enables separation of inflammatory adhesions and fluid loculations, facilitating mobilization of the appendix.

Occasionally, there are a number of adhesions that must be taken down sharply, in which case a Metzenbaum endoscopic scissors can be used. Bipolar electrosurgery enables careful division of the adhesions while cauterizing any blood vessels to minimize bleeding. Once the appendix is mobilized and its junction with the base of the cecum is clearly identified, the mesoappendix and appendix are divided.

The GIA stapler can be used to divide the mesoappendix and appendix. The device, after being placed through a 12 mm left lower quadrant port, allows the mesoappendix and appendix to be secured down to its junction with the cecum. One must be sure that the tip of the stapler is well identified and the line indicating the end of the cut is beyond the tissue. If the mesoappendix and appendix are divided in one application of the stapler, and the tissues are thick or inflamed, there may be a leak at the junction of the mesentery and the appendiceal stump. The jaws of the stapler are then closed; the surgeon must check to be certain of the stapler position and that there are no additional tissue(s) or loops or bowel engaged in the device. Once the proper position is certain, the safety latch is released and the stapler fired.

The appendix can then be extracted through the left lower quadrant 12 mm cannula so the inflamed or contaminated tissue never touches the cannula tract, which would add the risk of possible infection. If the inflamed appendix is so thick it cannot be removed through the cannula, a tissue sac can be inserted through the right lower quadrant port, the appendix placed within it, and the sac withdrawn into the cannula to its point of resistance (Fig. 18.3). The cannula should be withdrawn completely so the neck of the sac is outside the abdominal wall. After the sac is removed, the left lower quadrant trocar and cannula are reinserted, and the surgical bed is inspected for hemostasis and irrigated

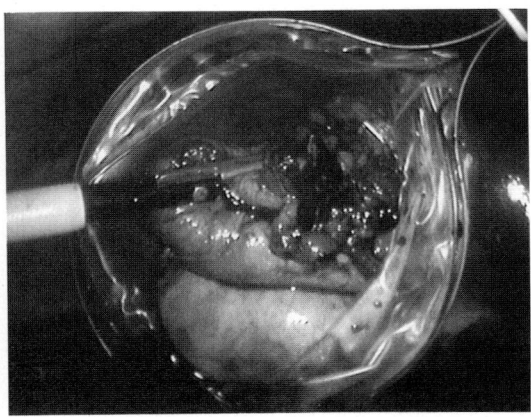

Figure 18.3. Extraction of the appendix using a sac. (Reprinted from *Pediatric Laparoscopy and Thoracoscopy*, 1st ed, Lobe TE, Schropp KE, eds. Philadelphia, W.B. Saunders Co., 1993, p 118, with permission)

as necessary. If the surgeon is uncomfortable leaving the appendiceal stump exposed, it can be inverted by placing Z stitch or purse-string stitch using standard laparoscopic suturing techniques.

Ruptured Appendix

With a ruptured or gangrenous appendicitis, the surgeon ought to identify friable segments of the appendiceal wall through which a fecalith may extrude. A fecalith lost in the peritoneal cavity may be a nidus for abscess formation, requiring subsequent intervention. In cases of ruptured appendicitis where one or more abscesses are found, a Luken's trap is attached to the end of the suction device to obtain material for culture. At the end of the procedure, copious irrigation of the peritoneal cavity with Ringer's lactate or saline followed by antibiotic-containing irrigation solution is recommended. In cases of intraabdominal inflammation (e.g., appendicitis) where frank pus is present, and irrigation is used to help cleanse the peritoneal cavity, one should be aware of the dependent position of the diaphragm or pelvis, depending on the procedure and the use of large quantities of irrigation fluid that are not adequately aspirated. There is the potential risk of loculation of the fluid and subsequent abscess formation. After laparoscopic appendectomy, in cases of ruptured appendicitis for which an abscess is drained and the abdomen irrigated, the patient is placed in reverse Trendelenburg position at the end of the procedure to allow the irrigation fluid to run into the pelvis, where it can be meticulously aspirated.

The laparoscopic procedure tends to take longer with ruptured appendicitis with abscess because it is necessary to dissect out the appendix and lyse adhesions and loculations. Occasionally, in cases of retrocecal appendicitis or where the tip of the appendix is markedly inflamed and involved in an inflammatory mass, retrograde removal of the appendix can be accomplished. Generally it is achieved through an incision into the mesoappendix near the normal base; the stapler is inserted at this juncture to divide the appendix or the appendix can be divided with a laser approximately 1.0–1.5 cm from its base and the ends secured with Surgitie (US Surgical Corp., Norwalk, CT) before grasping the resected end of the appendix and dissecting the appendix and its mesentery free, as described above.

After the procedure has been completed, the ports are removed and the incision closed. Patients with ruptured appendicitis remain on antibiotics and nasogastric suctioning, as is routine for open appendectomy. Patients with acute "simple" appendicitis may take a regular diet and resume normal activities as tolerated. They are discharged on the day of surgery or as soon thereafter as is feasible. Patients may return to unrestricted activities immediately upon discharge.

Meckel's Diverticulum

Generally, patients with Meckel's diverticulum fall into two categories: those who present with obstruction or inflammation and those with hemorrhage. Either group is usually diagnosed inadvertently at exploration. Those who present with hemorrhage are often diagnosed preoperatively by imaging studies that demonstrate acute hemorrhage or ectopic gastric mucosa.

When a Meckel's diverticulum is identified, it can be resected in one of two ways. If it is broad-based and its aberrant gastric mucosa is in its tip, rather than at its junction with the small bowel, it can be resected easily by transection across its base using the linear stapler. In these cases it is imperative that the surgeon inspect the removed specimen to ensure that the offending aberrant tissue is removed in its entirety.

When the diverticulum is short and broad-based, or aberrant tissue is suspected at its junction with the small bowel, bowel resection is required. This procedure is best accomplished by exteriorizing the diverticulum and performing the resection in a standard fashion, or with laparoscopic techniques using the linear stapler.

Cholecystectomy

The results of laparoscopic cholecystectomy in children compares favorably with the procedure performed on adult patients.[10–14] One technique for cholecystectomy in the child is described as follows.

The surgeon is positioned on the patient's left, with the scrub nurse on the opposite side. The first assistant is across from the surgeon, and the camera operator stands next to the surgeon (Fig. 18.4).

A pneumoperitoneum is created in the standard fashion. A four-cannula technique is preferred (Fig. 18.5). A 5 mm port is placed at the umbilicus for insertion of the laparoscope. Careful inspection of the liver and gallbladder allows optimal insertion of the three operating ports. Different functions are performed through the ports, the particular function determining cannula placement. The midclavicular port is placed initially. A grasper is inserted through this port and the fundus of the gallbladder grasped. The fundus is displaced over the anterior edge of the liver, exposing the triangle of Calot (Fig. 18.6). This port site may be altered depending on the position of the gallbladder; ideally it is positioned lower in the smaller child.

A 5 mm port is placed in the anterior axillary position. A grasper is positioned through this cannula and the gallbladder grasped at the junc-

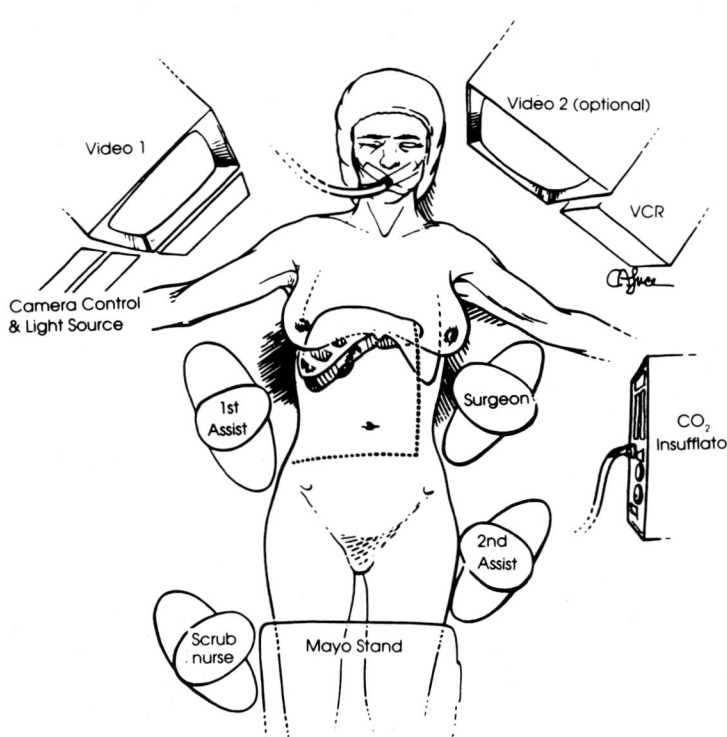

Figure 18.4. Operating room set-up for laparoscopic cholecystectomy. (Reprinted from Schirmer BD, et al: Laparoscopic cholecystectomy: treatment of choice for symptomatic cholelithiasis. *Ann Surg* 1991;213:665, with permission)

Figure 18.5. Extraction of gallbladder via laparoscopic cholecystectomy (From Davidoff et al.[12] Reprinted with permission.)

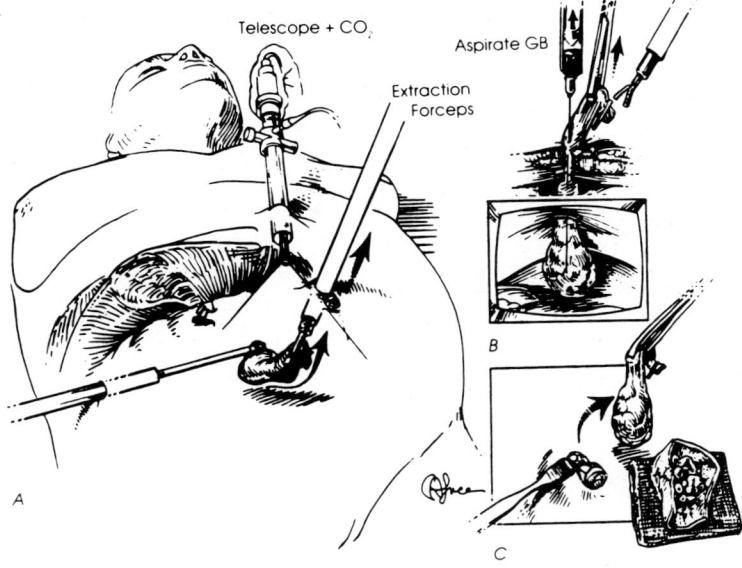

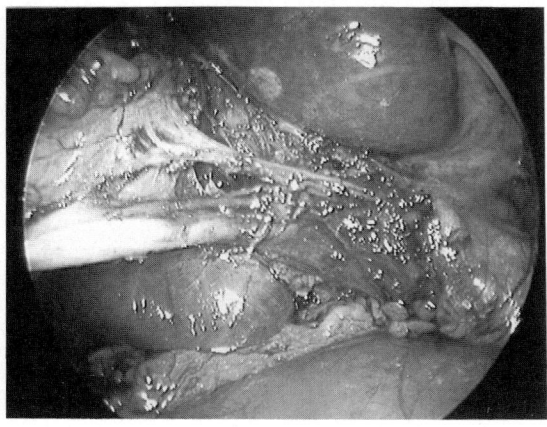

Figure 18.6. Triangle of Calot. Note the artery (top) and the cystic duct (bottom).

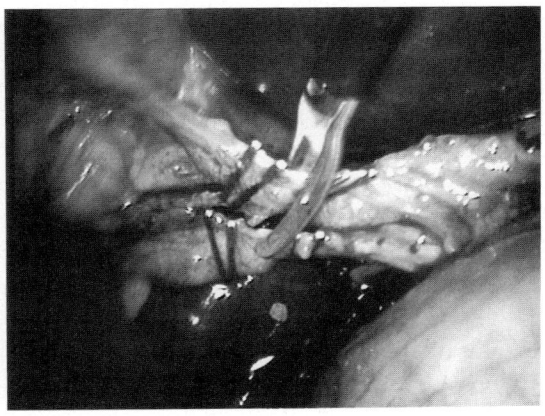

Figure 18.7. Exposure and division of the structures in the hepatocystic triangle. (From Davidoff et al.[12] Reprinted with permission)

tion of the body and neck. When this instrument is directed in a caudal and lateral direction, it exposes the structures in the hepatocystic triangle (Fig. 18.7). As with the midclavicular port, it may be necessary to adjust the position of this cannula for small patients. It is sometimes desirable to reverse the roles of the transfers in the anterior axillary and midclavicular ports when retracting the gallbladder. It is helpful to use ratcheted instruments in these ports to minimize the discomfort of the assistant.

The 10 mm port is placed in the subxiphoid position to the right of the falciform ligament in adult patients. Dissection and ligation of the cystic duct and artery are performed through this port, and the gallbladder is removed as well (Fig. 18.8). It is important that the instruments placed through the port intersect the cystic duct at a 60° or 90° angle. To obtain this angle, it may be necessary to place this port to the left of the falciform ligament in young patients. The dissector can be passed below the ligament, or the falciform ligament can be divided.

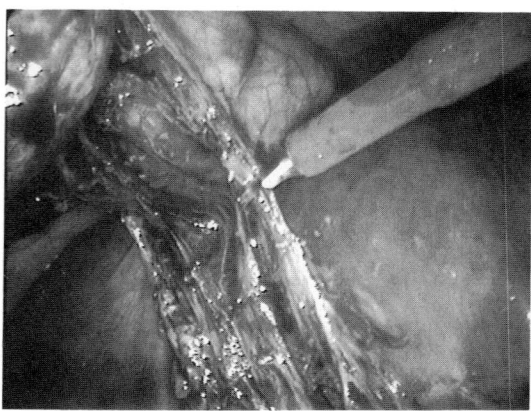

Figure 18.8. Electrosurgical application (Hook Tip) during cholecystectomy.

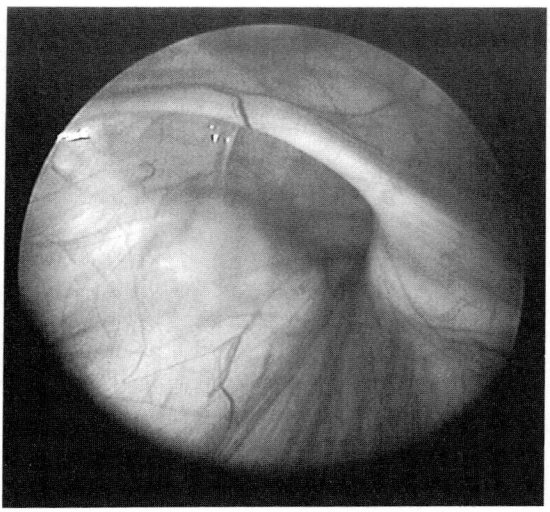

Figure 18.9. Examination of the liver bed for control of hemorrhage. (Reprinted from Schirmer BD, et al: Laparoscopic cholecystectomy: treatment of choice for symptomatic cholelithiasis. *Ann Surg* 1991;213:665, with permission)

Adhesions to the gallbladder are dissected free. The cystic artery is then separated from the cystic duct. It is imperative that the surgeon ensures that the cystic artery, duct, and right hepatic artery are clearly identified before any structure is divided. The cystic artery is ligated with the use of four clips and then divided between the two sets of clips. The cystic duct is separated from the surrounding structures by blunt dissection. Two clips are then placed on the distal cystic duct in preparation for a cholangiogram (Plate 30). Cholangiography may be performed by any one of several methods. There are commercial catheters that can be passed through a 5 mm port. Unfortunately, this method results in a loss of exposure, as one of the graspers must be removed (Fig. 18.9).

Inguinal Herniorrhaphy

Laparoscopic repair of inguinal hernias is an acceptable procedure in adults.[15] It has been less widely reported in the literature for the pediatric-adolescent patient. Repair consists in incising the peritoneum anterior to the hernial defect, excising the sac, inserting a roll of polypropylene mesh into the inguinal defect, tacking a piece of polypropylene mesh over the defect using a hernia stapler, and reperitonealizing the repair.

Laparoscopy usually proves useful for managing inguinal hernias in children to determine if a hernia is present on the asymptomatic contralateral side. A 3 mm cannula is inserted through an umbilical stab wound after insufflating the infant's abdomen to 8–10 mm Hg with CO_2. A 2 mm 0° telescope enables inspection of the lower abdomen. Hernias are obvious when they are identified (Fig. 18.10). A patent processus vaginalis or the neck of a small hernial sac can also be identified when present (Fig. 18.11).

Inguinal hernias have been repaired laparoscopically, and it seems to be a reasonable approach in older children. Essentially, the same principles of indirect inguinal hernial repair applies in children as are recommended in adults. The hernial sac is divided and the neck of the sac obliterated.

Repair is carried out with the patient in Trendelenburg position with three ports being placed. An umbilical cannula is used for laparoscope placement. The two other ports are inserted lateral to the rectus muscle, at or slightly above the level of the umbilicus, one on either side of the abdomen. The peritoneum is incised

18. Principles of Pediatric Laparoscopy

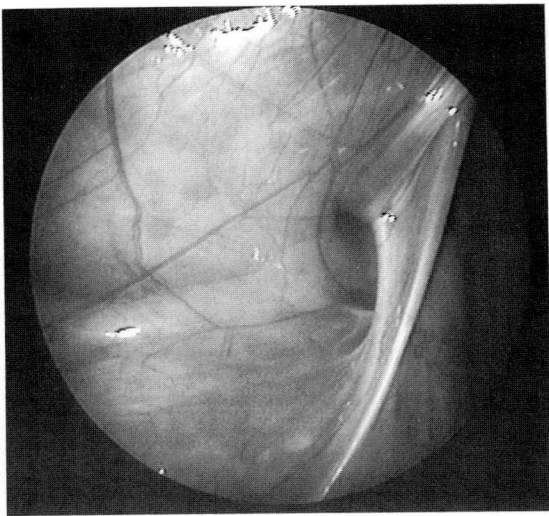

Figure 18.10. Large inguinal hernia. (Reprinted from *Pediatric Laparoscopy and Thoracoscopy*, 1st ed, Lobe TE, Schropp KE, eds. Philadelphia, W.B. Saunders Co., 1993, p 158, with permission)

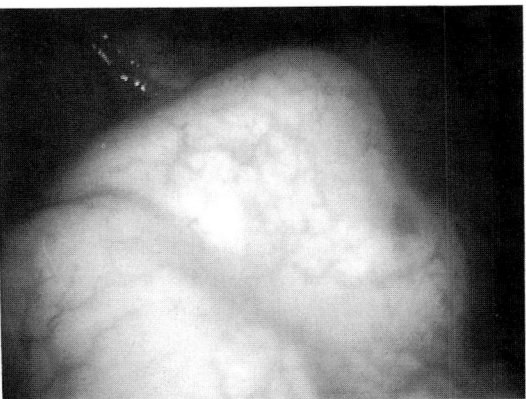

Figure 18.11. Patent processus vaginalis. (Reprinted from *Pediatric Laparoscopy and Thoracoscopy*, 1st ed, Lobe TE, Schropp KP, eds. Philadelphia, W.B. Saunders Co., 1993, p 158, with permission)

as for the adult repair. The hernial sac is then divided, taking care not to injure the cord structures, which are easily identified. The distal sac can be either removed or left in situ. The surgeon then closes the hernial defect using interrupted, nonabsorbable sutures. The peritoneum is then sutured. Patients are discharged on the day of surgery and instructed to return to unrestricted activities.

Mesenteric Cysts

Mesenteric cysts can be diagnosed preoperatively by means of diagnostic imaging. When a cyst is noted and it appears relatively free from surrounding structures, it is amenable to laparoscopic resection (Fig. 18.12).

Diagnostic laparoscopy through an umbilical cannula is initiated. If the cyst is large (obstructing the view), it is usually of low malignant potential. A needle can be inserted through the abdominal wall decompressing this cyst. If the cyst is on a pedicle, it can be easily excised using laser, electrosurgical techniques, endoscopic sutures, loop ligatures, or mechanical devices such as clips or staplers.

Cysts buried in the mesentery or omentum can be dissected free and similarly excised. Decompression of the cyst may help with its removal through the laparoscopic port. Rarely, a cyst is so intimately involved with an adjacent loop of bowel that a bowel resection may be necessary to remove the cyst. It too can be accomplished laparoscopically using linear staplers.

Hepatic and Splenic Cysts

Occasionally cystic lesions of the liver are observed and require intervention. Like other cystic lesions, they can be either excised or fenestrated using the techniques previously described. The cyst is unroofed and its lining obliterated. If infection is a concern, samples for culture can be obtained by use of a drainage tube placed directly, using the laparoscope as a guide.

Although splenic cysts are uncommon, simple epidermoid cysts are ideal for laparoscopic correction. A laparoscope is placed at the umbilicus to visualize the cyst. Two 5 mm ports are placed in the lower abdominal crease on either side of the rectus muscle to manipulate the tissues. An additional cannula may be required to complete the procedure, and ideally it is placed in the right midclavicular line midway between the umbilicus and the costal margin.

Once the cyst is inspected, and it appears to be a simple cyst without evidence of infection, a needle (e.g., spinal) is placed through a separate stab incision immediately over the presenting portion of the cyst or an aspiration needle is placed through a 5 mm port to puncture the wall and aspirate its contents. Serous fluid is extracted, further supporting the diagnosis of a simple cyst without infection. The cyst wall is then excised if necessary; cautery may be used and an effort made to remove the entire cyst wall. The cyst may be transected using an endoscopic GIA stapler. It is not worthwhile to attempt to strip the lining from the cyst for fear of inducing hemorrhage that might necessitate a splenectomy.

Pyloric Stenosis

Laparoscopic pyloromyotomy for idiopathic hypertrophic pyloric stenosis has been reported.[16] The technique requires an umbilical access after intraabdominal CO_2 insufflation has been established. Another port is inserted laterally from the left of the patient's midline. With the stomach decompressed it is easy to see the pyloric mass. Electrosurgical instrumentation is used to accomplish the pylorotomy through the pyloric muscle down to the mucosa, along the length of the pylorus. Another instrument is then used to spread the muscle and separate its two halves. Surgeons adept at the technique require 20–45 minutes to complete the procedure.

One problem is that the surgeon appears to have relatively little control of the pylorus during the procedure. Because of the high risk of perforation (approximately 10%) the procedure is still investigative.

Nissen Fundoplication

Dallemagne et al. first performed a laparoscopic Nissen fundoplication in Liege, Belgium in January 1991.[17] Later that year, Geagea performed a similar procedure in Nova Scotia.[18] Cuschieri and coworkers undertook laparoscopic antireflux surgery in 1989.[19]

Dallemagne et al. performed the procedure in patients ranging in age from 29 to 69 years.[17] The mean operating time has been reported to be 1.5–2.0 hours. Most patients are on a regular diet on the first postoperative day and are discharged on the second day. Results to date are similar to those achieved by laparotomy.[18] Some patients have early, transient dysphagia, but in general the postoperative course is benign and uneventful.

Indications for performing a laparoscopic antireflux procedure for gastroesophageal reflux in children are the same as those for the open approach. The theoretic advantages of the laparoscopic approach are related to the absence of a large abdominal incision. In obese patients an incision is more likely to develop a wound complication, and it may impair postoperative pulmonary function. In debilitated children, particularly those with severe mental retardation or those who cannot follow instructions, the incision may impair pulmonary function and predispose the patient to atelectasis or pneumonia.

One accepted technique involves placing 5 mm ports in the abdomen: one for viewing with the telescope, one for retracting the liver, two for tissue manipulation, and one for suturing. In essence, the operation is identical to that performed via laparotomy. The liver is retracted away from the esophageal hiatus, the esophagus is mobilized, the diaphragmatic crura are approximated with sutures, the short gastric vessels are divided as necessary, a 360° fundoplication wrap is sutured into position, and a gastrostomy tube is inserted as necessary.

The patient is best prepared for surgery by emptying the colon of gas and feces preoperatively, as a gas-distended colon makes the procedure difficult if not impossible. Under general anesthesia, the bladder is catheterized or emptied by means of a Credé maneuver, and a nasogastric tube is inserted. The patient is placed in the lithotomy position so the camera operator can stand between the patient's legs. A CO_2 pneumoperitoneum is established, and a 5 or 10 mm 0° laparoscope is passed by way of the

Figure 18.12. Endoscopic view of a mesenteric cyst.

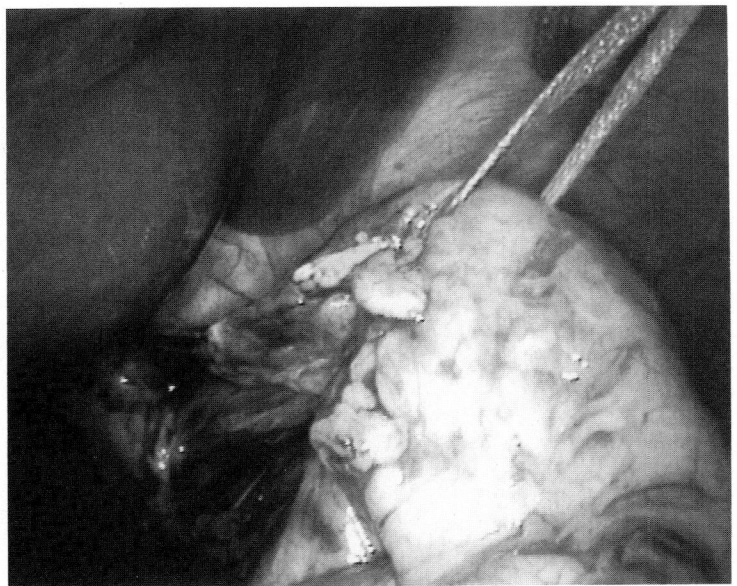

umbilicus. A 5 mm port is placed below the right costal margin in the midclavicular line and another in the epigastrium. A 10 mm port is placed in the left midclavicular line below the costal margin, and a 5 mm port is located in the left anterior axillary line below the costal margin. The liver is retracted via the epigastric cannula to expose the esophageal hiatus (Fig. 18.13).

In adult-sized adolescent patients a retractor may be necessary, whereas in small (pediatric adolescent) patients the cannula itself is sufficient to displace the liver. The short gastric vessels are divided between surgical clips as deemed necessary. Two medium-length clips on either side of the proposed line of division are feasible. Reticulating dissection instrumenta-

Figure 18.13. Exposure of esophageal hiatus for Nissen fundoplication. (Reprinted from ref. 20 with permission)

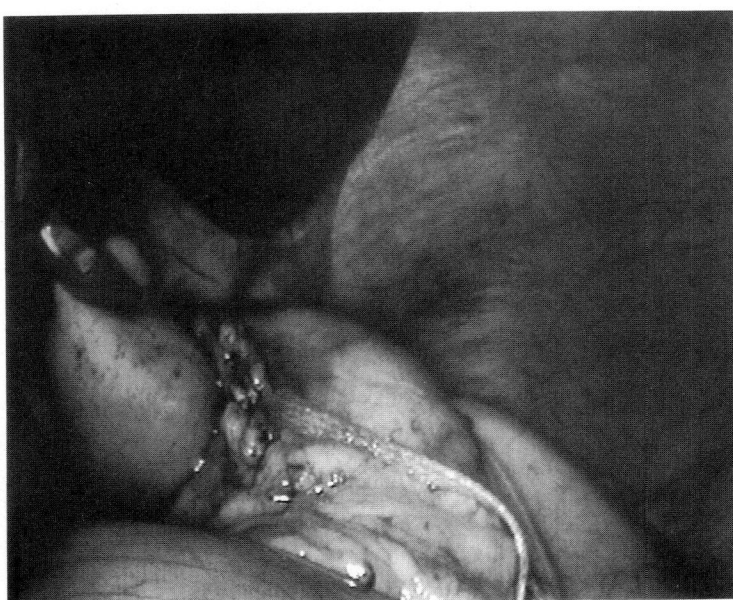

tion is ideal for isolating these vessels. The esophagus, with as large a bougie in place as can be accommodated, is mobilized and retracted using dissection instruments passed via the right and left lateral cannulas. A short segment of umbilical tape is then passed behind the esophagus. The exposed diaphragmatic crura are approximated to close the hiatus using interrupted 2-0 silk sutures that have been lubricated with mineral oil. (Extracorporeal knots are the easiest for secure tying under tension, although intracorporeal knot-tying is an option if one is sufficiently skilled with this technique.) The stomach is passed behind the esophagus from the patient's left to right. With the stomach held in position using an instrument passed from the right midclavicular line cannula, a back-handed suture is used to "snag" the stomach and complete the first (distalmost) suture of the wrap. This maneuver avoids having to place an additional port. The 3–5 cm wrap is then secured in place with interrupted 2-0 silk sutures, as for an open procedure (Plate 31). The esophageal bougie and the ports are then removed.

A percutaneous endoscopic technique can be used while observing the stomach with the laparoscope. Alternatively, the laparoscope is used to determine the optimal position of the gastrostomy, grasping the correct spot on the anterior gastric wall and externalizing the stomach through the subcostal midclavicular line trocar site. A gastrostomy is then sutured in place after the fundoplication is completed. Because of a lack of suitable small instrumentation, the procedure is difficult in infants weighing less than 3 kg, and we prefer the conventional approach in these patients.

Postoperatively, patients are provided a liquid diet on the evening of their surgery and a full diet (by tube or by mouth) on postoperative day 1. Generally, they are discharged 36–48 hours after surgery, at which time they return to unrestricted activities. No complications were noted in the series.[20] All of the patients were asymptomatic for gastroesophageal reflux at follow-up 18 months later, and the fundoplication remained intact in all.

References

1. SEMM K: Veress Weitere Entwicklungen in der gynakologischen Laparoskopie, Pelviskopie, Wysteroskopie, Fetoskopie. Baltimore, Urban & Schwarzenburg, 1978.
2. SEMM K: History. In Operative Gynecologic Endoscopy, Sanfilippo JS, Levine RL (eds). New York, Springer-Verlag, 1989, p 1.
3. GANS SL, BERCI G: Advances in endoscopy of infants and children. J Pediatr Surg 1981;6:199.
4. GANS SL, BERCI G: Peritoneoscopy in infants and children. J Pediatr Surg 1973;8:399.
5. GANS SL: A new look at pediatric endoscopy. Postgrad Med J 1977;62:91.
6. LOBE TE: The applications of laparoscopy and lasers in pediatric surgery. Surg Annu 1993;25:175.
7. GOTZ F, PIER A, BACHER C: Laparoscopic appendectomy: indications, technique and results in 653 patients. Chirurg 1991;62:253.
8. URE BM, SPANGENBERGER W, HEBEBRAND D, ET AL: Laparoscopic surgery in children and adolescents with suspected appendicitis: results of medical technology assessment. Eur J Pediatr Surg 1992;2:336.
9. GILCHRIST BF, LOBE TE, SCHROPP KP, ET AL: Is there a role for laparoscopic appendectomy in pediatric surgery? J Pediatr Surg 1992;27:209.
10. MOIR CR, DONOHUE JH, VAN HEERDEN JA: Laparoscopic cholecystectomy in children: initial experience and recommendations. J Pediatr Surg 1992;27:1066.
11. WARE RE, KINNEY TR, CASEY JR, ET AL: Laparoscopic cholecystectomy in young patients with sickle hemoglobinopathies. J Pediatr 1992;120:58.
12. DAVIDOFF AM, BRANUM GD, MURRAY EA, ET AL: The technique of laparoscopic cholecystectomy in children. Ann Surg 1992;215:186.
13. HOLCOMB GW III, OLSEN DO, SHARP KW: Laparoscopic cholecystectomy in the pediatric patient. J Pediatr Surg 1991;26:1186.
14. NEWMAN KD, MARMON LM, ATTORRI R, EVANS S: Laparoscopic cholecystectomy in pediatric patients. J Pediatr Surg 1991;26:1184.
15. LOBE TE, SCHROPP KP: Inguinal hernias in pediatrics: initial experience with laparoscopic inguinal exploration of the asymptomatic contralateral side. J Laparoendosc Surg 1992;2:135.
16. ALAIN JL, GROUSSEAU D, TERRIER G: Extramucosal pylorotomy by laparoscopy. J Pediatr Surg 1991;26:1191.

17. DALLEMAGNE B, WEERTS JM, JEHAES C, ET AL: Laparoscopic Nissen fundoplication: preliminary report. Surg Laparosc Endosc 1991;1:138.
18. GEAGEA T: Laparoscopic Nissen's fundoplication: preliminary report on ten cases. Surg Endosc 1991;5:170.
19. CUSHIERI A, SHIMI S, NATHANSON LK: Laparoscopic reduction, crural repair and fundoplication of large hiatal hernia. Am J Surg 1992;163:425.
20. LOBE TE, SCHROPP KP, LUNSFORD K: Laparoscopic Nissen fundoplication in childhood. J Pediatr Surg 1993;28:358.

19
Laparoscopic Suturing Techniques

Howard C. Topel

To perform laparoscopic surgical procedures a surgeon must learn new visual and tactile cues and develop hand–eye dexterity that is different from that needed for conventional open surgery. Whereas the transition to most laparoscopic techniques can be easily achieved, the mastery of endosuturing skills has required a greater level of practice and patience. Once mastered, however, the laparoscopic surgeon establishes a greater sense of confidence and accomplishment. Endosuturing and knot-tying become vital skills necessary for performing complex, advanced laparoscopic operations.

As with conventional laparotomy surgery, endosuturing techniques permit restoration of normal anatomic relations, organ reconstruction, approximation of tissue planes, and establishment of hemostasis. Three suturing methods (Endoloop, extracorporeal, intracorporeal) and their specific applications, limitations, and variations are described.

Endoloop Technique

The Endoloop (Ethicon, Somerville, NJ) is a simple endosuturing device designed to ligate tissue with a looped slipknot. It is currently available in a variety of suture sizes and materials. The loop can be precisely placed around tissue pedicles and blood vessels. Ligation and hemostasis are accomplished as the loop is constricted around the tissue and secured in place with the aid of a plastic knot-pusher (Fig. 19.1).

1. An Endoloop (Plain, chromic, or Polydioxanane sutures [PDS] (Ethicon, Somerville, NJ)) is back-loaded into a suture applicator (3 mm) until the entire loop disappears in the channel (Fig. 19.2).
2. The applicator is placed in the abdominal cavity through a 5 mm port or a larger trocar using a 5 mm reducer channel.
3. The Endoloop is then pushed out the end of the applicator channel until the loop is totally opened inside the abdominal cavity.
4. The loop is placed directly over the tissue to be ligated. To facilitate application, the loop should rest on the tissue.
5. A grasping instrument is passed through the loop. The tissue is grasped and gently pulled upward into the loop (Plate 32).
6. The tip of the endoloop is broken, and the plastic shaft slides downward, causing the loop to tighten over the tissue.
7. With the loop properly positioned, the ligature is completed by firmly pulling the end of the suture upward, as the plastic shaft is held against the knot. The shaft should be aligned perpendicular to the knot to prevent suture breakage as the loop is tightened.

19. Laparoscopic Suturing Techniques

Figure 19.1. Endoloop ligature.

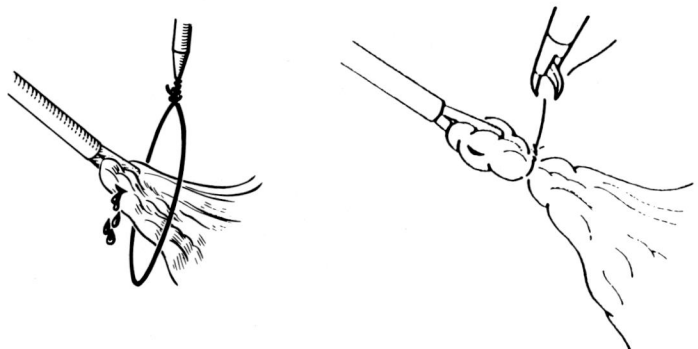

8. Endoscopic scissors are introduced through an ancillary trocar. The suture is then cut about 1 cm from the knot.
9. The plastic shaft, applicator, and excess suture are withdrawn from the abdominal cavity.
10. If the ancillary trocar is occupied, the plastic end is cut off and the shaft withdrawn. A scissors can then be introduced down the same port, and the suture is cut.
11. Often several Endoloops are placed across a structure to ensure good hemostasis. Each loop should be placed in a slightly different position, not directly on top of each other.

Advantages to the Endoloop technique are the relative ease of use, precision, and excellent hemostasis. One should always consider using an Endoloop when attempting to control bleeding. In contrast to electrocautery or metal clips, an Endoloop, when correctly applied, causes no lateral thermal injury or trauma to surrounding tissue. However, it can only be used to ligate a structure that can be fashioned into a pedicle, permitting complete encirclement.

Extracorporeal Endosuturing

Endoscopic suturing can be performed with a variety of suture and needle combinations. After introduction into the abdominal cavity, the needle is passed through tissue, and the suture can be ligated with several techniques. When the knot is formed within the abdominal cavity, using special graspers to manipulate the needle and suture, the technique is called intracorporeal suturing. When the suture material is brought outside, and the knot is formed and then reintroduced into the body, it is termed extracorporeal suturing.

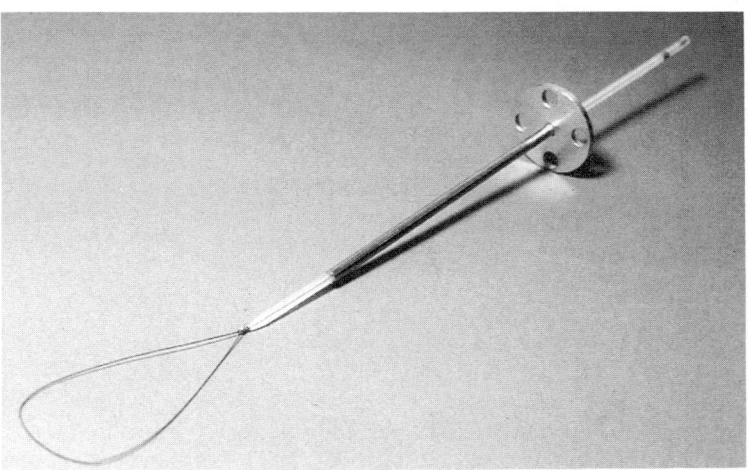

Figure 19.2. PDS Endoloop back-loaded into suture introducer.

Figure 19.3. Extracorporeal slipknot.

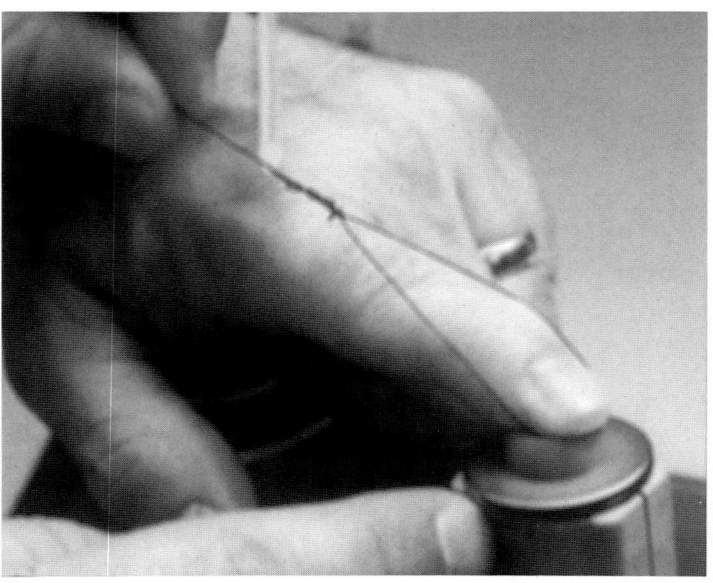

Special types of long (> 36 inches) sutures with straight, ski, and curved needles are available for extracorporeal suturing. A variety of slipknots have been developed that are tied on the outside, then reintroduced into the abdomen, and pushed down the trocar channel. In addition, several knot-pushers have been designed to guide the knot down the trocar and to tighten the knot against the sutured tissue.

Extracorporeal sutures with plastic knot-pushers (Endoknots) have been combined with straight, ski, and curved needles. Straight and ski

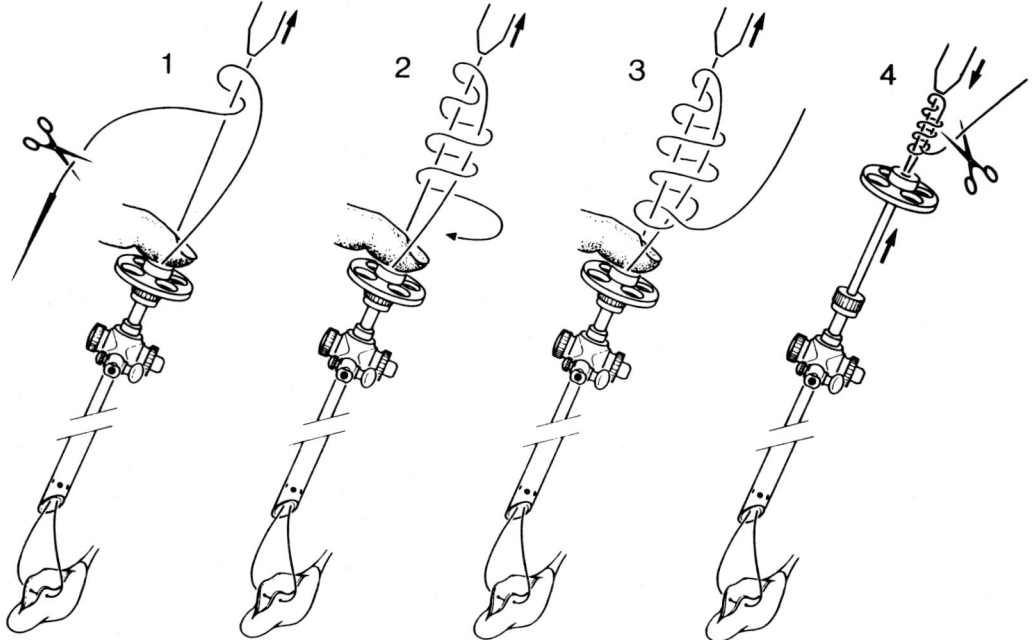

Figure 19.4. Extracorporeal knot for endosuture. From Osborne N (ed.) *Operative Laparoscopy for Gynecologists,* Parthenon/IDI Publications, 1993. Reprinted with permission.

19. Laparoscopic Suturing Techniques

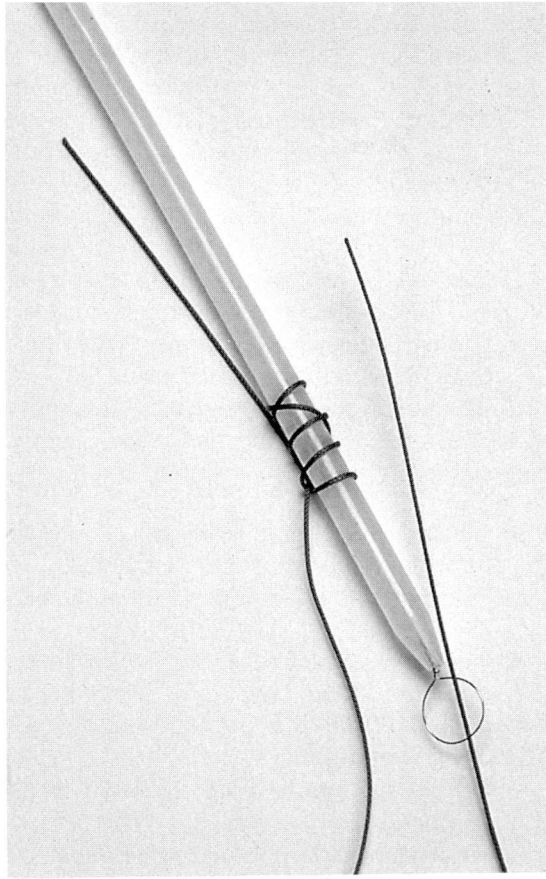

Figure 19.5. Pre-tied extracorporeal suture.

needles can be grasped near the swage point and directly inserted down a 5 mm trocar channel. Curved suture needles require a larger (> 10 mm) adapter channel for introduction.

The suture/needle is passed through the tissue with the aid of an endoscopic needle driver and a 5 mm grasper introduced from the contralateral port. After the suture is cut, the needle is removed from the abdomen under direct vision. Great care must be taken never to drop a loose needle during this extraction step. The excess suture length must be first brought down the trocar into the abdominal cavity and gently pulled through the tissue before the free cut end can be pulled up the trocar channel and exteriorized. After this step, both suture ends are now positioned outside the abdomen, through the same trocar port.

An extracorporeal slipknot, as shown in Figure 19.3, can be fashioned in numerous ways and then reintroduced into the abdomen (Fig. 19.4). The plastic knot-pusher is released at its distal end. The knot is directed down toward the tissue as the pusher secures the knot in place. It is essential that great care be exercised to minimize any tension on the suture line and to prevent the suture from evulsing through the tissue. After the knot is tightened, a scissors can be placed down the same port and the excess suture cut and removed.

The technique for extracorporeal knot-tying has been greatly simplified with the development of a pre-tied extracorporeal suture. Introduction and removal of the suture/needle follows the previously described steps. However, the exteriorized free suture end is now passed through a small wire loop located at the end of a plastic knot-pusher (Fig. 19.5). As the wire loop is pulled upward through the center of the pusher, the suture end is also pulled up this channel and out the distal end. A pre-tied knot, located around the shaft of the plastic pusher, is slipped down and tightened over the proximal portion of the suture line. The plastic rod pushes the pre-tied slipknot into the abdominal cavity and ligates the knot securely against the tissue. This pre-tied extracorporeal suture eliminates manual knot-tying and greatly expedites the entire process in a fast, consistent manner.

A variety of knot-pusher devices have been developed to facilitate extracorporeal suturing. One popular device is the Clarke-Reich knot-pusher, which permits successive placement of single-loop knots into the abdominal cavity. In addition, a laparoscopic Babcock instrument can serve as a simple, effective extracorporeal knot-pusher. After both suture ends are exteriorized, a double square knot is tied. The two free suture ends are threaded through the fenestrated ends of the Babcock (Fig. 19.6). While holding both ends in one hand, the Babcock slides the double tie down the trocar port into the abdominal cavity. With the suture passed through fenestrated ends, the suture line cannot slip off the pusher as the square knot is advanced down toward the tissue. The ligature

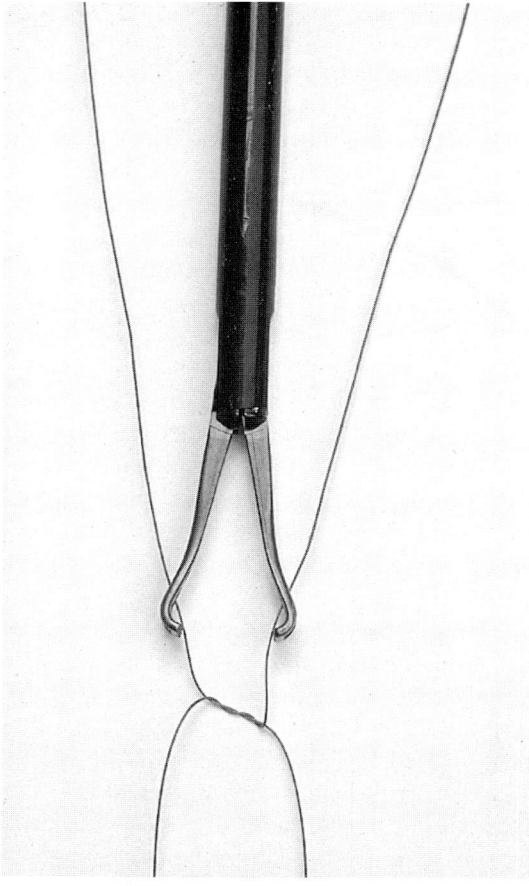

Figure 19.6. Extracorporeal Babcock knot-pusher.

can be precisely positioned and then tightened and secured by repeatedly opening and closing the Babcock. The advantages of this technique are a tight ligature, with multiple square double knots, using a variety of suture materials and sizes.

Intracorporeal Curved-Needle Suturing and Knot-Tying

Once limited to short, straight needles, laparoscopic suturing can be performed with curved suture needles and a wide variety of suture materials and sizes. When working from a two-dimensional video field, curved-needle suturing offers a surgeon greater versatility and more surgical options. Curved needles allow multiple placement choices, variable angulations, and multidirectional movement. Straight-needle endosuturing, in contrast, is significantly limited in both direction and tissue placement options. Needle drivers have been designed to firmly hold a curved needle with minimal instability at the distal tip (Plate 33). The rotational motion, so characteristic of open conventional needle drivers, can be now duplicated with endoscopic drivers. Tissue structures of varying thickness and consistency can be reconstructed with excellent approximation and hemostasis.

A curved needle and suture can be introduced into the abdominal cavity in the following manner.

1. Advance the curved needle driver through the 10 mm suture introducer channel.
2. Grasp the tail end of the suture in the needle driver jaws.
3. Pull the needle driver back through the suture introducer, allowing the suture needle (SH, CT-3) to hang freely beyond the end of the introducer.
4. Release the suture from the jaws of the needle driver.
5. While stabilizing the suture line inside the channel, advance the needle driver back down the introducer.
6. Secure the suture needle (at the needle–suture junction) in the needle driver jaws, keeping the needle curve parallel to the driver and suture introducer (Fig. 19.7).
7. Pull the suture taut (not tight), then withdraw the loaded needle driver into the introducer until the entire suture needle is inside the distal end.
8. Cut the excess suture, leaving approximately 1 inch or less exposed at the proximal end of the introducer. The critical suture length is 8–9 cm.
9. The loaded introducer is then readvanced through the 10- or 11-mm trocar into the abdominal cavity.
10. After needle placement in the tissue, the entire length of suture can be brought into the abdominal cavity, and the suture ends can then be equalized in length in preparation for tying.
11. For needle removal, grasp the suture within the jaws of the needle driver 2 cm from the

19. Laparoscopic Suturing Techniques

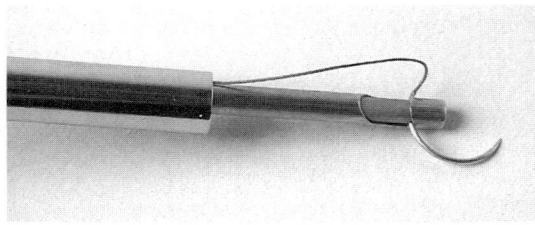

Figure 19.7. Curved needle being withdrawn into suture introducer.

needle, then cut the suture and withdraw the needle into the introducer channel (Plate 34).
12. The needle driver, suture needle, and introducer are all withdrawn at once through the trocar port, leaving the trocar in place.
13. The suture is now ready for intraabdominal knot-tying.

This technique for introduction and retrieval of the suture/needle is designed to control the curved needle at all times. The surgeon has total visual contact in order to prevent inadvertent tissue injury or accidental loss of the needle within the abdominal cavity.

Intracorporeal knot-tying can be a tedious, time-consuming, and often frustrating experience. However, with patience and a great amount of practice, intraabdominal knot-tying can be mastered and become a valuable endoscopic skill. Two types of intracorporeal knot-tying are discussed: the classic instrument tie and a new "twist" technique.

The classic instrument tie is demonstrated in Figure 19.8. This technique is similar to microsurgical knot-tying performed during open surgery.

A new intracorporeal "twist" knot-tying technique has greatly simplified endoscopic tying.

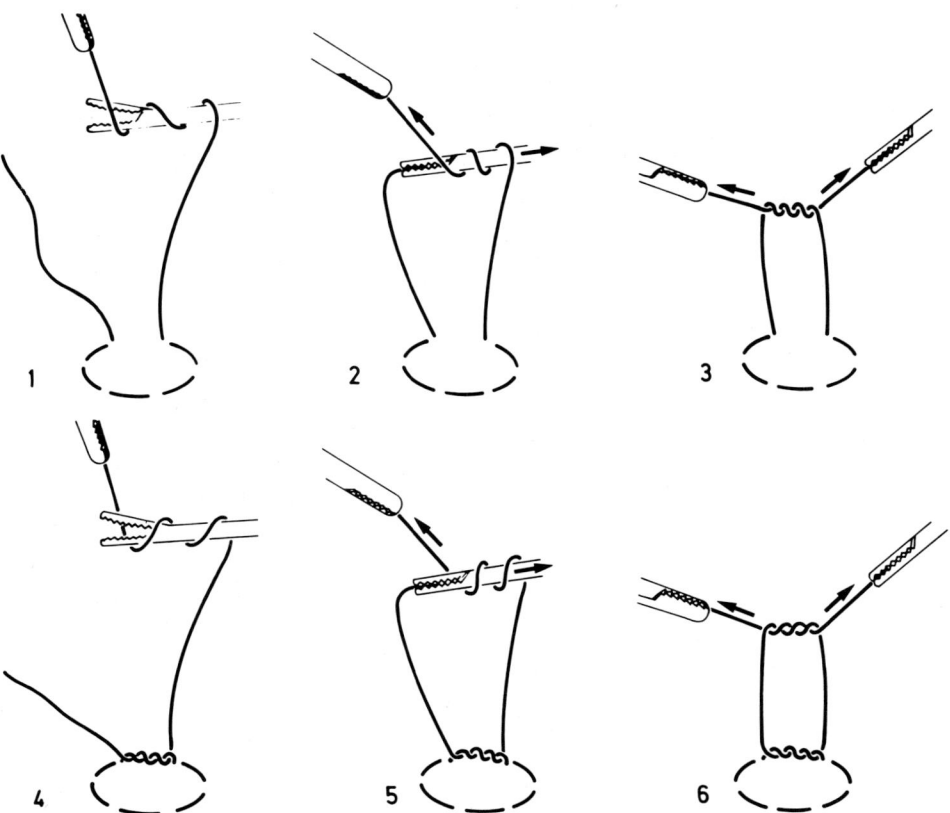

Figure 19.8. Classic instrument knot tie. Reprinted with permission from: Shirk, GJ, ed. *The Video Encyclopedia of Endoscopic Surgery for the Gynecologist.* Copyright © 1994, Medical Video Productions and the American Association of Gynecologic Laparoscopists.

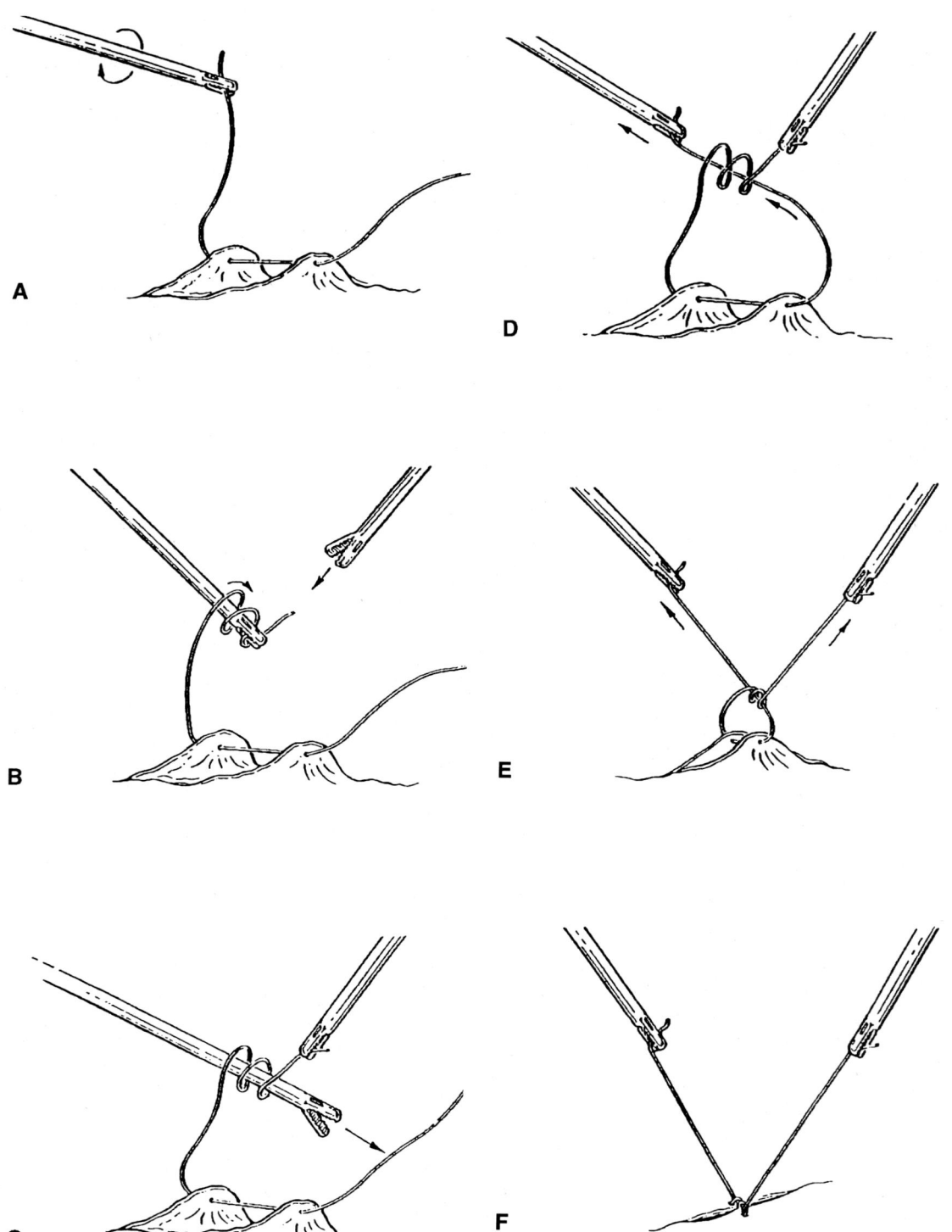

Figure 19.9a-f. Intracorporeal "twist" knot tying technique.

This technique is illustrated in Figure 19.9. It is applicable to all suture sizes and is designed to consistently form a square double "surgeon" knot with minimal slippage. One end of the suture is grasped and rotated up the shaft of a 5 mm instrument until three or four loops are formed. A second grasper removes the suture end from the jaws of the rotating grasper and slides the suture upward along the shaft of the instrument. The other free suture end is now grasped by the initial rotating grasper. As the two instruments are pulled in opposite directions, a square double knot is formed (Plate 35). The knot can be firmly tightened against the tissue surface and does not loosen as a second square knot is similarly fashioned and positioned in the tissue.

This "twist" technique provides excellent approximation of heavy tissue that is under tension, such as with uterine reconstruction following myomectomy. In addition, fine microsurgical knot-tying with delicate suture is readily accomplished with this technique. Suturing is often the method of choice to control bleeding. The "twist" knot-tie offers a reliable, consistent way to form a nonslipping knot and to establish hemostasis.

Laparoscopic surgery does not preclude the ability to perform continuous endosuturing. With the aid of a specially designed applier, a PDS clip called a Laparo-tye (Ethicon, Somerville, NJ) can be attached to the suture end. This clip serves to anchor the start of the suture line while a second PDS clip is placed to secure the end of the continuous locking closure (Plate 36). As demonstrated in Plates 37 and 38, this continuous technique, employing PDS clips, can approximate the large uterine defect following myomectomy with an excellent anatomic reconstruction.

Experienced endoscopic surgeons have recognized that neither energy sources, clips, nor staples can totally replace the need for sutures. Whether we perform an open laparotomy or a minimally invasive operation, suturing is a vital and necessary skill required for successful surgery. Future advancement of laparoscopic surgery will be driven by the development of new and innovative instrumentation. Devices such as pre-tied intracorporeal loop sutures, preloaded needle drivers, and automated "sewing" machines will make endosuturing more user-friendly. As a result, laparoscopic suturing will become more generally practiced by a greater number of surgeons performing more complex operations with fewer intraoperative complications.

20
Assisted Reproductive Technology Versus Tubal Surgery

Claudio A. Benadiva, Isaac Kligman, and Zev Rosenwaks

Significant advances in the field of human reproduction and reproductive surgery are responsible for a dramatic change in our approach to the infertile couple. Since the landmark report of Steptoe and Edwards in 1978,[1] in vitro fertilization (IVF) and other assisted reproductive technologies (ARTs) have evolved to assume a preeminent role in the management of infertility. IVF was originally developed to treat infertile women with irreversible tubal damage. In time it became evident that most causes of infertility unresponsive to conventional therapy could be treated with the various forms of ART, including IVF with intrauterine embryo transfer, gamete and zygote intrafallopian transfer (GIFT and ZIFT, respectively), and the micromanipulation of gametes and embryos. Technologic advances such as transvaginal ultrasonography have made the current procedures much less invasive, decreasing the risks to patients. New laboratory techniques have expanded the indications for IVF, allowing the clinician to reach a larger number of couples with complex infertility problems. Although variations of the basic procedure continue to be developed, the basic concept remains unchanged: assisting the fertilization process by combining the sperm and the egg in vitro, thereby bypassing any mechanical, immunologic, or unknown factors that might be impeding conception.

Following a parallel trend, the field of reproductive surgery and particularly operative laparoscopy has produced far-reaching advances in the recent past. The development of lasers and digital video equipment, as well as a large array of endoscopic instruments and stapling devices, have provided the substratum to a revolution in the way we approach gynecologic surgery, particularly reproductive surgery. Procedures that classically required a laparotomy can now be safely performed on an outpatient basis with lower cost, shorter hospital stay, and faster recovery. Despite the controversy these new surgical techniques have generated,[2] an increasing number of practitioners are endeavoring to acquire the skills necessary to perform complex endoscopic procedures.

Abnormalities of the uterine (fallopian) tube comprise one of the largest diagnostic groups presenting to most ART centers. Tubal disease accounts for approximately 25% of cases of infertility. Tubal damage or dysfunction may result from a variety of factors, including infection, intraabdominal surgery, and congenital malformations. In a series reported by Westrom[3] 12% of patients became infertile following a single episode of laparoscopically documented acute pelvic inflammatory disease (PID). After two episodes of infection this figure increased to 35% and after three or more episodes 75%. The overall infertility rate in women with a history of PID was 21% compared with only 3% for the control group in the same series. Pelvic infections that resulted in tuboovarian abscess formation led to infertility in 56% of affected women, with 11% ectopic gestations in the women who were able to conceive. Thus the increasing incidence of PID and other sexually transmitted diseases in the United States has led to a rise in tubal factor infertility. Numerous factors must be taken into consideration when choosing IVF or reconstructive surgery. Pertinent factors include the cause and extent of tubal disease, the woman's age, previous surgical therapy, the presence of associated infertility factors, physician bias, and the financial aspects of treatment.

The purpose of this chapter is to provide the reader with an understanding of the basic aspects of IVF and its role in the treatment of tubal disease, including the prognostic factors that have a significant impact on a successful outcome. Understanding the success rates, risks, and complications of tubal surgery and IVF permits the physician to provide appropriate guidance and more realistic expectations to the infertile couples suffering from tuboperitoneal disease. The appropriate decision regarding a surgical approach versus ART requires knowledge of the alternatives available, thereby facilitating counseling of the infertile couple.

Outcomes of Tubal Surgery

Salpingolysis and Ovariolysis

The introduction of laparoscopy into the field of gynecology has been invaluable for the diagnosis and treatment of pelvic adhesions. Peritubal adhesions may impair fertility by interfering with ovum pickup by the fallopian tube or by distorting the normal tuboovarian relations. Generally, adhesions are secondary to salpingitis, previous appendicitis, pelvic endometriosis, puerperal infection, or previous gynecologic surgery. Results obtained following lysis of adhesions depend on the presence of concurrent endosalpingeal damage and the severity of extratubal disease. Pelvic adhesions may be treated by laparotomy, macroscopically or microscopically, or by laparoscopy, using blunt or sharp dissection, electrocautery, or laser. The first question is whether adhesiolysis is efficacious in promoting pregnancy. Tulandi et al.[4] carried out a controlled study to evaluate the effect of salpingoovariolysis on subsequent fertility. The cumulative pregnancy rate in the group that underwent salpingoovariolysis was three times higher than in the nontreated group (32% versus 11% at 12 months and 45% versus 16% at 24 months). Their study strongly suggested that salpingoovariolysis is indeed associated with a higher pregnancy rate. Laparoscopic salpingoovariolysis as an initial procedure to promote fertility was popularized in North America by Gomel.[5] The intrauterine pregnancy rate after laparoscopic salpingoovariolysis was 62% and the ectopic pregnancy rate 5.4%.

The CO_2 laser has gained popularity for use in adhesiolysis. Advantages of the laser include precision, minimal bleeding, and minimal damage to adjacent tissue. In the animal model, the CO_2 laser resulted in less adhesion formation and less tissue injury when compared with electrocautery.[6] On the other hand, Tulandi[7] found no significant difference in the pregnancy rates or degree of periadnexal adhesions after salpingoovariolysis using the CO_2 laser versus the microdiathermy needle. Based on these and other studies, no technique appears to be superior for preventing adhesion reformation or improving pregnancy rates.

Finally, the issue of adhesiolysis by laparotomy versus laparoscopy has not been addressed in a prospective, well controlled manner. Luciano et al.,[8] in a study using rabbits, found that not only did laparoscopic adhesiolysis effectively reduce adhesions, de novo adhesion formation was greater after laparotomy than after laparoscopy. Thus laparoscopic salpingoovariolysis should be the first choice of surgical treatment for women with periadnexal adhesions. Because the disruption of tubal anatomy and function in these patients is generally minimal, one can expect a high rate of intrauterine pregnancy and a low rate of ectopic pregnancy. Patients with thicker, more vascular, more extensive adhesions have a much poorer prognosis after surgery.[9-11] Thus in the presence of adnexal adhesions, IVF should be reserved for those patients with severe disease or who have failed to conceive after approximately 1 year after surgical treatment.

Fimbrioplasty

Fimbrioplasty is defined as the lysis of fimbrial adhesions or dilatation of fimbrial phimosis. Fimbrial agglutination may interfere with oocyte pickup by the fallopian tube. The underlying process in most cases is PID; therefore involvement of the endosalpinx is frequently found. The pregnancy rates after fimbrioplasty are similar to those observed after salpingolysis or ovariolysis. In a review of the literature, Lavy et al.[12] concluded that the use of microsurgical technique has resulted in both an increase in intrauterine pregnancy (from 42% to 59%) and a decrease in the rate of ectopic pregnancy (from 14% to 6%) when compared with the rates reported for macrosurgery. Similar intrauterine pregnancy rates have been reported for laparoscopic fimbrioplasty, with ectopic pregnancy rates ranging between 5% and 14%.[5,13]

Salpingostomy

Distal tubal occlusion and varying degrees of dilatation of the distal tubal segment are usually a result of PID. The endosalpinx is often severely damaged as a result of the underlying disease process and the long-standing dilatation of the uterine tube that follows obstruction. Tubal function in these patients is generally severely compromised. The success of the repair depends on the size and thickness of the hydrosalpinx, the extent of disruption to the tubal mucosa, and the presence or absence of peritubal adhesions. Variation in reports of pregnancy rates after tubal reconstruction (17-44%) represents, at least in part, different degrees of intrinsic tubal damage associated with this condition and the duration of follow-up. In addition to an overall low pregnancy rate, the risk of ectopic pregnancy is higher than that observed after most other tubal procedures. Paradoxically, severe disease is reported to be associated with a lower ectopic pregnancy rate than is noted with moderate disease. Presumably, severe disease completely interferes with egg pickup, precluding any pregnancy, whereas with moderate tubal dysfunction there is a greater likelihood for ectopic pregnancy.

Schlaff et al.[14] reported on a series of 95 women who underwent microsurgical terminal neosalpingostomy for distal tubal obstruction. Pregnancy success was inversely related to the extent of tubal distortion and degree of adnexal adhesions. Interestingly, no significant difference in pregnancy outcome was observed compared to a group in whom microsurgical technique was not used. Microsurgical technique for salpingostomy resulted in a surprisingly high rate of ectopic pregnancy (7.8% versus 4.3%) when compared with that seen after macrosurgery, but the total pregnancy rate in the two groups was similar (27% versus 26%, respectively).[12] Perhaps the partial restoration of tubal function made possible by the new surgical technique allows ovum pickup, but the abnormal tube is unable to transport the embryo into the uterus properly, resulting in an ectopic pregnancy. The use of CO_2 laser for salpingostomy does not offer any clear advantages over electrocautery in terms of increasing the incidence of pregnancy or reducing the incidence of ectopic pregnancy.[15,16] As has occurred with microsurgery, laparoscopic salpingostomy seems comparable with the same procedure performed via laparotomy; and most of the conceptions occur within the first 18 months.[17] The use of laser surgery does not offer any advantage over other treatment modalities.[18,19]

Factors that influence the success of salpingostomy include the diameter of the hydrosalpinx, fimbrial appearance after eversion, presence of periovarian adhesions, and rugal pattern on hysterosalpingogram.[20] Only 7% of patients with preoperative hysterosalpingograms that indicated a poor prognosis (e.g., large diameter of hydrosalpinx, absence of rugal pattern) conceived in one series versus 70% of those in the good prognosis category.[21] More recently, salpingoscopy has been advocated as a method to assess the status of the tubal mucosa. Preliminary studies suggest that finding adhesions, agglutination, and flattened mucosa correlates with poor pregnancy outcome.[22] Most evidence seems to indicate that if pregnancy has not occurred within a reasonable time after surgery, the likelihood for a successful outcome is significantly diminished. Audibert et al.[23] studied 266 patients with distal tubal infertility who underwent microsurgical or laparoscopic procedures for correction. They concluded that pregnancy would most likely occur within 6–12 months after surgery and recommended IVF for all patients not achieving pregnancy during the first year. Based on what has been published to date, it appears that young patients with mild or moderate tubal disease should be offered tubal reconstructive surgery,[24] whereas those with severe disease in whom the potential benefit of tubal reconstruction is limited, should be treated primarily with IVF. Likewise, postoperative patients who have not conceived within the first year after surgery should be directed to IVF.

Proximal Tubal Occlusion

Tubocornual anastomosis is performed in cases of cornual obstruction. The outcome of this procedure was shown to depend on the etiology of the cornual block. Novy et al.[25] have shown by hysteroscopic tubal cannulation that hysterosalpingography misdiagnoses proximal tubal occlusion in approximately 50% of cases. Transcervical fallopian tube catheterization may be useful for elucidating false-positive results obtained by hysterosalpingography and for overcoming obstruction associated with a mucous plug or cornual synechiae.[26] Bilateral tubocornual anastomosis has been associated with intrauterine pregnancy rates ranging from 50%[27] to 71%[28] and ectopic pregnancy rates of 0%[27,28] to 40%.[29] Attempts to correct multiple occlusion sites of the fallopian tubes (bipolar tubal disease) have produced poor results. Patton et al.[30] reported the outcomes of tubal reconstructive surgery in 31 patients with both proximal and distal occlusions. The probability of conception at 2.5 years after surgery was 12%, but no live births were achieved. Thus multiple site tubal occlusion strongly suggests IVF therapy rather than surgical correction.

Reversal of Sterilization

Sterilization remains the most common method of contraception in the United States for women over age 30. Fortunately, tubal reanastomosis can often restore fertility. Success of tubal reversal procedures includes the following factors: length of each tube upon completion of the procedure,[31] type of sterilization procedure,[32] location of the anastomosis along the tube, age of the patient, and the presence of other coexisting tubal pathology. Henderson[33] found that the isthmus–isthmus anastomosis was the most successful in terms of pregnancy rates (81%), and that the length of the longest tube in centimeters multiplied by a factor of 10 provided a close approximation of the term delivery rate. Sterilization procedures associated with the least tubal damage (e.g. Silastic rings or clips) resulted in the most favorable outcome. The reversal of sterilization treated with unipolar cautery carries a notoriously high incidence of tubal gestation.[34]

When compared with the macrosurgical approach, the use of microsurgery has significantly improved the outcome of tubal anastomosis (62% versus 44%) and has significantly reduced the rate of ectopic pregnancy (2.3% versus 9.2%) (Table 20.1).[12] For the young patient in the good prognosis categories, microsurgical tubal reversal clearly offers excellent results and the opportunity for multiple conceptions. In contrast, reversal of sterilization in patients over age 40 is controversial. Trimbos-Kemper[35] achieved a 33% term pregnancy rate in patients 40 years of age and older, with a mean interval of 5.5 months from surgery to pregnancy. In 1992 the overall success rate for IVF in the United States for patients aged 40 years and over without a male factor was 7.2% (deliveries per retrievals).[36] Thus when normal ovarian function exists, treatment decisions should be made after a careful analysis of chances for success and the risks of each option. Needless to say, for patients who are poor candidates for reanastomosis because of inadequate tubal length, extensive cornual scarring, or distal fimbriectomy, IVF should be recommended. Special attention should be paid to the age factor, as with each year after age 40 fecundity

Table 20.1. Ectopic pregnancy after tubal surgery: summary

Technique	Pregnancy (%)		Ectopic pregnancy (%)	
	Mean	Range	Mean	Range
Salpingostomy				
Macrosurgery	42	35–65	3.4	1–20
Microsurgery	52	31–69	1.8	0–16
Fimbrioplasty				
Macrosurgery	42	36–50	14.0	10–18
Microsurgery	59	26–68	6.0	4–11
Neosalpingostomy				
Macrosurgery	27	20–38	4.2	2–20
Microsurgery	26	17–44	7.7	0–18
Tubal Anastomosis				
Macrosurgery	44	25–38	9.2	0–15
Microsurgery	62	35–78	2.3	1–6.2
Removal of ectopic pregnancy				
Salpingectomy	42	38–49	12.0	8–17
Salpingostomy	57	39–73	11.0	0–20

Adapted from Lavy et al.[12] Reprinted with permission of the publisher, the American Society for Reproductive Medicine (The American Fertility Society).

drastically decreases and IVF may afford an immediate chance for conception without the potential morbidity of abdominal surgery.

Ectopic Pregnancy and Tubal Reconstructive Surgery

The association of tubal surgery and ectopic pregnancy is well recognized. Tubal pregnancy results from a delay in the passage of the embryo through the fallopian tube. This delay can be caused by anatomic defects or tubal dysfunction. Tubal anatomy and function can be altered by tubal surgery or prior PID. The relative importance of these two factors is difficult to determine because both are often present in the same individual. The risk of ectopic pregnancy after tubal surgery varies greatly and depends on the prior condition of the tube, the nature of the surgical procedure performed, the technique utilized, and the surgeon's skill. Imperfect surgical repairs may lead to the formation of blind mucosal pouches, which in turn could entrap the ovum and thus predispose the patient to an ectopic pregnancy. Likewise, peritubal adhesions, which are a common sequela of surgery, may restrict tubal motility and thus interfere with ovum pickup or transport.

Patients with a history of ectopic pregnancy are at significant risk for recurrence. This risk is related to the underlying tubal disease that led to the initial ectopic pregnancy and to the surgical procedure performed for its removal. In a literature review that included 1083 women, Oelsner and Tarlatzis[37] calculated the risk of recurrent ectopic pregnancy after salpingectomy in women desiring pregnancy; they found that ectopic pregnancy occurred in 15.4% and intrauterine pregnancy in 36.5%.

Conservative procedures that endeavor to preserve the fallopian tube at the time of ectopic pregnancy removal are commonly utilized. Operative laparoscopy with a linear salpingostomy has become the procedure of choice for the treatment of ectopic pregnancy in the hemodynamically stable patient who desires to preserve her reproductive potential.[38,39] The rates of ectopic pregnancy recurrence are not different from those achieved after salpingectomy. A subgroup of special interest consists of women with one remaining patent oviduct after salpingostomy for ectopic pregnancy. In 15 such patients DeCherney et al.[40] have reported that 53% achieved intrauterine pregnancy and 20% a recurrent ectopic pregnancy. Of particular concern are women who have had multiple ectopic pregnancies. The high likelihood of repeat ectopic pregnancies and the low rates of intrauterine pregnancy[41,42] in this group strongly suggest that IVF should be the treatment of choice, with consideration given to prophylactic salpingectomy.

Outcomes of Assisted Reproduction

Cumulative Pregnancy Rates

To provide the couple with acceptable treatment alternatives, the gynecologic surgeon must be familiar with success rates of the various procedures as well as the variables involved in a realistic estimate of their chances of conception. The purpose of this section is to analyze the results of ART and the main prognostic factors that influence its outcome.

The most recent success rates reported by the Society for Assisted Reproductive Technology (SART) IVF-ET (embryos transferred) registry are summarized in Table 20.2.[36] In 1992 the delivery rates per retrieval following 37,164 stimulation cycles for IVF, GIFT, and ZIFT were 16.8%, 26.7%, and 22.8%, respectively. In addition, 5354 cryopreserved ET provided a delivery rate per retrieval of 11.5%. We have studied the cumulative pregnancy rates of couples with tubal factor infertility treated at our IVF program in relation to the patients' age and other associated infertility factors. The overall delivery rate per ET was 28.9% (303/1048) in 771 patients with a principal diagnosis of tubal factor infertility who underwent 1068 oocyte retrievals. Cumulative pregnancy rates for cycles 1 to 4 in patients with sole tubal factor were 32%, 59%, 70% and 77%, respectively (Fig 20.1). Delivery rates (28%, 55%, 62%, and 75% for cycles 1 to 4, respectively) did not differ significantly when compared with the notes from couples having other associated infertility factors [i.e., male factor, endometriosis, immunologic problems, diethylstilbestrol or (DES) exposure] in addition to tubal disease.

It is also of interest to note that neither the stage of tuboovarian disease nor any history of pelvic adhesions or tubal surgery seems to have a significant impact on the efficiency of IVF.[43] Nevertheless, a significant decline in pregnancy rates in patients with tubal factor infertility was observed in our IVF program when different age groups were compared: <30 years 48.4%,

Table 20.2. Reported outcomes for all ART procedures

Parameter	IVF	GIFT	ZIFT	Donor[a]	Cryopreserved ETs[b]
Cycles/procedures[c]	29,404	5,767	1,993	1,802	5,354
Cancellation (%)	15.4	16.2	15	5.2	NA
Retrievals	24,996	4,837	1,696	1,708	NA
Transfers	21,870	4,712	1,497	1,699	5,354
Transfers per retrieval (%)	87.5	97.4	88.3	99.4	NA
Pregnancies	5,279	1,621	488	625	820
Pregnancy loss (%)	20	16.9	21.1	14.9	23.8
Deliveries	4,206	1,273	386	534	619
Deliveries per retrieval (%)	16.8	26.7	22.8	31.3	NA
Singleton (%)	67.3	67.3	64.2	63.3	77.9
EPs	272	61	20	14	32
EP per transfer (%)	1.2	1.3	1.3	0.8	0.6
Birth defects per neonates delivered (%)[d]	1.9	2.4	2.5	1.7	1.3

Adapted from ref. 36. Reprinted with permission of the publisher, the American Society for Reproductive Medicine (The American Fertility Society).
NA, not available; EP, ectopic pregnancy.
[a]Donor includes known or anonymous, but not surrogate.
[b]Cryopreserved embryo transfer cycles not done in combination with fresh ETs and not with donor egg/embryo.
[c]Includes all cycles, regardless of age or diagnosis.
[d]Birth defect reporting did not account for all neonatal outcomes

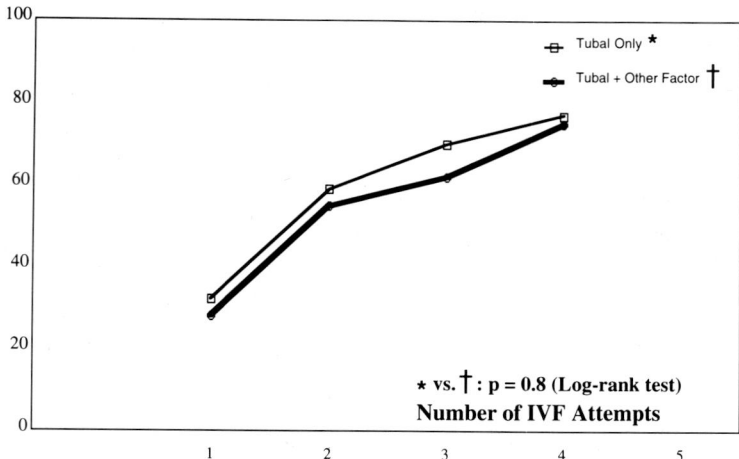

Figure 20.1. Life table analysis: cumulative pregnancy rates after four cycles of IVF in 771 patients with diagnosis of tubal factor ($n = 491$) and other associated factors in addition to tubal disease ($n = 280$) treated at New York Hospital–Cornell Medical Center from December 1989 through December 1992.

30–34 years 44%, 35–38 years 28%, 39–40 years 20%, 41–42 years 9%, and >42 years 4.3% (Fig 20.2).

Age Factor

One of the most important prognostic factors for fecundability in humans is the age of the female partner. The classic study is that of the Hutterites.[44] The Hutterites live in the Dakotas, Montana, and adjacent parts of Canada. Contraception is condemned, and because of the communal arrangement of their society there is no incentive to limit the size of their families. The average age at the time of the final pregnancy is 40.9 years, and there is a definite increase of infertility with age.[44]

The decline of fertility among married couples with advancing age has been documented repeatedly.[45] It is safe to say that about one-third of women who defer pregnancy until their mid to late 30s have an infertility problem, and at least one half of women over age 40 experience difficulty conceiving. This measurable decline in fecundity begins at least 15 years before menopause. During this period menstrual periods are regular, but there is an observed steady decrease in cycle length due to a shortened follicular phase.[46] Cycle lengths are shortest during the late thirties, an age when subtle but real increases in follicle-stimulating hormone (FSH) and decreases in in-

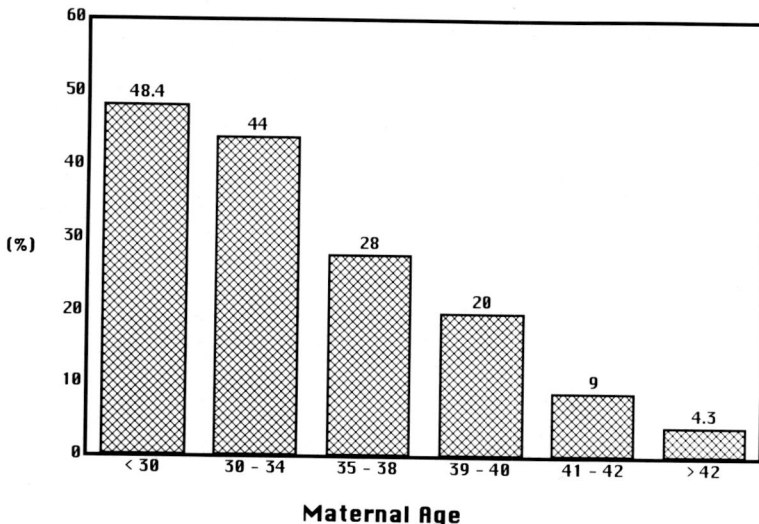

Figure 20.2. Pregnancy outcome (deliveries per transfer) by maternal age group in women with tubal factor infertility treated at New York Hospital–Cornell Medical Center from December 1989 through December 1992.

hibin levels are occurring.[47] This change is often manifested by accelerated follicular growth, although at the same time fewer follicles develop per cycle. Eventually menopause occurs because the supply of follicles has been depleted.

The decline in female fecundity has been observed with IVF and other assisted reproductive procedures.[48,49] These findings, however, are not confined to ART; women undergoing donor insemination because of a clear male factor exhibit a significant decline in fecundity with increasing age over 30 years.[50] Success rates associated with IVF decline significantly with the advancing age of the female patient. Many ART programs have established an age cutoff based on the markedly poorer prognosis for women over 40 owing to the reduced pregnancy rate and increased risk of spontaneous abortion.[51] Unlike their male partners, women are endowed with a finite and nonreplenishable complement of germ cells that peaks at midgestation.[52] From this point onward, no further gametogenesis occurs; ongoing follicular atresia eventually culminates in menopause. The absolute number and functional capacity of follicles and germ cells comprise what may be called the *ovarian reserve,* which affects a given patient's response to stimulation and her chance for success. A number of tests have been described to assess ovarian reserve indirectly, including the clomiphene citrate challenge[53] and leuprolide screening tests.[54] Patterns of response to either drug place the patient in good, intermediate, or poor prognosis groups. Patients in the poor prognosis group have fewer oocytes retrieved, lower peak estradiol (E_2) levels in response to ovarian stimulation, and decreased pregnancy rates. Another simple, highly predictive approach that is employed frequently in this age group consists in measuring basal levels of FSH and E_2 on day 3 of the menstrual cycle.[55,56] Serum FSH concentrations during the early follicular phase seem to rise at least 5–6 years before the onset of menopause.[57] This subtle elevation, signaling a decline in ovarian reserve in the regularly menstruating woman, is often manifested by a poor ovarian response to gonadotropin stimulation in women undergoing IVF.[58] The results of a study comparing stimulated cycles in young and older women[59] suggested that decreased serum inhibin levels are responsible for the elevation in FSH secretion. It is unknown, however, whether this decline in ovarian inhibin production is due to a reduction in the number of follicles or to impairment of the maximum ability of the granulosa cells to produce inhibin.[60]

The relation between elevated FSH concentrations and IVF outcome is striking. The effect is observed in the pattern of ovarian response to ovarian stimulation, pregnancy rates, and implantation efficiency. A review of our experience (January 1989 to June 1993) included 1249 stimulation cycles and 875 retrievals wherein the baseline serum FSH level was measured during the cycle of stimulation. It revealed that the mean peak E_2 level on the day of human chorionic gonadotropin (hCG) administration declines steadily with increasing FSH concentration. This fall in the hormonal response is paralleled by a similar decline in the mean number of oocytes retrieved per cycle. The ongoing pregnancy rate per retrieval in this series drops from 21.1% in women with day 3 FSH concentrations <10 mIU/ml to 8.3% in women with a basal FSH level exceeding 20 mIU/ml (Fig 20.3). More importantly, the per-embryo implantation rate (fetal heartbeat/embryo replaced) declines from 12–13% in women with FSH concentrations <20 mIU/ml to 6–7% in women with levels >20 mIU/ml (Fig 20.4). Analogous to the rise in FSH, an elevation of serum E_2 levels exceeding 75 pg/ml on day 3 of the menstrual cycle is, in our experience, a poor prognostic indicator and may be due to an increase in FSH secretion during the late luteal phase of the prior cycle.[56] The negative feedback of E_2 on the pituitary could be suppressing and potentially masking what would otherwise be a high FSH level. It is also likely that elevated day 3 E_2 concentrations are a consequence of early follicular recruitment, a phenomenon that may account for the shortening of the follicular phase seen during the perimenopausal transition.

It appears that the major obstacle to natural conception in the older woman is related to diminished embryo implantation. In our pro-

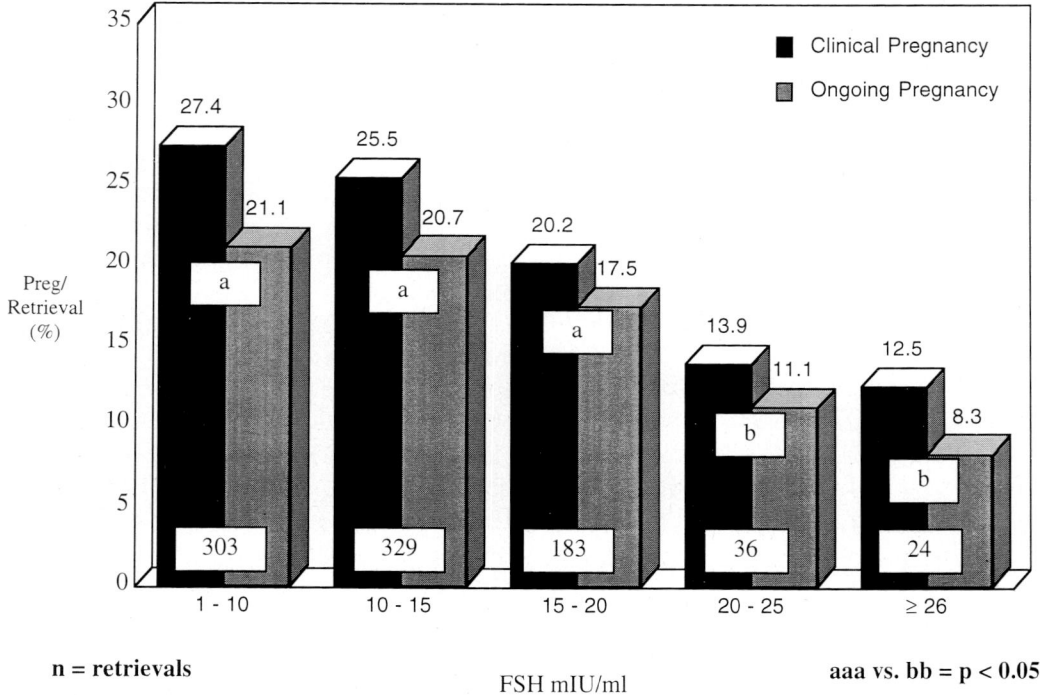

Figure 20.3. Clinical and ongoing pregnancy rates after 875 retrievals wherein the serum FSH level was measured during the cycle of stimulation at the New York Hospital–Cornell Medical Center from January 1989 through June 1993.

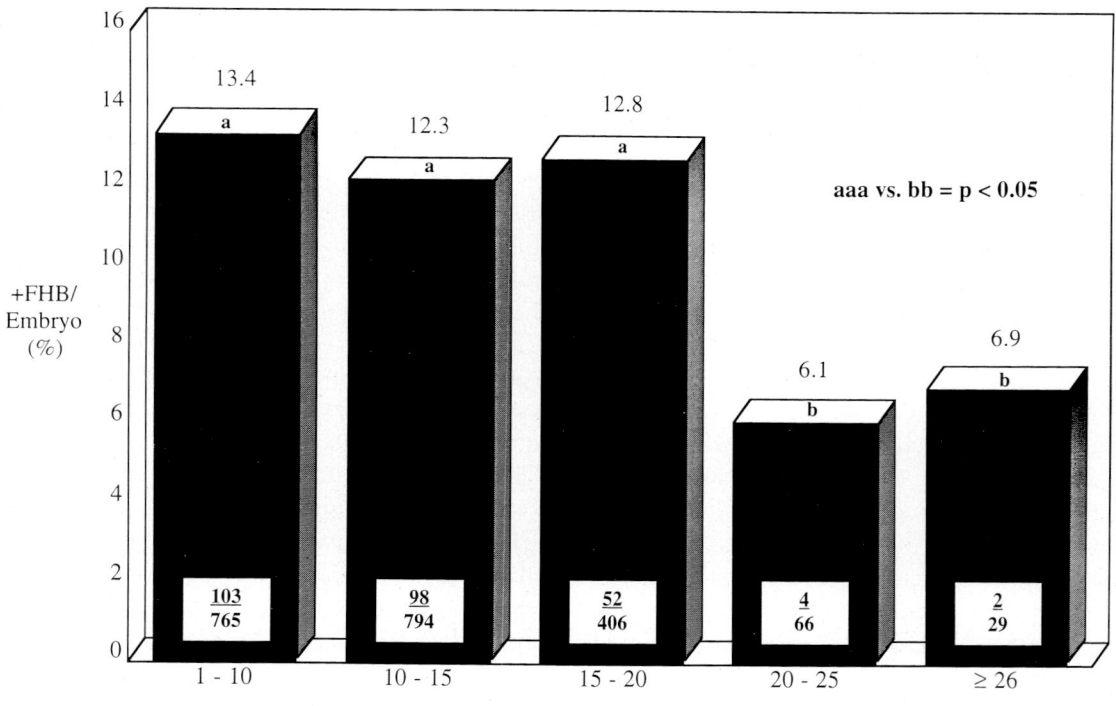

Figure 20.4. Implantation rate per transfer (number with fetal heartbeat detected on ultrasonography per embryos transferred) by day 3. FSH levels were measured during the cycle of stimulation at the New York Hospital–Cornell Medical Center from January 1989 through June 1993. aaa versus bb: $p < 0.05$.

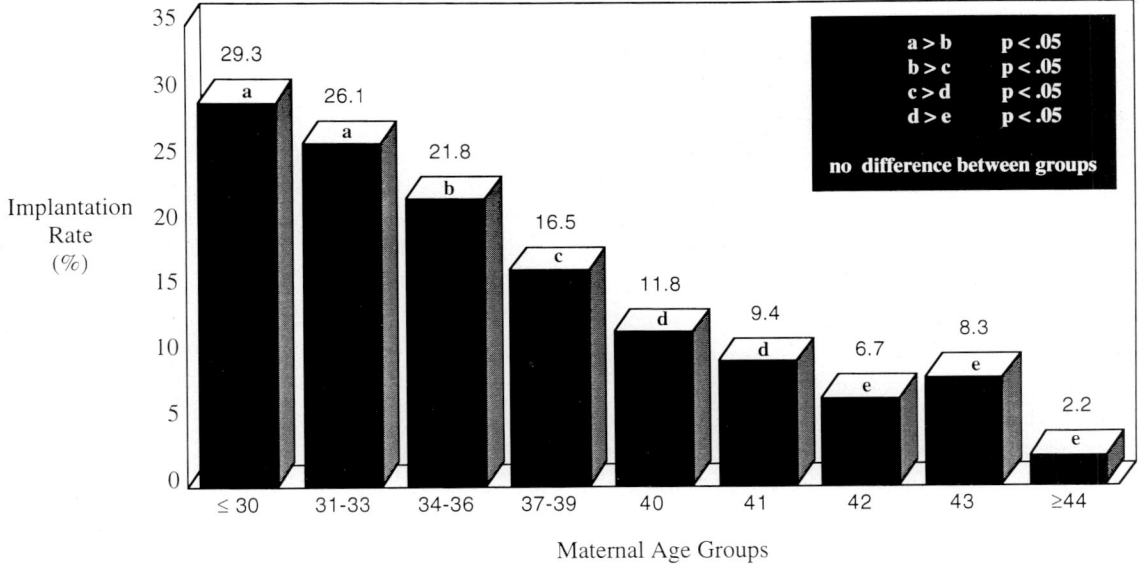

Figure 20.5. Implantation rate per embryo (number with fetal heartbeat detected on ultrasonography per embryos transferred) by maternal age group at the New York Hospital–Cornell Medical Center from January 1990 through June 1993. aaa versus bb: $p < 0.05$.

gram the mean number of embryos replaced is constant across all age groups, suggesting that embryo number per se is not the critical determinant of the decrease in success rates seen with advancing age. Indeed, the per-embryo implantation rate declines from 29.0% in women under 34 years to 21.8% at age 34, with a linear decline to 2.2% per embryo at age 44 (Fig 20.5). When agonadal women receive oocytes from younger donors, their pregnancy rates are among the highest observed in assisted reproduction, suggesting that the decreased implantation rate with advancing age is clearly related to poor oocyte quality.[61] Moreover, increasing evidence obtained from our preimplantation genetic diagnosis program suggests that embryos obtained from women over age 40 have a significantly higher frequency of aneuploidy than those from younger women.[62] These findings are consistent with observations seen in IVF patients, who display higher spontaneous abortion rates with advancing age.[63] This increased rate of spontaneous abortion is directly related to an increased rate of chromosomal abnormalities in the abortuses, probably because prolonged meiotic arrest in aged oocytes leads to nondysjunctional events.

Because of the rapid decline in fertility potential in women over age 40, the older patient should undergo an accelerated evaluation. Day 3 FSH and E_2 levels are helpful when counseling the patient regarding realistic goals or directing the patient with elevated gonadotropins toward ovum donation. Laparoscopy or surgical repair of diseased fallopian tubes should be seriously questioned in women approaching their late thirties in whom (even when baseline day 3 gonadotropin levels are normal on initial evaluation) ovarian reserve may decline precipitously along with their chance for a successful pregnancy. In this particular group of women, we believe efforts should be directed toward the ART methods that could provide the highest success during the shortest time interval. Although controversial, the combined therapy of controlled ovarian hyperstimulation (COH) and intrauterine insemination (IUI) has been introduced as an effective method for treating infertile couples with patent fallopian tubes when more traditional therapy has failed.[64,65]

Evidence suggests that cycle fecundity rates are significantly higher using a combination of COH and IUI than with either modality alone.[66] Nevertheless, the fecundity rate showed a significant decrease after three cycles. Consequently, the number of attempts should be limited to three or four and the patient directed toward IVF without further delay.

Techniques of ART

To provide proper counseling regarding treatment alternatives for tubal infertility, the gynecologist must be familiar with the results of contemporary surgical techniques as well as the clinical prognosis after assisted reproductive procedures. Treatment options should be guided also by careful comparisons of the steps involved and the risks and morbidity of the procedures being considered. This section describes the present approach and the state of the art clinical and laboratory aspects of IVF.

Initial Evaluation

At the outset the clinician should determine the appropriateness of IVF therapy with the aim of individualizing the treatment regimen. A thorough review of prior infertility evaluations and therapy is mandatory. Particular attention should be paid to previous IVF treatments, especially the type of ovarian stimulation protocols and responses. A complete history and physical examination should be performed for both partners. Examination of the woman should include a uterine trial transfer at the time of a uterine sounding to determine the depth of the cavity and to anticipate any potential technical difficulties prior to the embryo transfer. Cervical cultures for *Neisseria gonorrhoeae, Chlamydia trachomatis,* and *Mycoplasma* should be obtained. Ovarian reserve can be assessed by measuring baseline serum FSH and E_2 levels on day 3 of the menstrual cycle. Hysterosalpingographic films should be reviewed to evaluate intrauterine pathology, including submucous leiomyomas, polyps, synechiae, or the presence of a septum, which may interfere with embryo implantation or increase the risk of spontaneous abortion. In selected patients, vaginal ultrasonography of the endometrial cavity may be sufficient to rule out the presence of significant pathology that may interfere with implantation. Semen analysis [ideally, computer-assisted semen analysis (CASA)] along with a sperm separation technique should be performed by the IVF laboratory so as to select and anticipate the appropriate laboratory methods to be utilized on the day of egg retrieval. The procedural aspects of the IVF cycle should be reviewed, along with a detailed description of age- and case-specific success rates. The discussion should include a review of potential physical and psychological stresses, risks, and costs.

Ovarian Stimulation for IVF

Although the first human pregnancy following IVF resulted from a single fertilized oocyte obtained during a spontaneous menstrual cycle, it has subsequently become clear that success rates improve as the number of transferred conceptuses is increased. Given the relative inefficiency of single embryo transfer, in addition to the cumbersome need for around-the-clock monitoring most ART programs routinely utilize ovarian stimulation in an effort to attain multiple follicular development. Nonetheless, a renewed interest in natural-cycle ART has been advocated by some clinicians; use of the natural cycle obviates certain risks, including multiple gestations and ovarian hyperstimulation syndrome (OHSS). However, natural cycle IVF is associated with high cancellation rates and significantly lower pregnancy rates than are seen with stimulated cycles.[67] Gonadotropin-based regimens are commonly employed by most ART programs, usually combined with gonadotropin-releasing hormone agonists (GnRHa). The use of adjunctive GnRHa therapy has clearly affected IVF outcomes by reducing cycle cancellation rates[68] and preventing premature luteinizing hormone (LH) surges often associated with premature luteinization. More importantly, it is now generally accepted that the routine use of GnRHa in ovarian stimulation regimens also leads to an overall enhancement of pregnancy rates.[69] A meta-analysis of randomized, controlled trials supports the routine administra-

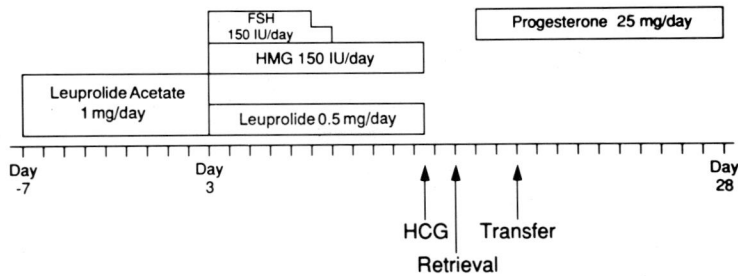

Figure 20.6. Standard *step-down* ovarian stimulation protocol for IVF at the New York Hospital–Cornell Medical Center (GnRH analogs and gonadotropins). (Reprinted from ref. 73, with permission)

tion of GnRHa in IVF and GIFT stimulation cycles.[70] It is not clear, however, whether the benefit of GnRHa in ART is due to improved oocyte or embryo quality or to an increase in the mean number of oocytes retrieved. Our analysis of 294 gonadotropin-only versus 449 gonadotropin–GnRHa cycles in our program supports the latter contention. The results revealed no significant difference in fertilization rates or in the per-embryo implantation and delivery rates, whereas the average numbers of oocytes recovered and embryos replaced were significantly increased during the GnRHa cycles.[71] When employed as an adjunct to COH, GnRHa may be administered via a long or a short protocol. With the long protocol, which is probably the most prevalent approach, GnRHa administration is initiated during the midluteal phase of the preceding cycle. Pituitary suppression usually occurs within 7–10 days, a phenomenon heralded by E_2 suppression and the onset of menstruation. Gonadotropin therapy is begun on cycle day 3 (Fig 20.6) or whenever adequate estradiol suppression is demonstrated. The GnRHa dosage is reduced by 50% and is discontinued on the day of hCG injection. We have favored a tapering step-down gonadotropin regimen, wherein the maximal dose of hMG or FSH (a total of four to six ampuls) is administered on days 3, 4, and 5 of the cycle followed by a dosage reduction to two ampuls as soon as follicular recruitment has been achieved. This approach to ovulation induction has proved clinically efficacious and is further supported by experimental evidence in a primate model suggesting that a step-down protocol results in improved synchronization of follicular maturation.[72]

Various strategies have been designed to individualized ovarian stimulation protocols. One of the major challenges of ART is the pursuit of effective approaches to the treatment of the low responder patient. In a significant proportion of cases, a poor response to ovarian stimulation is the result of diminished ovarian reserve, a consequence of advanced chronologic age or of premature oocyte senescence in the young patient. In these instances, a poor response to ovulation induction can often be predicted by an elevated FSH or E_2 level on day 3. Although intuitively sound, current evidence suggests that increasing the dose of exogenous gonadotropins is of limited value in the therapy of low-responder patients.[73,74] Another strategy in the management of this group of patients is to reduce the dose of adjunctive GnRHa. This approach is most useful for older women and those with a history of idiopathic hyporesponsiveness, in contrast to patients manifesting overt signs of incipient ovarian failure (high baseline FSH) who are likely to benefit from the elimination of GnRHa from their regimen so as to avoid oversuppression. Furthermore, the short GnRHa protocol (or "flare-up") may also improve the outcome for selected patients with a history of poor response by taking advantage of the agonistic phase of these agents. Management of the low-responder patient remains one of the most troublesome challenges of ART; and for many such women oocyte donation remains the only highly successful option. On the other end of the spectrum, women displaying a high response to ovarian stimulation enjoy a higher success rate following ART than do low-responders. A review of more than 1300 IVF cycles between January 1990 and December 1991 from our program revealed that high-responders (mean peak E_2 level >2000 pg/ml) had a delivery rate of 41% per transfer compared to the low-responders (mean peak E_2 <400 pg/ml), who experienced a delivery rate of 19.6% per transfer.[73] Women who manifest an exaggerated ovarian response to ovulation induction pose a unique challenge, however; a significant proportion of this subgroup of patients have either polycystic ovary syndrome (PCOS) or an elevated baseline LH/FSH ratio. They are at risk for cycle cancellation due to excessive E_2 levels, frequently in the setting of an inadequate number of mature preovulatory follicles. If hCG is administered, these women are placed at high risk for the development of severe OHSS, particularly if pregnancy occurs. We have developed what has so far proved to be a successful approach to the COH of high-responder patients, employing a dual approach to ovarian suppression with oral contraceptive pills (OCPs) and leuprolide acetate. OCPs are administered for 25 days, followed by subcutaneous leuprolide, 1 mg/day, overlapping with the final 5 days of OCP administration. Low-dose gonadotropin stimulation (two ampules per day) is initiated on the third day of withdrawal bleeding, at which point the dose of leuprolide is decreased to 0.5 mg/day. Among this difficult cohort of patients we observed delivery rates per embryo transfer of 73.3%, with a cycle cancellation rate of only 10%.[75]

Techniques of Oocyte Retrieval

Oocyte retrieval is performed 35 hours after hCG administration, an interval sufficient to allow oocyte maturation but prior to ovulation. Initially reported in 1983,[76] ultrasound-directed transvaginal follicle aspiration has virtually replaced the endoscopic approach, except in cases where cannulation of the fallopian tubes is required (i.e., GIFT). The patient is placed in the dorsal lithotomy position, and the vagina is prepared with an antiseptic solution followed by copious saline irrigation. Intravenous sedation is adequate for most transvaginal oocyte retrievals. Intravenous prophylactic antibiotics is recommended in high risk patients (i.e., those with a history of PID or tubal disease, or both). A transvaginal ultrasound probe housing a high-frequency transducer (5 or 7 MHz) is introduced in the vagina with a fixed needle guide. The maximum diameter of each follicle is aligned with the puncture line on the screen, and the needle is advanced into the follicle. A negative pressure of 100–120 mm Hg is applied to the needle just prior to follicle puncture; collapse of the follicle is visualized on the ultrasonography screen, and the needle tip may be used to curette the follicle. Following aspiration of each follicle, the needle may be advanced to the next follicle, removed and flushed, or kept in place until the oocyte is identified by the embryologist. We do not advocate routine flushing of follicles except in the rare circumstance in which oocytes are not found in the follicular aspirates. Advantages of the transvaginal approach include (1) ovarian accessibility in cases of laparoscopically inaccessible ovaries (e.g., severe pelvic adhesions); (2) reduced morbidity and easier patient recovery; (3) avoidance of general anesthesia; (4) decreased operative time and (5) avoidance of the need for CO_2 pneumoperitoneum. After oocyte retrieval, all patients in our program are treated with methylprednisolone (16 mg/day) and tetracycline (250 mg/6 hrs) for 4 days. Cohen et al.[77] have shown that low-dose immunosuppression during the first 4 days after oocyte retrieval improved implantation of partially zona dissected embryos, perhaps by diminishing the presence of immune cells and the inflammatory response of the endometrium.

Embryo Transfer

Embryo transfers are usually performed 48–72 hours after oocyte retrieval. Pregnancy rates improve as the number of embryos replaced is increased.[78] Beyond four embryos, the multiple gestation rate rises sharply; thus frequently the number of conceptuses transferred is limited to three in patients ≤ 34 years of age, four in the group 34–40 years, and up to five in patients > 40 years of age.

Embryo transfer is performed by the transcervical approach except in cases requiring tubal cannulation. A variety of transfer catheters are available. All are composed of nontoxic plastic, but they differ in length, caliber, stiffness, and location of the distal opening. Some catheters are inserted through a rigid introducer, whereas others are threaded directly into the uterus without an outer sheath. Preference for patient positioning also varies, although it has not been shown to affect success. Once the patient is positioned on the examining table, a sterile speculum is inserted, excess cervical mucus is aspirated, and the cervix is cleansed with culture medium. Although rarely necessary, a tenaculum may be used to straighten the uterine axis if difficulty is encountered negotiating the cervical canal. The embryos are loaded into a sterile catheter in a small volume of transfer medium. The embryologist delivers the loaded catheter to the physician, who inserts it transcervically toward the uterine fundus. The embryos are slowly injected using a small syringe attached to the catheter. It is important to minimize endometrial trauma, as it has been reported that fresh bleeding reduces implantation rates.[79] The catheter is returned to the embryologist, who examines it under the microscope; it is flushed with medium in an effort to identify any retained embryos. If the catheter is clean (i.e., all embryos are transferred), the patient is transferred to a holding area where she remains supine for 30 minutes prior to discharge. The length of this posttransfer resting period probably has no bearing on outcome.

After embryo transfer, most programs routinely implement exogenous luteal support. This policy is guided by the concern that ovulation induction can predispose the patient to luteal phase insufficiency, and that follicular aspiration may remove some of the granulosa cells lining the follicles. This philosophy is supported by clinical evidence that the incidence of histologic luteal phase defect is increased in canceled IVF cycles.[80] Our regimen consists in daily intramuscular progesterone in oil (25 mg) starting on the day after oocyte retrieval. The dose may be increased to 50 mg/day when the peak E_2 level is > 2000 pg/ml, in an effort to promote a more favorable luteal progesterone/E_2 ratio. Progesterone may also be administered as vaginal suppositories, or luteal support can be accomplished with supplemental injections of hCG, although this practice increases the risk of OHSS in some patients.[81] Pregnancy is documented by an elevated serum β-hCG level 10–11 days after embryo transfer. Serial titers may be obtained to demonstrate a normal rise. Ultrasound examination is performed 3 weeks later to assess fetal viability and the presence of multiple gestation. We generally discontinue luteal support at this time except in instances of egg donation, where in the absence of corpus luteum function endometrial support is required until documentation of adequate steroid production by the fetoplacental unit.

Embryo and Oocyte Cryopreservation

The first pregnancy achieved after the transfer of cryopreserved-thawed preembryos was reported in 1983 by Trounson and Mohr.[82] Prior to the availability of embryo cryopreservation most clinics inseminated only a few oocytes, wasting the potential of many viable eggs. Embryo cryopreservation allows insemination of all recovered oocytes, thus maximizing the chance of transferring an optimal number of embryos, with the ability to freeze "excess" embryos for future transfer during a natural cycle. In successful programs, cryopreservation increases the cumulative pregnancy rate per oocyte retrieval.[83]

Human embryos may be cryopreserved at virtually any developmental stage, from pronuclear (zygote) to blastocyst. To date, freezing mature human oocytes generally has resulted in poor cryosurvival, poor fertilization, and few live births,[84,85] probably due to cryoinjury to the zona pellucida and meiotic spindle. Transfer of frozen embryos is usually performed during the natural cycle, with close monitoring of serum or urine LH levels (or both) to detect the onset of the LH surge. Alternatively, the patient's ovarian function can be suppressed with a GnRHa and her endometrial maturation controlled with exogenous estrogen and progesterone replacement. The goal is to transfer the embryos into an endometrium synchronized with their postinsemination age. Overall, approximately 50% of cryopreserved-thawed embryos survive. Only embryos retaining 50% or more of their original blastomeres are transferred. Of the 5354 frozen embryo transfer cycles in the 1992 AFS-SART Registry, the clinical pregnancy and delivery rates were 15.3% and 11.6%, respectively.[36] It has been our experience that cryopreserved embryos provide approximately half of the pregnancy rates when compared with "fresh" embryo transfer cycles.

ZIFT, GIFT

The first successful pregnancy resulting from translaparoscopic placement of gametes (ovum and sperm) into the human fallopian tube was reported in 1984.[86] Although there is considerable overlap between the indications for GIFT and IVF, GIFT requires at least one normal fallopian tube. The major indications for GIFT are idiopathic infertility and mild male factor, although the use of the procedure has been expanded to treat immunologic infertility, endometriosis, DES exposure, cervical factor, and anovulation.[87] Patients with tubal factor infertility are not good candidates for a procedure in which fertilization takes place in the fallopian tube. Nevertheless, in those cases where either GIFT or IVF is appropriate, the decision should be made by the couple and their physician, after considering the various procedural aspects, risks, and benefits.

Stimulation protocols, monitoring follicular recruitment, and timing of hCG administration are similar to those for IVF. Although ultrasound-guided transcervical techniques for fallopian tube cannulation have been developed,[88] their practice is limited; and GIFT is generally performed laparoscopically or, less frequently, through a minilaparotomy. Follicular aspiration is performed laparoscopically or transvaginally prior to laparoscopic tubal cannulation. The GIFT catheter loaded with a mixture of gametes is inserted into each tube to a depth of 1.5–2.0 cm, and the mixture is injected. The luteal phase is managed in a manner similar to that following IVF. The 1992 SART Registry[36] reported a clinical pregnancy rate of 33.5% and a live birth rate per retrieval of 26.3%. A total of 61 ectopic pregnancies were reported, representing 1.3% of transfers performed and 3.6% of the total clinical pregnancies.

Investigators have suggested that GIFT has certain advantages over IVF: fertilization occurs in the fallopian tube, a more physiologic environment than a culture dish. In addition the embryo remains in the usual in vivo milieu rather than the laboratory. Moreover, extracorporeal culture allegedly requires a more sophisticated laboratory than is required for the GIFT procedure. GIFT may be more ethically acceptable to some religious groups on the basis that fertilization occurs in the human body rather than in the laboratory. On the other hand, GIFT is associated with some inherent disadvantages: (1) It requires laparoscopy with general anesthesia; (2) it does not provide information regarding fertilization unless concurrent IVF is performed; and (3) it is inappropriate in cases of maternal anti-sperm antibodies, tubal factor, extensive pelvic adhesions, or cases of severe male factor. Although reported success rates have been superior to those with IVF-ET, one must consider the differences in experience and efficiency between embryology laboratories as well as the selection bias inherent in directing patients toward one procedure or the other.

Tubal embryo transfer combines IVF with the intrafallopian tube replacement of fertilized oocytes.[89] These procedures include ZIFT, pronuclear stage tubal transfer (PROST), and tubal embryo transfer (TET). Indications and patient selection are similar to those for GIFT, and again at least one normal fallopian tube must be present. TET procedures combine the advantages of an intrafallopian tube milieu for early embryogenesis with the diagnostic information obtained by observing fertilization in vitro. Standard IVF procedures are applied to the gametes, and in general a maximum of four zygotes are transferred laparoscopically to the fallopian tubes. The 1992 AFS-SART Registry reported an overall success rate of 22.8 deliveries per retrieval. In addition, 20 ectopic pregnancies were reported, representing 1.3% of transfers.[36]

Male Factor Infertility: Assisted Fertilization

Approximately 40% of infertile couples have a primary male factor. Thus semen analysis should be performed early during the infertility evaluation. Normal parameters include sperm concentration $\geq 20 \times 10^6$/ml, motility $\geq 40\%$, and $\geq 60\%$ normal forms by standard criteria. An

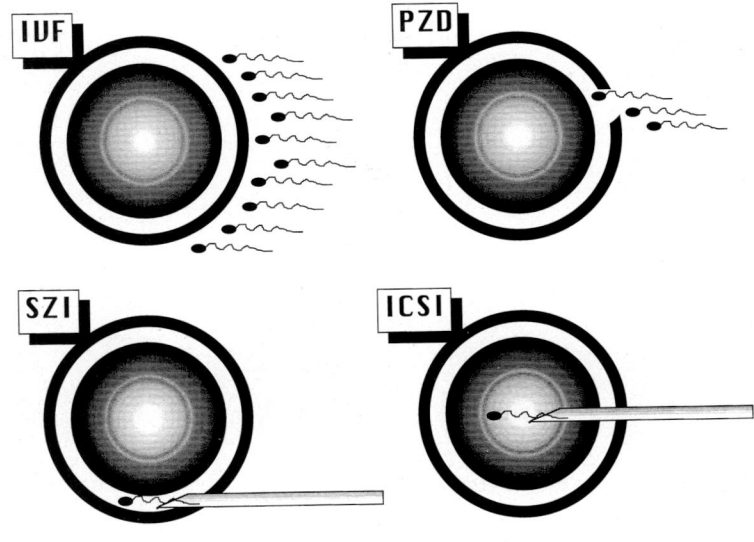

Figure 20.7. Methods of micromanipulation-assisted fertilization. Partial zona drilling (PZD) entails creation of an artificial breach in the zona pellucida, thereby allowing sperm direct access to the oolemma. Subzonal insertion (SZI): Spermatozoa are aspirated into a hollow microneedle and are deposited directly into the perivitelline space of the oocyte. Intracytoplasmic sperm injection (ICSI): A single spermatozoon contained within a microneedle is injected directly into the cytoplasm of the oocyte. (Adapted from J. Cohen, *Micromanipulation of Gametes and Embryoes,* p. 114. Reprinted with permission © 1992 by Raven Press)

alternate system of morphologic grading has been proposed by Kruger et al. that appears to be highly prognostic of IVF outcome.[90] Conventional IVF is useful for treatment of refractory male factor infertility. The ability to add high concentrations of motile sperm to oocytes in a small volume of medium increases the likelihood of fertilization. Moreover, IVF has significant diagnostic and prognostic value, as the ability of spermatozoa to fertilize oocytes can be assessed directly. Men who have severe asthenospermia (motility of < 10%), teratospermia (morphology of < 2% normal forms by strict criteria), or oligospermia (sperm density of $< 5 \times 10^6$ sperm/ml) have reduced chances for fertilization in vitro and may require assisted fertilization.[91] Assisted fertilization includes a variety of gamete microsurgical procedures aimed at promoting normal fertilization in couples at risk for fertilization failure following conventional insemination.

Four microsurgically assisted fertilization procedures have been described in humans (Fig. 20.7). The first of these methods involves creating an artificial gap in the zona pellucida, which allows motile spermatozoa to pass freely through the incision. With this "zona drilling" procedure, first developed in the mouse, a small volume of acidic solution is expelled from a microneedle onto a small area of the zona until it ruptures, followed by insemination.[92] Because application of zona drilling to clinical IVF was not successful, a mechanical procedure for introducing a gap in the zona was used as an alternative. This method, called partial zona drilling (PZD), resulted in the first human pregnancy from microsurgical fertilization.[93] The successful implementation of this technique was limited to male factor cases with sufficient spermatozoa (> 50,000/ml). However, excessive rates of polyspermy (> 20% per oocyte) reduced its clinical efficiency. A third procedure, subzonal insertion (SZI), was subsequently developed and involves the direct insertion of one or more sperm into the perivitelline space. Embryos derived from SZI implant at a significantly higher rate than those resulting from PZD.[94] The deposit of large quantities of sperm in the perivitelline space may increase the fertilization rate considerably—but at the expense of increasing the proportion of polyspermic embryos. Avoiding polyspermic fertilization has been accomplished by the development of the intracytoplasmic sperm injection (ICSI) procedure.[95] This new technique involves direct injection of a single spermatozoa into the cytoplasm of the

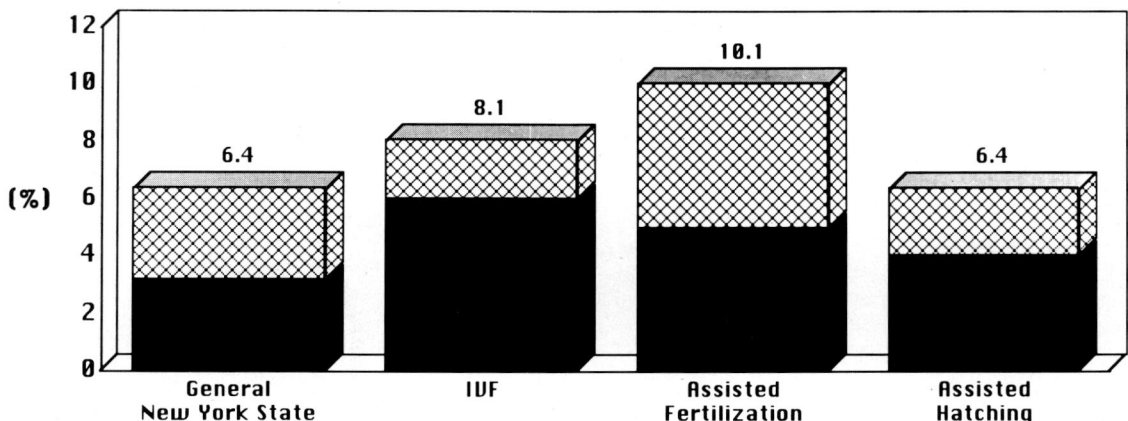

Figure 20.8. Comparison of the incidence of major and minor malformations after conventional IVF, assisted fertilization, and assisted hatching with the general population in New York State. (Courtesy of Dr. Gianpiero D. Palermo, The Center for Reproductive Medicine and Infertility, The New York Hospital–Cornell Medical Center, New York, NY)

oocyte. ICSI is presently reserved for treatment of infertile couples who have previously failed to fertilize via standard in vitro insemination or couples in whom the male partner has severely impaired semen parameters. In addition, ICSI offers excellent possibilities in cases of epididymal sperm aspiration or when the semen sample is produced by electroejaculation. Since its development, ICSI has resulted in overall fertilization rates of 55–65% per oocyte worldwide. The significant and consistent increase in fertilization achieved by ICSI, compared to SZI,[96] has led to the abandonment of all the previously utilized assisted fertilization procedures. The author's experience (at Cornell) from September 1993 to October 1994 involved treatment of 471 couples, 235 of whom had previously failed fertilization. The remaining 236 couples could not be treated by regular IVF because of poor semen parameters. Of 3991 microinjected mature oocytes, 67.1% displayed two pronuclei, with only 5 patients having no embryos for replacement. The clinical pregnancy rate (confirmed by a fetal heartbeat on transvaginal ultrasonography) was 41.4% per retrieval (195/471). Eleven of those patients had a spontaneous abortion between 7 and 11 weeks' gestation, resulting in an ongoing pregnancy rate of 39.1% per retrieval.

Data obtained regarding the rate of congenital malformations in infants conceived through standard IVF have not yielded any increase in the rate of congenital anomalies with basic IVF.[36] Despite this fact, our experience indicates a rise in the incidence of congenital anomalies following the microsurgical treatment of extreme male factor infertility patients and those with unexplained failure of fertilization. Information was obtained from a survey detailing the outcomes of pregnancies resulting from microsurgical fertilization.[97] Congenital malformations, both major and minor, were noted in 11 of 111 infants (9.9%), with major anomalies found in 6 (5.4%) (Fig 20.8). Although these data seem to indicate a higher rate of congenital malformations in children conceived through microsurgical fertilization, the interpretation of these initial data must be approached with caution. Not only is the rate for all congenital malformations in the general population difficult to assess, there is also controversy as to what constitutes major or minor malformations. Although initial reports on the incidence of congenital anomalies following ICSI are encouraging,[95] the evolution of pregnancies obtained by microinjection must be carefully assessed. It is our policy to routinely caution patients undergoing microsurgical fertilization about the potential slight increase in congenital anomalies. We advise strict monitoring of all pregnancies, including the ascertainment of karyotype by chorionic villus sampling (CVS) or amniocentesis, as well as obtaining high-level ultrasound scans during early pregnancy and careful pediatric follow-up after birth.

Assisted Hatching

Assisted hatching, the microsurgical creation of an opening in the zona pellucida prior to transfer, is based on the hypothesis that some embryos are unable to escape from their zona during blastocyst expansion.[98] The rationale for the development of assisted hatching was initially based on two clinical observations: (1) cleaved embryos displaying reduced zona thickness implanted more frequently than those with thick zonae;[99] and (2) microsurgically fertilized embryos with gaps in their zonae appeared to have higher rates of implantation than zona-intact embryos.[77] This finding led to the first clinical trial of assisted hatching: Cohen et al. undertook a prospective, randomized study comparing the outcome of transfers of four-cell embryos with small surgical incisions in their zonae (PZD) with replacement of zona-intact embryos and found a significant improvement in the per-embryo implantation rate in the assisted hatching group (22% versus 13% in the controls).[98] Assisted hatching has since been modified by the use of zona drilling with acidified Tyrode's solution, to create larger holes in the zona and by performing the procedure on 3-day-old embryos undergoing initial compaction because of the increased integrity that results from the formation of junctional complexes between the blastomeres. Randomized, controlled trials in 330 patients undergoing IVF at our institution revealed that assisted hatching is most efficacious when applied selectively to those embryos displaying thick zonae (>15 μm); the per embryo implantation rate in the selectively zona-drilled group was 25%, which was significantly higher than that seen with control embryos (18%).[100] It is of interest that when these results were analyzed according to age it was found that the most dramatic improvement in embryonic implantation rates following selective assisted hatching occurred in women older than 38 years (16% versus 3% in the controls). A randomized trial of selective assisted hatching in a small group of women (n = 30) with elevated FSH levels (>15 mIU/ml) on day 3, demonstrated an increased implantation rate in zona drilled embryos (26% versus 10% in controls).[101] These results suggest that selective assisted hatching facilitates implantation and leads to higher pregnancy rates in older patients and in patients with decreased ovarian reserve reflected by an elevated day 3 FSH level. It should be noted that these results require confirmation in larger studies. We have incorporated selective assisted hatching into our IVF procedure for those embryos with thick zonae, slow development, or excessive fragmentation (> 20%). Utilizing these criteria, selective assisted hatching appears to improve implantation through salvage of otherwise competent embryos. This concept is supported by a study in which serial serum β-hCG levels were measured during the luteal phase of patients randomized between control and assisted hatching groups.[102] Embryo implantation occurred significantly earlier in the assisted hatching group, suggesting that the procedure may enhance embryo implantation not only by mechanically facilitating the hatching process but also by allowing earlier embryo–endometrium contact.

Oocyte Donation

In women with ovarian failure, elevated day 3 gonadotropins, or a history of poor response to ovarian stimulation, ovum donation offers the ability to carry a pregnancy conceived with their partners' gametes. The oocyte donor may be anonymous or known (e.g., sisters), and the oocyte stove may include other IVF patients willing to donate excess oocytes. Potential donors must be thoroughly screened with a history and physical examination, including a genetic history and communicable disease evaluation identical to that used for sperm donors. The oocyte donor is stimulated using standard IVF protocols while the recipient's endometrium is simultaneously prepared with exogenous steroid hormones to receive the embryos. Patients without ovarian function require replacement with physiologic doses of exogenous steroids; patients with endogenous ovarian function are generally down-regulated with a GnRH analog followed by identical steroid replacement. Our current replacement regimen consists of graduated transdermal estrogen administration via estradiol patches, with the addition of intramuscular progesterone in oil commencing on cycle day 15, the day prior to oocyte retrieval in the donor. The donor's oocytes are retrieved, fertilized with the recipient partner's sperm, and transferred to the recipient. Embryo transfer is performed on day 19, within the established window of endometrial receptivity.[103] Estradiol and progesterone support are maintained after embryo transfer. If the patient conceives, the replacement regimen is continued until the "placental shift" has occurred and the appropriate increases in serum E_2 and progesterone levels have been documented.

Success rates following egg donation have been encouraging. The 1992 SART Registry reported an overall 36.6% clinical pregnancy rate and 31.3% live delivery rate/retrieval after 1699 transfers.[36] Data derived from our oocyte donation program reveal that implantation rates are closely related to the age of the donor. Pregnancy rates in excess of 50% per transfer can be expected, with an implantation rate per embryo of 30–35%.

Complications of ART

When counseling the infertile couple considering ART, the clinician must focus part of the discussion on the potential risks. Although generally safe, these techniques are not exempt from complications related to the medications used to induce multiple ovulation or the surgical procedures.[104] The main problem associated with the use of "fertility drugs" is hyperstimulation of the ovaries, mentioned later in the chapter. Retrieval of oocytes by the abdominal or transvaginal routes can also be associated with the dangers of anesthesia and the usual surgical risks associated with the establishment of a pneumoperitoneum and introduction of a trocar or needle into the peritoneal cavity. The transcervical transfer of embryos into the uterine cavity may also carry an increased risk of pelvic infection in the high risk patient. Pregnancies resulting from ovulation induction, with or without IVF or GIFT, are associated with higher ectopic and abortion rates, heterotopic pregnancies, and multiple gestations; each is associated with specific risks of complications during pregnancy or delivery. Another controversial danger is the future development of ovarian cancer, associated with ovulation induction.[105]

Multiple Gestation

The most common significant complication of ART is the increased incidence of multiple gestations. Multiple pregnancies reportedly comprise more than 22% of the clinical pregnancies in an IVF program, a rate that has remained fairly constant over the years.[106] Multifetal pregnancy should be considered a complication of ART because it exposes the woman to increased maternal morbidity and is associated with an increased perinatal morbidity and mortality. Multifetal pregnancies are known to be associated with increased incidence of preeclampsia, placenta previa and placental abruption, premature rupture of membranes, postpartum hemorrhage, and cesarean section. This risk is greatest for high-order multiple gestations: Triplet and quadruplet IVF pregnancies are associated with higher rates of obstetric and neonatal complications than are seen with IVF twins.[106] After reviewing the birth data on 1138 triplet gestations in the United States during 1984–1989, Elster et al. concluded that with modern obstetric care the average length of gestation for triplets was 33.8 weeks and the mean birth weight was 1911 g.[107] Elliot and Radin reported their experience with the management of 10 quadruplet pregnancies, delivered at a mean gestational age of 32.5 weeks and a mean birth weight of 1536 g.[108] Despite these encouraging results with modern obstetric care of high-order multiple gestations, morbidity and mortality rates are increased for the prematurely delivered neonate primarily because of respiratory distress syndrome and intraventricular hemorrhage. The social and economic difficulties are attributed to increased hospitalization of prematurely born infants and to the burden on families with three or more children, especially if one or more of them are physically disabled.

To prevent multifetal gestations and their undesired consequences, ovulation induction drugs should be used with extreme caution, and fewer embryos should be transferred, particularly in the young patient. The recent development of ultrasound-guided multifetal pregnancy reduction offers an alternative to couples with high-order multiple gestations.[109–112] Nevertheless, when 13 women with triplet pregnancies who underwent pregnancy reduction were compared with 11 women managed expectantly, no significant differences were found in regard to the gestational age at delivery or the incidence of newborn or obstetric complications.[113] Although fetal reduction techniques are associated with a low incidence of complications, they may be a source of distress for both parents and physicians, not to mention the social controversy that exists with regard to this subject.[114] The ultimate decision regarding fetal reduction should be made by the parents after careful consideration of all the medical, social, ethical, and religious issues involved.

Ectopic Gestation and IVF

The first human IVF pregnancy reported by Steptoe and Edwards in 1976 was ectopic.[115] Since then a large number of ectopic pregnancies have been reported after IVF, with an incidence ranging from 3.3% to 8.6% of clinical pregnancies.[116,117] The rates of ectopic pregnancy after ART obtained from the SART IVF-ET registry for the year 1992 are summarized in Table 20.2. Ectopic pregnancies per transfer after 37,164 stimulation cycles for IVF, GIFT, and ZIFT were 1.2%, 1.3%, and 1.3%, respectively.[36]

Most authors have identified preexisting tubal disease as the most important risk factor for ectopic pregnancy after IVF.[117–119] We examined the risk factors, stimulation characteristics, and future fecundity of IVF patients who developed ectopic pregnancies in our program.[119] Of 1123 pregnancies, 27 (2.4%) were ectopic following fresh IVF embryo transfers. Of 105 pregnancies 8 (7.6%) were ectopic following frozen-thawed embryo transfers. Thirty ectopic pregnancies were ampullary, two interstitial, two cervical, and one heterotopic. The interstitial pregnancies occurred in two patients with previous bilateral salpingectomy. Tubal factor was the cause of infertility in most (88.2%) of the ectopic pregnancies in our series. No difference was found between the ectopic pregnancies and matched controls in terms of stimulation and transfer characteristics, and during subsequent IVF cycles the intrauterine pregnancy rate of these patients was not decreased.

Heterotopic (combined intrauterine and extrauterine) pregnancy is a relatively rare condition. Fifty years ago, it was estimated to occur once in 30,000 pregnancies.[120] In recent years, however, combined pregnancy occurs more frequently in women undergoing ovulation induction with clomiphene citrate or gonadotropins.[121] Present evidence suggests that it occurs more often when pregnancy is achieved by IVF or GIFT than with natural conceptions. The first two heterotopic pregnancies resulting from IVF were described in 1985 by Yovich et al.[123] and Sondheimer et al.[124] The first GIFT heterotopic pregnancy was reported by Abdalla et al. in 1986.[125] In an international collaborative patient registry, 0.83% of 601 clinical pregnancies resulting from 2092 GIFT retrieval cycles were heterotopic.[125] After a review of the literature, Goldman et al.[127] summarized 34 published cases of combined pregnancy, 27 of which resulted from IVF and the rest from GIFT. For 1989, the U.S. IVF Registry reported that there were 20 heterotopic pregnancies after ART: 11 of 2811 (0.4%) clinical IVF pregnancies, 6 of 1112 (0.5%) GIFT pregnancies, and 3 of 139 (2.1%) resulted from combined IVF/GIFT pregnancies. The intrauterine gestation survived in 12 pregnancies (60%); 7 resulted in spontaneous abortion, and 1 patient elected to have a therapeutic abortion.[128] Overall, the reported incidence of multiple-sited pregnancies after ART has ranged between 0.9%[129] and 2.9%,[130] with most reports suggesting that the incidence of combined pregnancy after ART is approximately 1%.[131–133] The factors that predispose to heterotopic pregnancy seem to be similar to those involved in the pathogenesis of ectopic pregnancy. The development of combined pregnancy is probably related to ovarian stimulation and hence to ovulation of more than one oocyte. Because of the presence of an intrauterine gestation on ultrasonography, the diagnosis of this potentially fatal condition is often made at the time of surgery for rupture and onset of hemoperitoneum. Abdominal pain is the most frequent presenting symptom, followed by vaginal bleeding.[124] Serum hCG levels that are higher than expected for gestational age may indicate the presence of multiple pregnancy; in such cases, if only a single intrauterine sac is visible sonographically, heterotopic pregnancy must be considered. Routine ultrasonic scanning of the adnexa may improve the accuracy of diagnosis, but ultimately laparoscopy is the method of choice to confirm or exclude this hazardous condition.

In our series, interstitial pregnancy occurred in two patients despite previous uterotubal occlusion procedures. To prevent tubal pregnancy, several authors have recommended prophylactic bilateral salpingectomy or proximal tubal occlusion in patients who had failed tubal reconstructive surgery.[134] We prefer to perform salpingectomy only in patients who develop ectopic pregnancies following the IVF procedure with the hope of preventing recurrence during subsequent cycles.

Ovarian Hyperstimulation Syndrome

Ovarian hyperstimulation syndrome (OHSS) represents a spectrum of symptoms and signs ranging from benign abdominal discomfort to life-threatening complications. A revised classification system has been proposed by Golan et al.[135] that incorporates current diagnostic techniques. *Mild OHSS* is marked by abdominal distention and sonographic evidence of ovarian enlargement and may be associated with such gastrointestinal symptoms as nausea, vomiting, or diarrhea. These findings in addition to sonographic evidence of ascites are classified as *moderate OHSS*. In addition to features of moderate disease, the diagnosis of *severe OHSS* is characterized by secondary electrolyte, hematologic, renal, pulmonary, or liver abnormalities. Severe cases may present with massive ovarian enlargement, peritoneal irritation due to follicular rupture and hemorrhage, ovarian torsion, pleural effusion, hemoconcentration, oliguria, electrolyte imbalance, and a hypercoagulable state that may lead to life-threatening thromboembolic events. The pathogenesis of this syndrome may be explained by a sudden increase in capillary permeability possibly mediated by prostaglandins or the renin-angiotensin system, resulting in shifting of fluids from the intravascular compartment into the peritoneal and pleural cavities. The hemodynamic changes are those of a hypovolemic state, reflected by decreased renal perfusion and increased hemoconcentration.

We have implemented what has so far proved to be a successful approach to minimizing the risk of OHSS in our program.[136] A step-down gonadotropin regimen, combined with luteal phase leuprolide suppression was utilized in a series of 3333 IVF stimulation cycles. hCG was withheld when E_2 levels exceeded 4500 pg/ml; the dose was halved to 5000 IU during cycles where E_2 levels exceeded 2000 pg/ml, and it was further decreased to 3000 IU with E_2 levels higher than 2500 pg/ml. Fresh embryo transfers were withheld when the E_2 level was < 4000 pg/ml. With this approach, the incidence of OHSS requiring admission was significantly less than the general incidence in the United States (0.15% versus 0.50%, respectively), while still maintaining a high pregnancy rate. Nonetheless, OHSS cannot be altogether obviated unless hCG is withheld and the cycle canceled. Cycle cancellation should be considered when indicators such as markedly elevated E_2 levels and an exaggerated number of follicles prognosticate a high risk. If oocyte retrieval is undertaken during a high risk cycle, the embryos can be cryopreserved for future replacement, essentially eliminating the possibility of pregnancy during the stimulated cycle and thus reducing the likelihood of severe OHSS. It is conceivable that continuation of GnRHa treatment after oocyte recovery or the use of an aromatase inhibitor such as testolactone can further reduce the risk of OHSS in cycles in which all embryos are cryopreserved.

Risk of Cancer with Ovulation Induction

The association of some types of cancer with induction of ovulation, particularly ovarian cancer, has received considerable attention with resultant controversy.[136] Whittemore and colleagues[137] from the Collaborative Ovarian Cancer Group have published a combined analysis of three epidemiologic studies looking at the association of ovarian cancer and the use of fertility drugs. They found that white women who had used fertility drugs had three times the risk of developing invasive epithelial ovarian cancer as women without a history of infertility.[138] Among the nulligravidas, the corresponding relative risk was 27. They also reported that patients who had used fertility drugs had four times the risk of developing borderline ovarian tumors compared to women with no history of infertility.[139] The methodology and conclusions of the study have been questioned by most experts.[140] Indeed a previous report did not detect an increased risk of ovarian cancer among infertile women treated with various fertility drugs.[141] It is clear that although the findings of Whittemore et al. justify an increased level of concern about the possible causal relation between fertility drugs and ovarian cancer, more basic and epidemiologic research is needed to put this information into perspective. Until the issue is resolved, we suggest cautioning patients who receive fertility drugs about the possible increased risk of ovarian cancer.

Complications of Oocyte Retrieval

Today in most IVF units the ultrasound-guided follicular aspiration technique is used for oocyte retrieval, and laparoscopy is reserved for gamete or zygote transfer into the fallopian tube. Ultrasound-guided retrieval is rarely associated with pelvic or abdominal visceral or vascular injuries caused by the aspiration needle, but infection is a potential complication. Laparoscopic complications are related to the anesthesia, pneumoperitoneum, and injuries caused by trocar and other instrument insertion.[104] Dicker et al. reported a 0.38% incidence of severe complications after 3656 transvaginal oocyte retrievals, including acute abdomen, tuboovarian or pelvic abscess, rupture of endometriomas, and hemoperitoneum.[142] We have evaluated the incidence of pelvic infection requiring hospitalization after transvaginal oocyte retrieval for IVF in the New York Hospital–Cornell program.[143] Patients in the study group received oral tetracycline after retrieval and underwent povidone-iodine vaginal cleansing at the time of the procedure followed by saline irrigation. Patients with a history of PID or tubal disease received additional intravenous antibiotic prophylaxis with cefoxitin before the oocyte retrieval. There was a significantly lower incidence of pelvic infection in the study group than in a control group of patients who received no antibiotic prophylaxis and who had saline cleansing of the vagina. Thus we advocate utilizing sterile technique with povidone-iodine vaginal cleansing and prophylactic intravenous antibiotics for high risk patients.

Conclusion

The decision process for infertile couples who wish to pursue therapeutic options to infertility requires accurate comparative information with respect to pregnancy outcomes after either reconstructive surgery or IVF for their particular condition and age group. The "take-home baby" rate per cycle of IVF and the cumulative rate after multiple cycles must be provided. As the optimum number of repeated cycles of IVF is unknown, it seems reasonable to consider the cumulative pregnancy rate after four cycles. In addition, the clinician must counsel patients about the potential complications of the procedure and the risk of multiple gestation, spontaneous abortion, and ectopic pregnancy. Finally, the effect of frozen embryo replacement on the cumulative pregnancy rate must be computed in the analysis; it is imperative that such figures reflect results from the treating center rather than general results. Armed with this information, the couple is in a position to make logical choices, particularly when comparison is made with results of tubal surgery. Surgery, if successful, offers multiple cycles in which to achieve conception and the opportunity to have more than one pregnancy.

It appears that for young patients with mild to moderate tubal disease, tubal reconstructive surgery should be offered as their first treatment modality. For patients with severe disease accompanied with extensive pelvic adhesions, IVF should be the primary approach. Likewise, IVF clearly represents the only therapeutic option for patients with inoperable tubal disease (i.e., absent tubes or prior tuberculous salpingitis) and for couples in whom tubal disease is associated with severe male factor.

In addition to the medical aspects involved in the decision process, consideration should be given to the woman's age and the cost of the procedure. During this era when society's increasing concern seems to be focused on cost-containment, the calculated costs per live birth after tubal surgery compared with IVF are a central issue for discussion.[144] Comparisons are difficult, as cost calculations do not take into effect whether third-party insurance carriers reimburse patients for surgical or IVF expenses. In general, patients are more likely to be reimbursed for surgical procedures than for IVF.

The development of operative laparoscopy, microsurgery, and IVF since the 1970s has improved the outlook for couples suffering from tubal infertility. The goals for any infertile couple should be either a live birth or being able to believe that they have exhausted all reasonable attempts to achieve a pregnancy. For the infertile woman with tubal damage there are only two realistic options: reconstructive surgery or IVF. The choice of the primary and subsequent treatments depends on careful consideration of technical and nontechnical factors, individualized to the circumstances of the patient. The two options should not be regarded as competitive but, rather, complementary. The final decision rests with the couple and is influenced by their perception of the facts and their own internal value systems.

References

1. STEPTOE PC, EDWARDS RG: Birth after reimplantation of a human embryo. Lancet 1978;2:366.
2. PITKIN, RM: Operative laparoscopy: surgical advance or technical gimmick? Obstet Gynecol 1992;79:441.
3. WESTROM L: Effect of acute pelvic inflammatory disease on fertility. Am J Obstet Gynecol 1975; 121:707.
4. TULANDI T, COLLINS JA, BURROWS E, ET AL: Treatment-dependent and treatment-independent pregnancy among women with periadnexal adhesions. Am J Obstet Gynecol 1990;162:354.
5. GOMEL V: Salpingo-ovariolysis by laparoscopy in infertility. Fertil Steril 1983;40:607.
6. BELLINA JH, HEMMINGS R, VOROS JI, ET AL: Carbon dioxide laser and electrosurgical wound study with an animal model: a comparison of tissue damage and healing patterns in peritoneal tissue. Am J Obstet Gynecol 1984; 148:327.
7. TULANDI T: Salpingo-ovariolysis: a comparison between laser surgery and electrosurgery. Fertil Steril 1986;45:489.
8. LUCIANO AA, MAIER DB, KOCH EI, ET AL: A comparative study of postoperative adhesions following laser surgery by laparoscopy versus laparotomy in the rabbit model. Obstet Gynecol 1989;74:220.
9. SIEGLER AM, KONTOPOULOS V: An analysis of macrosurgical and microsurgical techniques in the management of the tuboperitoneal factor in infertility. Fertil Steril 1979;32:377.
10. CASPI E, HALPERIN Y: Surgical management of periadnexal adhesions. Int J Fertil 1981;26:49.
11. HULKA JF: Adnexal adhesions: a prognostic staging and classification system based on a five-year survey of fertility surgery results at Chapel Hill, North Carolina. Am J Obstet Gynecol 1982;144:141.
12. LAVY G, DIAMOND MP, DECHERNEY AH: Ectopic pregnancy: its relationship to tubal reconstructive surgery. Fertil Steril 1987;47:543.
13. FAYEZ JA: An assessment of the role of operative laparoscopy in tuboplasty: its relationship to tubal reconstructive surgery. Fertil Steril 1983; 39:476.
14. SCHLAFF WD, HASSIAKOS DK, DAMEWOOD MD, ET AL: Neosalpingostomy for distal tubal obstruction: prognostic factors and impact of surgical technique. Fertil Steril 1990;54:984.
15. TULANDI T, FARAG R, MCINNES RA, ET AL: Reconstructive surgery for hydrosalpinx with and without the carbon dioxide laser. Fertil Steril 1984;42:839.
16. MAGE G, BRUHAT MA: Pregnancy following salpingostomy: comparison between CO_2 laser and electrosurgery procedures. Fertil Steril 1983;40:472.
17. CANIS M, MAGE G, POULY JL, ET AL: Laparoscopic distal tuboplasty: report of 87 cases and a 4-year experience. Fertil Steril 1991;56:616.
18. DANIELL JF, HERBERT CM: Laparoscopic salpingostomy utilizing the CO_2 laser. Fertil Steril 1984;41:558.

19. DANIELL JF, DIAMOND MP, MCLAUGHLIN DS, ET AL: Clinical results of terminal salpingostomy with the use of the CO_2 laser: report of the intraabdominal laser study group. Fertil Steril 1986; 45:175.
20. ROCK JA, KATAYAMA KP, MARTIN EJ, ET AL: Factors influencing the success of salpingostomy techniques for distal fimbrial obstruction. Obstet Gynecol 1978;52:591.
21. YOUNG PE, EGAN JE, BARLOW J, ET AL: Reconstructive surgery for infertility at the Boston Hospital for Women. Am J Obstet Gynecol 1970;108:1092.
22. DEBRUYNE F, PUTTEMANS P, BOECKX W, ET AL: The clinical value of salpingoscopy in tubal infertility. Fertil Steril 1989;51:339.
23. AUDIBERT F, HÉDON B, ARNAL F, ET AL: Therapeutic strategies in tubal infertility with distal pathology. Hum Reprod 1991;6:1439.
24. MARANA R, QUAGLIARELLO J: Distal tubal occlusion: microsurgery versus in vitro fertilization—a review. Int J Fertil 1988;33:107.
25. NOVY MJ, THURMOND AS, PATTON P, ET AL: Diagnosis of cornual obstruction by transcervical fallopian tube cannulation. Fertil Steril 1988;50:434.
26. KERIN JF, SURREY ES, WILLIAMS DB, ET AL: Falloscopic observations of endotubal isthmic plugs as a cause of reversible obstruction and their histological characterization. J Laparoendosc Surg 1991;1:103.
27. GOMEL V: Tubal reanastomosis by microsurgery. Fertil Steril 1977;28:59.
28. MELDRUM DR: Microsurgical tubal reanastomosis: the role of splints. Obstet Gynecol 1981;57:613.
29. LAVY G, DIAMOND MP, DECHERNEY AH: Pregnancy following tubocornual anastomosis. Fertil Steril 1986;46:21.
30. PATTON PE, WILLIAMS TJ, COULAM CB: Results of microsurgical reconstruction in patients with combined proximal and distal tubal occlusion: double obstruction. Fertil Steril 1987;48:670.
31. SILBER SJ, COHEN R: Microsurgical reversal of female sterilization: the role of tubal length. Fertil Steril 1980;33:598.
32. ROCK JA, GUZICK DS, KATZ E, ET AL: Tubal anastomosis: pregnancy success following reversal of Falope ring or monopolar cautery sterilization. Fertil Steril 1987;48:13.
33. HENDERSON SR: The reversibility of female sterilization with the use of microsurgery: a report on 102 patients with more than one year of follow-up. Am J Obstet Gynecol 1984;149:57.
34. ROCK JA, BERGQUIST CA, ZACUR HA, ET AL: Tubal anastomosis following unipolar cautery. Fertil Steril 1982;37:613.
35. TRIMBOS-KEMPER TCM: Reversal of sterilization in women over 40 years of age: a multicenter survey in The Netherlands. Fertil Steril 1990;53:575.
36. SOCIETY FOR ASSISTED REPRODUCTIVE TECHNOLOGY, THE AMERICAN FERTILITY SOCIETY: Assisted reproductive technology in the United States and Canada: 1993 results generated from The American Fertility Society/Society for Assisted Reproductive Technology Registry. Fertil Steril 1994;62:1121.
37. OELSNER G, TARLATZIS BC: Radical surgery for extrauterine pregnancy. In Ectopic Pregnancy, DeCherney AH, (ed). Rockville, Md, Aspen Publishers, 1986:127–32.
38. DECHERNEY AH, ROMERO R, NAFTOLIN F: Surgical management of unruptured ectopic pregnancy. Fertil Steril 1981;35:21.
39. BRUHAT M-A, MANHES H, MAGE G, ET AL: Treatment of ectopic pregnancy by means of laparoscopy. Fertil Steril 1980;33:411.
40. DECHERNEY AH, MAHEAUX R, NAFTOLIN F: Salpingostomy for ectopic pregnancy in the sole patent oviduct: reproductive outcome. Fertil Steril 1982;37:619.
41. DECHERNEY AH, SILIDKER JS, MEZER HC, ET AL: Reproductive outcome following two ectopic pregnancies. Fertil Steril 1985;43:82.
42. HALLATT JG: Repeat ectopic pregnancy: a study of 123 consecutive cases. Am J Obstet Gynecol 1975;122:520.
43. OEHNINGER S, SCOTT R, MUASHER SJ, ET AL: Effects of the severity of tubo-ovarian disease and previous tubal surgery on the results of in vitro fertilization and embryo transfer. Fertil Steril 1989;51:126.
44. TIETZE C: Reproductive span and rate of reproduction among Hutterite women. Fertil Steril 1957;8:89.
45. MENKEN J, TRUSSELL J, LARSEN U: Age and infertility. Science 1986;233:1389.
46. SHERMAN BM, KORENMAN SG: Hormonal characteristics of the human menstrual cycle throughout reproductive life. J Clin Invest 1975;55:699.
47. LENTON EA, DEKRETSER DM, WOODWARD AJ, ET AL: Inhibin concentrations throughout the menstrual cycle of normal, infertile, and older women compared with those during spontaneous conceptions cycles. J Clin Endocrinol Metab 1991;73:1180.

48. SHARMA V, RIDDLE A, MASON BA, ET AL: An analysis of factors influencing the establishment of a clinical pregnancy in an ultrasound-based ambulatory in vitro fertilization program. Fertil Steril 1988;49:468.
49. PIETTE C, DE MOUZON J, BACHELOT A, ET AL: In vitro fertilization: influence of women's age on pregnancy rates. Hum Reprod 1990;5:56.
50. SCHWARTZ D, MAYAUX MJ, FEDERATION CECOS: Female fecundity as a function of age: results of artificial insemination in 2193 multiparous women with azoospermic husbands. N Engl J Med 1982;306:404.
51. ROMEU A, MUASHER SJ, ACOSTA AA, ET AL: Results of in vitro fertilization attempts in women 40 years of age and older: the Norfolk experience. Fertil Steril 1987;47:130.
52. PETERS H: Intrauterine gonadal development. Fertil Steril 1976;27:493.
53. NAVOT D, ROSENWAKS Z, MARGALIOTH EJ: Prognostic assessment of female fecundity. Lancet 1987;19:645.
54. PADILLA SL, SMITH RD, GARCIA JE: The Lupron screening test: tailoring the use of leuprolide acetate in ovarian stimulation for in vitro fertilization. Fertil Steril 1991;56:79.
55. SCOTT RT, OEHNINGER S, TONER JP, ET AL: Follicle stimulating hormone levels on cycle day 3 are predictive of in vitro fertilization outcome. Fertil Steril 1989;51:651.
56. LICCIARDI FL, LIN H-C, ROSENWAKS Z: Day 3 estradiol serum concentrations as prognostications of ovarian stimulation response and pregnancy outcome in patients undergoing in vitro fertilization. Fertil Steril 1995;64:991.
57. LENTON EA, SEXTON L, LEE S, ET AL: Progressive changes in LH and FSH and LH:FSH ratio in women throughout reproductive life. Maturitas 1988;10:35.
58. MUASHER SJ, OEHNINGER S, SIMONETTI S, ET AL: The value of basal and/or stimulated serum gonadotropin levels in prediction of stimulation response and in vitro fertilization outcome. Fertil Steril 1988;50:298.
59. HUGHES EG, ROBERTSON DM, HANDELSMAN DJ, ET AL: Inhibin and estradiol responses to ovarian hyperstimulation: effects of age and predictive value for in vitro fertilization outcome. J Clin Endocrinol Metab 1990;70:358.
60. PELLICER A, MARI M, DE LOS SANTOS MJ, ET AL: Effects of aging on the human ovary: the secretion of immunoreactive μ-inhibin and progesterone. Fertil Steril 1994;61:663.
61. NAVOT D, BERGH PA, WILLIAMS MA, ET AL: Poor oocyte quality rather than implantation failure is a cause of age-related decline in female infertility. Lancet 1991;337:1375.
62. MUNNÉ S, ALIKANI M, TOMKIN G, ET AL: Embryo morphology, developmental rates and maternal age are correlated with chromosome abnormalities. Fertil Steril 1995;64:382.
63. PADILLA SL, GARCIA JE: Effect of maternal age and number of in vitro fertilization procedures on pregnancy outcome. Fertil Steril 1989;52:270.
64. DODSON WC, WHITESIDES DB, HUGHES CL JR, ET AL: Superovulation with intrauterine insemination in the treatment of infertility: a possible alternative to gamete intrafallopian transfer and in vitro fertilization. Fertil Steril 1987;48:441.
65. SCORSON SL, BATZER FR, GOCIAL B, ET AL: Intrauterine insemination and ovulation stimulation as treatment of infertility. J Reprod Med 1989;34:397.
66. CHAFFKIN LM, NULSEN JC, LUCIANO AA, ET AL: A comparative analysis of the cycle fecundity rates associated with combined human menopausal gonadotropin and intrauterine insemination versus either hMG or IUI alone. Fertil Steril 1991;55:252.
67. CLAMAN P, DOMINGO M, GARNER P, ET AL: Natural cycle in vitro fertilization-embryo transfer at the University of Ottawa: an inefficient therapy for tubal infertility. Fertil Steril 1993;60:298.
68. DROESCH K, MUASHER SJ, BRZYSKI RG, ET AL: Value of suppression with a gonadotropin-releasing hormone agonist prior to gonadotropin stimulation for in vitro fertilization. Fertil Steril 1989;51:292.
69. MELDRUM DR, WISOT A, HAMILTON F, ET AL: Routine pituitary suppression with leuprolide before ovulation stimulation for oocyte retrieval. Fertil Steril 1989;51:455.
70. HUGHES EG, FEDORKOW DM, DAYA S, ET AL: The routine use of gonadotropin-releasing hormone agonists prior to in vitro fertilization and gamete intrafallopian transfer: a meta-analysis of randomized controlled trials. Fertil Steril 1992;58:888.
71. LIU H-C, LAI Y-M, DAVIS O, ET AL: Improved pregnancy outcome with gonadotropin-releasing hormone agonist (GnRH-a) stimulation is due to the improvement in oocyte quantity rather than quality. J Assist Reprod Genet 1992;9:338.
72. ABBASI R, KENIGSBERG D, DANFORTH D, ET AL: Cumulative ovulation in human menopausal gonadotropin/human chorionic gonadotropin-treated monkeys: "step-up" versus "step-down" dose regimens. Fertil Steril 1987;47:1019.

73. DAVIS OK, ROSENWAKS Z: The ovarian factor in assisted reproductive technology. In The Ovary, Adashi EY, Leung PCK (eds). New York, Raven Press, 1993, pp 545–560.
74. BENADIVA CA, BEN-RAFAEL Z, STRAUSS JF, ET AL: Ovarian response of individuals to different doses of human menopausal gonadotropin. Fertil Steril 1988;49:997.
75. NEAL GS, SULTAN KM, LIU H-C, ET AL: A successful approach to stimulation of the high responder patient using oral contraceptive pills, leuprolide acetate and menotropins [abstract]. Presented at the 8th World Congress of IVF-ET, Kyoto, 1993.
76. GLEICHER N, FRIBERG J, FULLAN N, ET AL: Egg retrieval for in-vitro fertilization by sonographically controlled vaginal culdocenteses. Lancet 1983; 2:508.
77. COHEN J, MALTER H, ELSNER C, ET AL: Immunosuppression supports implantation of zona pellucida dissected human embryos. Fertil Steril 1990;53:662.
78. MUASHER SJ, WILKES C, GARCIA JE, ET AL: Benefits and risks of multiple transfer with in vitro fertilization. Lancet 1984;1:570.
79. LEONARD G, BERKELEY A, ALIKANI M, ET AL: Difficulty of embryo transfer and IVF pregnancy outcome [abstract]. Presented at the 7th World Congress on In Vitro Fertilization and Assisted Procreation, Paris, 1991.
80. GRAF MJ, REYNIAK JV, BATTLE-MUTTER P, ET AL: Histologic evaluation of the luteal phase in women following follicle aspiration for oocyte retrieval. Fertil Steril 1988;49:616.
81. HERMAN A, RON-EL R, GOLAN A, ET AL: Pregnancy rate and ovarian hyperstimulation after luteal human chorionic gonadotropin in in vitro fertilization stimulated with gonadotropin-releasing hormone analog and menotropins. Fertil Steril 1990;53:92.
82. TROUNSON A, MOHR L: Human pregnancy following cryopreservation, thawing and transfer of an eight-cell embryo. Nature 1983;305:707.
83. COHEN J, DE VANE GH, ELSNER CW, ET AL: Cryopreservation of zygotes and early cleaved human embryos. Fertil Steril 1988;49:283.
84. CHEN C: Pregnancy after human oocyte cryopreservation. Lancet 1986;1:884.
85. VAN UEM JF, SEIBZEHURUBL ER, SCHUH B, ET AL: Birth after cryopreservation of unfertilized oocytes. Lancet 1987;1:752.
86. ASCH RH, ELLSWORTH LR, BALMACEDA JP, ET AL: Pregnancy after translaparoscopic gamete intrafallopian transfer. Lancet 1984;2:1034.
87. MASTROYANNIS C: Gamete intrafallopian transfer: ethical considerations, historical development of the procedure, and comparison with other advanced reproductive technologies. Fertil Steril 1993;60:389.
88. JANSEN RPS, ANDERSON JC, SUTHERLAND PD: Nonoperative embryo transfer to the fallopian tube. N Engl J Med 1988;319:288.
89. YOVICH JL, BRAECKLEDGE DG, RICHARDSON PA, ET AL: Pregnancies following pronuclear stage tubal transfer. Fertil Steril 1987;48:851.
90. KRUGER TF, ACOSTA AA, SIMMONS KF, ET AL: Predictive value of abnormal sperm morphology in in vitro fertilization. Fertil Steril 1988;49:112.
91. COHEN J, MALTER H, TALANSKY B, ET AL: Gamete and embryo micromanipulation for infertility treatment. Semin Reprod Endocrinol 1990; 8:290.
92. GORDON JW, TALANSKY BE: Assisted fertilization by zona drilling: a mouse model for correction of oligospermia. J Exp Zool 1986;239:347.
93. MALTER HE, COHEN J: Partial zona dissection of the human oocyte: a nontraumatic method using micromanipulation to assist zona pellucida penetration. Fertil Steril 1989;51:139.
94. COHEN J, ALIKANI M, MALTER HE, ET AL: Partial zona dissection or subzonal insertion: microsurgical fertilization alternatives based on evaluation of sperm and embryo morphology. Fertil Steril 1991;56:696.
95. PALERMO G, JORIS H, DEVROEY P, VAN STEIRTEGHEM AC: Pregnancies after intracytoplasmic injection of single spermatozoon into an oocyte. Lancet 1992;340:17.
96. PALERMO G, JORIS H, DERDE M-P, ET AL: Sperm characteristics and outcome of human assisted fertilization by subzonal insemination and intracytoplasmic sperm injection. Fertil Steril 1993;59:826.
97. COHEN J, WIEMER K, ALIKANI M: Advanced laboratory techniques for assisted reproduction. Infertil Reprod Med Clin North Am 1993;4:733.
98. COHEN J, WRIGHT G, MALTER H, ET AL: Impairment of the hatching process following in vitro fertilization in the human and improvement of implantation by assisting hatching using micromanipulation. Hum Reprod 1990;5:7.
99. COHEN J, INGE KL, SUZMAN K, ET AL: Videocinematography of fresh and cryopreserved embryos: a retrospective analysis of embryonic morphology and implantation. Fertil Steril 1989;51:820.
100. COHEN J, ALIKANI M, TROWBRIDGE J, ET AL: Implantation enhancement by selective assisted

hatching using zona drilling of embryos with poor prognosis. Hum Reprod 1992;7:685.
101. COHEN J, ALIKANI M, REING AM, ET AL: Selective assisted hatching of human embryos. Ann Acad Med Singapore 1992;21:565.
102. LIU H-C, COHEN J, ALIKANI M, ET AL: Assisted hatching facilitates earlier implantation. Fertil Steril 1993;60:871.
103. ROSENWAKS Z: Donor eggs: their application to modern reproductive technologies. Fertil Steril 1987;47:895.
104. SCHENKER JG, EZRA Y: Complications of assisted reproductive techniques. Fertil Steril 1994;61:411.
105. SPIRTAS R, KAUFMAN SC, ALEXANDER NJ: Fertility drugs and ovarian cancer: red alert or red herring? Fertil Steril 1993;59:291.
106. SEOUD MA-F, TONER JP, KRUITHOFF C, ET AL: Outcome of twin, triplet, and quadruplet in vitro fertilization pregnancies: the Norfolk experience. Fertil Steril 1992;57:825.
107. ELSTER AD, BLEYL JL, CRAVEN TE: Birth weight standards for triplets under modern obstetric care in the United States, 1984–1989. Obstet Gynecol 1991;77:387.
108. ELLIOT JP, RADIN TG: Quadruplet pregnancy: contemporary management and outcome. Obstet Gynecol 1992;80:421.
109. LYNCH L, BERKOWITZ RL, CHITKARA U, ET AL: First-trimester transabdominal multifetal pregnancy reduction: a report of 85 cases. Obstet Gynecol 1990;75:735.
110. ITSKOVITZ-ELDOR J, DRUGAN A, LEVRON J, ET AL: Transvaginal embryo aspiration—a safe method for selective reduction in multiple pregnancies. Fertil Steril 1992;58:351.
111. EVANS MI, MAY M, DRUGAN A, ET AL: Selective termination: clinical experience and residual risks. Am J Obstet Gynecol 1990;162:1568.
112. SHALEV J, FRENKEL Y, GOLDENBERG M, ET AL: Selective reduction in multiple gestations: pregnancy outcome after transvaginal and transabdominal needle-guided procedures. Fertil Steril 1989;52:416.
113. PORRECO RP, BURKE MS, HENDRIX ML: Multifetal reduction of triplets and pregnancy outcome. Obstet Gynecol 1991;78:335.
114. HOBBINS JC: Selective reduction—a perinatal necessity [editorial]? N Engl J Med 1988;318:1062.
115. STEPTOE PC, EDWARDS RG: Reimplantation of a human embryo with subsequent tubal pregnancy. Lancet 1976;1:880.
116. KARANDE VC, FLOOD JT, HEARD N, ET AL: Analysis of ectopic pregnancies resulting from in-vitro fertilization and embryo transfer. Hum Reprod 1991;6:446.
117. DUBUISSON JB, AUBRIOT FX, MATHIEU L, ET AL: Risk factors for ectopic pregnancy in 556 pregnancies after in vitro fertilization: implications for preventive management. Fertil Steril 1991;56:668.
118. HERMAN A, RON-EL R, GOLAN A, ET AL: The role of tubal pathology and other parameters in ectopic pregnancies occurring in in vitro fertilization and embryo transfer. Fertil Steril 1990; 54:864.
119. VERHULST G, CAMUS M, BOLLEN N, ET AL: Analysis of the risk factors with regard to the occurrence of ectopic pregnancy after medically assisted procreation. Hum Reprod 1993;8:1284.
120. PYRGIOTIS E, SULTAN KM, NEAL GS, ET AL: Ectopic pregnancies after in-vitro fertilization and embryo transfer. J Assist Reprod Genet 1994;11:79.
121. DE VOE RW, PRATT JH: Simultaneous intrauterine and extrauterine pregnancy. Am J Obstet Gynecol 1948;56:1119.
122. BERGER MJ, TAYMOR ML: Simultaneous intrauterine and tubal pregnancy following ovulation induction. Am J Obstet Gynecol 1972;113:812.
123. YOVICH JL, MCCOLM SC, TURNER SR, ET AL: Heterotopic pregnancy from in vitro fertilization. J In Vitro Fert Embryo Transf 1985;2:143.
124. SONDHEIMER SJ, TURECK RW, BLASCO L, ET AL: Simultaneous ectopic pregnancy with intrauterine twin gestations after IVF-ET. Fertil Steril 1985;43:313.
125. ABDALLA HI, AHUJA KK, MORRIS N, ET AL: Combined intra-abdominal and intrauterine pregnancies after gamete intrafallopian transfer. Lancet 1986;2:1153.
126. LI HP, BALMACEDA JP, ZOUVES C, ET AL: Heterotopic pregnancy associated with gamete intrafallopian transfer. Hum Reprod 1992;7:131.
127. GOLDMAN GA, FISCH B, OVADIA J, ET AL: Heterotopic pregnancy after assisted reproductive technologies. Obstet Gynecol Surv 1992;47:217.
128. PORTER JB, MANBERG PJ, HARTZ SC: Statistics and results of assisted reproductive technologies. Assist Reprod Rev 1991;1:28.
129. DOR J, SEIDMAN DS, LEVRAN D, ET AL: The incidence of combined intrauterine and extrauterine pregnancy after in vitro fertilization and embryo transfer. Fertil Steril 1991;55:833.
130. DIMITRY ES, SUBAK-SHARPE R, MILLS M, ET AL: Nine cases of heterotopic pregnancies in 4 years of IVF. Fertil Steril 1990;53:107.
131. MOLLOY D, DEAMBROSIS W, KEEPING D, ET AL: Multiple-sited (heterotopic) pregnancy after in

vitro fertilization and gamete intrafallopian transfer. Fertil Steril 1990;53:1068.
132. SVARE J, NORUP P, GROVE THOMSEN S, ET AL: Heterotopic pregnancies after in-vitro fertilization and embryo transfer—a Danish survey. Hum Reprod 1993;8:116.
133. RIZK B, TAN SL, MORCOS S, ET AL: Heterotopic pregnancies after in vitro fertilization and embryo transfer. Am J Obstet Gynecol 1991; 164:161.
134. ZOUVES C, ERENUS M, GOMEL V: Tubal ectopic pregnancy after in vitro fertilization and embryo transfer: a role for proximal occlusion or salpingectomy after failed distal tubal surgery? Fertil Steril 1991;56:691.
135. GOLAN A, RON-EL R, HERMAN A, ET AL: Ovarian hyperstimulation syndrome: an update review. Obstet Gynecol Surv 1989;44:430.
136. SULTAN KM, NEAL GS, DAVIS OK, ET AL: An approach to ovulation induction for IVF-ET which minimizes the incidence of ovarian hyperstimulation syndrome [abstract]. Presented at the 8th World Congress of IVF-ET, Kyoto, Japan, 1993.
137. WHITTEMORE AS, HARRIS R, ITNYRE J, ET AL: Characteristics relating to ovarian cancer risk: collaborative analysis of 12 US case-control studies. I. Methods. Collaborative Ovarian Cancer Group. Am J Epidemiol 1992;136:1175.
138. WHITTEMORE AS, HARRIS R, ITNYRE J, ET AL: Characteristics relating to ovarian cancer risk: collaborative analysis of 12 US case-control studies. II. Invasive epithelial ovarian cancers in white women. Collaborative Ovarian Cancer Group. Am J Epidemiol 1992;136:1184.
139. HARRIS R, WHITTEMORE AS, ITNYRE J: Characteristics relating to ovarian cancer risk: collaborative analysis of 12 US case-control studies. III. Epithelial tumors of low malignant potential in white women: Collaborative Ovarian Cancer Group. Am J Epidemiol 1992;136:1204.
140. INTERNATIONAL FEDERATION OF FERTILITY SOCIETIES: Fertility drugs and ovarian cancer. Fertil Steril 1993;60:406.
141. RON E, LUNENFELD B, MENCZER J, ET AL: Cancer incidence in a cohort of infertile women. Am J Epidemiol 1987;125:780.
142. DICKER D, ASHKENAZI J, FELDBERG D, ET AL: Severe abdominal complications after transvaginal ultrasonographically guided retrieval of oocytes for in vitro fertilization and embryo transfer. Fertil Steril 1993;59:1313.
143. SULTAN KM, NEAL GS, GRIFO JA, ET AL: Incidence of pelvic infection following transvaginal oocyte aspiration for IVF-ET [abstract]. Presented at the 8th World Congress of IVF-ET, Kyoto, Japan, 1993.
144. HOLST N, MALTAU JM, FORSDAHL F, ET AL: Handling of tubal infertility after introduction of in vitro fertilization: changes and consequences. Fertil Steril 1991;55:140.

21
Current Perspectives

Lothar W. Popp

The traditional competition between vaginal versus abdominal surgical procedures has acquired the facet of operative laparoscopy. Today, almost all gynecologic operations that previously required laparotomy are being performed endoscopically. A number of procedures (e.g., tubal sterilization) have obvious advantages and are commonly accepted as the method of choice. On the other hand, the best approach to procedures such as hysterectomy or ovarian surgery continue to be debated. A third group of laparoscopic interventions are merely new or nongynecologic at first glance and consequently are involved in a struggle for acceptance. This group includes such procedures as creation of a neovagina, appendectomy, and herniorrhaphy.

Simplification

The current trend of technical development is aimed toward more sophisticated and thus more expensive laparoscopic instrumentation. The large array of specialized instruments, lasers, high frequency devices, robotics, insufflators, and three-dimensional video systems are but a few of the latest innovations. This development not only tends to complicate simple procedures and lengthen otherwise short ones but also adds to the cost explosion in health care, placing laparoscopic surgery in the "unaffordable range" in many parts of the world. Simplification and cost-effectiveness for laparoscopic procedures is therefore a major priority. "Not only must the operation be associated with minimal complications, but it must also be simplified to the utmost." This basic surgical principle, proposed in 1891 by Tait[1] with respect to hernia repair, has gained a new application in laparoscopic surgery and may be acknowledged as Tait's law.

Logistics

Habits and basic tenets of the surgeon also play an important role. One example is catheterization of the urinary bladder prior to each laparoscopic procedure. Our patients are asked to void shortly before laparoscopy unless an extensive procedure is anticipated. In this way the time, cost, and patient discomfort are reduced, all of which factors are associated with catheterization. In addition, the risk of urinary tract infection is diminished. Many other procedures should be scrutinized for necessity and effectiveness (e.g., routine lithotomy positioning of the patient with placement of a cervical manipulator and the numerous sterile precautions that may not be necessary). Introducing logistics into the area of laparoscopic surgery that are widely accepted in many professional fields can certainly add to the time involved and reduce cost efficacy. Bearing in mind the simplification and logistics of laparoscopic surgery, three examples of currently innovative laparoscopic procedures are described.

Creation of a Neovagina

More than 100 surgical procedures have been reported for the creation of a neovagina in patients with Mayer-von Rokitansky-Kuster-Hauser syndrome.[2] Different parts of the gastrointestinal tract have been used for its creation. Free skin grafts, pediculated skin and peritoneal grafts, human amnion grafts, and preserved human dura mater cerebri have been applied to the wall of a bluntly formed tunnel in the vesicorectal space. Nonsurgical methods for dilating the vaginal dimple, including intercourse, have been used successfully.

According to the method of Vecchietti and Ardillo,[2] an "olive" pulled up into the vaginal dimple is used to create a neovagina. Two suture threads fixed to the olive are placed at the wall of the vaginal dimple and delivered through an abdominally formed tunnel in the vesicorectal space, through the preperitoneal space, and out through the wound edges of a Pfannenstiel incision; tension is applied to the threads for 14 days.

In 1991 Ghirardini and Popp performed the first laparoscopic modification of a Vecchietti procedure and proposed a new diagnostic and therapeutic management regimen to treat Mayer-von Rokitansky-Kuster-Hauser syndrome.[3,4] The diagnosis is established by physical examination, identification of normal secondary sex characteristics with absence of a vagina, and the ultrasound examination findings of normal ovaries, uterine agenesis, and primary amenorrhea. Management consists of appropriate counseling, with delay of the surgical procedure until the capability for intercourse is desired, at which time laparoscopic creation of a neovagina or use of a dilation method become the choices of therapy.

A segmented mold designed by Pelzer and Graf[5] may be used for laparoscopic creation of a neovagina. It is phallus-shaped and can be lengthened by attaching additional segments. At the time capability for intercourse is desired, operative endoscopy is performed (Plate 39). The patient is placed in a lithotomy position, preferably with a suprapubic catheter in place. An umbilical port is established for the laparoscope, and two 5 mm suprapubic ports are provided. Laparoscopic tunneling of the vesicorectal space, even though not absolutely necessary, facilitates placement of the suture threads. The sutures are fixed to the end-piece of the segmented mold and threaded through the eye at the tip of a blunt perforator, which is then passed from the vaginal dimple into the vesicorectal tunnel.

One of the suprapubic trocar sheaths is retracted until its abdominal opening comes to lie preperitoneally. The sheath is then advanced to the vesicorectal tunnel, one of the suture threads seized with a grasping forceps, and the thread pulled out through the suprapubic trocar sheath. The same procedure is performed on the opposite side as well. Traditionally, two suture threads are used; however, one-thread traction, which has been performed in one case,[6] may provide the same result.

Tourniquets (circumference 2 cm) on the abdominal wall provide compression of the vaginal dimple. The tourniquets are fixed to a protective plate utilized for wire sutures on the abdomen and secured with surgical tape. It may be advisable to allow the mold to protrude approximately 5 cm from the introitus and appropriately add segments as the mold is gradually drawn upward by tightening the tourniquets (Fig. 21.1). An additional dilatation effect can be achieved by having the patient sit on the protruding mold, as on a bicycle seat, three times daily.

The results of this otherwise unchanged Vecchietti-Ardillo procedure are theoretically similar to those achieved with the traditional procedure.[2] Patients profit from the novel logistics of diagnosis and preoperative management as well as from a simplified operative method.

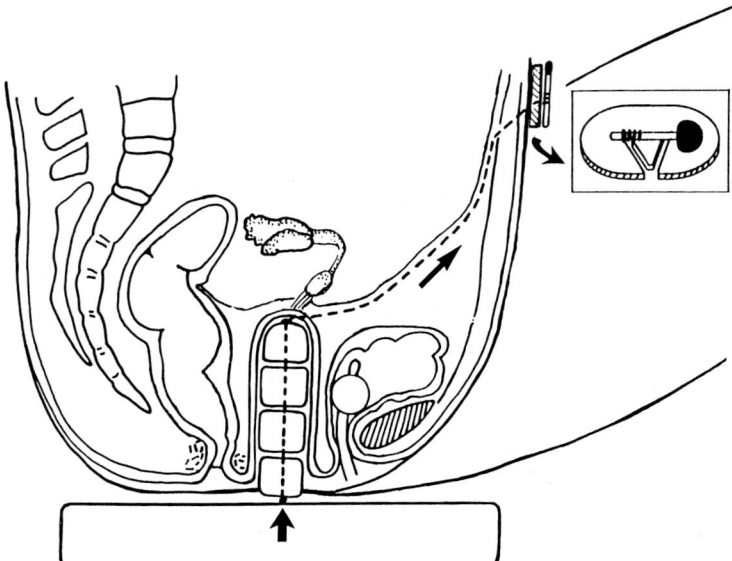

Figure 21.1. Laparoscopic creation of a neovagina using a segmented mold.

Appendectomy

Chronic appendicitis is one of the differential diagnoses of pelvic pain and may be detected during gynecologic laparoscopy. Although this subject is addressed elsewhere in this text, the controversial issue is whether it is the gynecologist's responsibility to proceed with incidental appendectomy or a general surgeon's expertise is required. A simple answer is that *expertise* is required, be it that of a general surgeon, a gynecologist, or a team. From a historical perspective, laparoscopic appendectomy was first performed in 1982 by Schreiber, a gynecologist in Mettmarn, Germany.[7] The organ is amenable to extraction through a 10 mm laparoscopic port.

One-Loop Technique

When diagnostic laparoscopy with use of a 5 mm right suprapubic port reveals chronic appendicitis, a 10 mm suprapubic port should be placed on the left. If adhesions are present, adhesiolysis of the appendix and mesoappendix is achieved. A grasping instrument, which has been introduced through an extraction tube in the left-sided 10 mm trocar sheath, is passed through a 5 metric catgut loop ligature introduced through the right-sided 5 mm trocar port.

The mesoappendix is grasped close to the middle of the appendix. As the appendix is elevated, it forms "equilateral legs of a triangle" with the mesoappendix at the base. The loop is brought to lie around the edge of the mesoappendix, and the tip of the loop applicator is maneuvered to the base of the appendix. The mesoappendix and the base of the appendix are ligated by securing the loop. The mesoappendix is released, and the suture is loop-clipped.

The mesoappendix is now regrasped close to the tip of the appendix. By pulling the appendix into the sleeve of the port and incising the mesoappendix close to the opening of the port, the appendix is skeletonized to its base. The appendix is then held under tension and incised directly at the opening of the port, approximately 1 cm distal to the loop ligature. Placement of iodine at the stump may be considered, as small amounts of the contents of the appendix may escape. Any remaining mesoappendix tissue may be resected.

Alternative Techniques

Clearly, an alternative method is use of a stapler device, which may be as efficient and quick as the single-loop technique. Its disadvantage is the larger port required, placement of nonresorbable material, and its high cost.

Use of any form of electrocoagulation for dissecting the mesoappendix or the base of the appendix is best avoided whenever possible, as there is a risk of thermal bowel damage. In a number of cases, burns of the cecal wall and subsequent bowel perforation, often first noted 1 week postoperatively, have been reported.

Application of metal clips is best avoided.[8] A second loop ligature on the appendix stump "for security" is often not necessary when reliable suture material is used and the loop is appropriately secured. If the "security loop" is not placed precisely on top of the first ligature,[8,9] the contaminated bowel segment between the loops may give rise to an abscess.

Placement of a purse string suture on top of a Z suture for burying the appendix stump, as with open appendectomy, is in all probability unnecessary. The laparoscopic one-loop technique as applied to treatment of chronic appendicitis with associated right lower quadrant pain may be the most advantageous procedure because it avoids the risks and hazards of more extensive operative procedures.

Herniorrhaphy

Abdominal wall hernia is part of the differential diagnosis for chronic abdominal pain. The diagnostic spectrum of a gynecologist who performs laparoscopy for pelvic pain should include direct and indirect inguinal hernia femoral, obturator, and incisional hernia. When obtaining a patient's history, symptoms specific for a hernia should be determined; physical examination should include consideration of abdominal wall hernia during examination of the groin with the patient in a standing position. Pain associated with hernia usually is localized, sharp, and aggravated by a change in position or straining. Relief is attained by ceasing the physical activity that precipitated it (see Chap. 32).

Diagnostic Laparoscopy

During diagnostic laparoscopy, the round ligament is followed to the internal inguinal ring, which may be closed or opened, forming the entrance to an indirect inguinal hernia (canal of Nuck). The inguinal fossa is inspected medial to the internal inguinal ring. This anatomic region is divided longitudinally by the lateral umbilical fold (containing the inferior epigastric artery and vein) forming the lateral and medial inguinal fossa. Direct inguinal hernias are primarily protrusions of the medial inguinal fossa. The rupture or bulging of the overlying transversalis fascia is generally broad-based with a dome shape.[10]

Acquired laxity of the transversalis fascia, which represents the only fibrotic abdominal wall layer in this area (Hesselbach triangle), may result in broad, deep inguinal fossae, which are expanded by the pneumoperitoneum during laparoscopy. Diagnostic criteria, their coincidence with pain, and the need for surgical repair are not well defined.[11]

A femoral hernia is a protrusion through the femoral ring, which is located below Cooper's ligament, medial to the femoral vein. Both structures can be identified by laparoscopy with the patient in the Trendelenburg position.

The rare but dangerous obturator hernia protrudes into the obturator canal located in continuation of the lateral umbilical fold, below the superior pubic ramus. Obturator hernias may contain ileum, with only a portion of the ileal circumference (Richter hernia) or an entire ileum loop incarcerated.[12]

Approximately 1% of all transparietoneal abdominal incisions result in a postoperative hernia.[13] At times the hernial defect is small, and a thick panniculus can prevent palpation of the defect. Patients may experience tenderness or vague discomfort, or they may describe a feeling of tearing in the area of an abdominal scar. During laparoscopic lysis of abdominal wall adhesions in the area of a former incision, care should be taken not to cut through the contents of an incisional hernia which may contain bowel wall (Richter hernia) or an incarcerated loop of bowel.

Operative Technique

A hernia may be repaired with suture closure, best termed herniorrhaphy, or by a prosthetic implant, termed hernioplasty or hernia patch repair. The first report on laparoscopic hernia

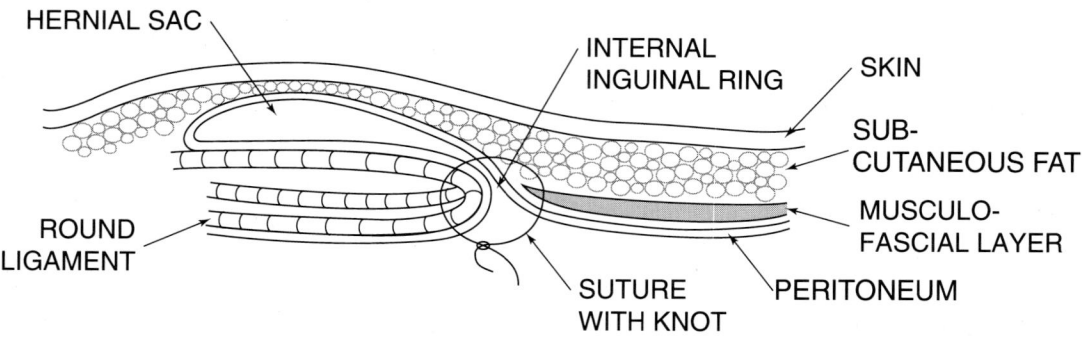

Figure 21.2. Laparoscopic occlusion of the open internal inguinal ring of an indirect hernia in a female patient.

repair was presented in 1989 by the gynecologist Bogolavjensky.[14] The type of laparoscopic hernia repair greatly depends on whether the peritoneum of the hernial sac is detachable, as it is with a direct inguinal hernia, or not detachable, as with an indirect inguinal hernia.

Herniorrhaphy of the Internal Hernial Ring

Endoscopic suturing with use of intra- or extracorporeal knot tying techniques may be the best means for occluding the internal inguinal ring with indirect inguinal hernias (Fig. 21.2). The round ligament may be included with suturing.[14,15] Obturator hernia and other types of hernia with a narrow neck may be approached in a likewise manner.

Alternatively, staples can be applied with a variety of instruments (e.g., the Herniatat®, Innovative Surgical Devices, Westbury, NY). Easier and perhaps faster occlusion of the internal hernial ring by stapling may be advantageous; the disadvantages are the unnecessary implantation of nonabsorbable materials and the higher cost.

Hernia Patch Repair

Patches composed of varying nonabsorbable and absorbable materials may be implanted laparoscopically, either intra- or preperitoneally. The first published case of laparoscopic hernia repair was one of combined herniorrhaphy and intraperitoneal patch repair of a direct inguinal hernia. A human dura mater transplant was fixed to the peritoneum around the hernia via laparoscopically placed sutures.[15] Intraperitoneal patch repair is not widely used today, even though it would be applicable to direct inguinal, umbilical, and incisional hernias. The fear of creating adhesions remains the primary concern.

Preperitoneal patch repair is the most commonly used method at the present time. Nonabsorbable Dacron mesh (the most common mesh) is implanted after laparoscopic dissection of large areas of the peritoneum. Transcutaneous or laparoscopic hydrodissection of the preperitoneal hernial sac[16,17] facilitates the procedure. Fixation of the implanted mesh is accomplished with staples or sutures. A preperitoneal mesh patch trapped by merely closing the peritoneum may have an effect similar to that of mesh sutured in place.

Hernioscopy

Transcutaneous inspection of the preperitoneal hernial sac is termed hernioscopy.[15] (Fig. 21.3; Plate 40). This procedure can only be applied to hernias with a sliding peritoneum in the hernial sac.

A beveled 5- or 10-mm trocar sheath with laparoscope is passed through an appropriate skin incision over the hernial protrusion. The musculofascial defect is gently explored with the tip of the trocar sheath; the resistance of the intact abdominal wall and the nonresistant gap of the hernia can thus be palpated. If no rupture but bulging of the transversalis fascia is present,

21. Current Perspectives

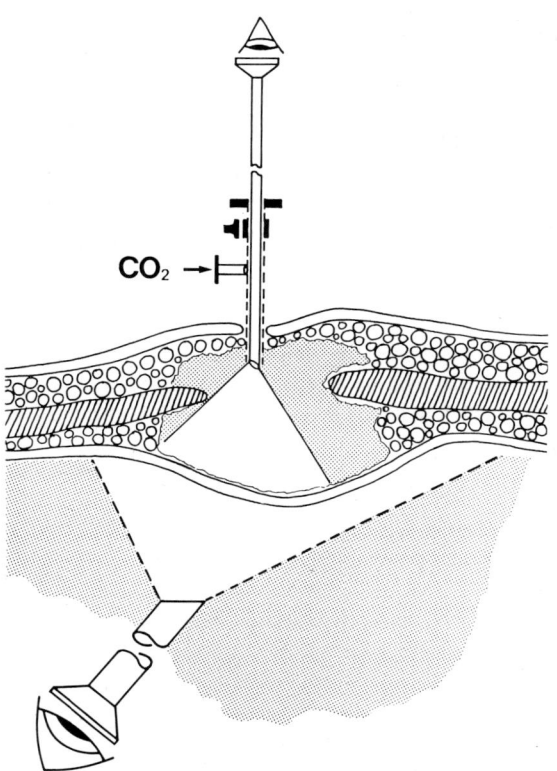

Figure 21.3. Hernioscopy in detail.

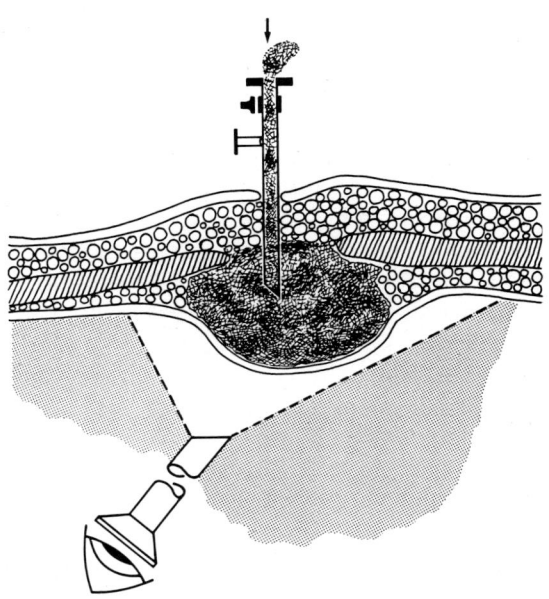

Figure 21.4. Hernioscopic stuffing repair.

the flimsy fascial layer can be penetrated by the beveled tip of the trocar sheath. By creating preperitoneal emphysema with a CO_2 insufflator, the peritoneum of the hernial sac is elevated toward the abdominal cavity at pressures of 12 mm Hg and the hernial sac can be inspected.

Hernioscopic Stuffing Repair

After hernioscopic dissection of the preperitoneal hernial sac, the laparoscope is removed and exchanged for an applicator tube loaded with a segment of absorbable mesh. The mesh is stuffed (load by load) into the preperitoneal hernial sac. In this way a plug of mesh that is larger in diameter than the hernial ring per se is formed beyond the hernial ring (Fig. 21.4). The hernial ring is plugged by the mesh, which may be regarded as a three-dimensional patch. Sufficient occlusion of the musculofascial defect can be achieved by the extensive scar formation induced by the gradually resolving patch material ("induction of stabilization"). Hence the possible disadvantages of permanent implants, are avoided.

Hernioscopic "stuffing repair" is indicated in small direct inguinal hernias. Its disadvantage is the need for laparoscopic control with an extraperitoneal procedure and the significant cost of the mesh. Refinements in selecting suitable patients (i.e., by high resolution ultrasonography diagnosis) may lead to hernioscopic stuffing repair without laparoscopic control, in which case the procedure may be accomplished with local anesthesia. Moreover, the plug of mesh may be replaced by an appropriate foam or sponge material that is easier to apply and possibly less expensive than the existing patch materials.

Conclusion

Diagnostic laparoscopy for pelvic pain requires expertise regarding the nature and clinical appearance of abdominal wall hernias. A gynecologist not focused on the possibility of hernia as the cause of pelvic pain and who does not evaluate the abdominal wall during diagnostic laparoscopy may easily miss the diagnosis. Consequently, a diagnosis of unexplained pelvic pain or even the suspicion of psychological causes for pelvic pain may result.

Hernias, when detected laparoscopically, are ideally repaired laparoscopically when feasible. Although the indications for laparoscopic hernia repair are still controversial, a hernia detected by the gynecologist during diagnostic laparoscopy for pelvic pain must clearly be repaired. Such repairs should be undertaken by a physician with appropriate expertise, be it a general surgeon or a gynecologist.

References

1. TAIT L: A discussion on treatment of hernia by median abdominal section. Gr Med J 1891;2:685.
2. VECCHIETTI G, ARDILLO L: La sindrome di Rokitansky-Kuester-Hauser. Fisiopathologia e Clinica Dell-aplasia Vaginale con Corni Uterini Rudimentali. Rome, Society Editrice Universo, 1970.
3. GHIRARDINI G, POPP LW: New approach to the Mayer-von Rokitansky-Kuster-Hauser syndrome. Adolesc Pediatr Gynecol 1994;7:41.
4. POPP LW, GHIRANDINI G: Creation of a neovagina by pelviscopy. J Laparoendosc Surg 1992;2:165.
5. PELZER V, GRAF M: Das gegliederte Steckphantom zur Bildung einer Neovagina nach Vecchietti. Geburtsh Frauenheilkd 1989;53:677.
6. POPP LW: Endoscopic creation of a neovagina using a segmented plexiglass mould—case report. Zentralbl Gynaekol 1993;115:570.
7. SCHREIBER JH: Early experience with laparoscopic appendectomy in women. Surg Endosc 1987;1:211.
8. REDDICK EJ, SAYE WB: Laparoscopic appendectomy. In Surgical Laparoscopy, Zucker KA (ed). St. Louis, Quality Medical Publishing, 1991.
9. BAJUSZ H, MCMAHON MJ: Laparoscopic appendectomy. In Minimal Access General Surgery, Rosin D (ed). Oxford, Radcliffe Medical Press, 1994.
10. SMEDBERG SGG, BROOME AEA: Herniography. In Hernia, Nyhus LM, Condon RE (ed). Philadelphia, Lippincott, 1989.
11. CONDON RE: The anatomy of the inguinal region and its relation to groin hernia. In Hernia, Nyhus LM, Condon RE (eds). Philadelphia, Lippincott, 1989.
12. SKANDALAKIS JE, GRAY SW: Strangulated obturator hernia. In Hernia, Nyhus LM, Condon RE (eds). Philadelphia, Lippincott, 1989.
13. BAKER RJ: Incisional hernia. In Hernia, Nyhus LM, Condon RE (eds). Philadelphia, Lippincott, 1989.
14. BOGOLAVJENSKY S: Laparoscopic Treatment of Inguinal and Femoral Hernia [video]. Presented at the 16th Annual Meeting of the American Association of Gynecological Laparoscopists, Washington, DC, 1989.
15. POPP LW: Endoscopic patch repair of inguinal hernia in a female patient. Surg Endosc 1990; 4:10.
16. POPP LW: Laparoscopic and hernioscopic diagnosis and repair of abdominal wall hernias. In Minimal Access General Surgery, Rosin D (ed). Oxford, Radcliffe Medical Press, 1994.
17. POPP LW: Improvement of endoscopic hernioplasty: transcutaneous aquadissection of the musculofascial defect, and preperitoneal endoscopic patient repair. J Laparoendosc Surg 1991;1:83.

Section IV
Hysteroscopic Techniques

22
Operative Hysteroscopy and Resectoscopy

Rafael F. Valle

Operative hysteroscopy was introduced simultaneously with diagnostic hysteroscopy when Pantaleoni attempted direct hysteroscopic treatment of bleeding endometrial polyps in a postmenopausal woman.[1] Nonetheless, technologic advances and appropriate instrumentation did not make it possible to operate inside a uterine cavity with a practical hysteroscopic method until the early 1970s, when appropriate instrumentation, safe and effective distending media, and adequate light sources were introduced.[2] Attention to operative hysteroscopy was focused on tubal sterilization by electrical thermal destruction of the intramural portion of the fallopian tubes. When these attempts proved unsatisfactory and risky, interest shifted to other aspects of the uterine cavity that could be treated endoscopically.[3] Innovations in operative hysteroscopes and energy sources have enhanced the capabilities of operating inside the uterine cavity safely and efficiently, supplanting traditional, more invasive surgical procedures (e.g., laparotomy and hysterotomy) for treating symptomatic uterine conditions.[4]

Instrumentation and Energy Sources

Hysteroscope

There are two types of hysteroscopes: rigid and flexible. The most commonly used operative hysteroscope is the rigid type.

The rigid hysteroscope has several components; a telescope 4 mm outer diameter (O.D.), with a fore-oblique view of 30° angle; the bridge, which connects to the telescope and permits insertion of operating instruments of a 7F caliber; and an outer sheath of 7–8 mm O.D. When assembled, these components permit infusion of a liquid distending medium and, to some degree, its recovery after lavaging the uterine cavity. Some hysteroscopes also have an obturator shaped like the dilator to introduce the outer sheath atraumatically. The telescope contains a rod lens system, which provides a wider angle of view and brighter image than the original "bead" lens. Most telescopes have a 30° fore-oblique angle to observe the uterine cavity, particularly the lateral portions of the uterotubal ostia, providing complete visualization. The depth of the visual field of the telescope is about 2–3 cm, with low-power magnification (4+ to 5+) using a liquid distending medium.

Hysteroscopes with a built-in double-channel system for injecting the distending medium and its recovery are available (Weck/Linvatec); others have a continuous-flow system for cleansing the uterine cavity intraoperatively (Olympus, Circon, Storz) (Figs. 22.1–22.3).

Ancillary operative instruments required for hysteroscopy are of three types: flexible, semirigid, and rigid. The most useful ancillary in-

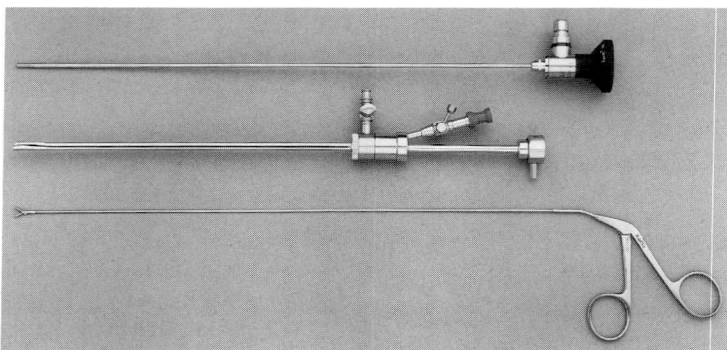

Figure 22.1. Unassembled operative hysteroscope. Top to bottom: telescope, operating bridge, semirigid grasping forceps (Wolf).

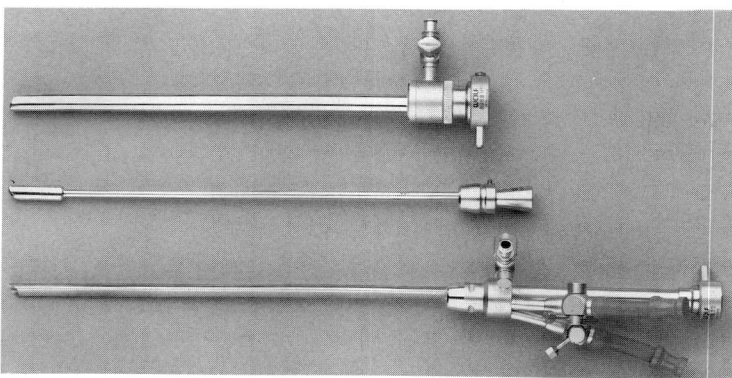

Figure 22.2. Outer cannula (top) with obturator (middle) and a double-channel cannula (bottom) (Wolf).

struments are semirigid (biopsy forceps, grasping forceps, scissors), permitting easier, more rapid manipulation than the flexible instruments. The rigid ancillary instruments, or so-called optic instruments, are fixed at the end of the hysteroscope. The whole hysteroscope must be moved to-and-fro to reach the desired area to be dissected, incised, or biopsied. It is important when using these rigid, fixed instruments to have a perfect panoramic view of the uterine cavity in order to avoid injuring the uterine walls. Introduction of these instruments through the cervical canal must be accomplished with caution to prevent injury and possible uterine perforation (Figs. 22.4–22.10).

The flexible and the steerable operative hysteroscopes have an outer diameter of 4.9 mm and an operating channel of 2.0 mm. These

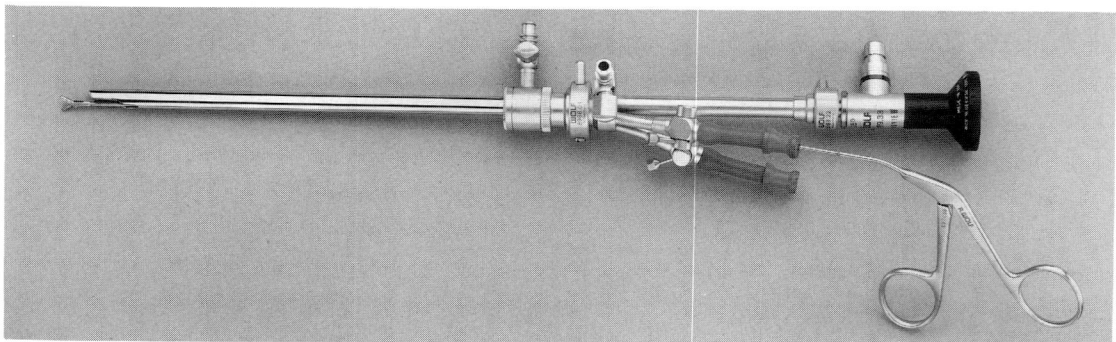

Figure 22.3. Assembled operative hysteroscope with biopsy forceps in place (Wolf).

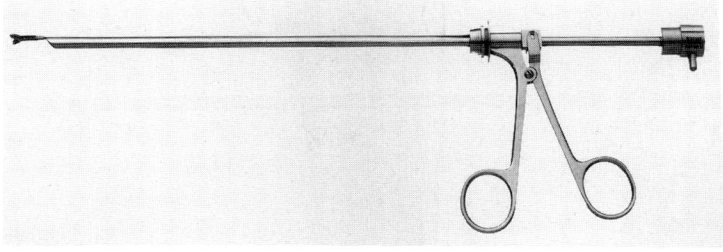

Figure 22.4. Optical, fixed hysteroscopic scissors.

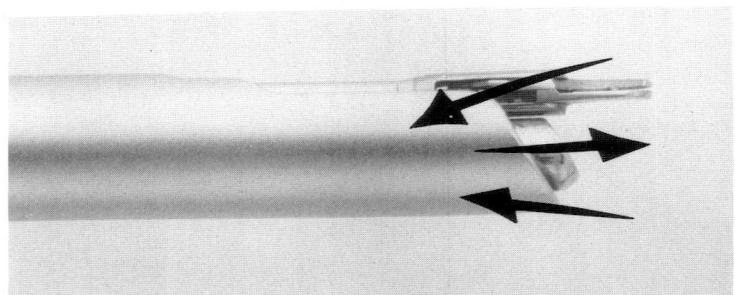

Figure 22.5. Fixed optical scissors adjacent to telescope and encased in sheath. Arrows mark the direction of fluid inflow (middle) and outflow, peripheral to telescope and scissors (Olympus).

hysteroscopes are delicate and require special care to avoid breaking the fibers that cross the full length of the hysteroscope. Only flexible instruments can be utilized when operating with this type of hysteroscope; and because of their small size they do not permit extensive manipulation(s). They are most useful when operating in the uterotubal cornual region, as the instruments can be steered atraumatically exactly to the point where the lesion, polyp, or adhesion is to be resected. They are most useful for tubal cannulation, as the catheter is soft and flexible and can be directed by steering the tip of the hysteroscope to the uterotubal junction, permitting easy insertion of these catheters with guidewires, directly into the fallopian tube. The drawbacks of the steerable operative hysteroscopes are the small size of the ancillary operating instruments, the granular aspect of the view obtained by the light-transmitting fibers, maintenance to

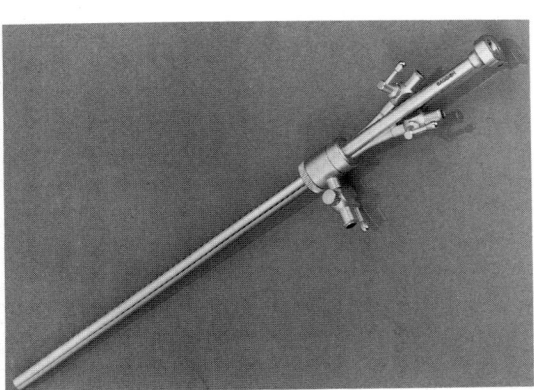

Figure 22.6. Operative, double-channel hysteroscopic sheath (Weck/Linvatec).

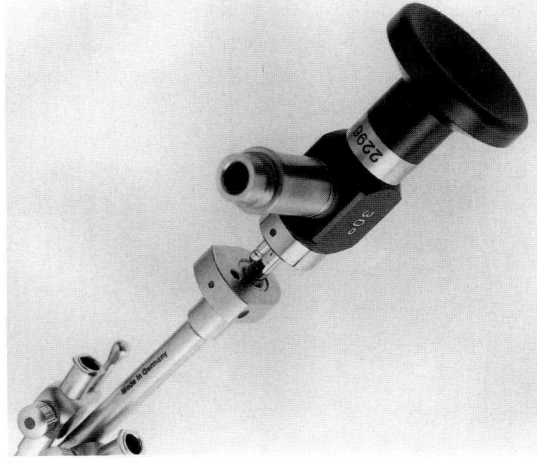

Figure 22.7. Close-up view of telescope inserted into sheath (Weck/Linvatec).

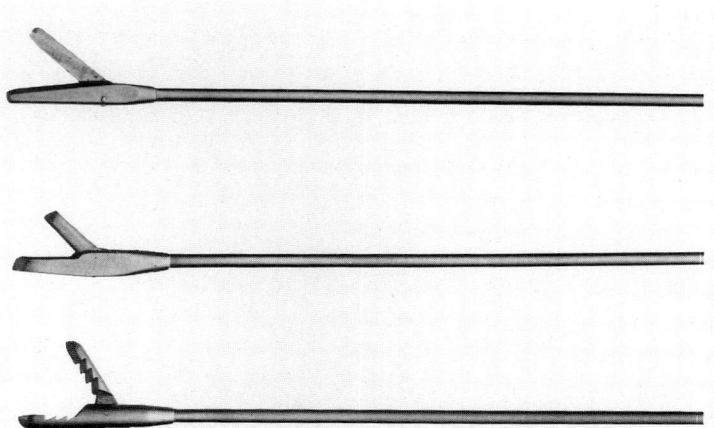

Figure 22.8. Semirigid hysteroscopic operative instruments. Top to bottom: scissors, biopsy forceps, grasping forceps (Storz).

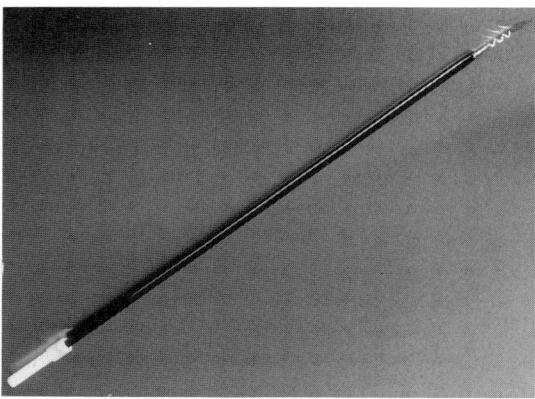

Figure 22.9. Corkscrew for fixation of submucous myomas (Cook Ob/Gyn).

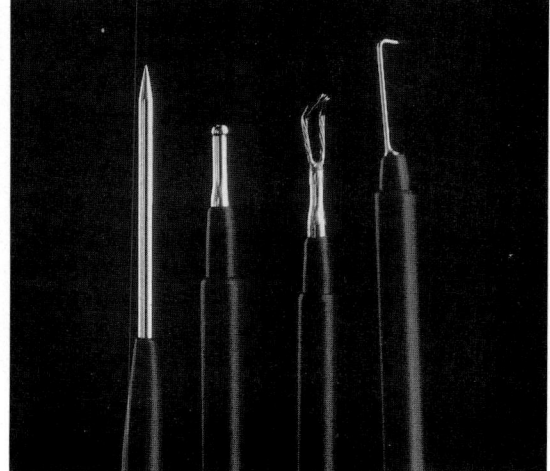

Figure 22.10. Electrodes for use with unipolar energy. Left to right: needle, ball-tip, loop-tip, hook-tip (Cook Ob/Gyn).

avoid breaking the fibers in the scope, and cost that is higher than that of the rigid hysteroscopes (Figs. 22.11, 22.12).

The advantages of using this type of instrumentation, particularly when the uterine cavity is distorted by pathology, are size and flexibility; the hysteroscope can be directed to the area in need of therapy, and insertion is easier when there is marked retroflexion or retroversion of the uterus.

Resectoscope

The gynecologic resectoscope was derived from the urologic resectoscope by modifying the size and shape of the outer sheath and adding a continuous-flow system. The resectoscope includes a telescope with a straightforward view (0°) or a slight fore-oblique view (15°–20°) and 3.5–4.0 mm O.D. Two concentric outer sheaths are required to provide a system of continuous flow. The outer sheath is 8–9 mm O.D. with distal fenestrations to permit exit of the fluid; a ceramic tip is added to insulate the loop, once it has been retrieved inside the sheath. The inner sheath fits snugly into the outer sheath and has an inflow port to permit uterine distention. A spring-loaded mechanism is adapted to the

22. Operative Hysteroscopy and Resectoscopy

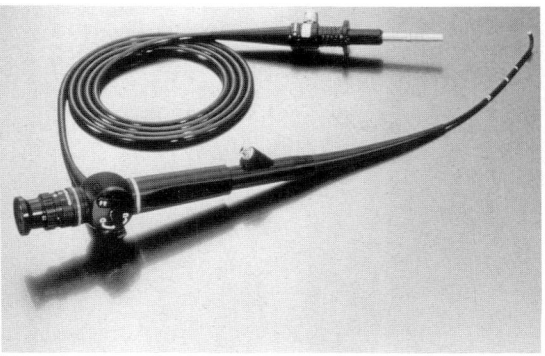

Figure 22.11. Flexible operative hysteroscope (Olympus).

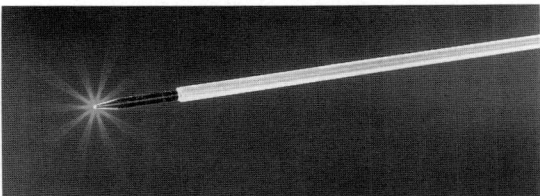

Figure 22.13. Quartz sculpted conical fiber for contact precise cutting and coagulating. Tip size 300 µm (Laser Sonics).

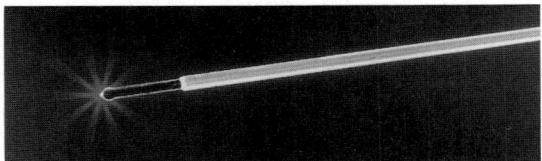

Figure 22.14. Quartz sculpted ball-tip fiber for enhanced coagulation. Tip size 1200 µm (Laser Sonics).

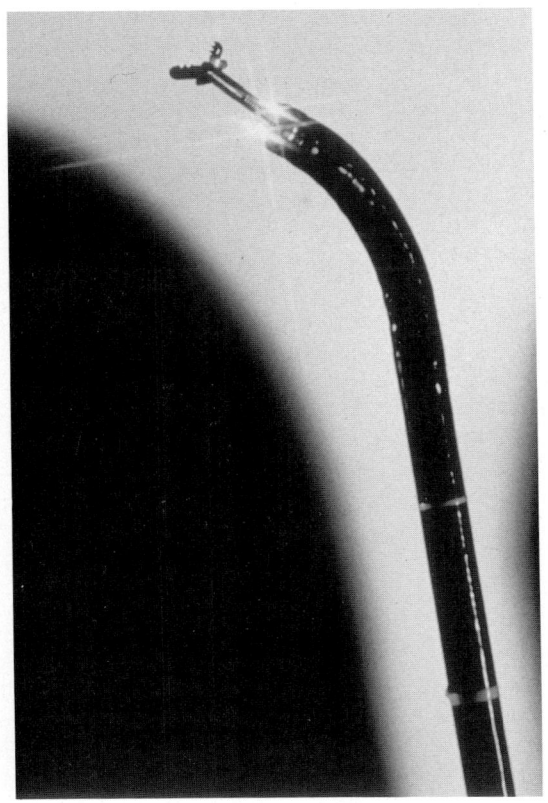

Figure 22.12. Distal tip of flexible operative hysteroscope with biopsy forceps in place (Olympus).

bridge to permit manipulation of electrodes, which can be fitted to this bridge. The spring-loaded mechanism of the bridge permits movement of the electrodes back and forth with 4 cm displacement into the field of view. The bridge has a special adaptor to connect the electrical cord of the high frequency electrosurgical unit. When the resectoscope is assembled, the port for the light source faces up with the electrode in a down position due to the fore-oblique view (Figs. 22.12–22.17).

Ancillary Instrumentation

In addition to the operating ancillary instruments necessary to perform intrauterine operations, the light source unit, preferably a xenon lamp, is necessary, particularly because the small-caliber telescope requires a potent light source for optimal visualization. An electrosurgical unit with wattage display monitoring and return electric monitoring system is important if electrosurgery should be required. Operative hysteroscopy and resectoscopy are best performed through a video monitor; a high resolu-

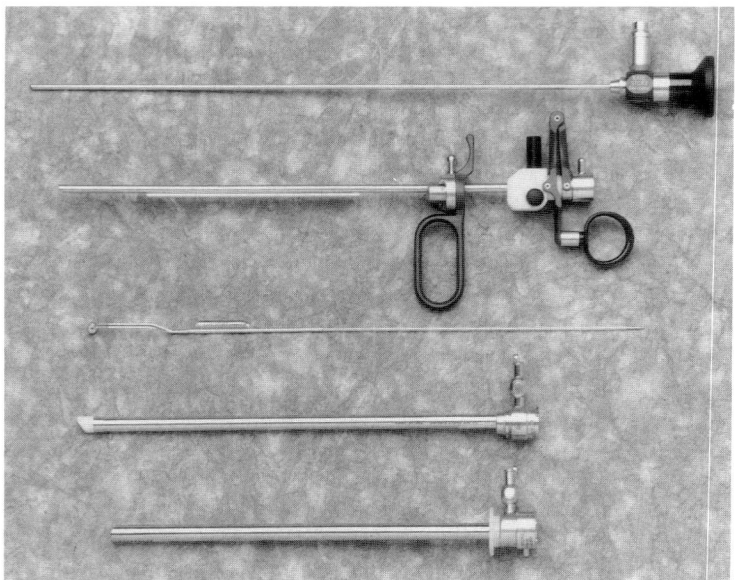

Figure 22.15. Unassembled gynecologic resectoscope. Top to bottom: telescope, spring-loaded bridge, electrode, inner sheath for inflow, outer sheath for outflow (Storz).

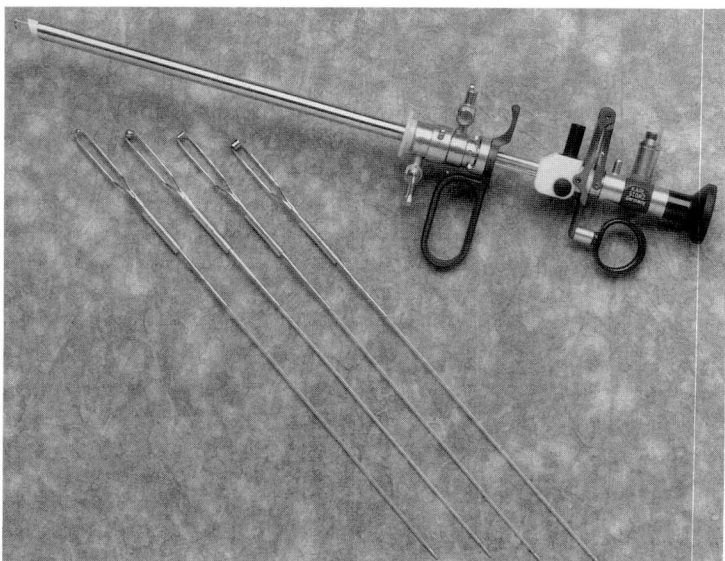

Figure 22.16. Assembled gynecologic resectoscope with various electrodes for coagulation (Storz).

tion camera allows sharing of information with assistants and other operating room personnel and is most useful for a team approach. Precision is improved, as the field of view increases and details of the target tissue are enhanced by the technology of the new cameras. Furthermore, comfort for the operator increases as the need for continued ocular–telescope contact is not required (Fig. 22.18).

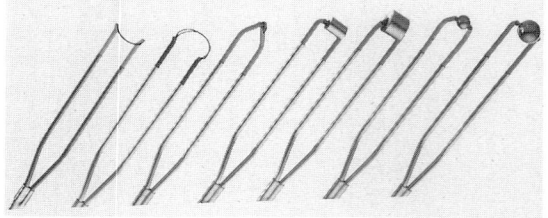

Figure 22.17. Electrodes for cutting and coagulating with resectoscope (Storz).

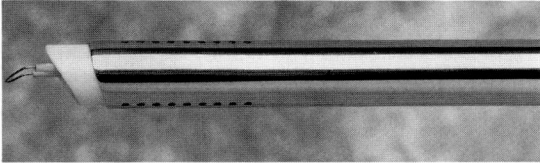

Figure 22.18. Close-up view of distal end of resectoscope with forward cutting loop in place. The outer cannula is fenestrated to permit retrieval of irrigating fluid (Storz).

Energy Sources

Many operations can be performed hysteroscopically with mechanical instruments, but the utilization of fiberoptic lasers and electrosurgery can enhance the applications of intrauterine surgery. Fiberoptic lasers can be introduced through the operating channel of the hysteroscope and deliver the laser energy transmitted through fluids that distend the uterine cavity without blockage. The most commonly used fiberoptic laser for intrauterine surgery has been the Nd:YAG laser, particularly for endometrial ablation, owing to its properties of (1) being attracted by the purplish tissue, destroying tissue protein by coagulation, and (2) scattering both frontally and laterally, which is useful for destroying the endometrium. Because this laser is located in the infrared portion of the spectrum with a 1064 nm wavelength, it is invisible and requires a helium beam guide to target the area to be treated.

When the fiberoptic lasers are used for purposes other than endometrial ablation, the depth of coagulation must be reduced. "Bare" fibers should be avoided. To concentrate and focus the laser to prevent scattering, new sculptured or extruded fibers have been introduced that permit dissection or cutting with little coagulation. These fibers can be used to divide a uterine septum, divide intrauterine adhesions, or dissect a pedunculated submucous leiomyoma. Sapphire tips have been attached to the quartz fiber of the Nd:YAG; these specific tips require continuous cooling, which can be accomplished with either fluid or gas medium.

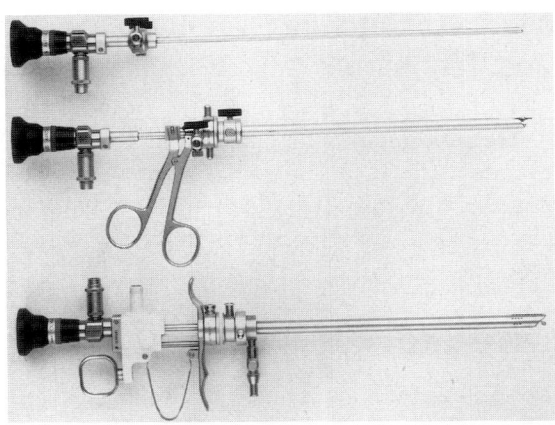

Figure 22.19. Telescope fitted to different sheaths permits various uses. Top to bottom: diagnostic hysteroscope, operative hysteroscope with fixed optical scissors, gynecologic resectoscope (Olympus).

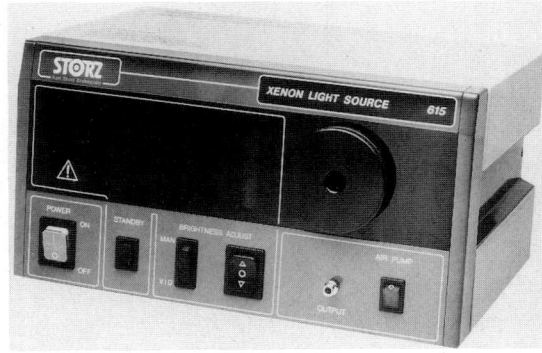

Figure 22.20. Xenon light source for illumination and video (Storz).

Fluids can be used safely, but they increase the probability of intravasation and fluid overload, as the quantity of fluids required to cool the fibers is significant. If cooling gases (including CO_2) are used for this purpose, gas embolus can occur. A high flow, about 1 L/min, is required to cool the sapphire tips. Sapphire tips cooled by gases or air should never be used in the uterine cavity (Figs. 22.19, 22.20).

Media for Uterine Distention and Techniques

There are primarily three media used to distend the uterus for diagnostic and therapeutic applications: low viscosity fluids with or without electrolytes, high viscosity fluids (Hyskon), and CO_2 gas.

Low Viscosity Fluids

Low viscosity fluids for uterine distention are of two types: fluids containing electrolytes and those devoid of electrolytes. An important condition for operating in the uterine cavity is adequate uterine distention and sufficient lavage of the uterine cavity to remove mucus, debris, and blood obscuring the view. Low viscosity fluids are most useful for this purpose. To obtain distention and good visualization with the hysteroscope, it is important to have a system that offers continuous flow. Most (operative) hysteroscopes do not have the perfect continuous flow provided by the resectoscope; therefore this system can be improvised by inserting a polyethylene catheter of adequate size through the operating channel of the hysteroscope and providing a siphoning effect to cleanse the uterine cavity prior to and during intrauterine surgery. These catheters provide targeted cleansing of the uterine cavity that even with hysteroscopes that offer some type of continuous flow (Olympus, Storz, Circon) this targeted effect may not be obtained as well as with the polyethylene catheter. The imperfect continuous flow most hysteroscopes provide does not permit accurate measurement of the retrieved fluid or an estimate of the fluid absorbed by the patient.

Low Viscosity Fluids with Electrolytes

Low viscosity with electrolytes, specifically sodium, are the most useful fluids for distending the uterus during operative hysteroscopy when no electrical energy is being utilized, such as when operating with mechanical ancillary instruments or fiberoptic lasers. Because there is no problem with conduction utilizing these modalities, the addition of electrolytes to the distending medium increases the threshold for fluid overload, as sodium may act as a diuretic by opposing the effect of antidiuretic hormone. This situation does not imply that excessive intravasated fluid may not cause fluid overload and pulmonary edema, but the threshold is substantially increased, permitting more fluid to be absorbed without serious sequelae than when utilizing fluids devoid of electrolytes.

Low viscosity fluids with electrolytes that can be used for operative hysteroscopy are (1) normal saline (0.9% NaCl); (2) 5% dextrose in half-normal saline ($D_5\frac{1}{2}SN$) (0.45 NaCl); and (3) Ringer's lactate, a balanced solution that also permits adequate visualization. Although these three media provide similar visualization when used as a distending medium, the most commonly used fluid is D_5S, which provides the advantages of dextrose, a crystalloid that may lyse erythrocytes should a small amount of bleeding occur. Should excessive fluid not be recovered (> 2 L), diuretics could be used more liberally, as hyponatremia does not occur with this type of fluid.

Low Viscosity Fluids Without Electrolytes

Because electrolytes are excellent conductors, they cannot be utilized in fluids that distend the uterine cavity when electrosurgery is performed. Electrosurgery applied in the uterus distended with fluids containing electrolytes behaves erratically and may cause unnecessary injury to adjacent organs due to the poor effect at the tissue contact when these fluids are utilized and the increase in power of the electrosurgical unit.

Low viscosity fluids without electrolytes are most commonly used during urologic procedures with a resectoscope, and similar fluids can be utilized during resectoscopy for gynecologic procedures. These fluids are 5% dextrose in water (D_5W), 1.5% glycine, 3% sorbitol, and Cytal (2.8% sorbitol plus 0.5% mannitol). D_5W has an osmolarity of 256 mOs/L. Because dextrose is packaged in plastic or glass 1 L containers, it cannot be used without a mechanical pump to provide adequate uterine distention. Alternatively, a plastic bag could be compressed with an appropriate wrapper to provide the positive pressure of 100–150 mm Hg required to maintain uterine distention. In the absence of a mechanical pump, two 1 L plastic bags can be prepared through Y-type tubing and used alternatively, one at a time. Glycine 1.5%, a substance composed of amino acids, is nonconductive with an osmolarity of 200 mOs/L and can also be used safely during intrauterine electrosurgery. Glycine, which is broken down to ammonia, serine, and glyoxalic acid, may precipitate oxalate crystals in the urine and can cause central nervous system (CNS) toxicity if excessive amounts are intravasated. Because it comes packaged in 3 L plastic bags, it does not necessarily require an infusion pump during resectoscopy, but using a high flow large-bore urologic tubing and elevating the 3 L plastic bag 3–4 feet above the patient provide sufficient pressure to distend the uterus and permit resectoscopy. Because glycine does not contain electrolytes, it is important to measure accurately the amount of fluid infused and the amount recovered, as the resectoscope provides a continuous-flow system. If the estimated deficit exceeds 700 ml, it is important to observe the patient's vital signs and pulse oximetry and determine the serum sodium level to prevent fluid overload and hyponatremia. If significant glycine decomposition is observed, the procedure should be aborted.

Sorbitol (5%), a reduced sugar with an osmolarity of 165 mOs/L, also can be used during resectoscopy and provides excellent visualization. Because this fluid does not contain electrolytes the same precautions should be taken as with glycine.

Cytal (2.8% sorbitol and 0.5% mannitol) or 5% mannitol alone (274 mOsm/L) also can be used during resectoscopy, with the advantage of causing slight diuresis. Nonetheless, diuretics must be used cautiously in these patients, particularly if hyponatremia exists, as diuretics (even osmotic diuretics) initially are also natriuretics and may exacerbate the condition should hyponatremia already exist.

High Viscosity Fluids (Hyskon)

Hyskon, a derivative of Dextran, is a 32% dextran solution (molecular weight 70,000 daltons) mixed in 10% dextrose in water; it is non-electrolytic solution that provides excellent visualization because of its crystal clear appearance. Because of its high viscosity it permits hysteroscopic surgery with small amounts of the solution (compared to high viscosity fluids). It has the advantage of not mixing with blood during operative hysteroscopy and providing "low magnification" as a distending medium, thereby improving visualization and facilitating the operative procedure. Because of its hyperosmotic properties, if intravasation of this fluid occurs during operative hysteroscopy it may draw fluids into the vascular tree that, if excessive, may cause pulmonary edema of noncardiogenic type. It may also cause a coagulopathy similar to disseminated intravascular coagulation. For this reason, the amount of Hyskon used should be carefully monitored, measuring the amount injected and calculating the amount that is retrieved so as to not permit more than 400–500 ml of Hyskon to be lost in the system.

Hyskon is most useful when performing operative hysteroscopy with mechanical tools and fiberoptic lasers; even with these methods, however, the time of the operation may be restricted by the caramelization of the dextran around the instruments. Its viscosity and stickiness, which makes use of the substance cumbersome for the operator and delivery of the substance mechanically with plastic syringes difficult, requires an assistant when a mechanical pump is not used. It is difficult to recover the Hyskon in the system, as it is difficult to estimate the amount of fluid that is lost on the drapes or occasionally on the floor. For this reason Hyskon must be used for short procedures with backup systems.

Hyskon does not contain electrolytes, and it can be used with electrosurgery. Its utilization with a resectoscope is cumbersome, as it cannot be retrieved from the outflow because of its viscosity. Therefore the continuous-flow system cannot be utilized to its full advantage.

CO_2 Gas

Carbon dioxide gas is an excellent medium for distending the uterus, particularly when utilizing small diagnostic endoscopes and when no manipulation of the uterine cavity is planned. For therapeutic applications, CO_2 gas can be somewhat cumbersome, particularly if bleeding produces bubbling and obscures the view. For this reason, CO_2 gas is preferable for diagnostic hysteroscopy and is seldom utilized for therapeutic uses.

Operative Hysteroscopy and Resectoscopy

Operative Hysteroscopy Technique

Whether utilizing local, regional, or general anesthesia, the technique of operative hysteroscopy is essentially the same. The patient is placed in the dorsal lithotomy position, and a bimanual examination is performed. The vulva, vagina, and cervix are then cleaned with an antiseptic solution. A vaginal speculum with an open side is introduced, and the anterior lip of the cervix is grasped with a single-tooth tenaculum. The endocervical canal is gradually dilated to the size of the operative hysteroscope being used, usually 7–8 mm. The hysteroscope attached to its light source and distending medium is then introduced atraumatically. If an obturator is used, insertion of the obturator and sheath simulates the insertion of a dilator up to the internal cervical os, where the obturator is removed and replaced by the telescope and bridge. When low viscosity fluids for uterine distention are used, a polyethylene catheter 2.4 mm O.D. and 1.6 mm inside diameter (I.D.) is introduced to the end of the hysteroscope before distention begins. Fluid under pressure is then allowed to enter the uterine cavity, permitting siphoning of the fluid through the polyethylene catheter. When the distending medium exiting through the catheter is clear from debris and blood clots, intrauterine visualization begins. Targeted areas of the uterine cavity are then aspirated with this polyethylene catheter to permit complete, unopposed visualization. If the operative hysteroscope has only one operating channel, the polyethylene catheter is removed, and the various ancillary instruments are inserted. The videocamera, if used, is attached to the ocular portion of the hysteroscope before the hysteroscope is inserted in the uterine cavity, and the colors are made uniform and the image focused. The correct orientation of the hysteroscope before insertion is with the fiber-optic cable conducting the light going downward, indicating that the fore-oblique view of the telescope is facing outward. The camera is kept in position without rotation; should rotation be required, only the hysteroscope is rotated clockwise or counterclockwise to observe the lateral aspects of the uterine cavity.

When low viscosity fluids are used for uterine distention, it is important to place a plastic pouch at the patient's buttock to collect the fluid that exits from the system. This technique aids in measuring the fluid intake and output and prevents fluid from wetting the floor.

If laparoscopy is used as an adjunct to monitor intrauterine surgery, it is preferable to insert the laparoscope first and then, aided by the laparoscopic view, perform the required uterine manipulation, such as cervical dilation or even introducing the hysteroscope. To monitor the hysteroscopic surgery, it is important to dim the light of the laparoscope to allow illumination of the hysteroscope through the uterine wall.

Resectoscopy Technique

The technique of resectoscopy is similar to the technique of operative hysteroscopy, but there are some important variations, particularly when activating and operating with the resectoscope. Most outer sheaths are 8–9 mm O.D., so they require prior endocervical dilatation. The resectoscope is assembled, and the connections are attached to the appropriate ports. The high flow urologic tubing for infusing the fluid is connected to the inner sheath port, and the outer port is connected to an exit tubing for collection of fluid. Usually the endocervical canal is dilated to at least 8–9 mm. It may be difficult to introduce the resectoscope without an obturator; therefore an obturator attached to the concentric cannulas already assembled is introduced and driven through the endocervical canal until the internal cervical os is reached. The obturator is then replaced with the telescope and operating bridge, already fitted with an appropriate electrode. Once the connections are in place, the inflow and outflow ports are opened simultaneously to permit washing of debris and blood clots out of the uterine cavity. This period of cleansing may require removing the bridge and telescope or the inner sheath occasionally to clear away blood clots that obstruct the continuous flow of the distending liquid medium. Once the uterine cavity is clean, uterine visualization and exploration begin. The electrical cord is attached to the resectoscope, and the operation may commence. It is important to check that the patient is properly grounded with the returning plate system to complete the circuit of monopolar surgery. Only fluids devoid of electrolytes can be used for resectoscopy. Several spare electrodes should be on hand because electrodes may collect debris that may impede their proper tissue effect when activated; although they may be cleaned, it is sometimes necessary to replace them with new electrodes.

Therapeutic Applications of Hysteroscopy

With the use of operative hysteroscopy and resectoscopy, the therapeutic applications have expanded, particularly because of new instrumentation, better methods of distending the uterine cavity, the use of high resolution videocameras, and the utilization of laser energies and electrosurgery through these endoscopes[4] (Table 22.1).

Table 22.1. Therapeutic applications of hysteroscopy

Targeted biopsies
Removal of endometrial polyps
Removal of submucous leiomyomas
Division of a uterine septum
Removal of a "lost" IUD and other foreign bodies
Lysis of intrauterine adhesions
Endometrial ablation (laser, electrosurgery)
Tubal cannulation (e.g., tubal obstruction)
Chorionic villus sampling
Tubal occlusion (electrocoagulation, cryocoagulation, chemical, mechanical)

Targeted Hysteroscope Biopsies

Although the sampling techniques already available in gynecology to detect abnormal (pathologic) endometrial changes are satisfactory when large areas of the endometrium demonstrate such lesions, visual appraisal of the uterine cavity can provide accurate targeting of focal lesions that may be missed by the mechanical or suction devices available today. Specifically, endometrial polyps can easily be detected and resected, and specific focal areas of the endometrium can be biopsied directly, particularly those located at the uterotubal ostia, where they may easily be missed by blind methods of evaluation. Lesions suspicious of malignancy are visually evaluated and the biopsy directed to a specific area that demonstrates abnormalities. Only small portions may be obtained with the present hysteroscopic ancillary biopsy instruments, and it may be necessary to obtain several samples of the same area to have adequate tissue for histopathologic evaluation.

Removal of Endometrial Polyps and Submucous Leiomyomas

The most important facet in the evaluation of endometrial polyps is to establish an accurate diagnosis, as removal can be accomplished by a variety of instruments, including forceps, curettes, and special polypectomy forceps. These instruments, introduced blindly into the uterine cavity, may fail to remove the polyps completely, particularly when they are pedunculated, as these structures are mobile and drift away from the forceps. Therefore the visual appraisal of the uterine cavity provided by the hysteroscope is of value during removal of polyps, as the polyps can be transected and removed completely. The sessile polyps are easily removed with a resectoscope using a cutting loop; the pedunculated ones can be removed by transecting the pedicle with semirigid scissors. Whatever method is used, it is important to confirm that the entire polyp has been removed.

There are several alternatives for removal of endometrial polyps, but to treat submucous leiomyomas these blind alternatives are not useful. Removal of these tumors must be accomplished via endoscopy, which requires expertise. There are several endoscopic hysteroscopic methods to remove submucous leiomyomas, depending on the type of leiomyoma present; for leiomyomas that are pedunculated and not > 3 cm in diameter, transection of the pedicle with mechanical tools is most advantageous, particularly because it saves time and the tumor can be easily removed once the pedicle is transected. When the pedicle of the leiomyoma is broad or the leiomyoma is sessile, the resectoscope offers the best alternative for resection. When a resecting loop is used, the leiomyoma is shaved systematically to the level of the uterine wall. This shaving is performed using blended monopolar current to permit incision and coagulation while the tumor is shaved or cut systematically. The resectoscope permits tactile appraisal of the tumor. The fibrous hard tissue of the leiomyoma is compared to the softer myometrial tissue surrounding it. The hysteroscopist can observe the whitish fibrous tissue of the leiomyoma and the fascicular aspect of the myometrial tissue. It is important not to dig into the myometrium with the cutting loop of the resectoscope; these tumors should be shaved only to the level of the uterine wall. The continuous contractions of the myometrium push the remaining leiomyoma so it becomes intraluminal; most of the tissue is removed by this shav-

Table 22.2. Hysteroscopic myomectomy for abnormal bleeding

Author	No. of patients	Type of myoma		Method	IUD	E/P	Antibiotics	Cure	Recurrence
		Pedunculated	Sessile						
Haning et al. (1980)	1	–	+	Resectoscope	–	+	+	1	–
DeCherney & Polan[8] (1983)	8	+	+	Resectoscope	Foley	+	+	8	–
Neuwirth[9] (1983)	28	+	+	Resectoscope	Foley	+	+	17 (60.7%)	8 (28.5%)
Lin et al. (1986)	13	+	–	Resectoscope (9); rigid scissors (4)	Foley	+	+	9 (69.2%)	4 (30.7%)
Hallez and Perino (1988)	300	+	+	Resectoscope	+	+	+	299[a]	–
Baggish et al.[13] (1989)	23	+	–	Nd:YAG laser	Foley (5 pts)	–	+	NR	NR
Valle and Sciarrá (1990)	52	+	–	Semirigid scissors	–	–	–	52 (100%)	NR
Donnez et al.[16] (1990)	60	48	12	Nd:YAG laser	–	–	–	48 (80.0%)	12 (20.0%)
Loffer[17] (1990)	53[c]	18	25[e]	Resectoscope	NR	–	–	40 (93.0%)	3 (6.9%)
Corson & Brooks[18] (1991)	92	92	–	Resectoscope	NR	–	+	65 (81.2%)[b]	15 (18.7%)[b]
Derman et al.[19] (1991)	94	94[d]	–	Resectoscope	Rubber balloon	+	+	69 (75.0%)	23 (24.5%)
Wamsteker et al.[20] (1993)	51	25	26[f]	Resectoscope	–	–	+	48 (94.1%)	3 (5.9%)
Total	775							656 (84.6%)	68 (8.7%)

IUD, intrauterine device; E/P, estrogen progestin; NR, not reported.
[a]One patient required laparotomy.
[b]From 80 patients.
[c]Ten were polyps.
[d]Two intraoperative laparotomies.
[e]Two patients had two procedures.
[f]Several patients had two or three procedures.

22. Operative Hysteroscopy and Resectoscopy

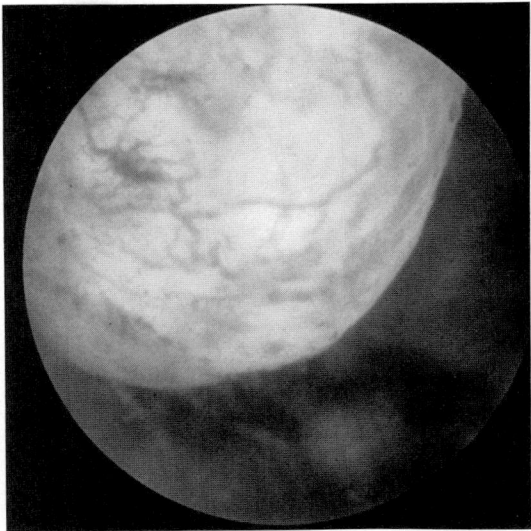

Figure 22.21. Hysteroscopic view of submucous myoma. Peripheral vascularization is visible throughout the atrophic endometrium.

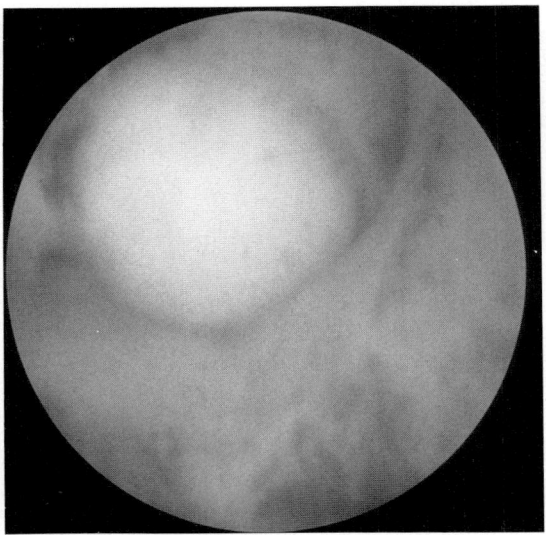

Figure 22.23. Hysteroscopic view of submucous myoma.

ing technique. As an alternative to mechanical tools, the Nd:YAG laser, argon laser, or KTP-532 laser can be used to transect a pedicle of a pedunculated submucous leiomyoma or to shave a broad-based submucous leiomyoma from the uterine wall. Morcellation of larger tumors can be accomplished with the Nd:YAG laser. Devitalization of remaining intramural tumors has also been accomplished via hysteroscopy[5-20] (Table 22.2; Figs. 22.21–22.28).

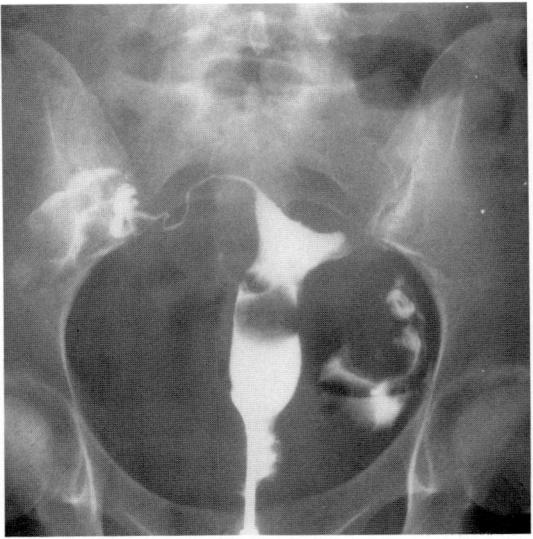

Figure 22.22. Hysterosalpingogram shows a lower segment submucous myoma distorting the symmetry of the uterine cavity.

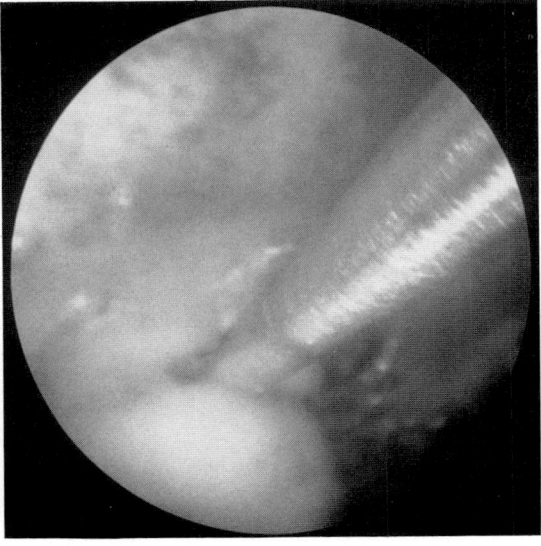

Figure 22.24. Hysteroscopic removal of myoma utilizing semirigid scissors.

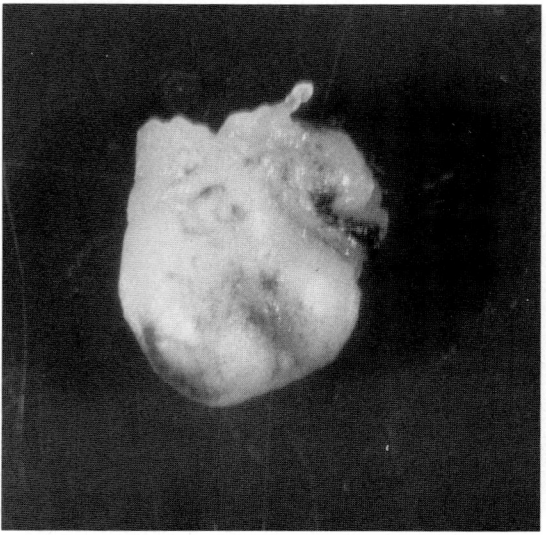

Figure 22.25. Myoma after removal.

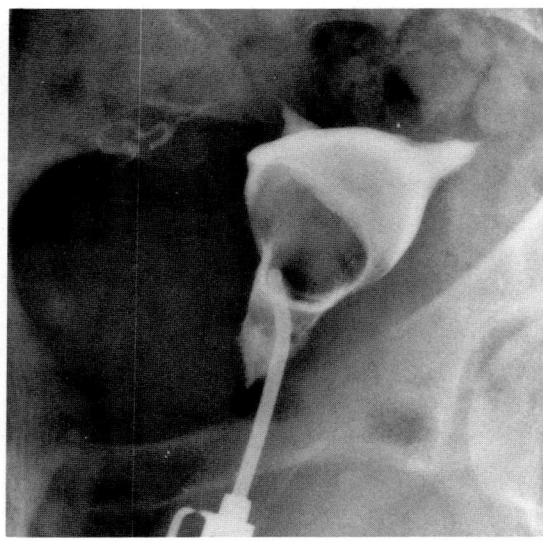

Figure 22.27. Hysterosalpingogram shows marked distortion of the uterine cavity by a submucous myoma.

Although concomitant laparoscopy is not mandatory during these procedures, it should be liberally applied, particularly when resecting large submucous tumors, when the landmarks of the endometrial cavity are somewhat distorted, and when the hysteroscopist doubts the safety of transcervical removal of the tumor(s).

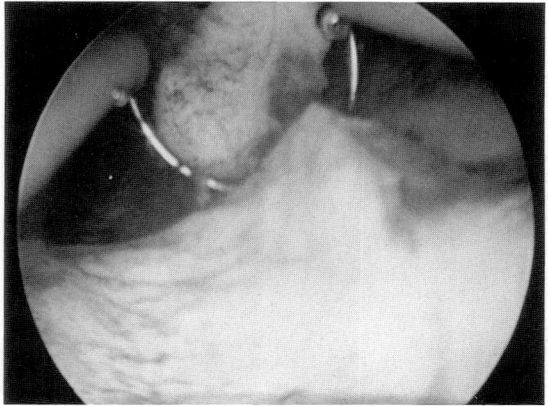

Figure 22.26. Submucous myoma in the posterior uterine wall has been removed with a cutting loop of the resectoscope.

Hysteroscopic Treatment of Symptomatic Uterine Septa

Most women with uterine septa reproduce successfully, but 20–25% have reproductive problems, particularly spontaneous abortions during the late first and early second trimesters of pregnancy. In the past, women with a poor obstetric history (second trimester) related to uterine septa were treated via laparotomy and hysterotomy. The uterine corpus was divided anteroposteriorly in the midline and the septum resected transcervically without removing any myometrial tissue (Tompkins procedure); alternatively, a wedge resection and excision of the fundal cuneiform portion of the uterine corpus, including the septum, was resected; and the remaining myometrium was reconstructed (Jones procedure). Because these procedures required a laparotomy and hysterotomy, hospitalization with prolonged recovery was prerequisite. Furthermore, these patients could not attempt pregnancy until 3–6 months after the procedure in order to permit "healing of the uterus." The reproductive outcome was good in approximately 82% of the patients treated, but there

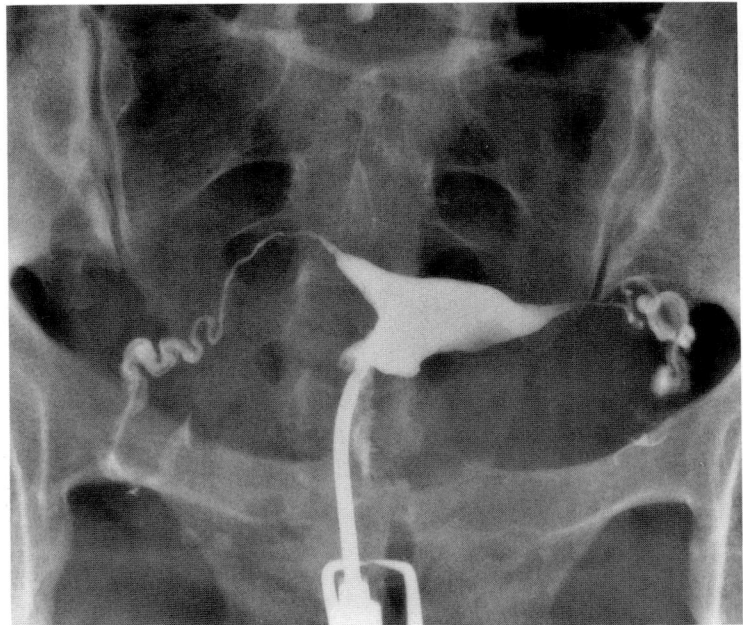

Figure 22.28. Uterus demonstrating normal anatomy after hysteroscopic removal of a myoma.

were patients who could not conceive after these procedures because of pelvic adhesions, particularly to the ovaries and fallopian tubes.[21–24]

Hysteroscopy permits intrauterine visualization and guided dissection within the uterine cavity. Hence the uterine septum can be treated transcervically when necessary by division of this embryologic remnant. Three instruments can be utilized to divide the uterine septum: (1) hysteroscopic scissors; (2) resectoscope; (3) fiberoptic lasers.

Most commonly the uterine septum is divided hysteroscopically with semirigid scissors. The septum is usually poorly vascularized, so the division is performed at the middle of the septum without drifting anteriorly or posteriorly, thereby avoiding vascularized areas. The division progresses from side to side systematically until the uterotubal ostia are well visualized. It is important to use concomitant laparoscopy during these procedures to monitor the operation and warn about thinning of the myometrium, which could result in perforation. The laparoscope is used with a dimmed light to permit transillumination of the hysteroscopic light through the myometrium. Upon reaching the fundal area, small arterial bleeders can be observed, indicating that the myometrium has been reached. Once the septal division is completed, and before the hysteroscope is removed, the uterine fundal area is observed hysteroscopically; the intrauterine pressure produced by the distending medium is decreased to observe any significant bleeding. In the presence of arterial bleeding, selective coagulation is performed[25–34] (Figs. 22.29–22.35).

This technique of dividing the septum with scissors is relatively simple and quick and can be applied to practically all septa. Because no electrical current is used, the media to distend the uterine cavity may safely contain electrolytes, which provides a safety margin for utilization of fluids, as more volume may be safely used than when fluids devoid of electrolytes are employed. Because the scissors are small they can easily become dull and loose, and they therefore must be exchanged periodically. The rigid, fixed optical scissors cut better than the semirigid scissors, but the risk of perforation increases with their use. They should be used under perfect panoramic view, with caution, particularly at the fundal area.

The second method for treating a uterine septum is with the gynecologic resectoscope and a

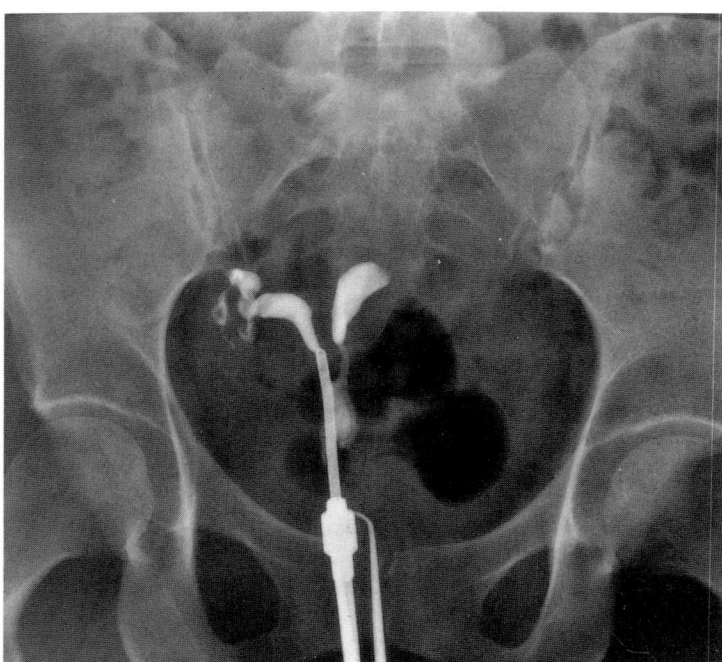

Figure 22.29. Hysterosalpingogram shows a complete uterine septum.

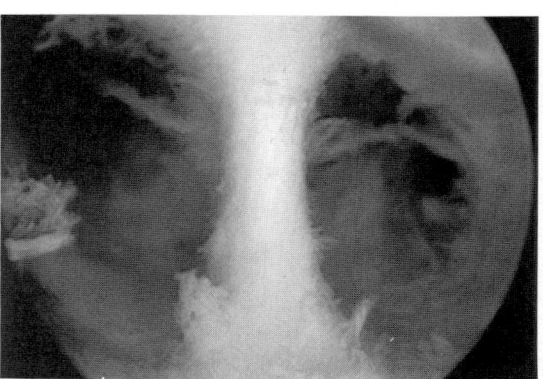

Figure 22.30. Hysteroscopic view of the uterine septum.

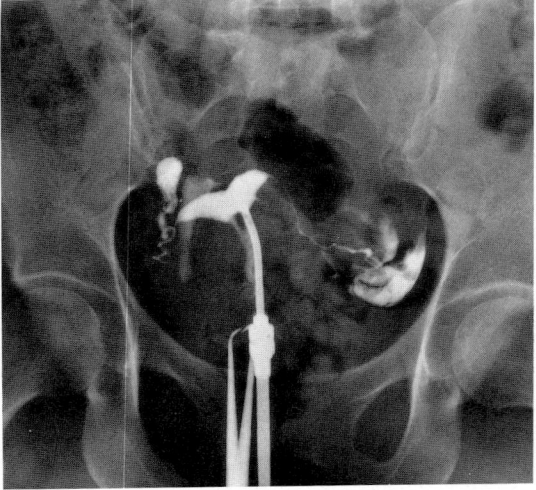

Figure 22.32. Hysterosalpingogram following hysteroscopic metroplasty shows a unified uterine cavity.

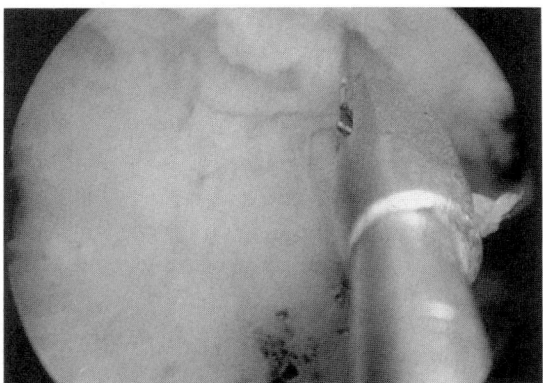

Figure 22.31. Hysteroscopic division of the uterine septum with semirigid scissors.

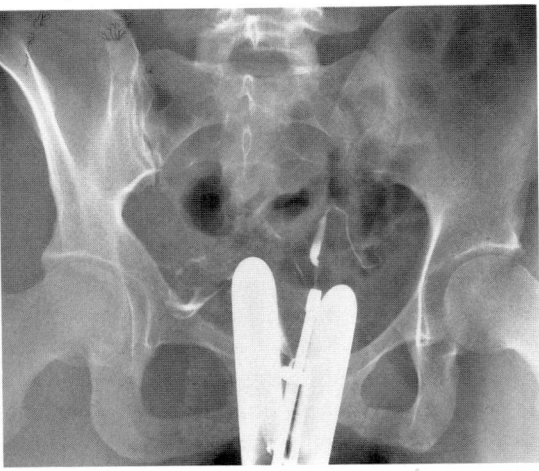

Figure 22.33. Hysterosalpingogram shows the left uterine horn in a patient with a complete uterine septum including the cervix.

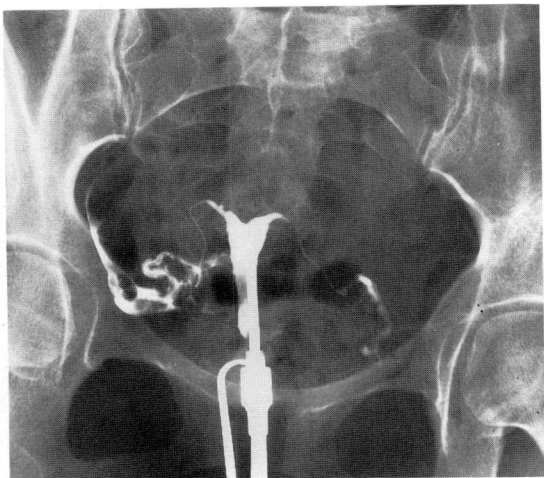

Figure 22.35. Uterine cavity is unified after hysteroscopic treatment of the septum.

thin electrode oriented forward, a cutting loop, or a knife electrode. A blended current is utilized and the septum transected systematically from its nadir to the fundal region. Because electrosurgery is used, only fluids devoid of electrolytes should be utilized. Sorbitol (3%) or 1.5% glycine is most useful for this purpose. Because the resectoscope provides a continuous-flow system, the uterine cavity is continuously irrigated clean of bubbles and debris that may form during the electrosurgical transection of the septum. Because the resectoscopic electrode also provides coagulation while the septum is incised, vessels at the fundal region may not bleed upon division, depriving the hysteroscopist of this landmark when the myometrium is reached. Special attention is important at the fundal area to avoid penetration of the myometrium. The uterotubal ostia serve as landmarks. Observation of the hysteroscopic light by an assistant with a dimmed light of the laparoscope are useful for preventing perforation[29,31] (Figs. 22.36, 22.37).

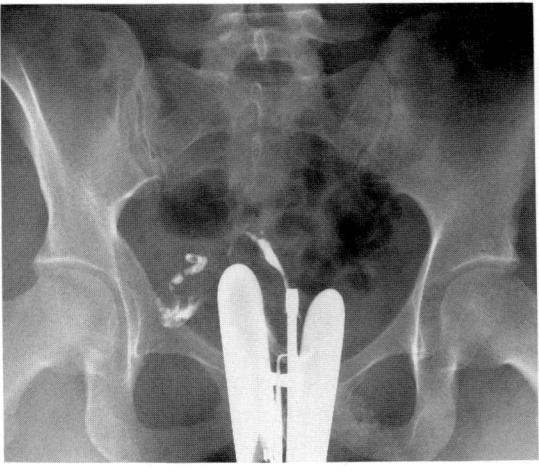

Figure 22.34. Hysterographic view of the right uterine horn.

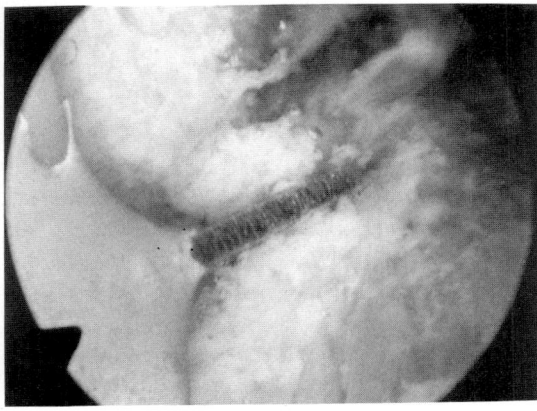

Figure 22.36. Resectoscopic division of the broad uterine septum with a knife electrode.

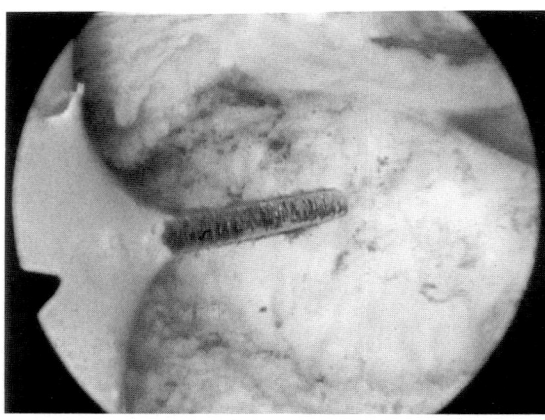

Figure 22.37. Knife electrode is completing division of the uterine septum.

The symmetry of the divided uterine septum should be noted and the uterine cavity from the internal cervical os periodically observed to avoid asymmetric division of the septum. Bleeding during resectoscopic division of the uterine septum is prevented by the monopolar current. The transection may be somewhat slower than with scissors, and theoretically the lateral scattering of the monopolar current may destroy the peripheral normal endometrium, which serves as a reservoir for reepithelialization of the denuded area.[33] Nonetheless, the most important consideration when resecting the uterine septum with the resectoscope is not to invade the uterine wall at the fundal region while septal transection is performed.

Fiberoptic lasers, particularly the Nd:YAG with sculpted or extruded fibers of the sharp point type, can be used to divide the uterine septum. Alternatively, the argon or KTP-532 laser can be used in this manner with sculpted fibers. In these situations, fluids containing electrolytes should be used to distend the uterine cavity. Normal saline, $D_5\frac{1}{2}NS$ or Ringer's lactate is useful for distending the uterine cavity and obtaining clear visualization. A continuous-flow hysteroscope or a hysteroscope with built-in inflow and outflow channels is advantageous for removing bubbles and debris produced by activation of the laser.[33-35]

The technique for dividing the uterine septum with fiberoptic lasers is similar to that used with a resectoscope. The septum is systematically divided from side to side. Special care should be taken upon reaching the fundal area to avoid damaging the juxtaposed myometrium. Concerns similar to those with the resectoscope apply to the fiberoptic lasers, as they may cause peripheral coagulation of the surrounding normal endometrium while performing the division. The coagulation produced by the lasers may obscure the fundal vascularization of the myometrium and may not warn the hysteroscopist of having completed the division of the fibrotic septum. It is important to evaluate patients with pregnancy wastage who also have uterine septa so as to rule out other possible causes for their reproductive wastage, such as genetic, endocrine, metabolic, or autoimmune/alloimmune problems.

The reproductive outcome after hysteroscopic treatment of a symptomatic septate uterus has surpassed the results obtained with traditional abdominal metroplasty, with more than 85% viable pregnancies. The patient is spared a laparotomy and hysterotomy, avoiding the potential for pelvic adhesions and the associated pain, disability, and expense. Patients treated hysteroscopically must wait only 4 weeks to attempt conception, and they do not require a mandatory cesarean section should pregnancy be carried to viability[36-40] (Table 22.3).

Hysteroscopic Treatment of Intrauterine Adhesions

Intrauterine adhesions or synechiae usually occur following trauma to the uterus (curettage) after a pregnancy. Curettage of the endometrial cavity performed 1-4 weeks after a delivery or an abortion may result in denudation of the basal endometrium and subsequent coaptation of the uterine walls, resulting in a permanent scar that bridges both uterine walls and produces distortion of its symmetry. Depending on the extent of the uterine cavity occlusion, patients afflicted with this condition may present with menstrual abnormalities such as amenorrhea or hypomenorrhea; and should pregnancy occur, they may suffer repetitive spontaneous abortions.[41-44] Blind manipulation to divide these adhesions has not been satisfactory for

Table 22.3. Hysteroscopic metroplasty

Author	No. of pts	Medium	Technique	IUD	E/P	Anti-biotics	Pregnancy			
							Term	Premature	Abortion	In progress
Edstrom (1974)	2	Dextran 70 (32%)	Rigid biopsy forceps	+	–	–	19 weeks	–	–	–
Chervenak and Neuwirth (1981)	2	Dextran 70 (32%)	Scissors adjacent to hysteroscope	+	+	+	1	–	–	–
Rosenberg et al. (1981)	1	Dextran 70 (32%)	Flexible scissors	NA	NA	NA	NA	–	–	–
Daly et al.[28] (1983)	25	Dextran 70 (32%)	–	–	–	–	7	–	1	2
Perino et al. (1985)	11	CO_2	Flexible, semirigid scissors	+	–	–	NA	–	–	1
De Cherney et al. (1986)	72	Dextran 70 (32%)	Resectoscope	–	–	–	58	–	4	4
Corson and Batzer (1986)	18	Dextran 70 (32%), CO_2	Resectoscope and rigid scissors	–	–	–	10	1	2	2
Fayez[37] (1986)	19	Dextran 70 (32%)	Rigid scissors	Foley catheter	–	+	14	–	–	–
March and Israel[29] (1987)	91	Dextran 70 (32%)	Flexible scissors	+	–	–	44	4	7	7
Valle (1987)	59	D5W/Dextran 70 (32%)	Flexible, semirigid rigid scissors	–	–	+	44	2	5	–
Choe and Baggish[35] (1992)	19	Dextran 70 (32%)	Nd: YAG with bare or sculptured fibers	Foley catheter (3 pts)	–	+	10	1	1	3
Fedele et al.[36] (1993)	102	Dextran 40 (10% in normal saline)	Semirigid scissors (80) argon laser (10) Resectoscope (12)	+(21)	+(39)	+	45	10	11	NA
Total	421						233	19	31	18

Adapted from Siegler and Valle.[10] Reprinted with permission of the publisher, the American Society for Reproductive Medicine (The American Fertility Society).
IUD, intrauterine device; E/P, estrogens/progestins; NA, not applicable.

restoring the normal architecture of the uterine cavity, and the reproductive performance of patients treated with such methods has remained disappointing. In contrast, hysteroscopy provides direct visual assessment of the uterine cavity, permitting selective division of these adhesions. The success in reestablishing normal menstruation and improving the reproductive outcome has made the hysteroscopic approach the standard method for treatment of intrauterine adhesions.[45–49]

The time of the early follicular phase of the menstrual cycle is chosen for treating patients who are menstruating and demonstrate intrauterine adhesions on hysterosalpingography. Based on the extent of uterine cavity occlusion demonstrated by hysterosalpingography, laparoscopy is used concomitantly in patients with extensive uterine cavity involvement, tubal occlusion, or both. An operative hysteroscope 7 mm O.D. may be used, and semirigid hysteroscopic scissors are utilized to divide the adhesions. Fluid containing electrolytes, specifically sodium, is preferred for uterine distention (e.g., D_5S or Ringer's lactate). Tubal patency is evaluated by injecting indigo carmine transcervically. An intrauterine splint is left in the uterus to keep the uterine walls separated. An indwelling 8F catheter is placed in the uterus with 3.0–3.5 ml of saline injected in the balloon and left in situ for a week. Concomitant prophylactic antibiotics are used during and after the procedure, particularly when splints are left in place, doxycycline (Vibramycin) 100 mg bid PO is given for a week or intraoperative cefazolin (Kefzol) 1 g IV, followed by cephalexin (Keflex) 500 mg qid PO for 7 days. To aid in reepithelialization of the denuded area, conjugated estrogens are prescribed. Conjugated estrogens 2.5 mg bid are prescribed for a 30- to 40-day cycle, with the addition of progesterone acetate 10 mg every day for the last 5–6 days of the cycle. At the conclusion of the hormonal treatment, hysterosalpingography is performed to assess the uterine cavity and determine whether further treatment is warranted or the patient may attempt conception. The reestablishment of normal menstruation in patients treated for intrauterine adhesions has been successful in more than 90%, although the reproductive outcome has paralleled the severity of the disease, with an overall pregnancy rate of 60–70%, defining a correlation of the extent of uterine cavity occlusion and the composition of the adhesions with the reproductive outcome; the more extensive the intrauterine adhesions and the thicker they are, the worse is the prognosis. Among 187 patients treated hysteroscopically by Valle and Sciarra,[49] removal of mild filmy adhesions in 43 had the best prognosis, with 35 (81%) term pregnancies; among 97 patients with a moderate degree of fibromuscular adhesions, 64 (66%) achieved term pregnancies; and in 47 with severe connective tissue adhesions, there were 15 (32%) term pregnancies. Overall restoration of normal menses occurred in 90% of the patients, and the term pregnancy rate was 79.7%. These results demonstrated far superior reproductive outcome than was previously obtained with nonvisualization methods of therapy. Other approaches to dividing intrauterine adhesions hysteroscopically have been described, such as with the resectoscope and with fiberoptic lasers. When using the resectoscope a special thin wire electrode is required. Special precautions are necessary when using electrosurgery, particularly to avoid uterine perforation and damage to healthy endometrium and myometrium. Fluids devoid of electrolytes are mandatory, and excessive coagulation should be avoided. With the utilization of fiberoptic lasers, only the sculptured fibers should be used to prevent lateral scattering and damage of the remaining healthy endometrium. Care should be taken to prevent coagulation and damage of the juxtaposed myometrium once the adhesions have been divided (Figs. 22.38–22.43).

Treatment of intrauterine adhesions utilizing the resectoscope has produced results similar to those obtained with mechanical instrumentation; postoperative complications may be serious and should be kept in mind when using this type of instrumentation.[50] Few series report lysis of adhesions with fiberoptic lasers; but when used appropriately, results should not vary from those reported with electrosurgery[51] (Table 22.4).

22. Operative Hysteroscopy and Resectoscopy

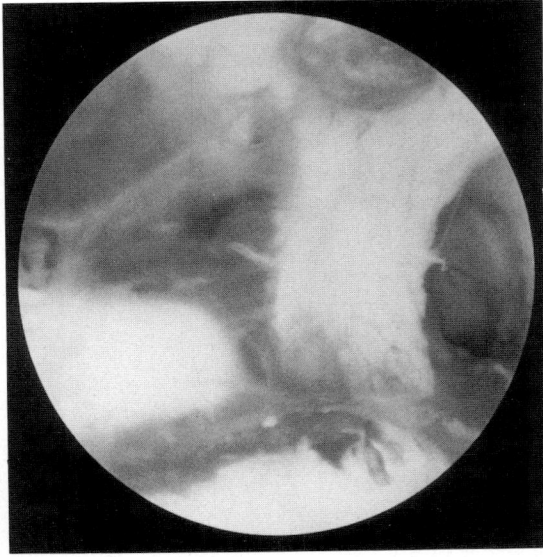

Figure 22.38. Extensive uterine cavity occlusion with thick, fibrotic adhesions.

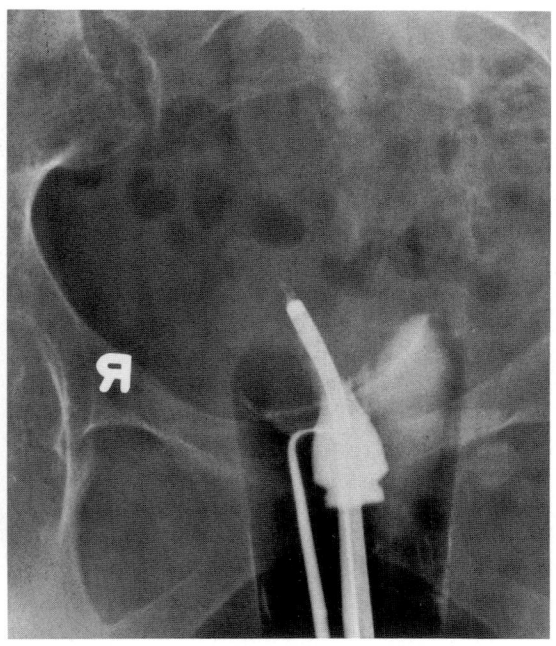

Figure 22.40. Hysterosalpingogram shows complete uterine cavity occlusion by adhesions.

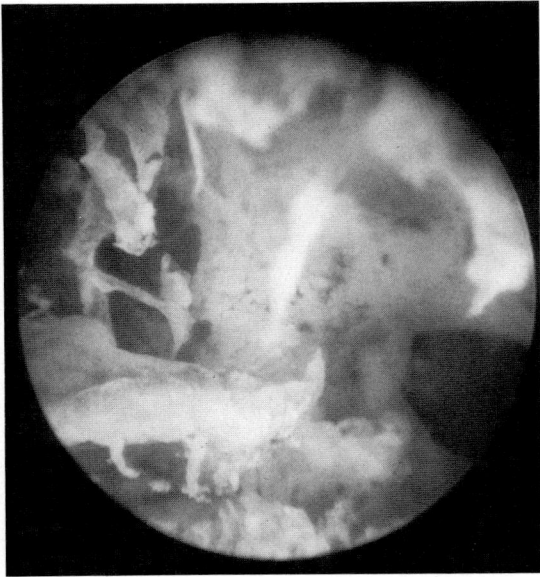

Figure 22.39. Central, thick, fundal adhesions simulating a uterine septum.

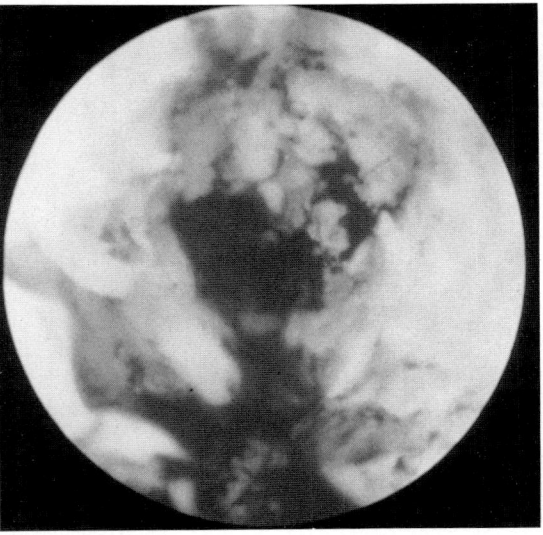

Figure 22.41. Remaining fibrotic stumps are visible after hysteroscopic lysis of adhesions.

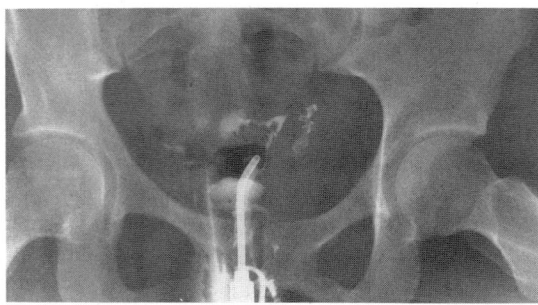

Figure 22.42. Hysterosalpingogram shows extensive uterine cavity occlusion by adhesions.

The use of hysteroscopy has facilitated not only the confirmation and treatment of intrauterine adhesions but evaluation of the type of adhesions present and, in conjunction with hysterosalpingography, the extent of uterine cavity occlusion. This evaluation has permitted a useful classification of these adhesions. Valle and Sciarra[49] proposed a three-stage classification of the extent and severity of intrauterine adhesions (mild, moderate, severe) based on degree of involvement as revealed by hysterosalpingography and the extent and type of adhesions found on hysteroscopy. Three stages of intrauterine adhesions are defined:

Mild adhesions: filmy adhesions composed of basal endometrium, producing partial or complete uterine cavity occlusion

Moderate adhesions: fibromuscular adhesions that are characteristically thick; still covered with endometrium that may bleed upon division; partially or totally occluding the uterine cavity

Severe adhesions: composed of connective tissue; lacking any endometrial lining and likely to bleed upon division; partially or totally occluding the uterine cavity

There has been no uniformity in defining these adhesions, making comparison of results difficult. The American Society for Reproductive Medicine (formerly the American Fertility Society) has proposed a classification of intrauterine adhesions based on hysterosalpingography and hysteroscopy, adding a correlation with menstrual patterns. This classification for intrauterine adhesions can increase our ability to report, evaluate, and compare results obtained by different treatments of intrauterine adhesions, particularly the results obtained by the hysteroscopic approach.[52-54]

Hysteroscopic Tubal Cannulation

Proximal fallopian tube obstruction is noted in 10–20% of women from whom hysterosalpingograms were obtained as part of an infertility evaluation. Approximately 20–30% of these occlusions are due to physiologic spasm. Pharmacologic agents have been used to minimize this occurrence (e.g., glucagon, isoxsuprine, or β-agonists such as terbutaline), but none has succeeded in consistently eliminating it. At present, laparoscopy under general anesthesia is the most effective method to rule out physiologic spasm and evaluate other fallopian tube or pelvic pathology. When proximal tube obstruction is confirmed by laparoscopy, surgical treatment has been used to resect the obstructed segment followed by microsurgical reconstruction. Patients operated for these conditions did not consistently show fibrosis or true occlusion of the affected area. In many cases simple occlusion or obstruction by debris or proteinaceous material plugging the tubal lumen was identified.[55] Tubal cannulation was introduced as the initial method to correct the obstruction.

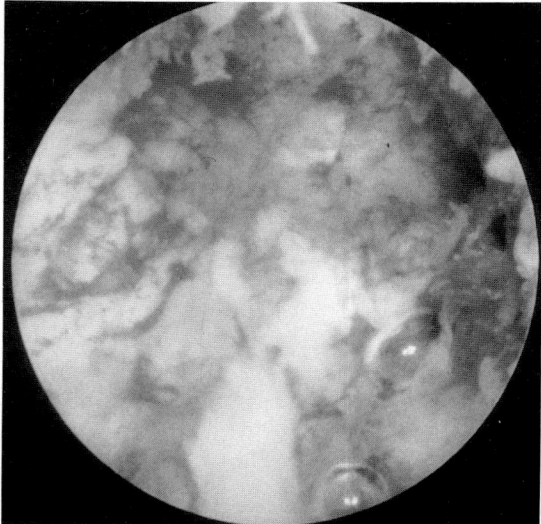

Figure 22.43. Small stumps from divided adhesions can be seen after hysteroscopic lysis of adhesions.

Table 22.4. Hysteroscopic lysis of intrauterine adhesions

Author	No. of pts.	IUD	E/P	Anti-biotics	Normal menses	Reproductive outcome	
						Pregnant	Term
Edstrom[2] (1974)	9	+	−	−	2	1	1
March et al. (1981)	38	+	+	+	38 (100%)	38 (100%)	34 (79.1%)
Neuwirth et al.[49] (1982)	27	+	+	+	20 (74.0%)	14 (51.8%)	13 (48.1%)
Sanfilippo et al. (1982)	26	+	+	−	26 (100%)	3 (50.0%)	
Siegler & Kontopoulos	25	Foley catheter	+	−	13 (52.0%)	11 (44.0%)	6 (24.0%)
Hamou et al. (1983)	69	+	+	−	59 (85.5%)	20 (51.3%)	15 (38.4%)
Sugimoto et al. (1984)	258	+	+	−	180 (69.7%)	107 (41.4%)	64 (24.8%)
Wamsteker (1984)	36	+	+	+	34 (94.4%)	17 (62.9%)	12 (44.4%)
Freidman et al.[51] (1986)	30	−	+	−	27 (90.0%)	24 (80.0%)	23 (76.6%)
Valle and Sciarra (1987)	187	+ Foley catheter	+	+	167 (89.3%)	143 (76.4%)	114 (60.9%)
Zuanchong and Yulian (1986)	70	+	+	+	64 (84.3%)	30 (85.7%)	17 (48.5%)
Total	775				630 (87.2%)	411 (60.3%)	302 (44.3%)

Adapted from Siegler and Valle[10] Reprinted with permission of the publisher, the American Society for Reproductive Medicine (The American Fertility Society).
IUD, intrauterine device; E/P, estrogens/progestin.

Although tubal cannulation was attempted for many years, a practical method of performing this procedure was not perfected until the late 1960s by Menken[56] and was made practical during the early 1970s by Quinones-Guerrero et al.[57] The catheters used maintained the rigidity required for ureteral catheterization, but it was difficult to introduce them atraumatically in the intramural portion of the fallopian tubes.[58] The development of soft, small-caliber catheters and the adaptation of angiographic techniques with coaxial catheters to cannulate the fallopian tubes have facilitated this procedure and renewed interest in this technique during the mid-1980s.[59] Although the fluroscopic approach has been used by radiologists, the hysteroscopic approach offers additional advantages that appeal to the gynecologist. It can rule out tubal spasm as performed under laparoscopic guidance, offering a direct view of the uterotubal junction, and it permits directing the catheter into the tubal lumen. Furthermore, the concomitant use of laparoscopy not only helps to assess tubal patency but provides an opportunity to evaluate and treat other pelvic conditions that may be present, such as pelvic adhesions, endometriosis, and minor distortion(s) of the tubal fimbriated end.

Borrowing from angiographic techniques, the catheters needed to perform tubal cannulations have been modified. Some are straight coaxial catheters, and others are fitted with the distal balloon that permits distention of the cornual tubal region once inserted. Experience has been gathered and reproductive outcome following these techniques assessed, and it has been found that the outcome does not vary with the two techniques, but the simplicity of coaxial catheters to cannulate the fallopian tubes makes them more appealing to the practitioner. The intramural portion of the fallopian tubes may not require dilatation. The fallopian tube offers enormous compliance and upon distention quickly recovers its normal anatomy. A truly fibrotic obstruction cannot be treated by tubal cannulation, and those patients still require microsurgical excision and reconstruction. Tubal cannulation clears the fallopian tube of proteinaceous material, mucous plugs, or debris that may simulate true occlusion[60–62] (Fig. 22.44).

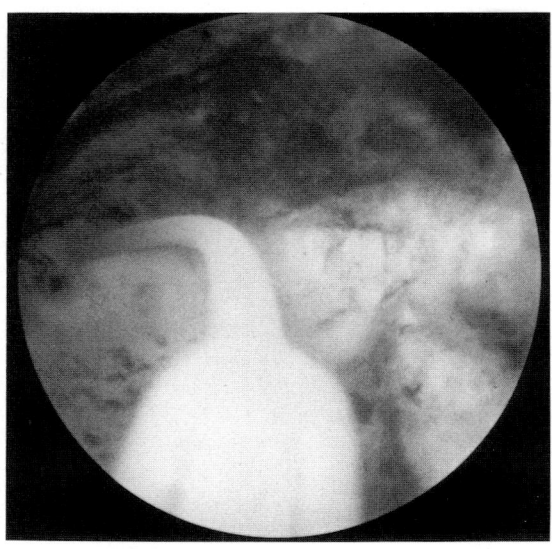

Figure 22.44. Tubal cannulation for intramural tubal obstruction.

teroscopes with 4.9 mm O.D. has facilitated tubal cannulation, particularly when the tubal openings are angulated and difficult to localize with rigid endoscopes or if anatomic variations in the uterine configuration make localization difficult, as may be the case in an acutely retroverted uterus. The steerability of these endoscopes facilitates tubal cannulation by aligning the endoscope in direct opposition with a proximal tubal ostium, simplifying the procedure and reducing the number of failures.

Endometrial Ablation

More than 700,000 women undergo a hysterectomy annually in the United States. Of these hysterectomies, 20–25% are performed for dysfunctional uterine bleeding unresponsive to hormonal therapy. Hysterectomy cures the symptomatology, but the patient must undergo an invasive procedure with its associated morbidity and occasional mortality. The inconvenience, disability, and cost involved are significant concerns to the patient. Because many of these women are at high risk of complications from a hysterectomy, alternative conservative methods have been sought without success.[71–81] Of late, however, endometrial ablation, or destruction of the endometrial lining, has drawn the attention of physicians and patients alike as a good alternative for treating abnormal uterine bleeding unresponsive to hormonal therapy short of hysterectomy.[82–86] There are two methods for obtaining endometrial ablation: (1) destruction of the endometrium with a fiberoptic laser and (2) endometrial ablation with electrosurgery utilizing the resectoscope.

The results of tubal cannulation are promising. Successful visualization of the fallopian tubes at cannulation by hysteroscopy has demonstrated 70–92% patency. The intrauterine pregnancy rate has been about 47%, with an ectopic pregnancy rate of 8% in patients followed for at least 12 months[62,70] (Table 22.5).

With this approach, only patients who fail tubal cannulation, demonstrating true fibrotic occlusion, require microsurgical tubal reconstruction. Most tubal cannulations can be performed with a rigid operative hysteroscope; nonetheless, the manipulations required may not permit tubal cannulation at the first attempt in some patients in view of the rigidity of the scope. Introduction of flexible operative hys-

Table 22.5. Results of hysteroscopic cannulation of proximal tubal obstruction

Author	Year	No of cases/failed	Catheter	Complications (perforation)	Pregnancies
Confino et al.[62]	1986	1/0	Balloon	1	—
Daniell & Miller[63]	1987	1/0	Urologic	0	1
Sulak et al.[64]	1987	2/0	Epidural	0	1
Confino et al.[65]	1988	12/5	Balloon	3	2
Novy et al.[66]	1989	10/1	Cornual set	1	2
Deaton et al.[67]	1990	11/4	Urologic	2	6 (3 ectopic)
Lin et al.[68]	1990	10/0	Urologic	—	5 (1 ectopic)
Flood & Grow[75]	1993	27/3	Cornual set	4	15
Total		74/13 (17.5%)		11 (14.8%)	32 (43.2%)

Laser Endometrial Ablation

The fiberoptic laser suited for this purpose is the Nd:YAG laser with a wavelength of 1064 nm, located in the near infrared (invisible) portion of the light spectrum, which permits deep destruction of tissue when used through a "bare" quartz fiber. The depth of penetration of this laser is 4–5 mm with associated scattering resulting in craters in the endometrium and penetrating the superficial portion of the myometrium.[82]

The 600 μm bare fiber is inserted through the operating channel of the hysteroscope, and the surface of the endometrium is systematically destroyed. Because it is imperative to destroy not only the total thickness of the endometrium but also the superficial layer (3 mm) of the myometrium, the endometrium must be thin and atrophic. This atrophy is induced hormonally by blocking ovulation and the production of gonadotropins. Danazol at a dose of 800 mg daily can be used preoperatively to obtain this effect. Alternatively, a GnRH analog such as leuprolide acetate (Lupron) can be used in a depot of 3.75 mg IM in two doses 1 month apart, with the operation being performed 2–3 weeks after the second injection. With this regimen more than 95% of patients have excellent gonadotropin suppression and atrophy of the endometrium. Although progestins such as medrodyprogesterone acetate have been used for this purpose, the response has not been satisfactory as they may cause a pseudodecidual reaction, which not only impairs visualization but impedes complete endometrial destruction.[83,84]

When the Nd:YAG laser is used for endometrial ablation, two techniques may be utilized: One is the *dragging procedure* or application of the quartz fiber on contact with the surface, producing furrows in the endometrium and turning the surface brown, which defines the areas that have been destroyed and those that have been left intact. The procedure begins at the cornual regions, where the thinnest portion of the myometrium is located, and systematically then moves to the fundal area, the anterior wall, the posterior wall, and finally the lateral recesses. Care is taken not to invade the endocervical canal so as to avoid cervical scarring. The second technique is the *blanching tech-*

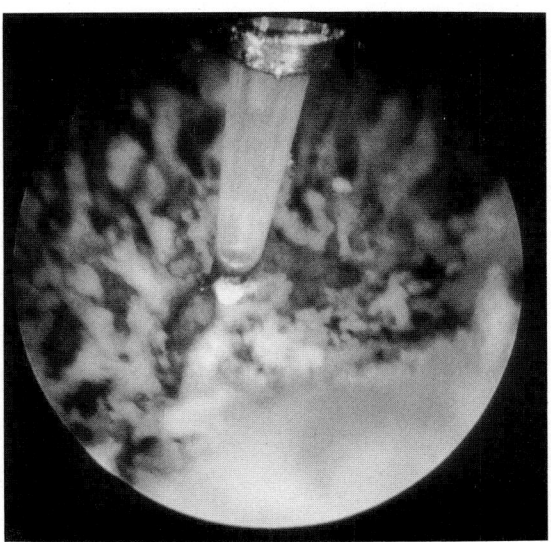

Figure 22.45. Endometrial ablation by a "dragging" contact technique with Nd:YAG bare quartz fiber. (courtesy of Dr. Richard Gimpelson)

nique, which permits coagulation of the endometrial surface by firing the laser 1–2 mm from the surface. This practice causes blanching of the surface, indicating coagulation. Because it is difficult to differentiate areas that have been treated from those that have not, several marking lines can be established to divide the uterine cavity in segments and then complete the procedure systematically. In general, these two techniques are combined utilizing the blanching technique for the cornual regions and fundal areas and the dragging technique for the remainder of the uterine cavity[85–91] (Figs. 22.45, 22.46).

When utilizing the Nd:YAG laser for endometrial ablation, fluids containing electrolytes are used: either D_5S or Ringer's lactate. The results of endometrial ablation utilizing the Nd:YAG laser have obtained 95% resolution of the abnormal bleeding (thus a 5% failure rate). The aim of the procedure is not to create amenorrhea but to resolve the abnormal, excessive uterine bleeding.

Endometrial Ablation with the Resectoscope

An alternative to laser endometrial ablation is to utilize the resectoscope with a loop electrode

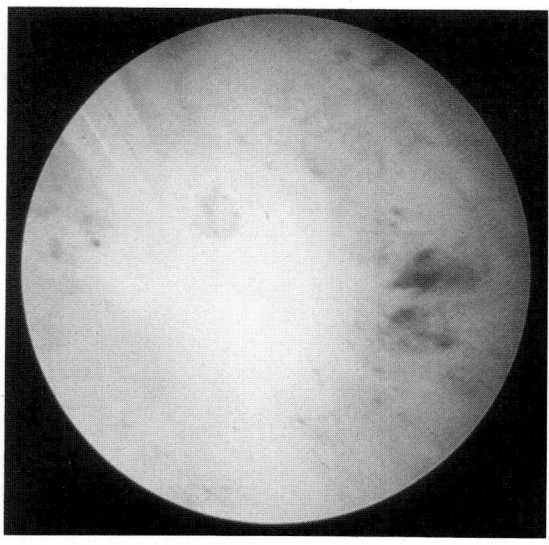

Figure 22.46. Endometrial ablation by "blanching," a noncontact technique with the Nd:YAG laser. (courtesy of Dr. Richard Gimpelson)

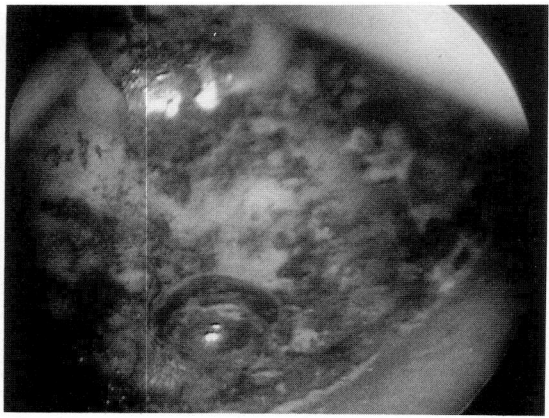

Figure 22.47. Resectoscopic roller-bar endometrial ablation.

to resect tissue and a ball or bar electrode to coagulate it. The initial attempt to produce destruction of the endometrium electrosurgically comprised resecting the endometrium, but difficulty was encountered when resecting areas at the cornual regions. The uniformity of resection cannot be kept precisely at the same depth; it requires experience and meticulous attention to the depth of penetration with this loop. Because by resecting the superficial portion of the myometrium vascular sinuses are open, fluid intravasation is a concern. On the basis of urologic experience with coagulation, other electrodes were tested, such as the roller-ball and the roller-bar electrodes. With these electrodes the surface of the endometrium is coagulated rather than resected. Because of the size and shape of the electrodes, destruction of the endometrium is faster than when using the Nd:YAG laser. The technique is simpler, faster, and as efficacious as resection. Because the instrumentation and electrical power units required to accomplish endometrial ablation by electrosurgery are less expensive and cumbersome than those required for laser ablation, this technique is highly appealing to practitioners. There are numerous variables involved in determining the depth destruction of the uterine wall (e.g., pressure, speed, shape and size of the electrode, tissue impedance, condition of the electrode), but in general pure coagulating current (30–40 watts) or, alternatively, pure cutting current (100–120 watts) can be used to accomplish this procedure. Because pure cutting current is more uniform and of lower voltage, produces less bubbling, and permits less debris to adhere to the electrode, it has been the waveform most commonly used. Indeed studies have demonstrated that this waveform may be more efficacious in accomplishing endometrial ablation[91-99] (Fig. 22.47).

When utilizing the resectoscope for endometrial ablation, only fluids devoid of electrolytes should be used; and grounding of the patient is necessary to complete the electrical circuit of the unipolar current. Because resectoscopes with continuous-flow systems allow exact measurement of fluids infused and the amount of fluids retrieved, it is imperative to follow these measurements accurately. In general, during endometrial ablation with the roller-ball or roller-bar electrodes there is no more than 200 ml of deficit fluid. If resection is performed, this deficit may be enhanced.

The results achieved with endometrial ablation by electrosurgery are similar to those obtained with the laser. The failure rate is slightly higher: 5–10%. This figure represents the inherent properties of electrosurgery, which is not as predictable as laser energy. Visual appraisal of the thermal damage cannot predict uterine wall penetration.[91-99] Both laser and electrosurgery are useful alternatives to hysterectomy for the treatment of dysfunctional uterine bleeding unresponsive to hormonal treatment.

Other Applications of Operative Hysteroscopy

The removal of misplaced or embedded IUDs was facilitated by the introduction of hysteroscopy, which remains the best method for removing these misplaced foreign bodies. Utilizing a rigid or semirigid grasping forceps, the operator grasps the device and withdraws the hysteroscope with the device fixed at the end of the endoscope. Unnecessary and dangerous trauma to the endometrium and uterine wall is thus avoided, particularly when the device is fragmented or partially embedded (Fig. 22.48).

Investigation of tubal sterilization by hysteroscopy continues. The methods so far explored have not provided acceptable success nor have they yielded significant failures and complications. Hysteroscopy offers an excellent platform to exploration of the uterine tubes, but high resolution endoscopes small enough to tranverse the intramural portion of the fallopian tubes atraumatically have impaired exploration of this area transcervically. Although faloposcopy performed in the distal portion of the fallopian tube has gained in acceptance because of the good resolution and excellent visualization obtained to determine normalcy and pathology of the tubal endothelium with large rigid endoscopes, the transcervical approach remains at the forefront of investigation. Owing to advances in techniques for tubal cannulation, reproductive technologies such as GIFT, ZIFT, and intratubal insemination are being actively explored guided by hysteroscopic control. Future developments in instrumentation and refinements in flexible hysteroscopes may further enhance these applications.

Useful Adjuncts to Operative Hysteroscopy

Ultrasonography

Intrauterine surgery requires evaluation of the entire uterus to assess pathology and determine the utility and appropriate use of endoscopic surgery. Because endoscopy can appraise topographic findings, it is important to evaluate the uterus by ultrasonography to determine not only the presence or absence of additional pathology but the invasion of a submucous tumor in the myometrium. It is important to determine the number, size, location, and relation of leiomyomas to the endometrial stripe. This information helps the practitioner arrive at the appropriate decision when performing hysteroscopic removal of submucous leiomyomas rather than to shave only a portion of a truly intramural leiomyoma.[100-102]

Magnetic Resonance Imaging

Magnetic resonance imaging (MRI) is useful for the evaluation of uterine leiomyomas, but the expense involved may not justify routine use.

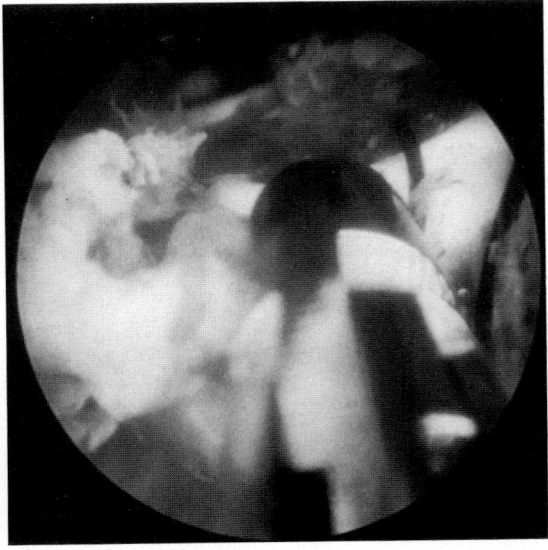

Figure 22.48. Hysteroscopic removal of a partially embedded intrauterine device (Lippes loop).

Leiomyomas are best visualized with this type of examination in view of its resolution compared to that of sonography, which involves different but similar echogenicity of tissues, which may confuse the examiner.[103]

Hysterosalpingography

Hysteroscopy is most accurate for detecting intrauterine lesions and affording their direct treatment. Subtle changes in uterine volume, distortion, and specifically fundal variations of the uterine symmetry can best be evaluated by hysterosalpingography (HSG), in view of the direction of access at which the image is projected. This different view is particularly true in the presence of intrauterine adhesions, where central adhesions may obscure the hysteroscopy view of the fundal aspects of the uterine cavity. Small uterine septa can best be evaluated from the perpendicular axis provided by the radiograph. Tubal patency and architecture cannot be evaluated by hysteroscopy and is best studied with HSG.[70]

Laparoscopy

Laparoscopy as an adjunct to operative hysteroscopy is of value when extensive intrauterine manipulations are required, such as treatment of extensive adhesions, division of a uterine septum, tubal cannulation, and removal of large submucous leiomyomas.

Complications

Like other surgical procedures, operative hysteroscopy may result in complications. With a background of appropriate indications, lack of contraindications, and meticulous attention to technique, these complications can be avoided. Should they occur, they can be recognized and appropriately treated.

The complications of operative hysteroscopy may be related to the technique per se, which may cause perforation of the uterine wall, excessive bleeding, or damage to adjacent organs. Following the techniques described and the landmarks for guidance during the operative procedures, these complications can often be avoided; furthermore when an extensive and difficult hysteroscopic procedure is foreseen, laparoscopy should be used as a guide to the hysteroscopist in conjunction with the hysteroscopic procedure, avoiding unnecessary injury to the uterus. Because the most serious complication related to the distending medium, particularly low viscosity fluids, is fluid overload and pulmonary edema, fluids used during the procedure should be carefully monitored. In this way there is an account of the fluid infused and the fluid recovered, and the deficit of these fluids can thus be measured serially. When the hysteroscopic operations are prolonged and require significant intrauterine dissections, it is important to measure urine output and monitor vital signs and pulse oximetry in consultation with the anesthesiologist. Prudent use of diuretics may be helpful, and the operation should be stopped if any of these variables is abnormal. Fluids must be used in accordance with the technique to be performed, and those fluids devoid of electrolytes should be reserved for procedures that utilize electrosurgery.[104-110]

Intraperative or postoperative bleeding is not a common occurrence, although it may happen during division of a uterine septum or dissection of a large submucous leiomyoma. In these situations coagulation should be accomplished before the operation is completed by selective coagulation and, if necessary, mechanical tamponade.

Although infection has not been a frequent occurrence following operative hysteroscopy, caution should nonetheless be taken when operating extensively in the uterine cavity, particularly in patients for whom fertility is a concern. Prophylactic antibiotics therefore should be individualized.

Operative hysteroscopy is best performed in the operating room with the patient under general anesthesia, except when minor interventions are performed, such as removal of an intrauterine device (IUD), biopsy of an endometrial lesion, or division of filmy adhesions that only partially abduct the uterine walls. Because laser energy and electrosurgery per se may cause additional tissue injury, these energies should be used only with the background and knowledge of their specific physical properties and their tissue interaction.

Safety measures should be taken to protect not only the operator but everyone in the room from back-scattering of the fiberoptic lasers. Appropriate eye shields or safety goggles (alternatively, video systems) provide protection from retinal injuries. This approach also protects patients from laser-associated trauma. Operative hysteroscopy requires a fundamental knowledge and experience in diagnostic hysteroscopy. Furthermore, the appropriate instrumentation should be available, as improvisation may be the source of unnecessary complications. To prepare the practitioner for the safe use of operative hysteroscopy, special laboratory exercises, tutorials, and preceptorships are of paramount importance to acquiring dexterity and confidence in the preparation for a practice of safe and effective use of hysteroscopic surgery. With a background of progressive preparation, selection of patients, and meticulous technique, operative hysteroscopy can be performed safely, effectively, and with few or no complications.

Conclusion

The therapeutic applications of hysteroscopy have proliferated owing to improvements in instrumentation, distending media, and surgical techniques. The use of the gynecologic resectoscope has also increased the capabilities of intrauterine surgery. The use of fiberoptic lasers continues to be explored in an effort to decrease thermal damage to tissues and operate with precision in the uterine cavity.

Most of the uterine conditions that in the past required invasive surgical procedures such as laparotomy and hysterotomy can be treated with minimally invasive surgery using the hysteroscope and resectoscope. Intrauterine adhesions, uterine septum resection, submucous leiomyomas, tubal cornual obstruction, and abnormal uterine bleeding unresponsive to hormonal therapy can be addressed efficiently by hysteroscopy, with decreasing morbidity, less inconvenience to the patient, less disability, and lower cost. Other therapeutic applications remain on the horizon, but the transcervical approach remains promising for procedures such as salpingoscopy. Reproductive technologic procedures such as ZIFT, GIFT, and intratubal insemination are now being explored via hysteroscopy. The quest for a simple, effective transcervical method for tubal sterilization may eventually find its answer in the hysteroscopic approach.

References

1. PANTALEONI DC: On endoscopic examination of the cavity of the womb. Med Press Circ (Lond) 1869;8:26.
2. EDSTROM KGB: Intrauterine surgical procedures during hysteroscopy. Endoscopy 1974;6:175.
3. SCIARRA JJ, BUTLER JC, SPEIDEL JJ (EDS): Hysteroscopic Sterilization. New York, Intercontinental Medical Book Corporation, 1974.
4. SIEGLER AM, VALLE RF, LINDEMANN HJ, MENCAGLIA L: Therapeutic Hysteroscopy: Indications and Techniques. St. Louis, Mosby, 1990.
5. VALLE RF: Therapeutic hysteroscopy in infertility. Int J Fertil 1984;29:143.
6. NEUWIRTH RS, AMIN HK: Excision of submuous fibroids with hysteroscopic control. Am J Obstet Gynecol 1976;126:95.
7. LIN B-L, MIYAMOTO N, AOKI R, IWATA Y: Transcervical resection of submucous myomas. Acta Obstet Gynaecol Jpn 1986;38:1647.
8. DECHERNEY AH, POLAN ML: Hysteroscopic management of intrauterine lesions and intractable uterine bleeding. Obstet Gynecol 1983;61:392.
9. NEUWIRTH RS: Hysteroscopic management of symptomatic submucous fibroids. Obstet Gynecol 1983;62:509.
10. SIEGLER AM, VALLE RF: Therapeutic hysteroscopic procedures. Fertil Steril 1988;50:685.
11. NEUWIRTH RS: A new technique for and additional experience with hysteroscopic resection of submucous fibroids. Am J Obstet Gynecol 1978;131:91.
12. HALLEZ JP, NETTER A, CARTIER R: Methodical intrauterine resection. Am J Obstet Gynecol 1987;156:1080.
13. BAGGISH MS, SZE EHM, MORGAN G: Hysteroscopic treatment of symptomatic submucous myomata uteri with the Nd:YAG laser. J Gynecol Surg 1989;5:27.
14. VALLE RF: Hysteroscopic removal of submucous leiomyomas. J Gynecol Surg 1990;6:89.

15. DONNEZ J, SCHOURS B, GILLEROT S, ET AL: Treatment of uterine fibroids with implants of gonadotropin-releasing hormone agonist: assessment by hysterography. Fertil Steril 1989;51:947.
16. DONNEZ J, GILLEROT S, BOURGONJOU D, ET AL: Neodymium:YAG laser hysteroscopy in large submucous fibroids. Fertil Steril 1990;54:999.
17. LOFFER FD: Removal of large symptomatic intrauterine growths by the hysteroscopic resectoscope. Obstet Gynecol 1990;76:836.
18. CORSON SL, BROOKS PG: Resectoscopic myomectomy. Fertil Steril 1991;55:1041.
19. DERMAN SG, REHNSTROM J, NEUWIRTH RS: The long-term effectiveness of hysteroscopic treatment of menorrhagia and leiomyomas. Obstet Gynecol 1991;77:591.
20. WAMSTEKER K, EMANUEL MH, DE KRUIF JH: Transcervical hysteroscopic resection of submucous fibroids for abnormal uterine bleeding: results regarding the degree of intramural extension. Obstet Gynecol 1993;82:736.
21. BUTTRAM VC, GIBBONS WE: Mullerian anomalies: a proposed classification (an analysis of 144 cases). Fertil Steril 1979;32:40.
22. VALLE RF: Clinical management of uterine factors in infertile patients. Semin Reprod Endocrinol 1985;3:149.
23. JONES AW, JONES GES: Double uterus as an etiologic factor in repeated abortions: indications for surgical repair. Am J Obstet Gynecol 1953;65:325.
24. TOMPKINS P: Comments on the bicornuate uterus and twinning. Surg Clin North Am 1962;42:1049.
25. DALY DC, WALTERS CA, SOTO-ALBORS CE, RIDDICK DH: Hysteroscopic metroplasty: surgical technique and obstetric outcome. Fertil Steril 1983;39:623.
26. VALLE RF, SCIARRA JJ: Hysteroscopic treatment of the septate uterus. Obstet Gynecol 1986;676:253.
27. PERINO A, MENCAGLIA L, HAMOU J, CITTADINI E: Hysteroscopy for metroplasty of uterine septa: report of 24 cases. Fertil Steril 1987;48:321.
28. DALY DC, TOHAN N, WALTERS C, RIDDICK, DH: Hysteroscopic resection of the uterine septum in the presence of a septate cervix. Fertil Steril 1983;39:560.
29. MARCH CM, ISRAEL R: Hysteroscopic management of recurrent abortion caused by septate uterus. Am J Obstet Gynecol 1987;156:834.
30. DECHERNEY AH, RUSSELL JB, GRAEBE RA, POLAN ML: Resectoscopic management of mullerian fusion defects. Fertil Steril 1986;45:726.
31. ROCK JA, MURPHY AA, COOPER WH: Resectoscopic techniques for the lysis of a class V: complete uterine septum. Fertil Steril 1987;48:495.
32. CANDIANI GB, VERCELLINI P, FEDELE L, ET AL: Repair of the uterine cavity after hysteroscopic septal incision. Fertil Steril 1990;54:991.
33. CANDIANI GB, VERCELLINI P, FEDELE L, ET AL: Argon laser versus microscissors for hysteroscopic incision of uterine septa. Am J Obstet Gynecol 1991;164:87.
34. DANIELL JF, OSHER S, MILLER W: Hysteroscopic resection of uterine septi with visible light laser energy. Colposc Gynecol Laser Surg 1987;3:217.
35. CHOE JK, BAGGISH MS: Hysteroscopic treatment of septate uterus with neodymium-YAG laser. Fertil Steril 1992;57:81.
36. FEDELE L, ARCAINI L, PARAZZINI F, ET AL: Reproductive prognosis after hysteroscopic metroplasty in 102 women: life-table analysis. Fertil Steril 1993;59:768.
37. FAYEZ JA: Comparison between abdominal and hysteroscopic metroplasty. Obstet Gynecol 1986;68:399.
38. DALY DC, MAIER D, SOTO-ALBORS C: Hysteroscopic metroplasty: six years experience. Obstet Gynecol 1989;73:201.
39. SIEGLER AM, VALLE RF, LINDEMANN HJ, MENCAGLIA L: Hysteroscopic metroplasty. In Therapeutic Hysteroscopy: Indications and Techniques. St. Louis, Mosby, 1990, pp 62–81.
40. HASSIAKOS DK, ZOURLAS PA: Transcervical division of the uterine septa. Obstet Gynecol Surv 1990;45:165.
41. ASHERMAN JG: Amenorrhea traumatic (atretica). J Obstet Gynaecol Br Emp 1948;55:23.
42. ASHERMAN JG: Traumatic intrauterine adhesions. J Obstet Gynaecol Br Emp 1950;57:892.
43. KLEIN SM, GARCIA CR: Asherman's syndrome: a critique and current review. Fertil Steril 1973;24:722.
44. SCHENKER JG, MARGALIOTH EJ: Intrauterine adhesions: an updated appraisal. Fertil Steril 1982;37:593.
45. MARCH CM, ISRAEL R, MARCH AD: Hysteroscopic management of intrauterine adhesions. Am J Obstet Gynecol 1978;130:653.
46. VALLE RF, SCIARRA JJ: Current status of hysteroscopy in gynecologic practice. Fertil Steril 1979;32:619.
47. SIEGLER AM, KONTOPOULOS VG: Lysis of intrauterine adhesions under hysteroscopic control:

a report of 25 operations. J Reprod Med 1981; 26:372.
48. NEUWIRTH RS, HUSSEIN AR, SCHIFFMAN BM, AMIN HK: Hysteroscopic resection of intrauterine scars using a new technique. Obstet Gynecol 1982;60:111.
49. VALLE RF, SCIARRA JJ: Intrauterine adhesions: hysteroscopic diagnosis, classification, treatment, and reproductive outcome. Am J Obstet Gynecol 1988;158:1459.
50. FRIEDMAN A, DEFAZIO J, DECHERNEY AH: Severe obstetric complications following hysteroscopic lysis of adhesions. Obstet Gynecol 1986; 67:864.
51. NEWTON JR, MACKENZIE WE, EMENS MJ, JORDAN JA: Division of uterine adhesions (Asherman's syndrome) with the Nd-YAG laser. Br J Obstet Gynaecol 1989;96:102.
52. MARCH CM, ISRAEL R: Gestational outcome following hysteroscopic lysis of adhesions. Fertil Steril 1981;36:455.
53. SIEGLER AM, VALLE RF, LINDEMANN HJ, MENCAGLIA L: Intrauterine adhesions. In Therapeutic Hysteroscopy: Indications and Techniques. St. Louis, Mosby, 1990, pp 82–105.
54. AMERICAN FERTILITY SOCIETY: Classifications of adnexal adhesions, distal tubal occlusion, tubal occlusion secondary to tubal ligation, tubal pregnancies, mullerian anomalies and intrauterine adhesions. Fertil Steril 1988;49:944.
55. SULAK PJ, LETTERIE GS, CODDINGTON CC, ET AL: Histology of proximal tubal occlusion. Fertil Steril 1987;48:437.
56. MENKEN FC: Endoscopic observations of endocrine process and hormonal changes. In Simposio Esteroids Sexuales, Albrecht FR, Ramirez Sanchez J, Willomitzer H (eds). Bogota, Museo Nacional, Berlin, Saladruck, 1969, pp 276–281.
57. QUINONES-GUERRERO R, ALVARADO-DURAN A, AZNAR-RAMOS R: Tubal catheterization: applications of a new technique. Am J Obstet Gynecol 1972;114:674.
58. VALLE RF: Tubal catheterization for sterilization purposes. In Tubal Catheterization Procedures, Gleicher N (ed). New York, Wiley, 1992, pp 139–160.
59. THURMOND AS, NOVY M, UCHIDA BT, ROSCH J: Fallopian tube obstruction: selective salpingography and recanalization. Radiology 1987; 163:511.
60. THURMOND AS, NOVY MJ: Transcervical fallopian tube catheterization for management of proximal tubal obstruction. In Diagnostic Imaging in Infertility. Winfield AC, Wentz AC (eds). Baltimore, Williams & Wilkins, 1992, pp 192–207.
61. CONFINO E, TUR-KASPA I, DECHERNEY A, ET AL: Transcervical balloon, tuboplasty: a multicenter study. JAMA 1990;264:2079.
62. CONFINO E, FRIBERG J, GLEICHER N: Transcervical balloon tuboplasty. Fertil Steril 1986;46:963.
63. DANIELL JF, MILLER W: Hysteroscopic correction of cornual occlusion with resultant term pregnancy. Fertil Steril 1987;48:490.
64. SULAK PJ, LETTERIE GS, HAYSLIP CC, ET AL: Hysteroscopic cannulation and lavage in the treatment of proximal tubal occlusion. Fertil Steril 1987;48:493.
65. CONFINO E, FRIBERG J, GLEICHER N: Preliminary experience with transcervical balloon tuboplasty. Am J Obstet Gynecol 1988;159:370.
66. NOVY MJ, THURMOND AS, PATTON P, ET AL: Diagnosis of cornual obstruction by transcervical fallopian tube cannulation. Fertil Steril 1988; 50:434.
67. DEATON JL, GIBSON M, RIDDICK DH, BRUMSTED JR: Diagnosis and treatment of cornual obstruction using flexible tip guidewire. Fertil Steril 1990; 50:232.
68. LIN BL, IWATA Y, LIU KH, VALLE RF: Clinical applications of a new Fujinon operating fiberoptic hysteroscope. J Gynecol Surg 1990;6:81.
69. FLOOD JT, GROW DR: Transcervical tubal cannulation: a review. Obstet Gynecol Surv 1993; 48:768.
70. VALLE RF: Hysteroscopy in the evaluation of infertility. In Diagnostic Imaging in Infertility, Winfield AC, Wentz AC (eds). Baltimore, Williams & Wilkins, 1992, pp 117–150.
71. BABCOCK WW: Chemical hysterectomy. Am J Obstet Gynecol 1924;7:693.
72. DROEGEMUELLER W, GREER B, MAKOWSKI E: Cryosurgery in patients with dysfunctional uterine bleeding. Obstet Gynecol 1971;38:256.
73. DROEGEMUELLER W, GREER BE, DAVIS JR, ET AL: Cryocoagulation of the endometrium at the uterine cornua. Am J Obstet Gynecol 1978; 131:1.
74. EASTERDAY CL, GRIMES DA, RIGGS JA: Hysterectomy in the United States. Obstet Gynecol 1983;62:203.
75. SCHENKER JG, POLISHUK WZ: Regeneration of rabbit endometrium following intrauterine instillation of chemical agents. Gynecol Invest 1973;4:1.
76. SCHENKER JG, NICOSIA SV, POLISHUK WZ, GARCIA C-R: An in vitro fibroblast-enriched sponge

preparation for induction of intrauterine adhesions. Isr J Med Sci 1975;11:849.
77. STEVENSON TC, TAYLOR DS: The effect of methylcyanoacrylate tissue adhesive on the human fallopian tube and endometrium. J Obstet Gynecol 1972;79:1028.
78. RICHART RM: The use of chemical agents in female sterilization. In Female Transcervical Sterilization, Zatuchni GI, Shelton JD, Goldsmith A, Sciarra JJ (eds). Hagerstown, MD, Harper & Row, 1983, pp 24–35.
79. ZIPPER J, MEDEL M, PASTENE I, RIVERA M: Intrauterine instillation of chemical cytotoxic agents for tubal sterilization and treatment of functional metrorrhagia. Int J Fertil 1969;14:289.
80. WINGO PA, HUEZO CM, RUBIN GL, ET AL: The mortality risk associated with hysterectomy. Am J Obstet Gynecol 1985;152:803.
81. GRANT J, HUSSEIN IY: An audit of abdominal hysterectomy over a decade in a district general hospital. Br J Obstet Gynaecol 1984;91:73.
82. GOLDRATH MH, FULLER TA, SEGAL S: Laser photovaporization of the endometrium for the treatment of menorrhagia. Am J Obstet Gynecol 1981;140:14.
83. VALLE RF: Endometrial ablation for dysfunctional uterine bleeding: role of GnRH agonists. Int J Gynecol Obstet 1993;41:3.
84. PERINO A, CHIANDRIANO N, PETRONIO M, CITTADINI E: Role of leuprolide acetate depot in hysteroscopic surgery: a controlled study. Fertil Steril 1993;59:507.
85. LOMANO JM: Photocoagulation of the endometrium with the Nd:YAG laser for the treatment of menorrhagia: a report of ten cases. J Reprod Med 1986;31:148.
86. DANIELL J, TOSH R, MEISELS S: Photodynamic ablation of the endometrium with Nd:YAG laser hyseroscopically as a treatment of menorrhagia. Colposc Gynecol Laser Surg 1986;2:43.
87. LOFFER FD: Hysteroscopic endometrial ablation with Nd:YAG laser using a noncontact technique. Obstet Gynecol 1987;69:679.
88. DECHERNEY AH, DIAMOND MP, LAVY G, POLAN ML: Endometrial ablation for intractable uterine bleeding: hysteroscopic resection. Obstet Gynecol 1987;70:668.
89. LOMANO JM: Dragging technique versus blanching technique for endometrial ablation with the Nd:YAG laser in the treatment of chronic menorrhagia. Am J Obstet Gynecol 1988;159:152.
90. GIMPELSON RJ: Hysteroscopic Nd:YAG ablation of the endometrium. J Reprod Med 1988; 38:872.

91. BAGGISH MS, BALTOYANNIS P: New techniques for laser ablation of the endometrium in high risk patients. Am J Obstet Gynecol 1988;159:287.
92. RANKIN L, STEINBERG LH: Transcervical resection of the endometrium: a review of 400 consecutive patients. Br J Obstet Gynaecol 1992; 99:911.
93. DWYER N, HUTTON J, STIRRAT GM: Randomized controlled trial comparing endometrial resection with abdominal hysterectomy for the surgical treatment of menorrhagia. Br J Obstet Gynaecol 1993;100:237.
94. MAGOS AL, BAUMANN R, LOCKWOOD GM, TURNBULL AC: Experience with the first 150 endometrial resections for menorrhagia. Lancet 1991; 337:1074.
95. VANCAILLE TG: Electrocoagulation of the endometrium with the ball-end resectoscope. Obstet Gynecol 1989;74:425.
96. TOWNSEND DE, RICHART RM, PASKOWITZ RA, WOOLFORK RE: "Rollerball" coagulation of the endometrium. Obstet Gynecol 1990;76:310.
97. MCLUCAS B: Endometrial ablation with the roller ball electrode. J Reprod Med 1990; 35:1055.
98. DANIELL JF, KURTZ BR, KE RW: Hysteroscopic endometrial ablation using the rollerball electrode. Obstet Gynecol 1992;80:329.
99. ONBARGI LC, HAYDEN R, VALLE RF, DEL PRIORE G: Effects of power and electrical current density variations in an in vitro endometrial ablation model. Obstet Gynecol 1993;82:912.
100. TIMOR-TRISCH IE, BAR-YAM Y, ELGALI S, ROTTEM S: The technique of transvaginal sonography with the use of a 6.5 mHz probe. Am J Obstet Gynecol 1988;158:1019.
101. SYROP CH, SAHAKIAN V: Transvaginal sonographic detection of endometrial polyps with fluid contrast augmentation. Obstet Gynecol 1992;79:1041.
102. FEDELE L, BIANCHI S, DORTA M, ET AL: Transvaginal ultrasonography versus hysteroscopy in the diagnosis of uterine submucous myomas. Obstet Gynecol 1991;77:745.
103. BINKOVITZ LA, KING BF, CORFMAN RS: Advances in gynecologic imaging and intervention. Mayo Clin Proc 1991;66:1133.
104. WITZ CA, SILVERBERG KM, BURNS WN, ET AL: Complications associated with the absorption of hysteroscopic fluid media. Fertil Steril 1993; 60:745.
105. GARRY R, HASHAM F, KOKRI MS, MOONEY P: The effect of pressure on fluid absorption during endometrial ablation. J Gynecol Surg 1992; 8:1.

106. ARIEFF AI, AYUS JC: Endometrial ablation complicated by fatal hyponatremic encephalopathy. JAMA 1993;270:1230.
107. BAGGISH MS, BRILL AI, ROSENWEIG B, ET AL: Fatal acute glycine and sorbitol toxicity during operative hysteroscopy. J Gynecol Surg 1993; 9:137.
108. MCLUCAS B: Hyskon complications in hysteroscopic surgery. Obstet Gynecol Surv 1991; 46:196.
109. PETERSON HB, HULKA JF, PHILLIPS JM: American Association of Gynecologic Laparoscopists 1988 membership survey on operative hysteroscopy. J Reprod Med 1990;35:590.
110. HULKA JF, PETERSON HB, PHILLIPS JM, SURREY MN: Operative hysteroscopy: American Association of Gynecologic Laparoscopists 1991 membership survey. J Reprod Med 1993; 38:572.

23
Abnormal Uterine Bleeding and Endometrial Ablation

Richard J. Gimpelson

More than 600,000 hysterectomies are performed each year in the United States, with many having little or no pathology and no workup other than dilatation and curettage. Most of these hysterectomies are performed for abnormal uterine bleeding.[1] This problem can be divided into three categories: systemic causes, disease of the reproductive tract, and dysfunctional uterine bleeding.[2]

Bleeding from systemic causes such as hepatic disease, renal disease, blood dyscrasia, thyroid abnormality, or other medical conditions that alter blood-coagulating mechanisms are usually referred to the gynecologist for treatment. If medical therapy is unsuccessful or contraindicated, endometrial ablation is often a viable and safer alternative to hysterectomy for resolving the bleeding problem or improving the quality of the patient's life.

Diseases of the reproductive tract can be secondary to pregnancy-related causes, exogenous hormones, intrauterine contraceptive devices, malignant and premalignant conditions of the cervix and endometrium, pelvic infection, leiomyomas, and endometrial polyps. These conditions warrant specific treatment that usually corrects the resultant bleeding problem; however, in women who have completed their childbearing, endometrial ablation may be combined with the treatment of endometrial polyps and leiomyoma to reduce the incidence of recurrent bleeding problems.

Dysfunctional uterine bleeding occurs without a specific anatomic etiology and can often be treated medically with good results. In those patients whose medical therapy is unsuccessful, undesired, or contraindicated, endometrial ablation is an effective treatment and an excellent alternative to hysterectomy.

Endometrial ablation includes a variety of techniques whose common endpoint is thermal destruction of the endometrium and superficial myometrium with resultant marked reduction or elimination of uterine bleeding. The basic techniques have evolved from the use of either the Nd:YAG laser[3] or a loop[4] or roller[5] electrode. The single most important development that contributed to the ease and safety of endometrial ablation was the continuous-flow sheath, which enhanced visualization of the uterine cavity and reduced the risk of fluid overload for all operative hysteroscopic procedures.[6] Endometrial ablation should be performed only with a continuous-flow hysteroscope.

Indications and Contraindications

The indications for endometrial ablation were set forth by Goldrath et al. in the first paper on endometrial ablation.[3] "Twenty-two patients were carefully selected for this procedure. All had excessive and disabling uterine bleeding and were unable or unwilling to use other methods for control. All could be candidates for hysterectomy. All patients had stated that future childbearing was not desired." These words of wisdom are still guidelines worth following today.

Contraindications to endometrial ablation are endometrial cancer or endometrial hyperplasia, which can develop into endometrial cancer.[7] Relative contraindications are an enlarged uterus with leiomyomas, although a number of papers have reported successful treatment of patients using combined myomectomy and endometrial ablation.[8-11] However, if a portion of an intramural leiomyoma remains, the patient may require repeat myomectomy or hysterectomy.[12,13] Adenomyosis, which is a relative contraindication, has also been successfully managed with endometrial ablation.[8,11]

The patient must be informed that although endometrial ablation can markedly inhibit the ability to achieve pregnancy, it is not a method for permanent sterilization nor is it reversible. The patient must continue to use a method of contraception or have permanent sterilization for her or her partner. Although not published at this time, discussions with other gynecologists indicate that pregnancies following endometrial ablation have a higher incidence of complications, such as ectopic implantation, premature labor, need for cesarean section, and problems with placental implantation. One case of a ruptured ectopic pregnancy has been reported.[14]

Technique

All patients who desire or are candidates for endometrial ablation should undergo a thorough history and physical examination. Preoperative uterine assessment should be by hysteroscopy, although transvaginal ultrasonography and curettage may provide adequate information prior to ablation to minimize unexpected findings, such as hyperplasia, malignancy, leiomyomas, or polyps.

Preoperative suppression of the endometrium is utilized to thin the endometrium to less than 3 mm and allow thorough penetration into the superficial myometrium. This preoperative suppression is accomplished medically by the use of danazol[3] or leuprolide acetate[2] or mechanically by suction curettage.[15] In some cases the electrical loop has been utilized to resect the endometrium, and then the roller electrode is used to coagulate the remaining uterine cavity surface.[16]

Danazol is administered as 600–800 mg PO daily for 4–8 weeks. For this short time the androgenic and anabolic effects are usually tolerated by the patient, and rarely does the medication need to be discontinued prior to surgery. Weight gain and joint pain seem to be the predominant side effects. Medical therapy is usually not continued postoperatively.

Leuprolide acetate (Lupron) depot is given as 3.75 mg IM for one or two injections 4 weeks apart. If one injection is administered, the endometrial ablation is performed 4 weeks later. If two injections are chosen, the ablation can be performed 2–4 weeks after the second injection. The first injection can be given any time during the menstrual cycle, although giving it during the early luteal phase in patients who are ovulatory minimizes the bleeding that occurs. Leuprolide acetate is not usually administered postablation; however, if the procedure is performed 2 weeks after the second injection, there is a residual effect from the medication for 2–3 weeks. An alternative method is to give 7.5 mg of leuprolide acetate depot 4 weeks prior to the ablation as a single dose. Medroxyprogesterone acetate has also been used as a preparatory medication, but it tends to produce a secretory-type endometrium that is more difficult to ablate and results in less success of the procedure.[17]

Suction curettage is easily performed as a method of thinning the endometrium prior to ablation. A 7 mm Milex suction curette (Milex Corporation, Chicago, IL) is inserted into the uterine cavity just prior to ablation, and thorough curettage for 2–3 minutes can adequately denude the endometrium in preparation for endometrial ablation. This mechanical preparation is more easily accomplished during the late menstrual to midproliferative phase of the cycle. However, because many patients are anovulatory these clearly defined stages of the cycle

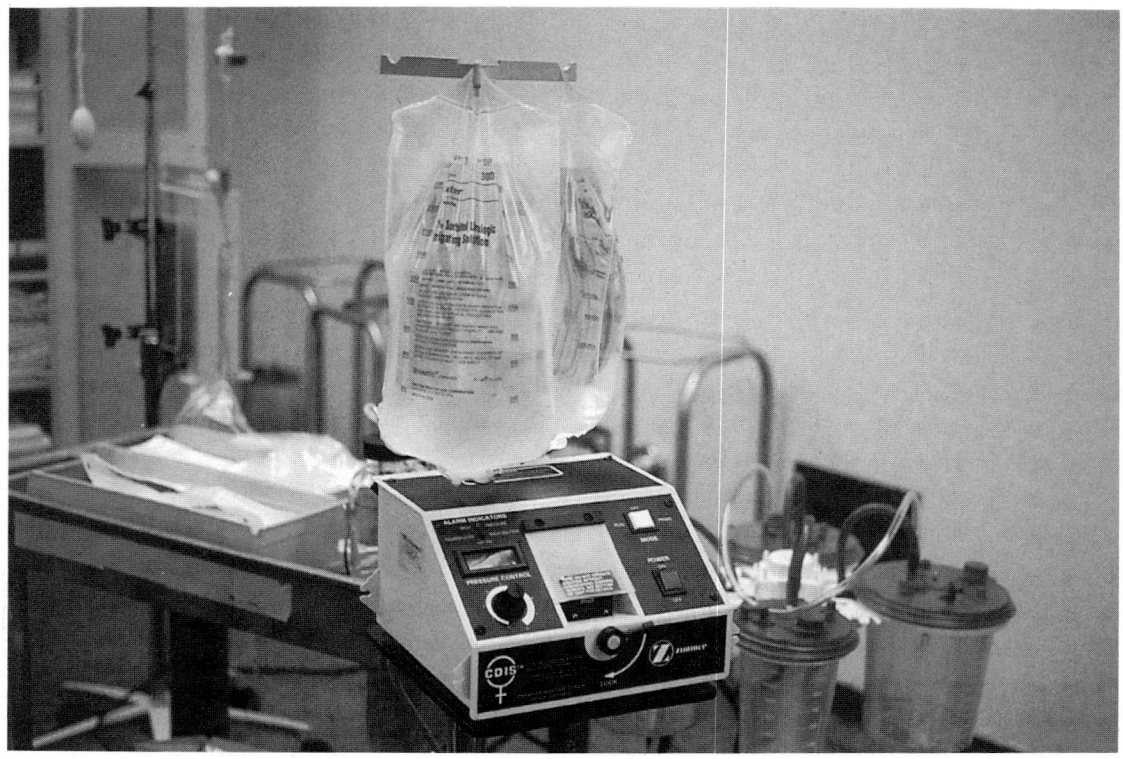

Figure 23.1. Controlled distension irrigation system (Zimmer Patient Care Products, Dover, OH).

are not present, and even in ovulatory patients mechanical preparation has been successful at any time during the menstrual cycle, which makes scheduling easy for the patient. Furthermore, some gynecologists advocate resection of the endometrium as preparation followed by roller ablation without mechanical or medical preparation.

Anesthesia for this procedure can be general, regional, or local. For local anesthesia (with sedation), the patient is first prepared, draped, and positioned in the operating room. Sedation is then administered by the anesthesiologist or anesthetist. Once the patient is adequately sedated a paracervical block is provided with 0.25% bupivacaine with 2 U of vasopressin for each 10 cc of local anesthetic. Usually 10–20 cc of local anesthesia is used. This local anesthetic is given even with general anesthesia to reduce the postoperative cramping that occurs, reduce bleeding and intravasation of fluid, and allow easier entry of the hysteroscopic sheaths. The anesthesiologist or anesthetist must be familiar with the potential for fluid overload and keep intravenous instillation of fluids at a minimum. Endometrial ablation is almost always accomplished as outpatient surgery, with hospital observation or admission limited to those patients with medical conditions that warrant such care.

Some gynecologists prefer dilatation of the cervix with *Laminaria* or synthetic dilatation prior to the procedure.[18,19] *Laminaria* are usually inserted into the cervical canal the night prior to surgery, although most physicians use mechanical dilators. In the mechanically prepared endometrium, insertion of the diagnostic sheath, followed by the operative sheath, and then placement of the resectoscope allows entry without blind dilatation in most patients. If the laser is used through an operative sheath, the uterine cavity can be entered without need for blind dilatation in 90% of cases.[15] Once again, it is important to emphasize that only continuous-flow instrumentation should be used for endometrial abla-

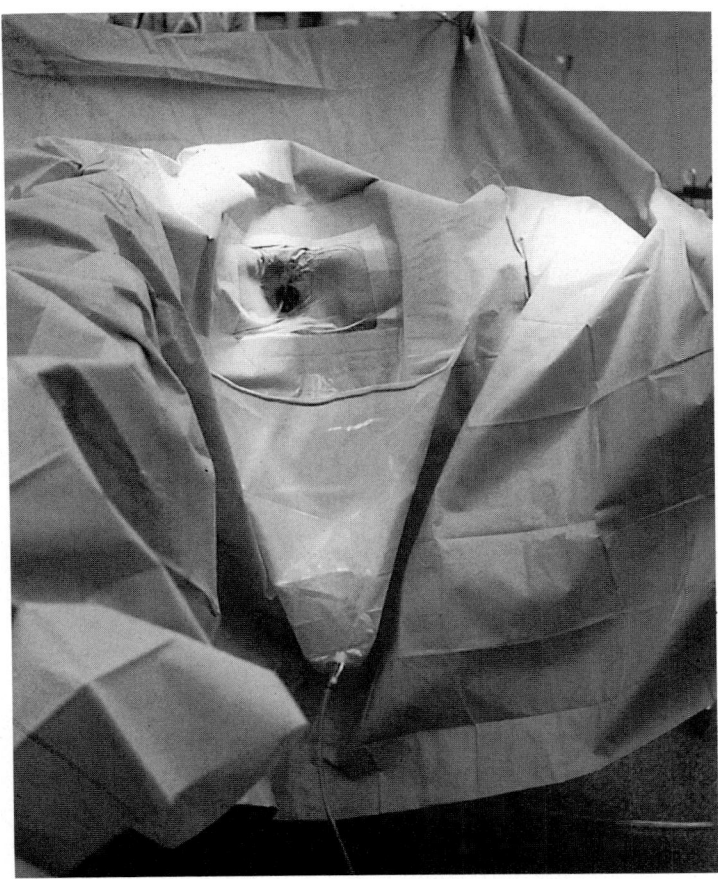

Figure 23.2. Lingemann percutaneous procedure drape (Lingemann Medical Products, Indianapolis, IN).

tion or for any operative hysteroscopic procedure during which more than 2 L of low viscosity fluids are used with a high flow technique.

Although 32% dextran 70 has been used for endometrial ablation, low viscosity, high flow liquids such as lactated Ringer's solution, normal saline, sorbitol, glycine, or mannitol have a wide margin of safety and should be utilized instead of 32% dextran 70. The low viscosity liquids do not cause the instrument valves to stick as does 32% dextran 70, and they are easier to manage if too much is instilled. These low viscosity liquids are best infused through controlled pressure devices, such as the CDIS (controlled distention irrigation system; Zimmer Patient Care, Dover, OH) (Fig. 23.1). These devices allow a preset pressure of instillation, are at a comfortable height for changing fluid bags, and allow monitoring of the inflow easier than when infusion bags are placed 3–4 feet above the patient (gravity feed) or when pressure cuffs are used, which must be removed to assess the fluid used in each bag. The fluid instilled circulates through the uterine cavity and is removed through the outflow channel of the continuous-flow sheath. This fluid is then delivered to collection canisters by means of a collecting funnel (Fig. 23.2), and the outflow is measured. Because fluid monitoring is the most important safety factor for successful completion of the endometrial ablation, attempts should be made to collect all outflow. Whatever does not exit through the outflow channel of the hysteroscope may be noted coming out of the cervix and the vagina. This fluid, which may run down the buttocks, can be carried to the floor by a plastic drape under the patient. A suction floor mat (Aqua Vac; Arthroplastics, Chagrin Falls, OH) (Fig. 23.3) has proved convenient for containing and collecting flow spill-

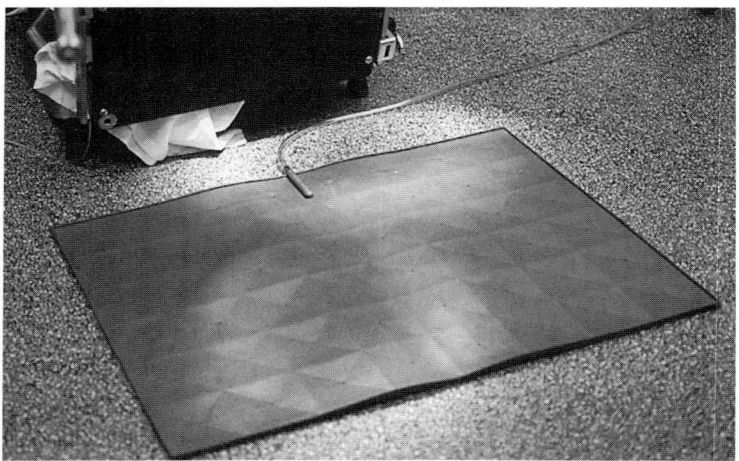

Figure 23.3. Aqua Vac floor mat (Arthroplastics, Chagrin Falls, OH).

age and transporting this fluid to the collection canisters. At least every 10 minutes, or more frequently, the circulating nurse announces the amount of fluid intake and output and records this information. A measurement should also be performed each time a fluid bag is changed, which sometimes results in a measurement at less than the 10 minute interval. The nurse should not be solely responsible for measuring any discrepancy between inflow and outflow, but by tracking total inflow and outflow all personnel in the operating room are aware of fluid balance. Endometrial ablation is presently being performed with both the Nd:YAG laser and electrical energy, each of which has specific requirements and is discussed separately.

Nd:YAG Laser

The Nd:YAG laser was the first energy source used for endometrial ablation and has been utilized for about two decades.[3] Power is set at 40–60 watts, and the laser is applied in either a dragging[3] (touch) or blanching[20] (nontouch) technique through a 6000- or 1000-μm fiber. In both cases, one starts at the fundus or cornual areas and works toward the internal cervical os. Individual preference guides one to work a long axis or side to side. In either case, the hysteroscope with the laser fiber is moved a fixed distance outside the sheath rather than moving the fiber in and out of the sheath. With the dragging technique, the laser fiber is applied to the surface of the endometrium and held against the surface as the laser is fired. This method creates grooves or furrows in the endometrium that usually extends about 2 mm in depth; it then destroys another 2 mm by radiated heat (Plate 41). The surgeon proceeds until the entire endometrial cavity has been furrowed.

The blanching technique involves holding the laser fiber approximately 1 mm off the surface of the endometrium and firing the laser without touching the surface, achieving permanent thermal damage to a depth of 4–5 mm. The visual endpoint of the nontouch technique is a white, blanched appearance (Plate 42). Often a combination of dragging and blanching is required to fully ablate the endometrium. One must be cautious in the cornual areas where the uterine wall thickness is less than 1 cm.

Any distention fluid can be used with laser energy, although normal saline or lactated Ringer's solution is usually chosen because either maintains the electrolyte balance. Bags of 3 L capacity are the most efficient and require less changing by the circulating nurse.

Electrosurgery: Roller Electrode

Electrical energy for endometrial ablation was first used in 1983 with a wire loop.[4] In 1988 the first roller electrode was used in Japan,[5] and in 1989 it was introduced to the United States.[21] Since 1989 the roller electrode has surpassed the Nd:YAG laser in usage for endometrial ablation; however, the guidelines for electrical usage are not as clear as those for the Nd:YAG laser. The energy used ranges from 30 watts[4] to 125 watts,[8] and the waveform has been reported as a cutting (undamped), coagulating (damped), or combination (blend) waveform. For the most part, the roller electrode is applied to the surface of the endometrium with some pressure to indent the surface to achieve adequate depth of thermal injury. If one just barely touches the surface, superficial fulguration occurs, and the procedure fails. In addition, one must move the roller electrode slowly to allow adequate penetration of electrical energy into the tissue. The roller electrode should always be directed in the long axis of the uterus except for the fundal area, which may be ablated in a side-to-side rolling action. The visual endpoint is a brownish cobblestone appearance that is characteristic of "burned" myometrium (Plate 43).

Only nonconductive media can be used with the roller electrode, otherwise the energy is so dispersed there is no effect. Nonconductive media utilized include sorbitol, glycine, and mannitol. As with the conductive medium, these fluids should be utilized in 3 L bags for ease of handling.

Wire Loop

Endometrial resection has been the most recent method advocated for endometrial ablation. With endometrial resection, a loop electrode is utilized to resect the endometrium along with the superficial myometrium (Plate 44). The power settings utilized are 80–210 watts (cutting current).[8,10,16] One must be careful with this technique not to go over the same area too vigorously, as perforation can occur. Often the surgeon resects the endometrium and then applies the roller electrode as previously described to complete the endometrial ablation. With the loop electrode, as with the roller electrode, nonconductive distention medium is used.

Is laser or electrosurgery the better energy source for endometrial ablation? This question has not been answered, as proponents seem to have comparable success with the two methods.

Postoperative Care

Most patients require minimal postoperative care. If pain occurs it is usually mild to moderate cramping for several days and usually responds well to nonsteroidal antiinflammatory drugs (NSAIDs). Patients may have several weeks of serosanguineous discharge. Heavy bleeding at the end of a procedure can usually be treated by inserting a catheter with 10–15 cc in the balloon for tamponade and drainage. The catheter can be removed within 2–6 hours.

Infection is rare, and postoperative antibiotics are not routinely required; however, if the patient presents with a low-grade fever or more uterine cramping and tenderness than expected, ampicillin or doxycycline for 7–10 days appears to resolve the problem.

Sounding at 2–6 weeks postoperatively is advocated by most physicians to reduce the risk of hematometra by enhancing patency of the cervical canal. Postoperative suppression of endometrial growth by medroxyprogesterone acetate or leuprolide acetate has been advocated by some authors,[19,22,23] but at present long-term results do not seem to show a difference when these patients are compared with those receiving no postablation suppression. Furthermore, suppression delays the time to evaluate surgical success or failure. By 3 months after operation the patient has a good idea of the results, although full healing and menstrual pattern may not be complete for 6 months.

Repeat Ablations

Roller electrodes may be slightly less expensive for the patient. However, the Nd:YAG laser is recommended for repeat ablations because the uterus has contracted, and this laser is much easier to insert and use through a 21F operating hysteroscope than the larger resectoscopes.[24]

Complications

Complications of endometrial ablation have the potential to be serious, but awareness of the possibility of such complications can minimize the untoward results. Fluid overload, uterine perforation, hemorrhage, air embolism, infec-

INTAKE AND OUTPUT FOR ZIMMER PUMP USE				
EVERY 10 MINUTES TIME	FLUIDS IN	FLUIDS OUT	PUMP PRESSURE	COMMENTS
TOTALS:				
OTHER TOTAL FLUIDS:				
I.V.s:				
Urine:				

Figure 23.4. Flow sheet for fluid monitoring.

tion, and the masking of cancer are all complications over which the surgeon has some control in preventing.

Fluid overload can occur quickly, so the entire operating room team must be cognizant of the patient's fluid balance. When using lasers, the fluids utilized are saline or lactated Ringer's solution, both of which contain electrolytes. With electrosurgical generators the fluid must be electrolyte-free (e.g., sorbitol, glycine, mannitol). All fluids have the potential for intravasation and if used in large amounts possible pulmonary edema and hyponatremia can result. The safety measures include use of continuous-flow instrumentation exclusively, intrauterine pressure < 80 mm Hg, and careful monitoring of the intake and outflow of fluids including those given by the anesthesiologist (mandatory). Fluids are monitored and recorded (Fig. 23.4). A procedure is stopped if one cannot account for 1500–2000 ml of electrolyte-containing fluids or 1000–1500 ml of electrolyte-free fluids. If excess intravasation of fluids is suspected, serum electrolytes must be measured immediately, and furosemide is usually administered parenterally. Management of fluid overload depends on the amount and type but should be initiated promptly.

Uterine perforation can be minimized by using the hysteroscope and sheath as a dilator. One first inserts a diagnostic sheath, followed by an operative sheath, then the resectoscope. This technique eliminates the need for dilators in more than 50% of all procedures and reduces the risk of perforation because of the dilatation under direct vision. If perforation occurs without the laser or electrical generator activated, one may observe it, stop the procedure, and in some cases perform laparoscopy to assess uterine damage. If the laser or electrical generator is being activated at the time of the perforation, ideally one proceeds with a laparotomy to explore for intraabdominal injury to bowel or blood vessels.

Hemorrhage can occur if one goes too deeply into the uterine or cervical wall. If bleeding occurs, a Foley catheter with a 30 cc balloon may be inserted and inflated with 10–20 ml of saline for tamponade. Usually the bleeding stops within several hours.

Fatal air embolism has been reported when coaxial laser fibers were used for endometrial ablation.[25] If these fibers are not used and liquid distention medium is utilized, the probability of this complication appearing is low.

Infection is an unlikely occurrence following any hysteroscopic surgery, including endometrial ablation. If it does occur, it usually responds to appropriate antibiotics and the patient has no sequelae.

The potential masking of or delay in the diagnosis of endometrial carcinoma is unknown at this time, although there are two such cases in the literature.[26] Endometrial ablation was performed with a prior diagnosis of hyperplasia. In one case the patient discontinued her prescribed progestin, and when she presented with recurrent bleeding she was immediately evaluated and the cancer identified.

Premenstrual Syndrome

Several studies[28,29] have demonstrated alleviation of premenstrual tension syndrome (PMS) following endometrial ablation, but additional studies by other authors are needed to confirm these findings.

Partial Resection

Partial resection of the endometrium has been performed,[8] but the results are not as consistent as after complete ablation. Therefore the technique cannot be recommended at this time.

Author's Technique

Preoperatively, hysteroscopic evaluation assesses the presence of any submucous leiomyomas or polyps and enables the gynecologist to rule out hyperplasia or other endometrial abnormality. In addition, transvaginal ultrasonography may be performed.

Most of my patients are scheduled for endometrial ablation without medical preparation, and the procedure is completed at any point during the cycle. Vigorous suction curettage with a 7 mm suction Milex curette for 2–3 minutes is performed just prior to endometrial ablation. Medical preparation including either two injections of leuprolide acetate depot 3.75 mg IM 4 weeks apart with the surgical procedure being performed 2–4 weeks after the second injection or one dose of 7.5 leuprolide acetate depot and the procedure performed 4 weeks later. In general, medical preparations are reserved for patients with an enlarged globular uterus or one proved to have adenomyosis on biopsy. In addition, medical preparation is used in patients with anemia to allow return of hemoglobin to the normal range or if the ablation is to be scheduled more than 1 month after the diagnostic procedure.

Patients receive ampicillin 1 g, cefonicid 1 g, or doxycycline 100 mg parenterally (intravenously) prior to the procedure. A paracervical block with 0.25% bupivacaine and 2 U vasopressin per 10 cc of anesthetic is administered at the onset of the procedure (usually 21 cc total). This paracervical block is given whether the surgery is performed under local (with sedation) or general anesthesia, as the consensus is that it allows easier cervical dilatation and decreases bleeding and fluid absorption. A Foley catheter is inserted in the bladder, and a percutaneous procedure drape (Lingemann Medical Products, Indianapolis, IN) is applied to the perineum. A plastic drape is put under the buttocks and an AquaVac mat (Arthroplastics, Chagrin Falls, OH) on the floor. A CDIS (Zimmer) pump with 3% sorbitol is set up, and under video guidance the 5 mm diagnostic sheath and 4 mm telescope are inserted into the uterine cavity for initial assessment. The diagnostic sheath is removed, and an operative sheath is inserted to further dilate the cervical canal. Most of the time this step can be accomplished without dilators, and thus the chance of perforation is minimized. Once the uterine cavity is evaluated, suction curettage is carried out if the patient did not undergo preoperative medical preparation. The suction curette has centimeter markings so the depth of the uterus can be measured. At this point, the resectoscope with roller electrode can be inserted without dilators more than 50% of the time. Pratt dilators are used if needed, with care taken not to overdilate the cervix as the visualization is much better if one works with a tight cervical seal.

The power is set at 60 watts coagulating current and 85 watts pure cutting current. The cutting current is used first, as there are fewer bubbles produced, and the entire endometrial cavity is ablated from the fundus to the internal os. The anterior wall is ablated first because it is where most bubbles collect and is the easiest to judge the tissue effect of the electrode. If it appears that adequate thermal destruction is achieved, the endometrium is then ablated from the middle of the anterior wall with each overlapping stroke lateral until the cornua are ablated. All strokes are from fundus to internal os in the long axis of the uterus. Once the anterior wall is completed, the lateral walls are then ablated and finally the posterior wall. Two or more passes of the roller electrode are made until the cavity appears ablated; then a final pass is made with the coagulating current. At this point the procedure is terminated, and the patient is taken to the recovery room if she had general anesthesia or to the outpatient area if she had local anesthesia.

If a submucous leiomyoma is present, the endometrial ablation is completed first as fluid absorption is much less likely with ablation than with myomectomy. The myomectomy is then performed with a wire loop electrode at a current setting of 85–90 watts. Once the myomectomy is completed, the rest of the ablation is carried out as noted above.

Most patients are discharged within 1–2 hours with a nonsteroidal analgesic being prescribed as the only analgesic required. Unless the patient has a medical condition that warrants specific coverage, no further antibiotics are administered. The patient is instructed to return in 4 weeks at which time the uterus is sounded to break up synechiae and minimize the occurrence of hematometra.

Of 228 patients who underwent endometrial ablation between May 1986 and December 1993, only 14 (6%) have had to undergo hysterectomy. A total of 114 (50%) of the 228 were amenorrheic, 60 (26%) had spotting, and 40 (18%) had light to normal flow. Twenty patients (9%) elected to undergo repeat ablation and 18 were able to avoid hysterectomy. Of the 20 with repeat ablation, 13 (65%) were amenorrheic, 3 (15%) had spotting, and 2 (10%) had light to normal flow. Two of these women (10%) underwent subsequent hysterectomy.

Those patients undergoing repeat ablation fall into five categories: improved but still heavy or prolonged flow; initial procedure not completed because of leiomyomas; physical or mental disability (amenorrhea desired); amenorrhea probably desired by patient despite achieving normal flow; and unimproved.[24] Ideally, repeat ablations are done with the Nd:YAG laser because it is easier to insert into the contracted postablation cavity. The uterus is evaluated by transvaginal ultrasonography to note the overall length and myometrial thickness. Ablation is carried out at 50 watts with nontouch technique. Repeat ablation has resulted in 65%

amenorrhea and 90% success (unpublished data). No preoperative suppression is required, as suction curettage is adequate for preparing the cavity. Postoperative care is the same as for initial ablation. To date, a third ablation has not been performed on any patient, and only two hysterectomies have been needed (unpublished data).

Conclusion

A quote from Goldrath et al.[3] is appropriate: "We have demonstrated an effective alternative to hysterectomy for the control of excessive uterine bleeding in patients where other modalities of treatment have failed, are contraindicated, or are otherwise undesirable." If one follows those recommendations and has the appropriate skill level, one can expect more than 90% successful responses. For those patients in whom initial ablation is less than satisfactory, the procedure can often be repeated, with an expected success rate with regard to menstrual flow of more than 90%.

References

1. EASTERDAY CL, GRIMES DA, RIGGS JA: Hysterectomy in the United States. Obstet Gynecol 1983; 62:203.
2. VALLE RF: Endometrial ablation for dysfunctional uterine bleeding: role of GnRH agonists. Int J Gynecol Obstet 1993;41:3.
3. GOLDRATH MH, FULLER TA, SEGAL S: Laser photovaporization of endometrium for the treatment of menorrhagia. Am J Obstet Gynecol 1981; 140:14.
4. DECHERNEY A, POLAN ML: Hysteroscopic management of intrauterine lesions and intractable uterine bleeding. Obstet Gynecol 1983;61:392.
5. LIN BL, MIYAMOTO N, TOMOMATU M, ET AL: The development of a new hysteroscopic resectoscope and its clinical applications on transcervical resection and endometrial ablation. Jpn J Gynecol Obstet Endosc 1988;4:56.
6. HALLEZ JP, NETTER A, CARTIER R: Methodical intrauterine resection. Am J Obstet Gynecol 1987; 156:1080.
7. COOPERMAN AB, DECHERNEY AH, OLIVE DL: A case of endometrial cancer following endometrial ablation for dysfunctional uterine bleeding. Obstet Gynecol 1993;82:640.
8. MAGOS AL, BAUMANN R, LOCKWOOD GM, TURNBULL AC: Experience with the first 250 endometrial resections for menorrhagia. Lancet 1991; 337:1074.
9. GARRY R, ERIAN J, GROCHMAL SA: A multi-center collaborative study into the treatment of menorrhagia by Nd:YAG laser ablation of the endometrium. Br J Obstet Gynaecol 1991;98:357.
10. SERDEN SP, BROOKS PG: Treatment of abnormal uterine bleeding with the gynecologic resectoscope. J Reprod Med 1991;36:697.
11. BROOKS PG, SERDEN SP: Endometrial ablation in women with abnormal uterine bleeding aged fifty and over. J Reprod Med 1992;37:682.
12. LOMANO J: Endometrial ablation for the treatment of menorrhagia: a comparison of patients with normal, enlarged and fibroid uteri. Lasers Surg Med 1991;11:8.
13. INDMAN PD: Hysteroscopic treatment of menorrhagia associated with uterine leiomyomas. Obstet Gynecol 1993;81:716.
14. LAM AM, AL-JUMAILY RY, HOLT EM: Ruptured ectopic pregnancy in an amenorrheic woman after transcervical resection of the endometrium. Aust NZ J Obstet Gynaecol 1992;1:81.
15. GIMPELSON RJ, KAIGH J: Mechanical preparation of the endometrium prior to endometrial ablation. J Reprod Med 1992;37:691.
16. WORTMAN M, DAGGETT A: Hysteroscopic endomyometrial resection: a new technique for the treatment of menorrhagia. Obstet Gynecol 1994; 83:295.
17. SERDEN SP, BROOKS PG: Preoperative therapy in preparation for endometrial ablation. J Reprod Med 92;37:679.
18. BENT AE, OSTERGARD DR: Endometrial ablation with the neodymium:YAG laser. Obstet Gynecol 1990;75:923.
19. TOWNSEND DE, RICHART RM, PASKOWITZ RA, WOOLFORK RE: "Rollerball" coagulation of the endometrium. Obstet Gynecol 1990;76:310.
20. LOFFER FD: Hysteroscopic endometrial ablation with the Nd:YAG laser using a non-touch technique. Obstet Gynecol 1987;69:679.
21. VANCAILLIE TG: Electrocoagulation of the endometrium with the ball-end resectoscope. Obstet Gynecol 1989;74:425.
22. GOLDRATH MH: Use of danazol in hysteroscopic surgery for menorrhagia. J Reprod Med 1990; 35:91.
23. GOLDFARB HA: A review of 35 endometrial ablations using the Nd:YAG laser for recurrent

menometrorrhagia. Obstet Gynecol 1990;76: 833.
24. GIMPELSON RJ, KAIGH J: Endometrial ablation repeat procedures: case studies. J Reprod Med 1992;37:629.
25. BAGGISH MS, DANIELL JF: Catastrophic injury secondary to the use of coaxial gas-cooled fibers and artificial sapphire tips for intrauterine surgery: a report of five cases. Lasers Surg Med 1989;9:581.
26. DWYER N, HUTTON J, STIRRAT GM: Randomized controlled trial comparing endometrial resection with abdominal hysterectomy for the surgical treatment of menorrhagia. Br J Obstet Gynaecol 1993;100:237.
27. COOPERMAN AB, DECHERNEY AH, OLIVE DL: A case of endometrial cancer following endometrial ablation for dysfunctional uterine bleeding. Obstet Gynecol 1993;82:640.
28. LEFLER HT, LEFLER CF: Endometrial ablation: improvement in PMS related to the decrease in bleeding. J Reprod Med 1992;37:596.
29. FRASER IS, ANGSUWATHANA S, MAHMOUD F, YEZERSKI S: Short and medium term outcomes after rollerball endometrial ablation for menorrhagia. Med J Aust 1993;158:454.

Section V
Supportive Techniques and Procedures

24
Anesthesia

Linda F. Lucas and Benjamin M. Rigor

Advanced operative laparoscopy has become a commonly accepted procedure. General, regional, and local anesthesia have all been used widely and safely for laparoscopy in hospitals and medical centers throughout the world. Advancements in anesthetic and surgical techniques have decreased complications and recovery time while increasing patient acceptance of endoscopic procedures on an outpatient basis. The choice of anesthetic technique varies with the requirements of the surgeon, the health status and preference of the patient, the type of facility, and the availability of well trained professionals, support personnel, and equipment. Such choices can be made intelligently only when the physiologic changes that accompany the procedure are known and the surgeon and anesthesiologist are familiar with them.

Physiologic Changes During Laparoscopy

The complications of laparoscopy are relatively low[1,2] (Table 24.1). Increased understanding of the physiologic changes that occur during anesthesia for endoscopy can further decrease the incidence of complications. Trendelenburg position and pneumoperitoneum have been shown to alter respiratory and circulatory mechanics.

Effects of Positioning

The patient, as noted in Chapters 2 and 3, is placed in the Trendelenburg position (15°–20°) so the abdominal viscera are moved cephalad. The steep Trendelenburg position in combination with the lithotomy position is known to impair ventilation and pulmonary mechanics.[3-5] In healthy, conscious patients placed in this position, vital capacity and functional residual capacity are decreased by 18.0% and 14.5%, respectively, as a result of compromised diaphragmatic excursion and increased pulmonary blood volume.[6] Under general anesthesia, the lithotomy position alone causes a 3% decrease in tidal volume; when combined with a 20° Trendelenburg position, there is a 15% decrease in tidal volume.[7,8] Pulmonary compliance is also altered,[9] especially in the obese patient.[10] This fact, in combination with alterations in the distribution of inspired air within the lungs[11] and a diminished functional residual capacity, predisposes the patient to postoperative pulmonary atelectasis and pneumonia. Other investigators have measured a reduction in functional residual capacity without consistent alterations in tidal volume, respiratory rate, minute volume, or oxygen consumption in conscious patients[11] and young, healthy women undergoing short, minor gynecologic procedures under light general anesthesia.[12] This maintenance of homeo-

Table 24.1. Complications of gynecologic endoscopy

Surgical complications affecting anesthetic management
Major vessel injury/hemorrhage
Bowel injury
Perforation of the uterine fundus
Abdominal wall hematoma
Anesthetic complications
Cardiac arrythmias
Hypotension
Hypertension
Hypoxia
Hypercarbia
Acid-base disturbance
Pneumothorax/pneumomediastinum (barotrauma)
Pulmonary aspiration
Gas embolism
Gastric dilation/perforation
Prolonged artificial ventilation/apnea

static respiratory function may be compromised under deeper general anesthesia, especially with longer procedures.[13]

In most cases the respiratory alterations produced by lithotomy and combined lithotomy and Trendelenburg positions in the patient undergoing general anesthesia can be corrected with the use of a modified lithotomy position, a cuffed endotracheal tube, and assisted or controlled ventilation. Reduced respiratory volumes can then be restored to normal and compressed basal lung areas ventilated to counteract the deleterious effects of positioning.

Effects of Pneumoperitoneum

Air, carbon dioxide, and nitrous oxide with intraabdominal pressures of 12–16 mm Hg are used to facilitate laparoscopy. Carbon dioxide is preferred because it decreases the incidence of gas embolism. It has been shown that carbon dioxide used in experimental animals is at least five times safer than oxygen.[14] The toxicity of the gas appears to correlate inversely with its solubility in blood. Carbon dioxide is the most soluble; nitrous oxide is only 68% as soluble as carbon dioxide in blood.[15] Although carbon dioxide appears to be more effective than nitrous oxide or air for reducing the incidence of gas embolism, it has been reported to cause increased intraoperative discomfort in awake patients undergoing procedures with local anesthesia.[16] This discomfort probably results from the combination of carbon dioxide with peritoneal fluid, forming carbonic acid, which irritates the diaphragm and peritoneal lining.[17]

In early studies, following insufflation of carbon dioxide, patients who were breathing spontaneously and had been anesthetized with halothane and a nitrous oxide/oxygen mixture demonstrated a significant increase in expired carbon dioxide concentrations and an increase in respiratory rate by as much as 75–100%.[16] Minute ventilation was increased despite reduced tidal volumes.[16,18,19] The findings were consistent with the depressant effects of inhalational anesthetics on respiratory drive, the depressant effects of premedicants, and further depression produced by increased intraabdominal pressure due to carbon dioxide insufflation.

A tendency toward respiratory and metabolic acidosis was demonstrated by a significant decrease in arterial pH.[11,14,20,21] Decreases in arterial oxygen tension were reported, with values occasionally as low as 46–64 mm Hg when the inspired oxygen concentration was less than 40%.[22] Another study demonstrated no evidence of hypoxia when ventilation was controlled with a gas mixture containing at least 30% oxygen. When nitrous oxide was used as the insufflating medium, no increases were noted in arterial carbon dioxide tension, and pH values were unchanged, suggesting that intraperitoneal insufflation of carbon dioxide contributed to the acidosis. Absorption of peritoneal carbon dioxide added approximately 8 mm Hg to the arterial carbon dioxide tension when compared with controls using nitrous oxide intraperitoneally.[23] No significant difference was identified between the two groups—one using carbon dioxide and the other nitrous oxide—in terms of base deficit or oxygen tension values.

Absorption of peritoneal nitrous oxide may contribute to postoperative diffusion of this gas into the alveolar space resulting in hypoxia.[24] This diffusion hypoxia, however, may be avoided with the postoperative administration of supplemental oxygen during recovery, which is recommended for all patients. Rare complications of nitrous oxide administration include entry of the gas into hollow viscera, such as emphysematous bullae of the lungs, resulting in spontaneous pneumothorax and, on one occasion, diffusion into an ovarian cyst.[25]

Spontaneous Versus Controlled Ventilation

Hypercarbia occurs in spontaneously ventilating patients undergoing laparoscopy with carbon dioxide insufflation and may contribute to acidosis and cardiac arrhythmias.[18,23,26] Even in intubated patients with controlled ventilation, airway peak and plateau pressure increased by about 75%, and end-tidal carbon dioxide levels rose by 2–19 mm Hg (mean 9 mm Hg) over preinsufflation levels with carbon dioxide insufflation. These increases correlated with the rate and overall volume of carbon dioxide insufflation.[27] Increases in carbon dioxide tension may be avoided by using mild to moderate hyperventilation with assisted or controlled ventilation to an initial end-tidal CO_2 of 4 kPa.[28] Moderate hyperventilation sufficient to eliminate excess carbon dioxide in an adequately relaxed patient has been suggested as a means of maintaining respiratory and acid-base homeostasis[22,24,29] as well as avoiding cardiovascular instability attributed to changes in arterial chemistry.[18] Ventilatory techniques used during gynecologic endoscopy should have little effect, however, on the hypercarbia that occurs after initial release of the pneumoperitoneum.[19]

Respiratory Changes Under Local Anesthesia

Minor laparoscopic procedures under local anesthesia with an awake, spontaneously ventilating patient are commonly performed safely with experienced personnel. With the patient in the Trendelenburg position, a slight increase in minute ventilation is caused by an increase in respiratory frequency. The tidal volume remains essentially unchanged. During pneumoperitoneum a large increase in minute ventilation results from an increase in respiratory rate with a small decrease in vital capacity. Vital capacity, however, remains sufficient for patients to increase tidal volume, if necessary.[19] Arterial carbon dioxide tension, pH, and base excess are not changed significantly during the procedure. Mean arterial carbon dioxide tensions and pH in the awake patient are consistent with an acute hyperventilatory state and respiratory alkalosis. Mechanical compression of the lung by diaphragmatic elevation due to Trendelenburg position and pneumoperitoneum may alter pulmonary stretch receptors, causing the increased workload and increased respiratory rate.[29] Pain and anxiety also may contribute to the altered pattern of breathing and arterial blood gas values.

Respiratory depression may occur when the awake patient is premedicated with intravenous diazepam or narcotics.[1] A general decrease in arterial carbon dioxide tension with no significant change in pH or arterial carbon dioxide tension,[29] or mild respiratory acidosis consistent with an elevated arterial carbon dioxide tension, is seen when compared with values prior to sedation.[17]

Cardiac Arrhythmias

Cardiac arrhythmias are a frequent complication of laparoscopy. Bradyarrhythmias, including asystole, may be life-threatening and have been observed in as many as 47% of women undergoing laparoscopy. Thirty percent of all arrhythmias were bradyarrhythmias, nearly all of which occurred during carbon dioxide insufflation with traction on pelvic structures.[30] Episodes of sinus tachycardia, ventricular arrhythmias, and asystole unrelated to previous bradycardia are also frequent occurrences.[18,19,26] Although electrocardiographic changes occur most commonly during pneumoperitoneum with rising carbon dioxide tension[28] and during the preinsufflation period,[2] carbon dioxide tensions have been observed to be highest after completion of the surgical procedure following release of the pneumoperitoneum in spontaneously breathing patients.[19]

Other causes of arrhythmias include hypoxia and vasovagal reflexes due to peritoneal stimulation and distention, light anesthesia, or tracheal stimulation from the presence of an endotracheal tube. Vasovagal reflex stimulation resulting in hypotension and bradycardia occurs in 3.4–14.0% of awake, sedated patients undergoing laparoscopic sterilization under local anesthesia.[22]

Patients with paracervical block in addition to local infiltration rarely develop bradycardia. Vagal stimulation arising from uterine motion and tubal compression is presumably abolished by the paracervical block. Atropine may be given prophylactically to block vasovagal reflexes, but it appears to have no advantage over prompt symptomatic administration. Vasopressors may also be indicated in the awake patient who experiences nausea in association with hypotension resulting from vasovagal stimulation. Antiemetics are seldom indicated, as this complication promptly responds to cessation of the stimulation.

Hemodynamic Alterations

Other changes in hemodynamic and cardiovascular parameters have been observed. Although pulse rate and systolic pressure remain steady in the supine patient during spontaneous ventilation with halothane,[19] significant increases in mean arterial pressure, pulse rate, and central venous pressure have been reported in association with the Trendelenburg position.[20] With pneumoperitoneum, hypotension has also been reported as a result of cardiac arrhythmias and excessive intraabdominal distention. Compression of the inferior vena cava impedes venous return especially in patients who are already hypovolemic, such as during the immediate postpartum period. Decreases in systolic pressure, pulse pressure, central venous pressure, and cardiac output may result from intraabdominal pressures above 20 cm H_2O.[21]

Trendelenburg position, however, favors venous return and improved cardiac output, which may counteract some of the deleterious effects of pneumoperitoneum. Cardiovascular changes associated with Trendelenburg position and pneumoperitoneum are affected by the degree of head-down tilt, intravascular volume status, mode of ventilation, anesthetic drugs, and the patient's age and concomitant cardiac disease. It has been demonstrated that healthy, normovolemic subjects placed in 15° Trendelenburg position have minimal (1.8%) central displacement of blood volume, causing insignificant hemodynamic changes.[31] Pricolo et al. also found small (10%) but insignificant increases in cardiac index, without elevation of central venous pressure, pulmonary capillary wedge pressure, heart rate, or systemic vascular resistance in healthy, normotensive patients in a 15° head-down position.[32] Normotensive patients with coronary artery disease, however, had significant decreases in cardiac index with concomitant rises in central venous pressure and pulmonary capillary wedge pressure with Trendelenburg positioning.[32]

High intraperitoneal pressure may elevate the intrathoracic pressure, causing decreased chest wall compliance, increased peak airway pressures, and increased intrapulmonary vascular resistance. For these reasons, laparoscopy may be contraindicated in the patient with severe cardiorespiratory disease, such as ischemic heart disease, mitral valve insufficiency, or other congenital or acquired cardiac conditions with pulmonary hypertension and low or fixed cardiac output.

Gas embolization should be suspected in a patient with sudden, profound hypotension or cardiovascular collapse. It may result from intravascular administration of air through the Verres needle or direct injection of air that is absorbed by the uterine venous sinuses.[33] Although carbon dioxide has been substituted for air for the pneumoperitoneum to decrease the danger of air embolism, circulatory collapse has been reported in women undergoing laparoscopy, probably caused by massive carbon dioxide embolism.[34] Auscultation of precordial "mill wheel" murmur, elevation of central venous pressure, detection of air bubbles by ultrasonography, and decreased end-tidal carbon di-

Plate 30. Cholangiogram catheter passed through percutaneously placed angiocath. (Courtesy of Ethicon Endo-Surgery, Cincinnati, OH)

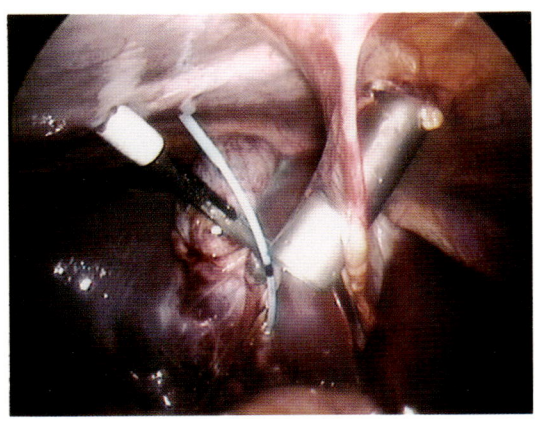

Plate 31. Sutures placed in stomach to secure 360° wrap (From Lobe TE, Schropp KP, Lunsford K. Laparoscopic Nissen fundoplication in childhood. J Pediatric Surg 1993;28:358, 1993, with permission)

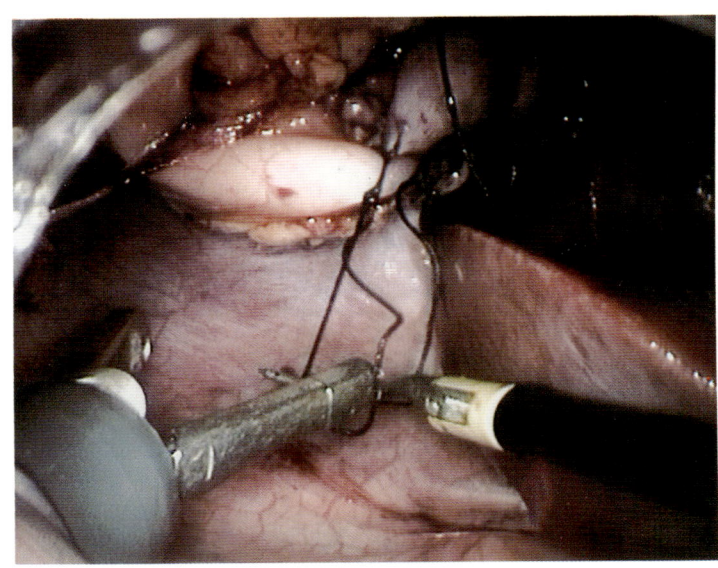

Plate 32. Endoloop ligature around ovarian vessels.

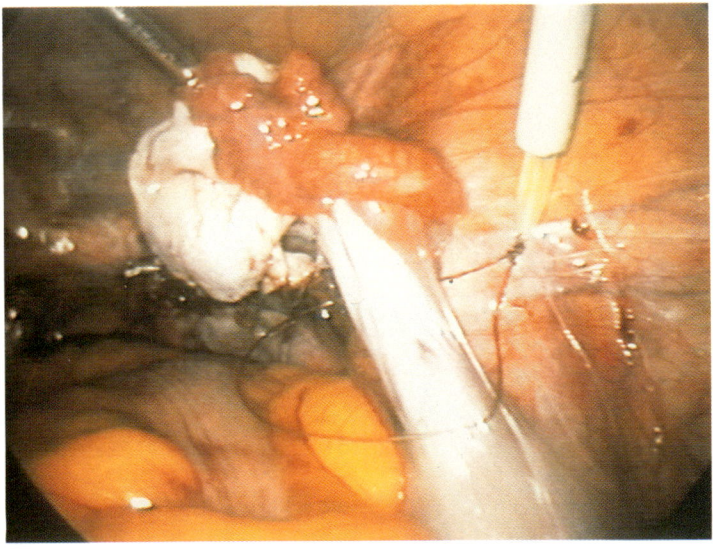

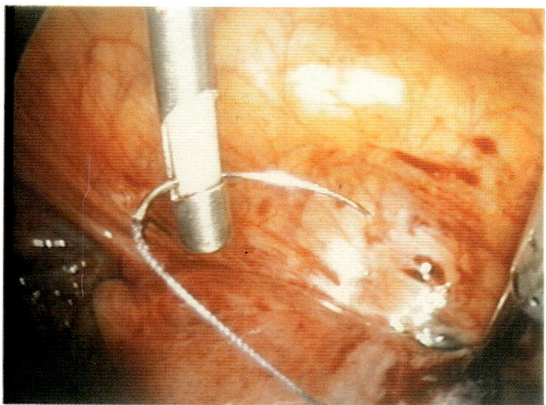

Plate 33. Curved needle driver.

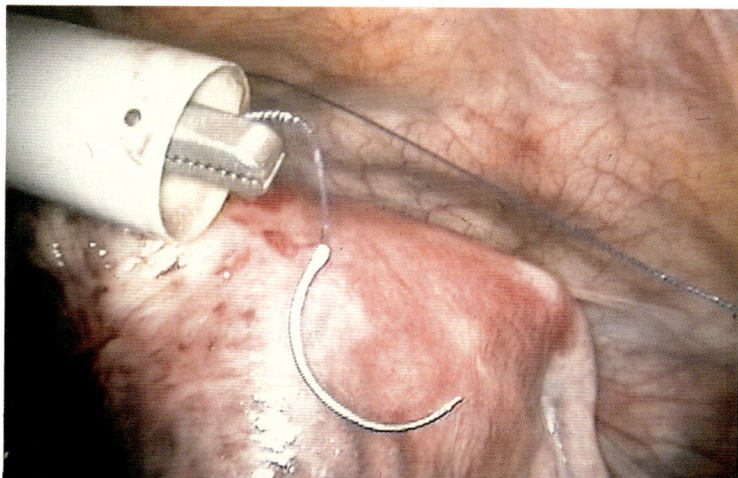

Plate 34. Suture needle removed from abdominal cavity through trocar.

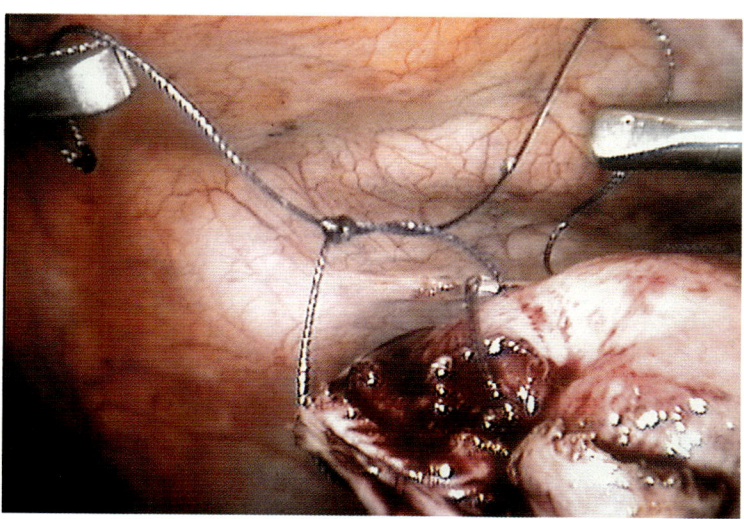

Plate 35. Intracorporeal square double knot.

Plate 36. PDS clip applier.

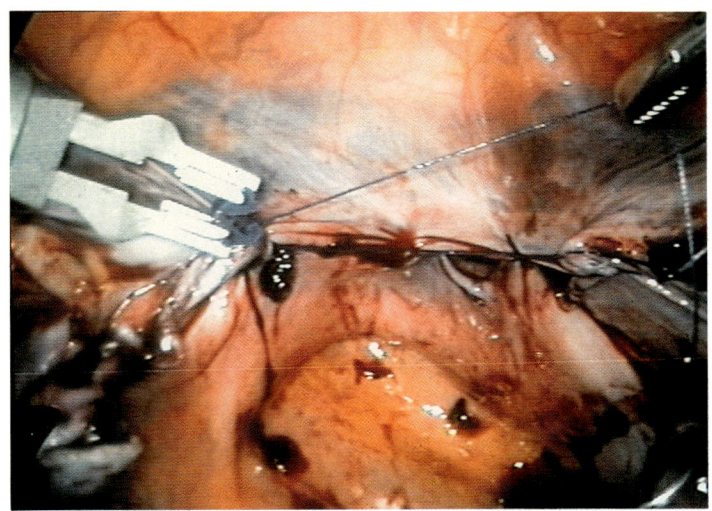

Plate 37. Large leiomyoma removed from uterus.

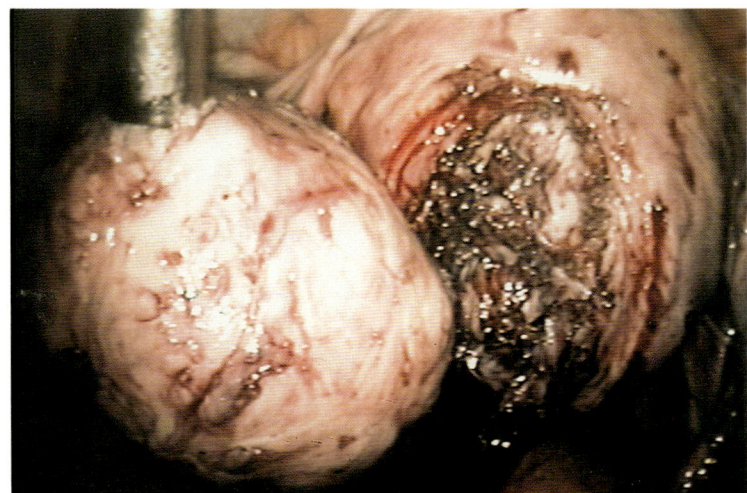

Plate 38. Uterus reconstructed with a continuous "laparo-tye" endosuture.

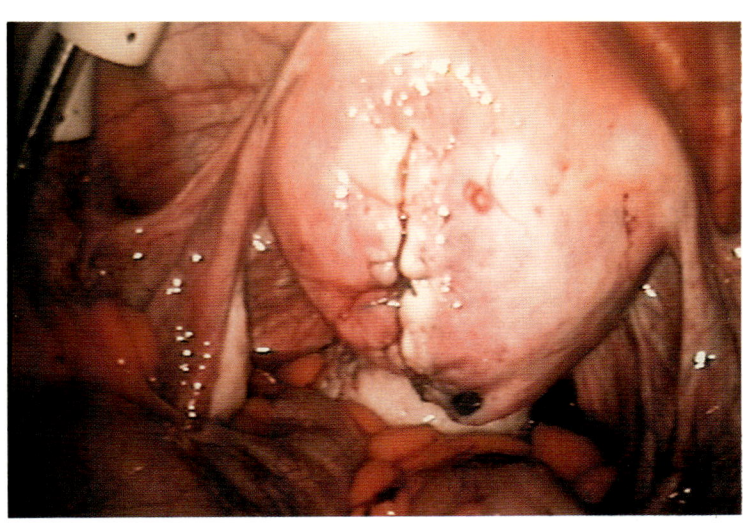

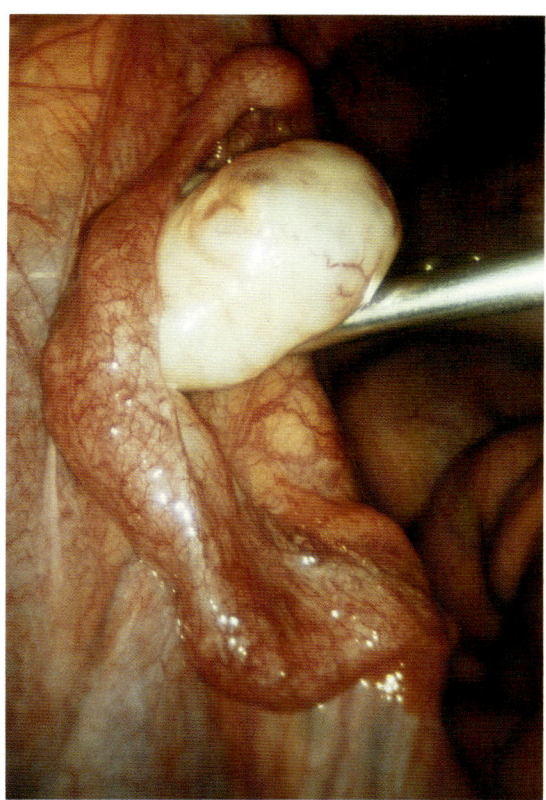

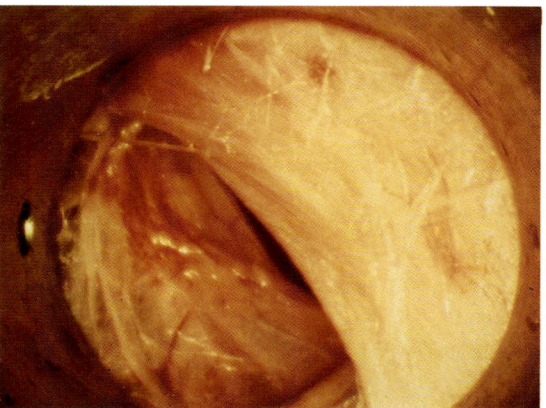

Plate 40. Hernioscopic view into direct inguinal hernia.

Plate 39. Laparoscopic view of Mayer-von Rokitansky-Kuster-Hauser syndrome visualizing the uterine bud and normal tube and ovary.

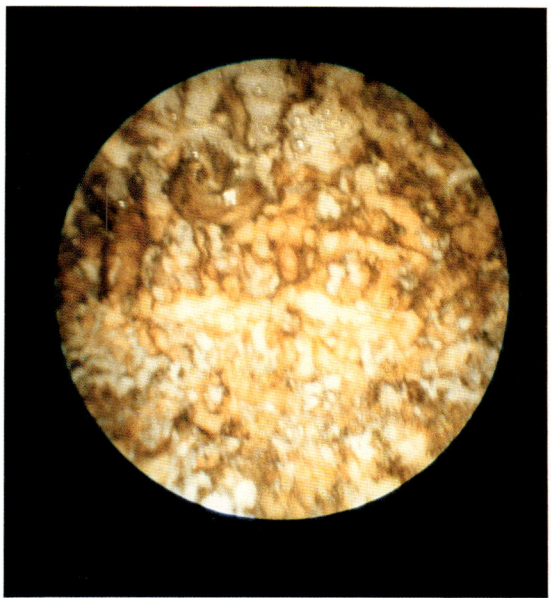

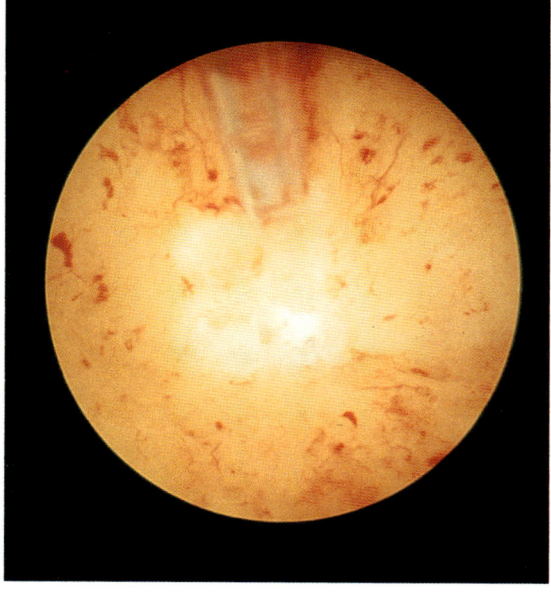

Plate 41. Dragging technique (Nd:YAG laser).

Plate 42. Blanching technique (Nd:YAG laser).

Plate 43. Roller ablation.

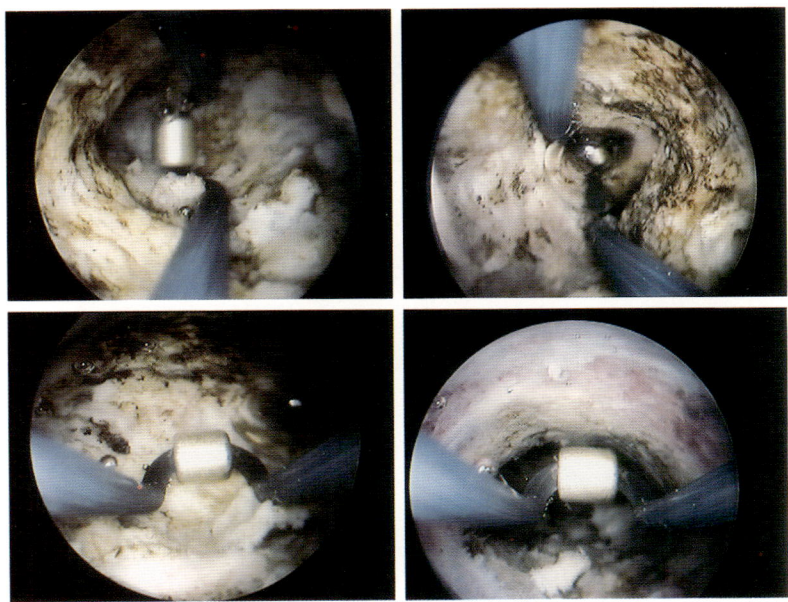

Plate 44. Endometrial resection.

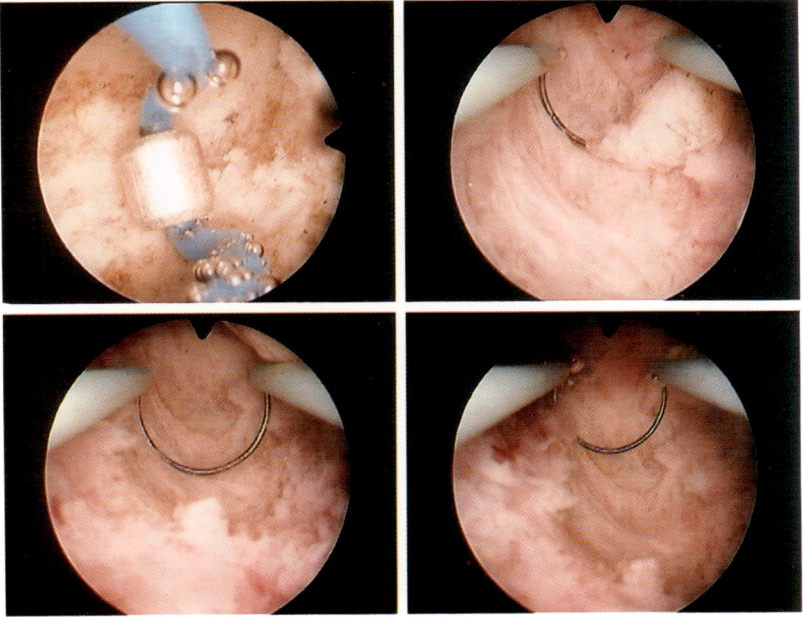

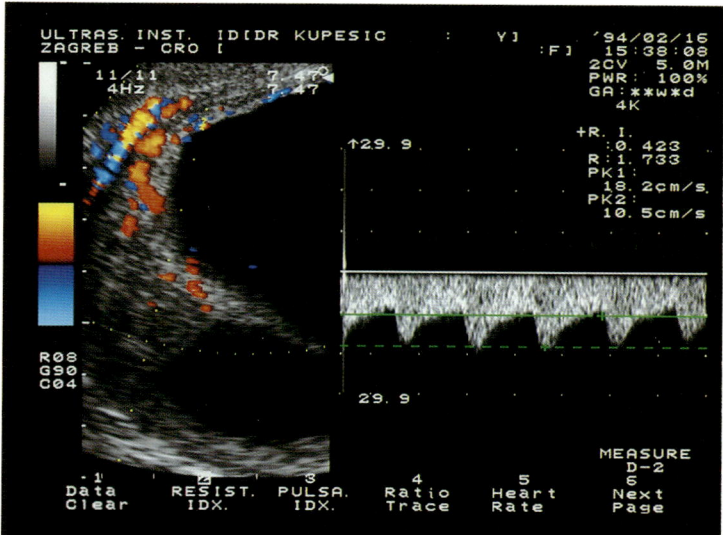

Plate 45. Transvaginal color Doppler scan of a bilocular (malignant) cystic structure. (Courtesy of Dr. Asim Kurjak, Ultrasound Institute, Zagreb, Croatia)

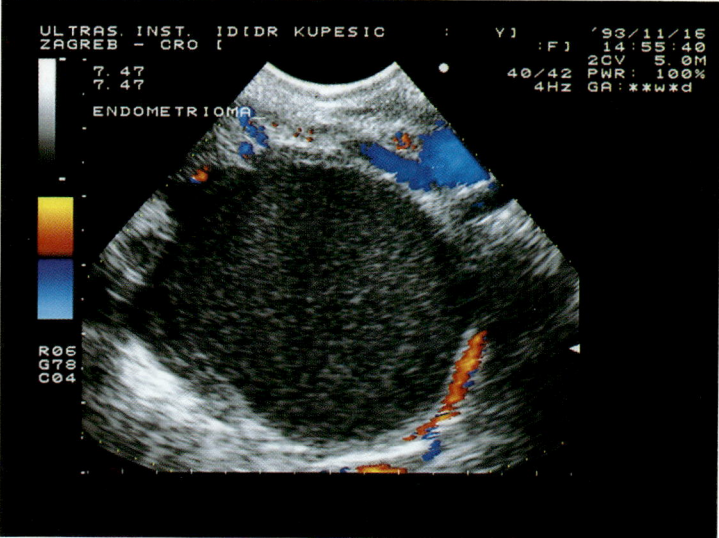

Plate 46. Transvaginal color Doppler scan of a (benign) cystic structure. (Courtesy of Dr. Asim Kurjak, Ultrasound Institute, Zagreb, Croatia)

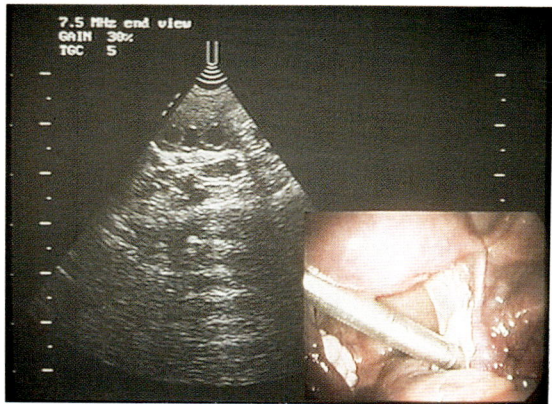

Plate 47. Submucosal uterine fibroid detected by laparoscopic probe.

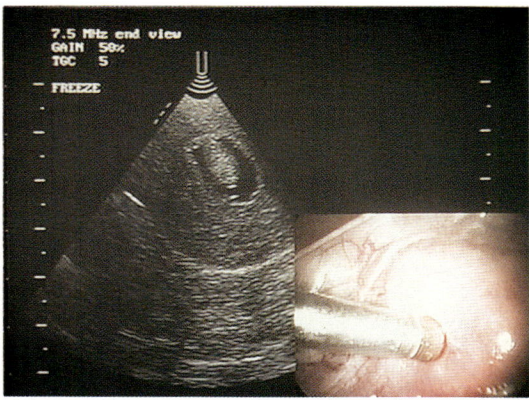

Plate 48. Polycystic ovary shown by laparoscopic ultrasound probe.

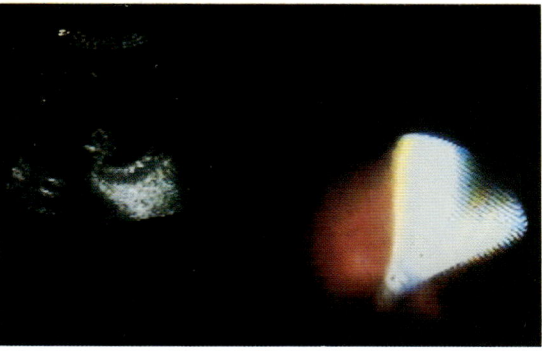

Plate 49. Simultaneous display of sonographic and endoscopic image in a single monitor using a video mixer. Coordination of the operating instruments is greatly facilitated.

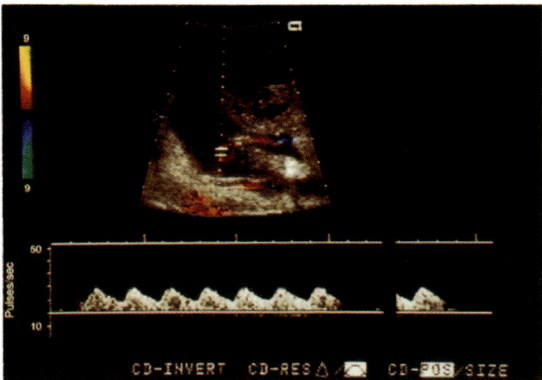

Plate 50. Color and pulsed Doppler demonstration of reverse arterial perfusion in a case of acardiac twin.

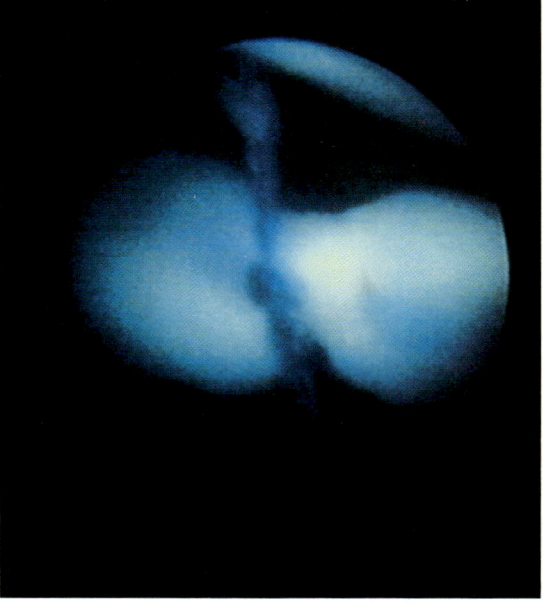

Plate 51. Endoscopic view of the knot placed on the umbilical cord of an acardiac twin. (From Quintero RA, Reich H, Puder KS, et al., N Engl J Med 1994;330:469. Reprinted with permission.)

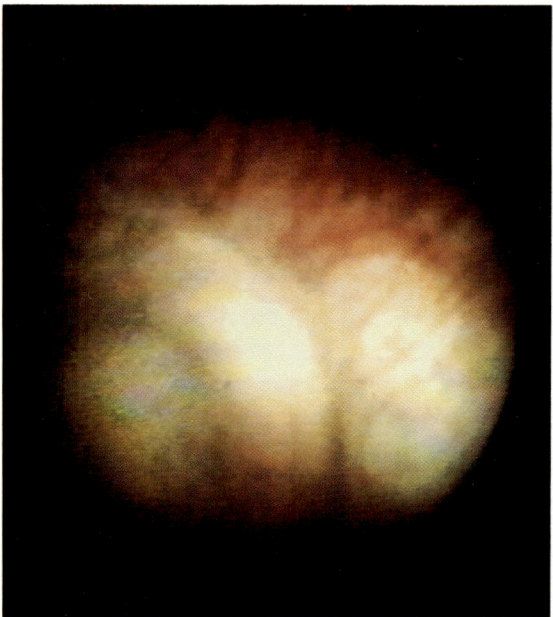

Plate 52. Endoscopic visualization of a dilated posterior urethra in a fetus with posterior urethral valves.

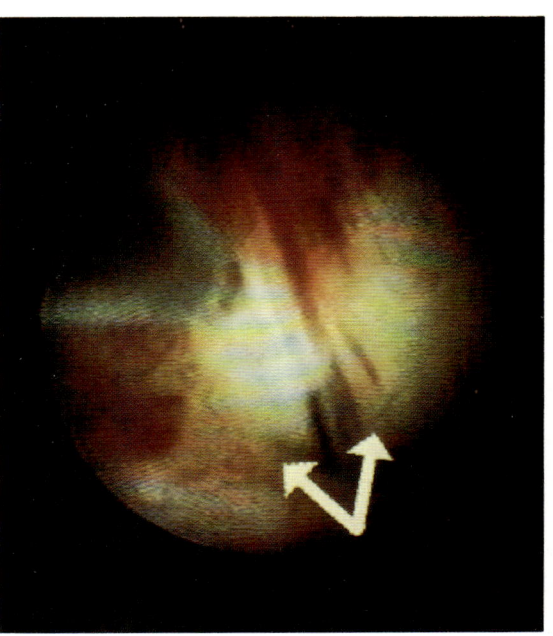

Plate 53. In utero endoscopic ablation of posterior urethral valves. Leaflets of the valves are identified (arrow). (From Quintero RA, Hume R, Smith C, et al., Am J Obstet Gynecol 1995;172:206. Reprinted with permission.)

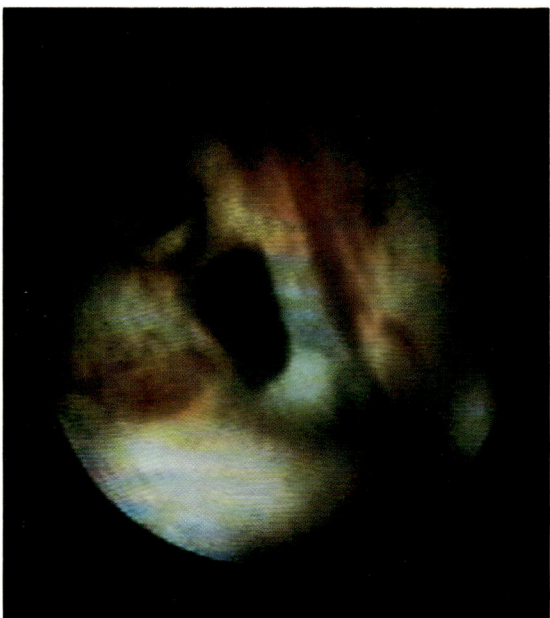

Plate 54. Electrode has been fired against the valve, and a small opening has been created. (From Quintero RA, Hume R, Smith C, et al., Am J Obstet Gynecol 1995;172:206. Reprinted with permission.)

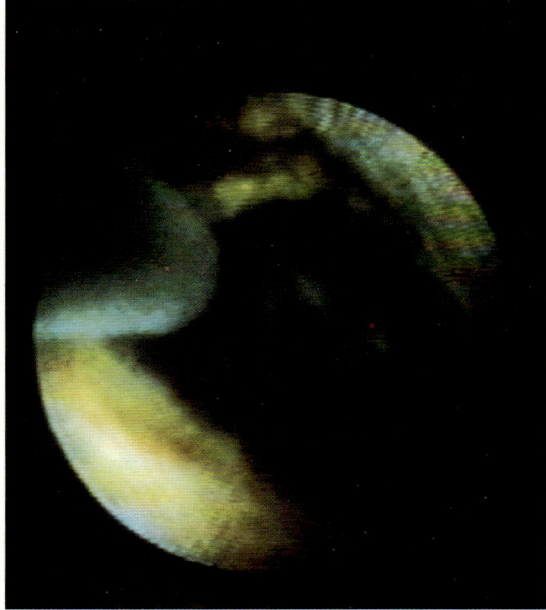

Plate 55. Completion of the ablation of the valves is accomplished with gentle rotation of the endoscope. Urethral permeability has been established. (From Quintero RA, Hume R, Smith C, et al., Am J Obstet Gynecol 1995;172:206. Reprinted with permission.)

Table 24.2. Gas embolism

Diagnosis
    Circulatory collapse
    Precordial "mill wheel" murmur
    Elevation of central venous pressure
    End-tidal CO_2 decreased
    Air bubbles detected with ultrasonography

Management
    Place patient in left lateral decubitus position
    Aspirate gas from right atrium (central venous catheter)
    Discontinue N_2O
    Administer 100% O_2

---

oxide as measured by capnography confirm the diagnosis in suspected cases. If embolization occurs, the patient must be turned to the left lateral decubitus position to reduce right ventricular outflow obstruction until the gas is absorbed or aspirated from the right atrium through a central venous catheter. Nitrous oxide should be discontinued, and administration of 100% oxygen is mandatory (Table 24.2).

Hypoxia may be associated with hypotension in cases of low inspired oxygen tension and spontaneous ventilation with inhalational agents or intravenous anesthesia, nitrous oxide, and oxygen. An oxygen concentration > 35% and continuous oximetry should be used at all times. Young women may develop hypoglycemia, which intensifies the hypotensive response to moderate hypoxia. Patients should therefore be scheduled for surgery early in the morning if possible. If surgery is to be performed in the afternoon, a small amount of clear liquid may be consumed up to 6 hours prior to surgery.

Selection of Anesthetic Technique

The anesthetic technique for a given surgical procedure should be as safe as possible, be the least likely to cause physiologic disturbance, and involve the shortest possible recovery time. As stated previously, the choice of technique is determined by the personal preferences of the anesthesiologist and surgeon, condition of the patient, extent of surgery, available facilities, and presence of support services and personnel. Until the early 1970s in the United States, most surgical procedures in obstetrics and gynecology were performed under general, spinal, or epidural anesthesia in hospital operating and delivery rooms. With concern for safety and economy, gynecologists are now performing an increasing number and variety of procedures in outpatient or ambulatory facilities. Laparoscopy is commonly performed under general, regional, or local anesthesia.

General Anesthesia

Advantages Versus Disadvantages

Most gynecologic endoscopic procedures are still performed under general anesthesia. This type of anesthesia may be performed safely in free-standing and outpatient surgical units, as well as in traditional inpatient facilities. Advantages include complete analgesia, amnesia, a quiet surgical field, and excellent muscle relaxation. Ventilation may be assisted or controlled to prevent atelectasis and hypercarbia, especially in obese individuals. The patient's airway can also be protected against vomiting and aspiration with a cuffed endotracheal tube.

The anxious patient may prefer to be unconscious, and some surgeons consider an asleep patient ideal for laparoscopic and pelviscopic procedures. General anesthesia is suitable for the novice as well as the experienced endoscopist and is preferable for the initial training of residents until smooth, gentle control of equipment and viscera can be accomplished.

Disadvantages of general anesthesia include prolonged recovery and an increased incidence of major and minor sequelae. Gastric dilation may occur with poor mask fit or vigorous ventilation prior to intubation. Pneumothorax or barotrauma may also result from increased airway pressure during controlled ventilation, especially in the emphysematous patient with pulmonary blebs. Perioperative aspiration may occur even in the presence of an endotracheal tube.

Hoarseness, sore throat, and muscle pains are frequent sequelae to intubation. Minor postoperative complaints include prolonged recovery, nausea, vomiting, lethargy, and weakness. These complaints generally resolve within 24–48 hours. Postoperative morbidity is highest in female patients undergoing their first anesthesia, especially if it lasts more than 20 minutes or requires endotracheal intubation.[35]

General anesthesia is more costly than local anesthesia. Specially trained personnel and equipment are required during the procedure and the recovery period.

Patient Selection

Patient selection for general anesthesia most appropriately includes patients suspected of having dense adhesions due to intrapelvic pathology or previous surgery or those requiring extensive endoscopic surgery, especially when a second or third incision is to be made to introduce an additional trocar. Patients with excessive fear of pain or awareness during surgery or patients who cannot relax or cooperate for office examination may require general anesthesia. This group includes patients with a language barrier, mental handicap, severe hearing loss, or physical anomalies that make pelvic relaxation or positioning difficult.[36]

General anesthesia may be the optimal choice for obese patients. There is severe respiratory impedance following insufflation for the pneumoperitoneum, even in the well ventilated, nonobese patient.[23] Such impedance can be expected to be even greater in the obese patient who already has decreased respiratory compliance and increased airway pressure at a given lung inflation volume.[24] Patients with decreased lung volumes, particularly those with decreased vital capacity and functional residual capacity producing a restrictive pulmonary defect, are at increased risk of acute respiratory insufficiency and postoperative atelectasis. Some young obese patients do not tolerate the Trendelenburg position comfortably. Absorption of intraperitoneal carbon dioxide used for insufflation may further compromise the patient suffering from obese hypoventilation syndrome (pickwickian syndrome) or supine hypotension secondary to obesity.[22]

The preference of the surgeon is also an important consideration, although it is understood that pelviscopic surgery and laser laparoscopy often require general anesthesia. General anesthesia, with controlled ventilation, is most often employed for laser laparoscopy because it provides most effectively a motionless operative field for delicate surgical procedures. Spinal anesthesia has been recommended for patients undergoing procedures related to infertility[37] because of concerns that anesthesia may impair fertility. Reports, however, indicate an increased secretion of ovarian hormones, possibly via activation of the hypothalamus-pituitary-ovarian axis in women receiving general anesthesia for laparoscopic procedures.[38]

Although local and regional anesthetic techniques are gaining increased surgeon and patient acceptance,[39,40] some surgeons object to local or regional anesthesia for short laparoscopic cases because their training or inexperience with awake patients makes them more comfortable when the patient is asleep. The surgeon may be unwilling to subject patients to even slight discomfort. To succeed with local anesthesia for laparoscopy, the gynecologist must be able to perform various procedures with gentleness, confidence, and skill. He or she must be sensitive to the physiologic and psychologic needs of the patient. Many physicians wish to avoid the distraction of communicating with the patient during surgery. If laparoscopy is performed in a training institution, it is much easier to demonstrate techniques and procedures when the patient is asleep. The surgeon and anesthesiologist may find local anesthesia cumbersome and may want to avoid the extra minutes spent administering local or regional anesthesia.

Often the previous experience of the surgeon or anesthesiologist plays a role in the decision to use a particular anesthetic technique. Local anesthesia, with monitored anesthesia care, sedation, and analgesia, is often chosen for critically ill patients. Attempts at local techniques in these high-risk patients under less than optimal conditions may result in failure and loss of confidence in local anesthetic techniques. The surgeon and anesthesiologist may then be placed in the difficult and dangerous position of inducing general anesthesia after the procedure has been initiated. Increasingly, laparoscopic procedures under general anesthesia have been advocated for high-risk and elderly patients owing to the low incidence of morbidity and mortality experienced in this patient population.[41] In fact, patients with moderate pulmonary dysfunction undergoing laparoscopic procedures with general anesthesia seem to benefit with improved postoperative pulmonary function when compared with patients undergoing similar open procedures.[42]

Premedication

Realistic goals of premedication are to reduce anxiety, nausea, and vomiting; augment induction; produce reliable sedation, amnesia, and analgesia; and reduce anesthetic requirements. Choice of premedicants is influenced by the anesthetic technique utilized, emotional and physical condition of the patient, and preference of the anesthesia team. Premedicants generally include anxiolytics, narcotics, antihistamines, hypnotic sedatives, antacids, antiemetics, and other pharmacologic agents (Table 24.3).

Almost all patients are anxious preoperatively. There is no substitute for counseling and reassurance by the surgeon, nursing staff, and anesthesiologist concerning expectations for the conduct of the procedure, pain relief, and type of anesthesia. Such counseling should be accomplished in the surgeon's office and in the preoperative preparation area by empathetic, considerate, confident, and experienced staff.

Although barbiturates were once widely utilized as preoperative oral medications, intravenous benzodiazepines have become the mainstay of preoperative anxiolytic therapy. They are generally administered immediately before

Table 24.3. Premedication for adults undergoing gynecologic endoscopy[a]

Drug	Dosage (mg)	Route of administration
Anticholinergics		
Atropine sulfate	0.4–0.8	IM or IV
Scopolamine	0.4–0.6	IM or IV
Glycopyrrolate (Robinul)	0.2–0.4	IM or IV
Gastric antisecretagogues		
Cimetidine (Tagamet)	200–400	PO, IM, or IV
Ranitidine (Zantac)	50–150	PO, IM, or IV
Famotidine	10–20	IV, PO
Antiemetics (antinauseant)		
Droperidol (Inapsine)	0.0625–0.1250	IM or IV
Promethazine (Phenergan)	7.5–25.0	PO, IM, or IV
Metaclopramide (Reglan)	10–20	PO, IM, or IV
Sedatives and anxiolytics		
Diazepam (Valium)	5–20	IV
Hydroxyzine (Vistaril)	25–100	IM
Midazolam (Versed)	2.5–5.0	IV, IM
Analgesics (narcotics-opiates)		
Alphaprodine (Nisentil)	15–45	IM or IV
Fentanyl (Sublimaze)	0.050–0.150	IM or IV
Meperidine (Demerol)	25–100	IM or IV
Morphine sulfate	5–10	IM or IV

[a]Typical 70 kg ASA class I or II patients; geriatric patients require a dose reduction up to one-third of the above-mentioned dosages.

Table 24.4. Side effects of midazolam (Versed)

Water-soluble
Shorter duration
Less vascular irritation
Thrombophlebitis
Somnolence
Apnea

and upon arrival in the operating room. Until recently diazepam (Valium) has been the most popular agent, but it is being replaced by the newer, water-soluble shorter-duration agent midazolam (Versed). Midazolam, like diazepam, is an excellent anxiolytic and amnestic drug. There is less vascular irritation, burning on injection, and thrombophlebitis (Table 24.4), which are commonly reported with diazepam. Postoperatively, however, there may be no difference in speed of recovery of psychomotor function.[43]

An additional advantage for premedication with the benzodiazepines for cases involving local or regional anesthesia is their anticonvulsive effect, which may raise the toxic or seizure threshold of local anesthetic agents.[44] It must be remembered, however, that benzodiazepines have no analgesic effect and must therefore be combined with a narcotic. Morphine, meperidine (Demerol), fentanyl (Sublimaze), sufentanil (Sufenta), and alfentanil (Alfenta) are suitable. The occasional disinhibitory effect of the benzodiazepines must also be considered, as it may cause some patients to become garrulous, restless, or uncooperative. Other reported problems with midazolam are somnolence and occasional apnea in awake patients.[45]

Because laparoscopy is often performed as an outpatient procedure, it must be emphasized that outpatients presenting for surgery and anesthesia have an increased risk of aspiration and subsequent pneumonitis due to higher gastric volumes and lower gastric pH levels compared to those of inpatients undergoing similar procedures.[46] At particular risk are obese patients, pregnant patients, diabetics, patients with hiatal hernia, and individuals who have recently eaten solid foods or particulate liquids. Premedication with metoclopramide (Reglan), antihistaminic agents (H_2 antagonists) such as nizatidine (Axid) famotidine (Pepcid), ranitidine (Zantac), cimetidine (Tagamet),[47] or a nonparticulate antacid such as sodium citrate (Bicitra) should decrease the incidence and morbidity associated with gastric acid aspiration.

Metoclopramide,[48] droperidol[49,50] (Inapsine) and other butyrophenones, phenothiazines (Compazine, Phenergan), and various antihistamines (H_1 antagonists) such as hydroxyzine[51] (Vistaril) may also be useful for sedation and prevention or treatment of perioperative nausea and vomiting.[52] These drugs may be given preoperatively, intraoperatively, or postoperatively in small doses as needed. In large doses, however, they may delay recovery and ambulation.

Short-duration narcotics such as fentanyl[53] or narcotic agonist-antagonists such as nalbuphine (Nubain) and butorphanol (Stadol)[54] are gaining wide acceptance. Rapid recovery and the absence of respiratory depression by agonist-antagonists make them useful in the outpatient setting. In combination with small doses of benzodiazepines, these drugs can be expected to provide sedation, analgesia, and amnesia for operative events without delaying recovery and ambulation. Indeed, such premedicants may shorten the recovery time by reducing the dosage of the anesthetic agent required.

Techniques

Frequently anesthesia is induced with a rapidly acting intravenous agent (Table 24.5). Until recently, methohexital (Brevital) was popular in the outpatient setting because it allows more rapid awakening and recovery than does the traditionally administered barbiturate thiopen-

Table 24.5. Induction of anesthesia

Barbiturates
   Thiopental: prolonged recovery
   Methohexital: hiccoughs, myoclonus

Nonbarbiturates
   Propofol (Diprivan): antiemetic, rapid recovery
   Etomidate: nausea and vomiting, involuntary motor activity, suppression adrenocortical activity
   Ketamine (Ketalar): dissociative anesthetic, psychomimetic effects

Table 24.6. Anesthesia for laparoscopy

General anesthetic techniques
  Inhalational anesthesia
  Total intravenous

Regional anesthetic techniques
  Spinal
  Epidural

Local anesthetic techniques—field block
  With/without paracervical block
  With/without intraperitoneal block
  With/without local anesthetic block
  Single versus multiple incisions

---

tal. It does, however, produce a high incidence of adverse side effects, such as pain on injection, hiccoughs, and myoclonus. Thiopental, when utilized, must be administered judiciously to avoid delayed or prolonged recovery. Etomidate (Amidate) compares favorably with methohexital for outpatient induction of anesthesia.[55,56] However, etomidate causes a high incidence of nausea, vomiting, and involuntary motor activity; and it may produce transient suppression of postoperative adrenocortical function.[57] Ketamine hydrochloride (Ketalar) has been shown to produce undesirable psychomimetic effects in patients undergoing minor gynecologic procedures[58] (Table 24.6). Propofol (Diprivan), a rapid-acting, nonbarbiturate induction agent has revolutionized outpatient procedures of all types. Propofol is particularly useful for outpatient gynecologic laparoscopic procedures because of its antiemetic effects and rapid patient emergence and recovery.[59] Propofol has few side effects when administered to young, healthy patients. Induction of anesthesia with propofol is associated with more rapid emergence from anesthesia than after induction with thiopental. Although maintenance of anesthesia with propofol does not improve overall recovery times when compared to maintenance with inhalational agents, such as enflurane, it significantly reduces nausea and vomiting.[60]

All patients undergoing gynecologic endoscopy are at risk for aspiration pneumonitis as a result of passive or active regurgitation and subsequent hypoxia or cardiovascular collapse. A cuffed endotracheal tube should be properly placed and secured to protect the airway. It is also advisable to pass an orogastric or nasogastric tube and aspirate the stomach contents prior to gas insufflation for pneumoperitoneum. The tube should be suctioned intermittently to relieve gastric dilation resulting from assisted ventilation with an anesthesia face mask prior to intubation or to relieve gas absorbed into the stomach from the pneumoperitoneum.

Maintenance of anesthesia can be provided with inhalational agents or intravenous agents. Fluothane (Halothane), enflurane (Ethrane), isoflurane (Forane), and desflurane (Suprane) have been used successfully. Although enflurane is a potent respiratory and cardiovascular depressant, its use is generally preferred for outpatient procedures because of rapid recovery and fewer side effects.[61] Fluothane may predispose the patient to life-threatening arrhythmias,[18,19,26] particularly when a local anesthetic solution containing epinephrine is administered by the surgeon or when it is administered to a patient who has elevated levels of endogenous plasma catecholamines due to anxiety, hypercarbia, and acidosis. Enflurane and isoflurane are associated with fewer arrhythmias in the presence of increased circulating catecholamines.[2] Desflurane, an inhalational anesthetic, is particularly promising for outpatient procedures, as recovery of consciousness and orientation are more rapid in patients whose anesthesia was maintained with desflurane than with propofol. There is, however, no difference in psychomotor function test scores at 30 minutes[62] (Table 24.7).

Fentanyl and a shorter-duration narcotic derivative alfentanil (Alfenta) appear to be safe and effective for total intravenous anesthesia or a balanced technique. In a balanced anesthetic technique with nitrous oxide and oxygen, fentanyl is commonly used for both inpatient and outpatient procedures. Its popularity is due to its potent analgesic properties, rapid elimination or reversal, and cardiovascular stability.[63] Narcotic and other total intravenous techniques may be preferred to inhalational techniques when increased intravascular fluid volumes are to be avoided, as during hysteroscopic endome-

Table 24.7. Maintenance of anesthesia

Generic name	Trade name	Comment
Inhalation agents		
Fluothane	Halothane	Cardiac arrhythmias
Enflurane	Ethrane	Rapid recovery, fewer side effects in outpatients, potent respiratory and CNS depressant
Isoflurane	Forane	? Increased nausea/dizziness in outpatients
Desflurane	Suprane	
Intravenous agents		
Fentanyl	Sublimaze	
Sufentanil	Sufenta	
Alfentanil	Alfenta	

trial laser ablative procedures. In addition, inhalational anesthesia alone may inhibit hypoxic pulmonary vasoconstriction, thereby decreasing oxygen saturation.[64]

Concerns about the safety of fentanyl during outpatient surgery result from the likelihood of postoperative respiratory depression and nausea and vomiting commonly associated with opiate analgesics. When used alone in moderate doses with nitrous oxide and oxygen, the respiratory depression produced by fentanyl often requires reversal with an antagonist such as naloxone (Narcan) or a combined agonist-antagonist such as nalbuphine or butorphanol to avoid the need for postoperative controlled ventilation and delayed recovery.

Alfentanil may be used for induction and maintenance of anesthesia with either bolus or continuous infusion without postoperative respiratory depression and the complications associated with narcotic reversal. Fentanyl and alfentanil anesthesia produce less cardiovascular depression and can be used safely in high risk and healthy patients. Alfentanil administration, however, may be associated with a particularly high incidence of nausea and vomiting.[65] Although outpatients who receive a balanced anesthetic technique incorporating short-acting narcotic agents develop a high incidence of early postoperative morbidity, the postdischarge incidence of complications does not differ significantly from those in inpatients receiving inhalational agents alone.[66] The use of nitrous oxide has also been implicated as a cause of postoperative nausea and vomiting.[67] Outpatients have a high incidence of minor side effects (e.g., nausea and vomiting) for up to 48 hours postoperatively regardless of the general anesthetic technique employed.[68]

Adequate muscle relaxation is important during laparoscopic procedures to limit the increase in intraabdominal and intrathoracic pressures, which alter vascular and respiratory homeostasis (Table 24.8). The choice of muscle relaxants as adjuncts to general anesthesia for short procedures was limited prior to the introduction of the intermediate- and short-duration drugs. Succinylcholine (Anectine), a depolarizing muscle relaxant, is commonly used in bolus form for rapid intubation and as an infusion (0.1–0.2%) for maintenance of muscle relaxation. Succinylcholine provides optimal intubating conditions more rapidly than any other muscle relaxant in clinical use today. It causes frequent minor side effects, such as muscle soreness, and occasional serious complications, including bradycardia, hyperkalemia, myoglobinemia, malignant hyperthermia, and rarely prolonged apnea in patients with plasma cholinesterase deficiency.[68] These problems can be avoided with the use of nondepolarizing agents.

Until recently, however, there were no agents suitable for short surgical procedures. Intermediate-duration agents, such as atracurium (Tracrium) have a reasonably rapid onset of action for adequate intubating conditions and provide hemodynamic stability.[69] Atracurium, however, may cause histamine release-induced broncho-

24. Anesthesia

Table 24.8. Muscle relaxants

Generic name	Trade name	Side effects
Succinylcholine	Anectine	Bradycardia, hyperkalemia, myoglobinemia, malignant hyperthermia, prolonged apnea
Atracurium	Tracrium	Histamine related hypotension and bronchospasm
Vecuronium	Norcuron	Cumulative effects, prolonged action when used in patients receiving steroids
Mivacurium	Mivacron	Histamine related hypotension, prolonged apnea
Rocuronium	Zemuron	No significant adverse effects

spasm and hypotension. Vecuronium (Norcuron) can also provide satisfactory muscular relaxation without cardiopulmonary side effects and has a medium duration of action appropriate for cases lasting 20–30 minutes or longer.[70,71] Mivacurium (Mivacron) offers advantages over atracurium in that there are no histamine side effects, and it has a shorter effective duration of action (20–25 minutes). In one clinical study, however, it offered no apparent advantages over succinylcholine for outpatient laparoscopy.[72] Satisfactory conditions for rapid intubation may be accomplished with these agents when the priming principle is used. The priming principle involves administration of a subparalyzing dose of a nondepolarizing muscle relaxant 3–4 minutes before induction and paralysis. A larger dose of the muscle relaxant is then administered with a reduction in the time to neuromuscular blockade for intubation.

Regional Anesthesia

Advantages Versus Disadvantages

Regional anesthesia, including epidural and spinal, has been used successfully for laparoscopy but has not gained popularity when compared with general or local anesthetic techniques. Most of the procedures described in this text are not amenable to regional or local anesthesia. Aribarg[73] and Bridenbaugh and Soderstrom[74] have reported the successful use of epidural anesthesia during laparoscopy. Epidural anesthesia has been advocated as a safe alternative to general anesthesia for patients undergoing short laparoscopic procedures including assisted reproductive technologic procedures such as gamete intrafallopian transfer (GIFT), as it does not contribute to ventilatory depression.[75] Advantages include an awake patient who can give information that may lead to early treatment of complications such as pneumothorax, gas embolism, arrhythmias, and concomitant respiratory insufficiency. Nausea and vomiting occur less frequently than with general anesthesia. Regional anesthesia provides a quiet surgical field and good muscle relaxation. It also provides postoperative pain relief, which decreases the need for narcotic analgesics and sedatives. Fewer pharmacologic agents are used, reducing the possibility of allergy, toxicity, and other adverse drug reactions.

Spinal anesthesia may be performed more simply, more quickly, and with less expense than epidural anesthesia. As a complication, however, postdural puncture headache may occur. By using a small-gauge needle (25 or 26 gauge) and by limiting spinal anesthesia to older patients (≥ 65 years of age), the incidence of postspinal headache may be reduced to < 1%.[76]

Because epidural anesthesia is accomplished without dural puncture, the need for treatment of spinal headache is minimized. Postspinal headache is a significant complication, particularly in the outpatient setting, where the patient may require an epidural blood patch or admission to the hospital for intravenous fluid therapy, analgesics, and supportive care.

Another annoying complication of spinal anesthesia is urinary retention requiring catheterization of the bladder, which often delays discharge from outpatient facilities. Prolonged sympathetic blockade may cause orthostatic hypotension and may also delay discharge.

Generally, the patient is free from the risk of orthostatic changes when sensory function has returned.[77]

Disadvantages of regional anesthesia include hypotension, the possibility of failed or inadequate block, systemic local anesthetic toxicity, and the need for skillful, well trained anesthesia personnel. Local anesthetics are administered in large volumes for epidural blocks and for many local anesthetic techniques and may result in seizures, apnea, arrhythmias, or cardiovascular collapse. The level of the block must be high enough to eliminate peritoneal discomfort. It is also contraindicated for most pelviscopic surgery because of the need for prolonged pneumoperitoneum at relatively high pressure. In patients with pulmonary disease, the T4–T6 sensory level required may decrease ventilatory function, restrict cough, and increase the possibility of atelectasis. Inadvertent subarachnoid block during epidural anesthesia may lead to a total spinal or cephalad extension of paralysis, causing respiratory insufficiency, cardiovascular collapse, and neurologic sequelae. The incidence of both major and minor anesthetic complications is reduced when a skilled and experienced anesthesiology staff is employed.

Regional anesthesia may delay a busy operating schedule when the anesthesiologist does not have the opportunity to initiate the block prior to the surgeon's readiness to start the procedure. Depending on the local anesthetic used, it may take 15–30 minutes for neural blockade after the anesthetic solution has been injected into the epidural space. As a solution to this problem, some facilities provide a separate holding or anesthetic induction room where the patient may receive intravenous fluids and have the block performed with standard monitoring and resuscitation equipment available. This procedure reduces operating room cost and saves time. Recovery from regional anesthesia is slower, however, than recovery from local anesthesia, and the cost for epidural anesthesia is not significantly different from that for general anesthesia.[74] Epidural anesthesia requires intravenous fluid administration of 1.0–1.5 L prior to initiation of anesthesia to prevent hypotension due to the loss of sympathetic tone and peripheral vasodilation. Spinal and epidural blocks are contraindicated in the volume-depleted woman suffering from marked dehydration or hemorrhage, as may occur during the postpartum period.

Other contraindications to spinal and epidural anesthesia include a history of neurologic disease, peripheral neuropathy, coagulopathies, infection at the site of needle insertion, previous allergic reaction to local anesthetics, patient refusal, and an inexperienced anesthesiologist. Prolonged epidural block with 2-chloroprocaine (Nesacaine CE) has been reported in a patient with plasma cholinesterase deficiency, as the drug is metabolized by this enzyme.[78] Vertebral and neurologic pathology are also relative contraindications to spinal and epidural anesthesia.

Premedication

Patients undergoing gynecologic endoscopy under regional anesthesia require less intravenous sedation and analgesia than do patients receiving general or local anesthesia. Benzodiazepines are commonly used for amnesia and may be administered in small, incremental doses alone or in combination with narcotics such as morphine or fentanyl. Premedication with ondansetron (Zofran)[79] and metoclopramide have proved effective for reducing nausea and vomiting in outpatients undergoing gynecologic laparoscopy.[80] Ondansetron is particularly effective for patients with a history of postoperative emetic symptoms.[81] Atropine 0.4–0.6 mg may be given intravenously just prior to incision to minimize bradycardia due to uterine manipulation, or it may be administered intraoperatively, if necessary, for management of vagovagal reflexes.

Lumbar epidural anesthesia involves the deposition of a local anesthetic solution within the potential space surrounding the lumbar dura and its contents. Various techniques have been described.[73,74,82] The local anesthetic solution may be deposited in the peridural space through the epidural needle once the space is entered and a test dose given. Alternatively, a catheter may be threaded through the needle and left in place when the needle is withdrawn to provide a conduit for additional anesthetic administration.

The onset and duration of the epidural block depend on the local anesthetic and adjuvant agents used. Lidocaine 1.5% is commonly effective in volumes of 20–25 ml.[82] Because of its rapid onset and short duration, 2-chloroprocaine has also been used, particularly for outpatient procedures. Although 2-chloroprocaine produces less systemic toxicity than lidocaine, Nesacaine CE, with its low pH and bisulfite preservative, has been implicated in several cases of neurologic sequelae when inadvertently injected into the subarachnoid space.[78,83–85] A bisulfite-free 2-chloroprocaine solution (Nesacaine MPF) has now been marketed to eliminate this complication. Epinephrine in a 1:200,000 concentration may be added to lidocaine to reduce systemic vascular uptake and resultant toxicity and to prolong the anesthetic block. It is seldom used for gynecologic endoscopy, however, because the prolonged duration of anesthesia with prolonged motor and sympathetic impairment is unsuitable for outpatient anesthesia. Longer-duration agents such as bupivacaine (Marcaine) are useful for longer pelviscopic surgical procedures.

For spinal anesthesia, hyperbaric lidocaine (Xylocaine), bupivacaine (Marcaine), or tetracaine (Pontocaine) may be used. Lidocaine, with the most rapid onset and shortest duration, is most appropriate for outpatient procedures lasting 30–45 minutes. The addition of epinephrine 1:200,000 provides anesthesia lasting approximately 1.5 times this duration for longer procedures.

Local Anesthesia

Local anesthesia with sedation for gynecologic endoscopy is attaining acceptance among surgeons and patients,[39,40] especially in free-standing clinics and ambulatory surgical units. This method of anesthesia currently is advocated primarily for diagnostic procedures and sterilizations, although it has also been advocated for hysteroscopy[86] and GIFT.[87] Local anesthesia offers maximum safety, minimum physiologic disturbance, and rapid recovery.[36] The incidence of serious complications is significantly lowered by the use of local anesthesia, as most of the untoward events that occur during endoscopic procedures are related to general anesthesia. Complications related to local anesthesia are far less frequent than those with general anesthesia and are rarely critical.[88] They include excessive sedation and systemic toxicity due to absorption or intravascular injection of local anesthetic agents.

Local anesthesia is most suitable for the cooperative and well informed patient. The patient with whom communication can be established and who can cooperate adequately for pelvic examination should obtain adequate analgesia with local anesthetic administration and supplemental intravenous sedation.[36] The importance of preoperative counseling and intraoperative reassurance by confident, considerate, experienced staff cannot be overemphasized. Gynecologic endoscopy under local anesthesia

Table 24.9. Commonly used local anesthetics for diagnostic laparoscopy

Drug and drug classification	Route of administration[a]	Dosage form and preparation	Maximum dose (mg)
Esters			
Procaine (Novocain)	I, S	10, 20, 100 mg/ml solution	1000
Chloroprocaine (Nesacaine)	I, N, E	10, 20, 30 mg/ml solution	1000
Tetracaine (Pontocaine)	S	10 & 20 mg/ml solution (niphanoid crystals)	200
Amides			
Lidocaine (Xylocaine)	I, N, T, S, E	10, 15, 20, 50 mg/ml solution; with/without 1:200,000 epinephrine 2.0% jelly, viscous 2.5%, 5.0% ointment	500
Mepivacaine (Carbocaine)	I, N, E	10, 15, 20 mg/ml solution	500
Bupivacaine (Marcaine)	I, N, S, E	2.5, 5.0, 7.5 mg/ml solution; with/without 1:200,000 epinephrine	200
Etidocaine (Duranest)	I, N, E	2.5, 5.0, 10.0 mg/ml solution	300

[a] I, local infiltrate; N, peripheral nerve block; T, topical; S, spinal; E, epidural.

requires smooth, effective teamwork, a minimum of extraneous operating room conversation and activity, and a gentle, precise, skillful surgeon.

The most common operations performed under local anesthesia are sterilization and diagnostic procedures. More extensive procedures require major regional or general anesthesia. Thus local anesthesia is generally unsuitable for pelviscopic surgery because of the length of time required, patient movement, and surgical components (Table 24.9).

Recovery and Discharge

Assessment

Throughout the recovery period, vital signs (including pulse, blood pressure, and respirations) must be closely monitored. If the patient has received a narcotic antagonist for reversal of narcotic anesthesia or sedation, she should be monitored for 2–3 hours postoperatively to avoid unrecognized renarcotization and respiratory depression.

Recovery following local anesthesia is generally more rapid than that after regional or general anesthesia, provided excessive sedation is avoided. Patients are often awake, alert, and ambulatory within 1 hour of the conclusion of surgery. Recovery times for regional and general anesthesia may be expected to average 1 hour 43 minutes and 2 hours 56 minutes, respectively.[76] Various tests have been used to assess psychomotor recovery from anesthetic agents.[89–92] It has been demonstrated that return of psychomotor function following intravenous and inhalational agents may take up to 48 hours.[93]

Outpatient Discharge

All outpatients, regardless of anesthetic technique utilized, should be discharged in the company of a responsible adult who accompanies the patient home. Preferably, this adult, as well as the patient, is informed of postoperative instructions, as the amnestic effect of anesthetic agents may impair the patient's memory and compliance. Travel time to the patient's home should be reasonable. The patient should be warned against operating an automobile or other equipment, taking nonprescribed medications, consuming alcohol, or making important decisions for at least 24–48 hours.[92] If the patient received general anesthesia with intubation, she and her escort are instructed to watch for signs of stridor related to laryngeal edema. The patient is given instructions and appropriate telephone numbers in case an emergency arises.

Safety

Positioning and Monitoring

Modified lithotomy position allows more adequate diaphragmatic excursion and less pulmonary atelectasis and compromise than does the traditional lithotomy position (Fig. 24.1). Monitoring requires continuous electrocardiography, intermittent blood pressure, pulse or cutaneous oximetry, and in-line oxygen sensors for general anesthesia equipment. Pulse oximetry is rapidly becoming the most popular instrument for continuous monitoring of capillary oxygen saturation. Oxygen saturation and hypoxia have been documented following extubation in healthy, young women undergoing routine laparoscopic procedures with carbon dioxide insufflation, even when no significant changes in arterial carbon dioxide tension were observed intraoperatively. Possible causes include diffusion hypoxia produced by nitrous oxide used as a general anesthetic agent, gas embolism, or postoperative hypoventilation as a central response to carbon dioxide diffusion from the pneumoperitoneum into the vascular system.[94] Monitoring of the patient's oxygen saturation should therefore be continued for at least 20 minutes into the postoperative period.

Capnography is particularly useful for the patient undergoing general anesthesia for laparoscopic procedures with carbon dioxide insufflation because the degree of vascular absorption of carbon dioxide and hypercarbia are not predictable.[95] It is also necessary for the rapid diagnosis of pulmonary gas embolism. Capnography is useful for patients receiving

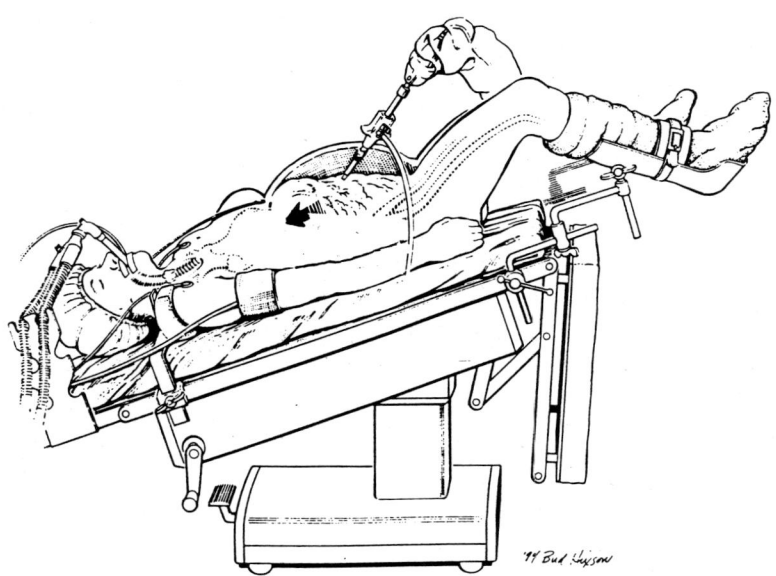

Figure 24.1. Trendelenburg and lithotomy positions limit diaphragmatic excursion and increase pulmonary blood flow. (Reprinted from Lucas LF, Asher EF, Schroeder JA, Rigor BM: Anesthesia for laparoscopic general surgery. In *Laparoscopic Surgery: An Atlas for General Surgeons,* Vitale G, Sanfilippo JS, Perissat J, eds. Philadelphia, Lippincott, 1995, with permission)

general anesthesia with or without controlled ventilation. The capability for blood gas determinations should be readily available in all anesthetizing locations.

Intraoperative temperature monitoring is advisable for all patients undergoing general anesthetic laparoscopic procedures. Artificial ventilation with anesthetic gases may cause significant respiratory heat loss. Although malignant hyperthermia is a rare anesthetic complication, its early recognition is key to patient survival. Hypothermia also occurs as a result of heat loss created by carbon dioxide peritoneal cavity insufflation, particularly if unwarmed gases are used.

Resuscitation Equipment

Pelviscopic surgery and laser laparoscopy involve potential risks, including hemorrhage due to injury to major vessels or bowel, gastric perforation, abdominal wall or visceral hematoma, and pneumothorax.[36,96–104] Gynecologic endoscopy utilizing a Verres needle for insufflation is ideally performed in a hospital or surgical center where emergency laparotomy may be performed under general anesthesia.[36] Therefore resuscitation equipment and trained personnel must be readily available, including a suctioning device, oxygen, defibrillator, emergency pharmacotherapeutic agents, and instruments for airway management. Such equipment should be regularly inspected and maintained.

Laser

Special safety considerations must be observed for laparoscopic laser procedures as presented in Chapter 3. It is of the utmost importance that all personnel in the operating room be equipped with protective eyewear, preferably with side shields when the CO_2 laser is in use. The patient's eyes must also be protected by either protective glasses or goggles or by moistened eye pads during general anesthesia.

Outpatient Laparoscopy

The desire for a low-cost, efficient setting for gynecologic surgical procedures will continue to increase the number of patients undergoing gynecologic endoscopy as outpatients. The safety and acceptability of outpatient sterilization has been well documented. Most patients presenting for endoscopy are potential candidates for outpatient anesthesia and surgery. Ambulatory surgical centers routinely admit young, healthy individuals, ASA class I (American Society of Anesthesiologists' classification) and patients with minor systemic conditions (ASA II). In many centers patients who have stable chronic illnesses (ASA III) may be considered for outpatient surgery, in consultation with the anesthesiologist. These patients must be capable and willing to comply with routine instructions for fasting, medication, discharge, and postoperative care.

Patients in whom complications may be expected should be admitted to the hospital the evening prior to or the morning of surgery. These patients include any patient with ASA II or III disease or medication requirements that preclude ambulatory anesthesia or surgery. Obese patients, those with a history of peritonitis, those suspected of having significant pelvic adhesions or ectopic pregnancy, or any other patient who may require laparotomy should be treated in a facility that has close access to a hospital in the event postoperative hospitalization becomes necessary.

Conclusion

In no other gynecologic procedure is an understanding of physiologic alterations and anesthetic requirements more important than for gynecologic endoscopy. The outpatient setting, requirements for pneumoperitoneum, electrical systems, and application of laser technology increase the hazards and potential for complications associated with endoscopic surgical procedures. The requirements for safe, judicious patient management create an interdependence between the surgeon and the anesthesiologist. Each must be knowledgeable and experienced in routine and emergency preparation and the procedures to be used in the patient undergoing pelviscopic surgery.

References

1. DIAMANT M, BENUMOF JL, SAIDMAN LJ, ET AL: Laparoscopic sterilization with local anesthesia: complications and blood-gas changes. Anesth Analg 1977;56:335.
2. HARRIS MN, PLANTEVIN OM, CROWTHER A: Cardiac arrhythmias during anaesthesia for laparoscopy. Br J Anaesth 1984;56:1213.
3. WOOD-SMITH FF, HORNE GM, NUNN JF: Effect of posture on ventilation of patients anaesthetized with halothane. Anaesthesia 1961;16:340.
4. SWAIN J: The case for abandoning the Trendelenburg position in pelvic surgery. Med J Aust 1960;47:536.
5. MARTIN JT: Positioning in Anesthesia and Surgery. Philadelphia, Saunders, 1987, pp 57–59.
6. CASE EH, STILES JA: The effect of various surgical positions on vital capacity. Anesthesiology 1946;7:29.
7. JONES JR, JACOBY J: The effect of surgical positions on respiration. Surg Forum 1954;5:686.
8. HENSCHEL AB, WYANT GM, DOBKIN AB, HENSCHEL EO: Posture as it concerns the anesthesiologist: a preliminary study. Anesth Analg 1957;36:69.
9. SHARP JT: The effect of body position change on lung compliance in normal subjects and in patients with congestive heart failure. J Clin Invest 1959;38:659.
10. WALTEMATH CL, BERGMAN NA: Respiratory compliance in obese patients. Anesthesiology 1974; 41:84.
11. ALTSCHULE MD, ZAMCHECK N: Significance of changes in subdivisions of the lung volume in the Trendelenburg position. Surg Gynecol Obstet 1942;74:1061.
12. SCOTT DB, LEES MM, TAYLOR SH: Some respiratory effects of the Trendelenburg position during anaesthesia. Br J Anaesth 1966;38:174.
13. SCOTT DB, SLAWSON KB: Respiratory effects of prolonged Trendelenburg position. Br J Anaesth 1968;40:103.
14. GRAFF TD, ARBEGAST NR, PHILLIPS OC, ET AL: Gas embolism: a comparative study of air and carbon dioxide as embolic agents in the systemic venous system. Am J Obstet Gynecol 1959; 78:259.
15. SCOTT DB: Some effects of peritoneal insufflation of carbon dixoide at laparoscopy. Anaesthesia 1970;25:590.
16. SHARP JR, PIERSON WP, BRADY CE III: Comparison of CO_2 and N_2O-induced discomfort during peritoneoscopy under local anesthesia. Gastroenterology 1982;82:453.
17. ALEXANDER GD, GOLDRATH M, BROWN EM, SMILER BG: Outpatient laparoscopic sterilization under local anesthesia. Am J Obstet Gynecol 1973;116:1065.
18. DESMOND J, GORDON RA: Ventilation in patients anaesthetized for laparoscopy. Can Anaesth Soc J 1970;17:378.
19. LEWIS DG, RYDER W, BURN N, ET AL: Laparoscopy—an investigation during spontaneous

ventilation with halothane. Br J Anaesth 1972; 44:685.
20. YOUSSEFF AR, IBRAHIM MM, ABDEL-ALIM MS, ALY AY: Some physiological changes during anesthesia for laparoscopy. Middle East J Anaesthesiol 1982;6:219.
21. MOTEW M, IVANKOVICH AD, BIENIARZ J, ET AL: Cardiovascular effects and acid-base and blood gas changes during laparoscopy. Am J Obstet Gynecol 1973;115:1002.
22. SEED RF, SHAKESPEARE TF, MULDOON MJ: Carbon dioxide homeostasis during anaesthesia for laparoscopy. Anaesthesia 1970;25:223.
23. ALEXANDER GD, NOE FE, BROWN EM: Anesthesia for pelvic laparoscopy. Anesth Analg 1969; 48:14.
24. MAGNO R, MEDEGÅRD A, BENGTSSON R, TRONSTAD SE: Acid-base balance during laparoscopy: the effects of intraperitoneal insufflation of carbon dioxide and nitrous oxide on acid-base balance during controlled ventilation. Acta Obstet Gynecol Scand 1979;58:81.
25. WHITWAM JG, SCOTT RB, SUNSHINE I: Entry of nitrous oxide into a giant gas-filled ovarian cyst: a case report. Br J Anaesth 1965;37:976.
26. HODGSON C, MCCLELLAND RM, NEWTON JR: Some effects of the peritoneal insufflation of carbon dioxide at laparoscopy. Anaesthesia 1970;25:382.
27. WALDVOGEL HH, SCHNECK HJ, FELBER A, VONHUNDELSHAUSEN B: Anesthesia relevant features of laparoscopy: the value of capnometry. Anestheziol Reanimatol 1994;19:4.
28. VEGFORS M, ENGBORG L, GUPTA A, LENNMARKEN C: Changes in end-tidal carbon dioxide during gynecologic laparscopy; spontaneous versus controlled ventilation. J Clin Anesth 1994;6:199.
29. BROWN DR, FISHBURNE JI, ROBERSON VO, HULKA JF: Ventilatory and blood gas changes during laparoscopy with local anesthesia. Am J Obstet Gynecol 1976;124:741.
30. MYLES PS: Bradyarrhythmias and laparoscopy: a prospective study of heart rate changes with laparoscopy. Aust NZ J Obstet Gynaecol 1991; 31:171.
31. BIVINS HG, KNOPP R, DOS SANTOS PA: Blood volume distribution in the Trendelenburg position. Ann Emerg Med 1985;14:641.
32. PRICOLO VE, BURCHARD KW, SINGH AK, ET AL: Trendelenburg versus PASG application: hemodynamic response in man. J Trauma 1986;26:718.
33. PHILLIPS JM, CORSON SL, KEITH MD, YUZPE AA: Laparoscopy. Baltimore, Williams & Wilkins, 1977, p 73.
34. CROZIER TA, LUGER A, DRAVECZ M, ET AL: Anaesthesiol Intensiomed Notfallmed Schmerzther 1991;26:412.
35. FAHY A, MARSHALL M: Postanaesthetic morbidity in out-patients. Br J Anaesth 1969;41:433.
36. PENFIELD AJ: Gynecologic Surgery Under Local Anesthesia. Baltimore, Urban & Schwarzenberg, 1986, pp 1–190.
37. SILVA PD, KANG SB, SLOANE KA: Gamete intrafallopian transfer with spinal anesthesia. Fertil Steril 1993;59:841.
38. CHOW WP, LOGANATH A, PEH KL, ET AL: Response of ovary in young women experiencing laparoscopy under general anesthesia. Med J Malaysia 1993;48:56.
39. MUNK T, KJER JJ: Laparoscopic sterilization under local anesthesia. Acta Obstet Gynecol Scand 1994;73:347.
40. RAEDER JC, BORDAHL PE, NORDENTOFT J, ET AL: Ambulatory laparoscopic sterilization: should local analgesia and intravenous sedation replace general anesthesia? A comparative clinical trial. Tidsskr Nor Laegeforen 1993;113:1559.
41. DUBOIS F, BERTHELOT G, LEVARD H: Laparoscopic cholecystectomy: historical perspective and personal experience. Surg Laparosc Endosc 1991; 1:52.
42. KLOCKGETHER-RADKE A: Anesthesiologic aspects of minimally invasive surgery - preoperative assessment. Zentralbl Chir 1993;118:588.
43. KORTTILA K, TARKKANEN J: Comparison of diazepam and midazolam for sedation during local anaesthesia for bronchoscopy. Br J Anaesth 1985;57:581.
44. MUNSON ES, WAGMAN IH: Diazepam treatment of local anesthetic-induced seizures. Anesthesiology 1972;37:523.
45. Midazolam (Versed). In Physicians Desk Reference. 50th ed. Montvale, NJ, Medical Economics, 1996, p 2170.
46. ONG BY, PALAHNIUK RJ, CUMMING M: Gastric volume and pH in out-patients. Can Anaesth Soc J 1978;25:36.
47. RAO TLK, SUSEELA M, EL-ETR AA: Metoclopramide and cimetidine to reduce gastric juice pH volume. Anesth Analg 1984;63:264.
48. CLARK MM, STORRS JA: The prevention of postoperative vomiting after abortion: metoclopramide. Br J Anaesth 1969;41:890.
49. COHEN SE, WOODS WA, WYNER J: Antiemetic efficacy of droperidol and metoclopramide. Anesthesiology 1984;60:67.
50. ABRAMOWITZ MD, OH TH, EPSTEIN BS, ET AL: The antiemetic effect of droperidol following outpa-

tient strabimus surgery in children. Anesthesiology 1983;59:579.
51. MCKENZIE R, WADHWA RK, UY NT, ET AL: Antiemetic effectiveness of intramuscular hydroxyzine compared with intramuscular droperidol. Anesth Analg 1981;60:783.
52. CHEN LH, WATKINS ML: Antiemetic premedication in outpatient anesthesia. Anesthesiology 1981;55:A280.
53. HORRIGAN RW, MOYERS JR, JOHNSON BH, ET AL: Etomidate vs thiopental with and without fentanyl—a comparative study of awakening in man. Anesthesiology 1980;52:362.
54. MURPHY MR, HUG CC JR: The enflurane sparing effect of morphine, butorphanol, and nalbuphine. Anesthesiology 1982;57:489.
55. BORALESSA H, HOLDCROFT A: Methohexitone or etomidate for induction of dental anesthesia. Can Anaesth Soc J 1980;27:578.
56. MILLER BM, HENDRY JG, LEES NW: Etomidate and methohexitone: a comparative clinical study in out-patient anaesthesia. Anaesthesia 1978;33:450.
57. WAGNER RL, WHITE PF: Etomidate inhibits adrenocortical function in surgical patients. Anesthesiology 1984;61:647.
58. FIGALLO EM, MCKENZIE R, TANTISIRA B, ET AL: Anesthesia for dilation, evacuation and curretage in outpatients: comparison of subanaesthetic doses of ketamine and sodium methohexitone-nitrous oxide anaesthesia. Can Anaesth Soc J 1977;24:110.
59. DING Y, FREDMAN B, WHITE PF: Recovery following outpatient anesthesia: use of enflurane versus propofol. J Clin Anesth 1993;5:443.
60. SUKHANI R, LURIE J, JABAMONI R: Propofol for ambulatory gynecologic laparoscopy: does omission of nitrous oxide alter postoperative emetic sequelae and recovery? Anesth Analg 1994;78:831.
61. TRACEY JA, HOLLAND AJ, UNGER L: Morbidity in minor gynaecological surgery: a comparison of halothane, enflurane and isoflurane. Br J Anaesth 1982;54:1213.
62. GRAHAM SG, AITKENHEAD AR: A comparison between propofol and desflurane anaesthesia for minor gynaecological laparoscopic surgery. Anaesthesia 1993;48:471.
63. CHEN LH, BERMAN ML: Fentanyl vs enflurane in outpatient anesthesia. Anesthesiology 1979;51:S51.
64. CROZIER TA: Anesthesiologic aspects of minimally invasive surgery. Zentralbl Chir 1993;118:571.
65. OKUM GS, COLONNA-ROMANO P, HORROW JC: Vomiting after alfentanil anesthesia: effect of dosing method. Anesth Analg 1992;75:558.
66. HENEGHAN C, MCAULIFFE R, THOMAS D, ET AL: Morbidity after outpatient anesthesia: a comparison of two techniques of endotracheal anesthesia for dental surgery. Anaesthesia 1981;36:4.
67. FELTS JA, POLER SM, SPITZNAGEL EL: Nitrous oxide, nausea, and vomiting after outpatient gynecologic surgery. J Clin Anesth 1990;2:168.
68. LEMAIRE WJ, NAGEL EL, SMITH JC: Plasma cholinesterase deficiency: a possible complication during anesthesia. Obstet Gynecol 1972;39:552.
69. WOOLNER DF, GIBBS JM, SMEELE PQ: Clinical comparison of atracurium and alcuronium in gynaecological surgery. Anaesth Intensive Care 1985;13:33.
70. CALDWELL JE, BRAIDWOOD JM, SIMPSON DS: Vecuronium bromide in anaesthesia for laparoscopic sterilization. Br J Anaesth 1985;57:765.
71. VARGA J: Muscle relaxation with Norcuron in patients undergoing obstetrical-gynaecological operation. Ther Hung 1992;40:37.
72. POLER SM, WATCHA MF, WHITE PF: Mivacurium as an alternative to succinylcholine during outpatient laparoscopy. J Clin Anesth 1992;4:127.
73. ARIBARG A: Epidural analgesia for laparoscopy. J Obstet Gynaecol Br Commonw 1973;80:567.
74. BRIDENBAUGH LD, SODERSTROM RM: Lumbar epidural block anesthesia for outpatient laparoscopy. J Reprod Med 1979;23:85.
75. CIOFOLO MJ, CLERGUE F, SEEBACHER J, ET AL: Ventilatory effects of laparoscopy under epidural anesthesia. Anesth Analg 1990;70:357.
76. MULROY M, BRIDENBAUGH LD: Regional anesthetic techniques for outpatient surgery. In Ambulatory Anesthesia Care, Wood SW (ed). Boston, Little Brown, 1982, pp 71–80.
77. PFLUG AE, AASHEIM GM, FOSTER C: Sequence of return of neurological function and criteria for safe ambulation following subarachnoid block. Can Anaesth Soc J 1978;25:133.
78. RAVINDRAN RS, BOND VK, TASCH MD, ET AL: Prolonged neural blockade following regional analgesia with 2-chloroprocaine. Anesth Analg 1980;59:447.
79. SUNG YF, WETCHLER BV, DUNCALF D, JOSLYN AF: A double-blind, placebo-controlled pilot study examining the effectiveness of intravenous ondansetron in the prevention of postoperative nausea and emesis. J Clin Anesth 1993;5:22.
80. MALINS AF, FIELD JM, NESLING PM, COOPER GM: Nausea and vomiting after gynaecological laparoscopy: comparison of premedication with

80. oral ondansetron, metaclopramide and placebo. Br J Anaesth 1994;72:231.
81. RAPHAEL JH, NORTON AC: Antiemetic efficacy of prophylactic ondansetron in laparoscopic surgery: randomized, double-blind comparison with metoclopramide. Br J Anaesth 1993;71:845.
82. MOORE DC: Regional Block (4th ed). Springfield, IL, Charles C Thomas, 1975, pp 412–427.
83. COVINO BG, MARX GF, FINSTER M, ET AL: Prolonged sensory/motor deficits following inadvertent spinal anesthesia [editorial]. Anesth Analg 1980;59:399.
84. MOORE DC, SPIERDIJK J, VAN KLEEF JD, ET AL: Chloroprocaine neurotoxicity: four additional cases. Anesth Analg 1982;61:155.
85. WANG BC, SPIEDHOLZ NI, HILLMAN DE, ET AL: Subarachnoid sodium bisulfite (the antioxidant in Nesacaine) causes chronic neurological deficit. Anesthesiology 1982;57:A194.
86. FINIKIOTIS G, TSOCANOS S: Outpatient hysteroscopy: a comparison of 2 methods of local analgesia. Aust NZ J Obstet Gynaecol 1992;32:373.
87. MILKI AA, HARDY RI, EL DANASOURI I, ET AL: Local anesthesia with conscious sedation for laparoscopic intrafallopian transfer. Fertil Steril 1992;58:1240.
88. FISHBURNE JI JR, FULGHUM MS, HULKA JF, MERCER JP: General anesthesia for outpatient laparoscopy with an objective measure of recovery. Anesth Analg 1974;53:1.
89. NEWMAN MG, TRIEGER N, MILLER JC: Measuring recovery from anesthesia—a simple test. Anesth Analg 1969;48:136.
90. STEWARD DJ, VOLGYESI G: Stabilometry: a new tool for the measurement of recovery following general anaesthesia for out-patients. Can Anaesth Soc J 1978;25:4.
91. KORTTILA K, LINNOILA M, ERTAMA E, ET AL: Recovery and simulated driving after intravenous anesthesia with thiopental, methohexital, propanidid or alphadione. Anesthesiology 1975;43:291.
92. TRIEGER N, LOSKOTA WJ, JACOBS AW, NEWMAN MG: Nitrous oxide—a study of physiological and psychomotor effects. J Am Dent Assoc 1971;82:142.
93. HERBERT M, HEALY TE, BOURKE JB, ET AL: Profile of recovery after general anaesthesia. BMJ 1983;286:1539.
94. NAKATSUKA I, OKADA M, KONISHI M, NOGUCHI J: Blood gas changes after laparoscopy. Masui 1991;40:1616.
95. WEYLAND W, CROZIER TA, BRAUER A, ET AL: Specifics of anesthesiology in the operative phase of laparoscopic surgery. Zentralbl Chir 1993;118:582.
96. PENFIELD AJ: Laparoscopic sterilization under local anesthesia: 1200 cases. Obstet Gynecol 1977;49:725.
97. REYNOLDS RC, PAUCA AL: Gastric perforation, an anesthesia-induced hazard in laparoscopy. Anesthesiology 1973;38:84.
98. WHITFORD JH, GUNSTONE AJ: Gastric perforation: a hazard of laparoscopy under general anaesthesia. Br J Anaesth 1972;44:97.
99. ESPOSITO JM: Hematoma of the sigmoid colon as a complication of laparoscopy. Am J Obstet Gynecol 1973;117:581.
100. DOCTOR NH, HUSSAIN Z: Bilateral pneumothorax associated with laparoscopy: a case report of a rare hazard and review. Anaesthesia 1973;28:75.
101. PENFIELD AJ: How to prevent complications of open laparoscopy. J Reprod Med 1985;30:660.
102. SMILER BG, FALICK YS: Complication during anesthesia and laparoscopy. JAMA 1973;226:676.
103. SODERSTROM RM, BUTLER JC: A critical evaluation of complications in laparoscopy. J Reprod Med 1973;10:245.
104. STEPTOE P: Hazards of laparoscopy. BMJ 1973;3:347.

25
Complications

Barbara S. Levy

Endoscopic procedures are associated with the potential for a unique set of complications. The increased use of endoscopic techniques has been accompanied by the unspoken belief that this surgery is simple and without significant risk. Although the length of hospital stay (due to avoidance of laparotomy) has decreased, the complexity of procedures attempted continues to increase. In the past many of these procedures were performed on medically low risk patients who required little preoperative evaluation. The indications for complex endoscopic procedures have been liberalized, and many of these procedures are now being performed on an outpatient basis in patients with complicated problems. Although the short hospitalization appears to be cost-effective and operative laparoscopy may reduce overall complications, it also often demands that the surgeon complete an extensive preoperative outpatient evaluation of the potential operative candidate. The primary safeguard against an unexpected outcome is a thorough understanding of the patient's medical history with a complete physical examination and laboratory assessment. As in all other areas of medicine, indications and contraindications for these procedures must be considered. We must remember that not all surgical patients are candidates for endoscopic procedures. The health and well-being of our patients and the optimal surgical outcome must be considered of primary importance when assessing the approach to a particular surgical procedure.

If adequate technical expertise is developed by a surgeon and adequate tools are available, almost any procedure performed at laparotomy can be converted to an endoscopic approach. Untoward events that occur as a result of the technique used to accomplish a particular operation are considered complications of laparoscopic surgery. As difficult anatomic dissections are accomplished and more complex procedures are approached endoscopically, it is to be expected that we will see more unavoidable complications, as is observed at laparotomy. The objective of this chapter is to address those issues unique to endoscopic surgery in an effort to avoid serious injury.

Surgeons are trained to perform operative procedures using numerous techniques. With laparotomy the operative field is usually seen in three dimensional space, and tissues may be palpated. Structures are thus recognized by their appearance, their feel, and their relation to other structures. Endoscopic surgery reduces the visual aspect of a procedure to a two-dimensional field. The direct tactile aspect of the surgical procedure is eliminated. Knowledge of new instrumentation complemented by the acquisition of new skills is required for mastery of this arena.

Abdominal Entry

Blind entry into the abdominal cavity using a sharp instrument can cause major vessel injury and damage to adjacent vital intraperitoneal structures. Before beginning any endoscopic procedure, the surgeon must be familiar with the anatomy pertinent to the procedure and perhaps unique to the individual patient. The aorta and both iliac crests must be palpated to properly place the Veress needle or the umbilical trocar.[1] Correct technique with respect to insertion of the Veress needle is essential. One technique requires that the needle be placed in the abdominal cavity (this is necessary) with the stopcock in the open position to allow room air to enter the abdominal cavity as the needle tip enters the peritoneal space. The rush of room air entering the abdominal cavity through the needle as it passes through the abdominal wall theoretically displaces vital structures away from the tip. The needle should be placed with a careful smooth motion in order to avoid impaling structures against the sacral promontory. Awareness of the patient's position on the operating table is crucial for preventing injuries. When the patient is in the Trendelenburg position, the sacral promontory is rotated anteriorly. The angle of insertion must therefore be shallow to avoid damage to the retroperitoneal vessels (Figure 25.1).[2] Alternate sites for placement of the Veress needle should be considered if difficulty is encountered at the umbilicus. Left upper quadrant insufflation, transvaginal insufflation through the cul de sac, or transuterine placement of the Veress needle may be considered.[3] Alternatively, an open laparoscopic method with direct placement of a trocar sleeve may be used. Once the needle is in position, its proper placement must be verified, which can be accomplished by attaching a syringe to the needle, injecting 10–20 ml of physiologic solution, and aspirating. Should small bowel contents be aspirated, the needle may be removed and replaced in an adjacent location. Areas of injury may be visualized once the laparoscope has been safely placed in the abdominal cavity. Under most circumstances the muscular wall of the small intestine heals such small (≤ 1 mm) holes, and further treatment is not required.[4] Monitoring insufflation pressure carefully ensures proper placement of the Veress needle.

If blood is unexpectedly aspirated into the Veress needle, the needle is left in place to minimize hemorrhage, and immediate laparotomy is performed.[5] A large midline incision is required

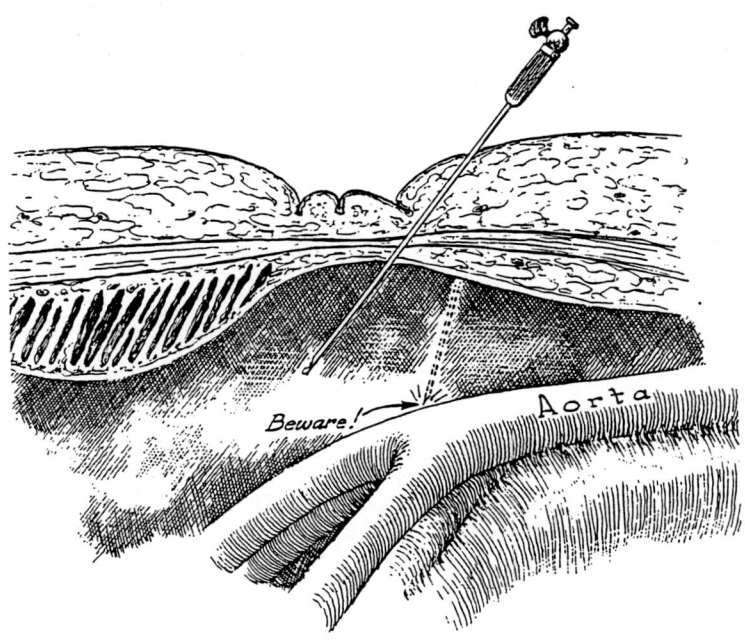

Figure 25.1. Angle of insertion of the Veress needle is essential. It must be shallow to avoid damage to the retroperitoneal vessels. (From Hulka et al.[2] Reprinted with permission)

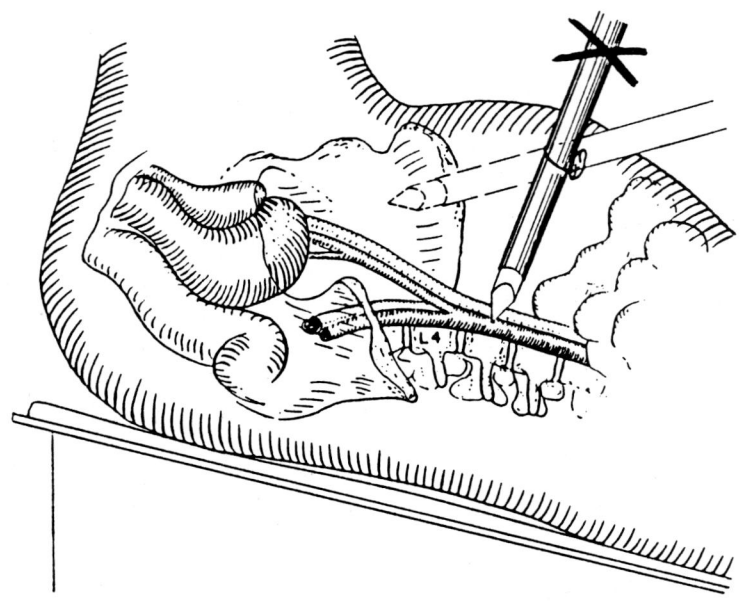

Figure 25.2. Retroperitoneal vessels may be in jeopardy if trocar insertion proceeds at an angle toward the umbilicus. (Reprinted from Phillips JM: *Laparoscopy*. Baltimore, Williams & Wilkins, 1977, with permission)

for adequate visualization and to control retroperitoneal bleeding. Immediately upon entering the abdomen, the surgeon's hand is used to occlude the aorta proximal to its bifurcation. If a retroperitoneal vessel has been injured, this maneuver allows resuscitation while appropriate assistance is obtained. Do not release the pressure on the aorta until vascular repair is under way, ideally with a vascular surgeon physically present. (Increasing damage to retroperitoneal vessels associated with a marked increase in morbidity occurs when surgeons repeatedly move the needle in an effort to change or verify its location.)

At closed laparoscopy primary trocar insertion is the final blind process during which major injuries can occur. Use of a sharp trocar is important to allow smooth, steady pressure for gently dividing the fibers of the fascia and allowing entry into the abdominal cavity. The use of disposable trocars with "safety shields" does not prevent injury to vital structures. If the pneumoperitoneum has already been established, additional elevation of the abdominal wall is not useful.[6] The surgeon's nondominant hand may be used to guide the trocar in a slow, steady fashion, thereby preventing sudden popping into the peritoneal cavity.

All accessory trocars are then placed under direct vision. Visualization may be lost as the peritoneum is tented during ancillary trocar insertions. Several techniques may be used to puncture the peritoneum before visualization is lost. A small, blunt instrument may be placed through the trocar sleeve and used to penetrate the peritoneum sharply. The secondary trocar tip must be angled toward the fundus of the uterus or toward the cul-de-sac. The retroperitoneal vessels may be in jeopardy if trocar insertion proceeds at an angle toward the umbilicus (Figure 25.2).[1]

The inferior epigastric vessels may be damaged during insertion of the accessory trocars. In some patients these vessels can be visualized intraabdominally prior to trocar insertion, but visualization may be difficult in other patients. Constant dripping of blood around the trocar sleeve is observed if these vessels have been injured. Hemostasis must be achieved before the vessels retract into the abdominal wall. It can be accomplished by threading a Foley catheter through the trocar sleeve, inflating the bulb, and using it to tamponade these vessels.[7] Alternately, unipolar or bipolar forceps may be introduced through another site and used to coapt the vessels. Finally, a large needle may be placed transabdominally and used for suture-ligation. All accessory trocar sleeves should be removed under direct vision at the end of the procedure to ensure adequate hemostasis in the abdominal wall.

The open laparoscopic technique has been used to avoid major vessel injury during umbilical trocar insertion. This technique, however, cannot prevent all injuries to the small or large bowel.[8] The small incision and compromised visibility may predispose to injury of underlying structures despite the open technique. Patients with a history of inflammatory bowel disease or those who have undergone multiple previous intraabdominal procedures are at increased risk for intestinal perforation at the time of trocar insertion. These patients should be advised that laparotomy may be required. Removal of the laparoscope with its sleeve at the end of a procedure while observing the abdominal wall layers ensures that a loop of bowel was not adherent underneath the insertion site. If the lumen of the small intestine is encountered as the trocar sleeve is withdrawn, the sleeve is left in situ, the incision extended slightly, and the loop of bowel pulled up through the incision. The bowel can then be repaired and replaced into the abdominal cavity. Care must be taken to avoid compromise of the lumen.

Isolated Bleeding

As more complex procedures are accomplished endoscopically there is an increased chance that venous and arterial bleeding may be encountered at sites of dissection. On occasion the instrumentation for attaining hemostasis malfunctions. The surgeon must anticipate the possibility of intraoperative hemorrhage and must be skilled in techniques available to achieve hemostasis. Mechanical, electrosurgical, laser, and suturing techniques have all been used successfully by skilled endoscopists to control bleeding. Each technique has its appropriate use depending on the size of the injured vascular structure and its proximity to vital organs. The pressure provided by the pneumoperitoneum during endoscopic surgery helps in obtaining hemostasis, but the surgeon must remain aware that this pressure may occlude venous, capillary, and even small arterial sources of bleeding. The combination of Trendelenburg position and pneumoperitoneum may therefore obscure bleeding. At the conclusion of the procedure, the patient must be taken out of Trendelenburg position and gas allowed to escape slowly while the surgeon monitors the operative field for previously unidentified bleeding sources. Some surgeons have chosen to place the abdomen "under water" using lactated Ringer's solution. After extensive endoscopic dissection where postoperative bleeding is more likely, a low-suction drain may be placed in the pelvis and the patient observed. Young, healthy patients may be slower to demonstrate clinical signs of hypovolemic shock. Therefore serial blood counts should be undertaken prior to discharge. Operative laparoscopy deserves the same respect as laparotomy, with monitoring of patients during the recovery period. Although major vessel injury is fortunately rare, it is essential to be able to perform emergency laparotomy and place digital pressure or vascular clamps across the aorta and other retroperitoneal vessels. The threshold for proceeding to laparotomy or for admitting the patient to the hospital for observation must not be compromised by the fact that these procedures are sometimes done in free-standing outpatient facilities.

Cardiovascular Complications

Gas embolism is a rare but potentially lethal complication of operative endoscopic procedures.[9] The U.S. Food and Drug Administration (FDA) has issued an alert regarding the use of air-cooled YAG laser tips during hysteroscopy.[10] This document also comments on the possibility of gas embolism at laparoscopy. The diagnosis is made on the basis of a sudden drop in arterial pressure, a fall in end-tidal CO_2, and an associated "millwheel" murmur across the precordium. Treatment includes immediate cessation of insufflation, turning the patient to the left lateral decubitus position, providing appropriate resuscitation, and placing a central venous catheter in the right ventricle to withdraw the gas.[11] Modern methods of "gasless" laparoscopy may eliminate this concern.

Cardiac arrhythmias and particularly vagal stimulation are not uncommon with initial insufflation of the abdomen. Rapid high pressure insufflation should be avoided in order to allow the self-regulatory mechanisms within the cardiovascular system to adjust for increased pressure on the venous structures. Although anesthesiologists treat these conditions and with appropriate monitoring they should not become a significant problem, care and proper surgical technique may allow their avoidance in most circumstances.

Intestinal Complications

Injury to the large or small intestine is one of the most serious and common complications of operative laparoscopy (Figure 25.3).[8] Intestinal damage occurs by mechanical means via insertion of primary or secondary trocars or during dissection of adhesions. In addition, bowel injuries may be caused by the use of any energy source within the abdomen. The most worrisome injury to the bowel is inadvertent unipolar coagulation, as the extent of damage may be 2–5 cm beyond the area of apparent injury. Necrosis, delayed bowel perforation, and peritonitis can result. Wide resection of the bowel is prudent when unipolar coagulation injury occurs. Superficial blanching caused by laser or bipolar instruments is more discrete and may be managed more conservatively.

The problem of injury secondary to capacitance coupling is relatively unique to endoscopic surgery when unipolar instrumentation is used. A capacitor is a device capable of storing electrical energy (Figure 25.4).[2] The laparoscope becomes a capacitor when insulated unipolar instruments are used through an operating channel, and it may discharge electrical energy when it touches the intestine. It is possible for this event to occur outside the operator's visual field. Metal trocar sleeves allow the current

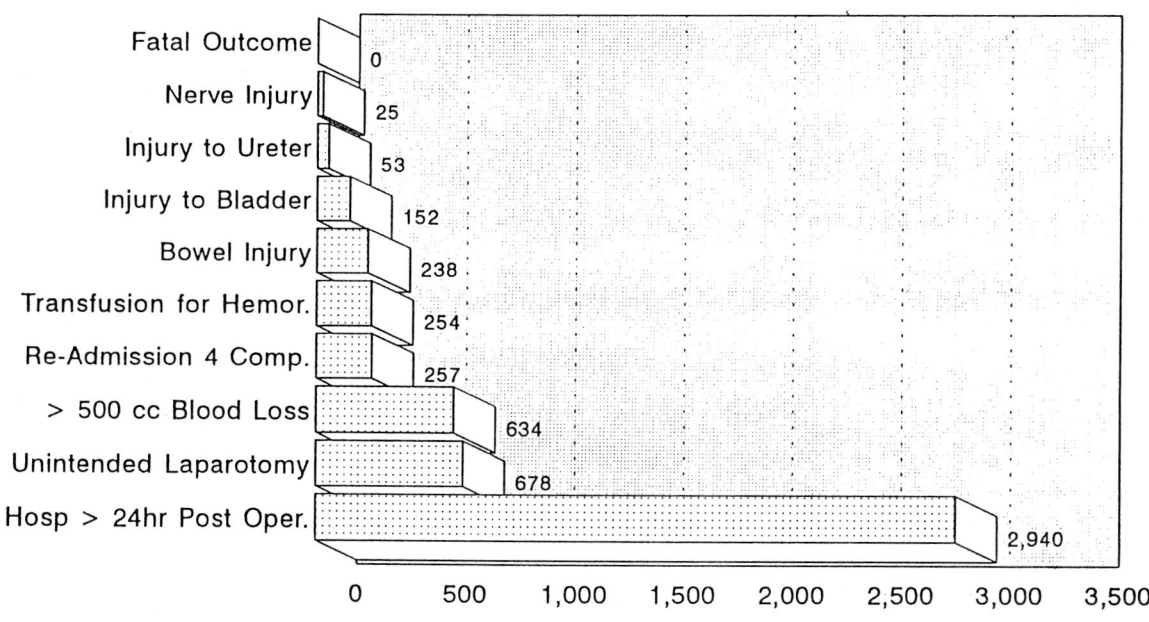

Figure 25.3. 1993 Operative laparoscopy complications survey from the AAGL. Note that injury to the large or small intestine is one of the most serious and common complications of operative laparoscopy. There were 80,031 total cases reported.

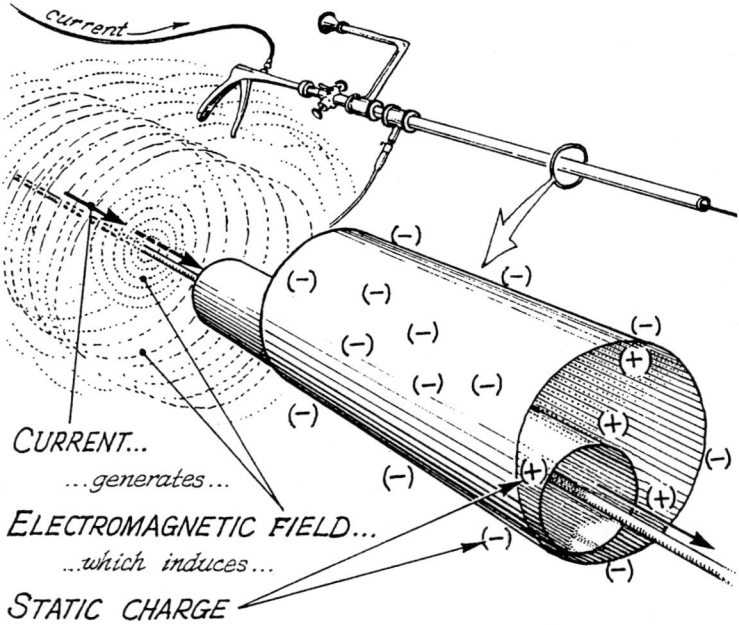

Figure 25.4. Unipolar induction of capacitance. The capacitor is a device capable of storing electrical energy. (From Hulka et al.[2] Reprinted with permission)

stored within the laparoscope to exit the abdominal cavity, pass through the abdominal wall, and travel back to the return electrode without being stored intraabdominally. The potential for injury increases, however, when hybrid trocar sleeves are used. If the metal instruments are isolated from the abdominal wall by an intervening plastic anchoring sleeve, sufficient energy may be stored in the laparoscope to cause inadvertent bowel injury.

Traumatic injury to the intestine can be managed by oversewing the area of perforation, which can be accomplished in one of two ways: (1) endoscopically suturing the tissues; or (2) extending the incision slightly, elevating the damaged bowel outside the abdomen, and performing a repair. The bowel wall opposite the area of perforation must also be inspected. Through-and-through perforation, especially with sharp disposable instruments is not uncommon.

The act of touching the bowel with a recently activated electrical instrument usually does not cause harm. However, unipolar or bipolar energy applied to the bowel wall while lysing adhesions or coagulating vessels may cause an extensive area of necrosis. Should a persistent blanched area be identified, resection of the bowel is indicated. When doubt exists about a possible bowel injury, the patient must be observed carefully during the postoperative period. Any increase in pelvic or abdominal pain, temperature elevation, or increase in abdominal distension should evoke strong consideration for immediate evaluation and possible surgical exploration. Classic laboratory and routine imaging studies may not be helpful for diagnosing bowel injuries. The presence of free air under the diaphragm is confusing in a patient who has recently undergone an endoscopic procedure with pneumoperitoneum. The classic findings—leukocytosis and elevated temperature—may not be present. Failure to recognize this complication and treat it expeditiously has led to several deaths.[12]

Bladder Perforation

Bladder perforation occasionally occurs during insertion of the secondary trocar.[13] This injury usually occurs in the dome of the bladder and can be managed simply by placing an indwelling catheter for a period of 7–14 days. The small, clean-edged wound tends to heal spontaneously. Laparoscopic sutures may also be placed; however, an indwelling catheter is still required for the same duration of time. The bladder is at risk as well during laparoscopic hysterectomy. Significant scarring may be present, most commonly due to previous cesarean sections or pelvic endometriosis, and may make bladder dissection difficult. Recognition of a bladder injury intraoperatively permits appropriate management under the same anesthetic. The use of indigo carmine administered intravenously aids in the identification of urinary tract trauma. Methylene blue should not be used in that it appears to be associated with methemoglobinemia.

Ureteral Injuries

The ureter is at risk primarily at three locations within the pelvis: at the pelvic brim as it travels medially to the ovarian vessels; at the level of the uterine arteries when it travels just underneath them; and at the level of the uterosacral ligaments prior to entering the posterior wall of the bladder. Fortunately, these injuries are relatively uncommon.[14,15] Strict adherence to proper surgical technique, ureteral dissection, and appropriate use of traction and countertraction help maintain ureteral integrity. Lighted ureteral stents may be placed preoperatively for easier visualization of the ureter in cases where difficult retroperitoneal dissection is anticipated. Thermal injury and late necrosis of the ureter may occur with either laser or electrosurgical techniques. Coagulation of endometriosis along the pelvic side wall and uterosacral nerve ablation place the ureters at increased risk. Lateral thermal spread of energy occurs even with bipolar coagulation techniques or CO_2 lasers. Unless careful ureteral dissection has been accomplished, use of a linear stapling device is risky. Its size makes it difficult to see the entire length of the two jaws, and the ureter may be transected inadvertently. With injury to only one ureter, symptoms may be subtle. Patients usually complain of flank pain or ascites. An intravenous pyelogram may not demonstrate a small perforation within the ureter. The diagnosis may be verified by injecting 5 ml of indigo carmine intravenously and performing culdocentesis or an abdominal tap 1–2 hours later. Small pinpoint injuries to the ureter may be managed conservatively. If it is possible to thread a ureteral catheter past the area of injury, a small perforation may close spontaneously without a need for laparotomy and ureteral reanastamosis. When the diagnosis has been significantly delayed, epithelialization may have occurred, and this technique will not be successful. Transection of the ureter or a larger defect requires surgical repair.

Delayed Complications

Delayed bleeding can follow any operative procedure. Temporary tamponade of vessels may have been produced by the pneumoperitoneum or with the use of intraoperative vasoconstrictors. Small vessels may also retract between the staple rows of linear cutting devices and lead to a large retroperitoneal hematoma. Injury to the inferior epigastric vessels may have been obscured by the trocar sleeve intraoperatively and may present with bleeding in the recovery room. Many of these patients do not present the usual signs and symptoms of hypovolemic shock until a large volume of blood has been lost. Monitoring fluid requirements and performing serial blood counts in the recovery room is frequently more useful than relying on routine vital signs for prompt identification of postoperative bleeding. This choice may permit earlier reexploration and perhaps avoidance of blood transfusion.

Life-threatening, delayed complications such as pulmonary embolus are rare but do occur. Unrecognized damage to the bowel, bladder, or ureter may not become symptomatic for 7–10 days postoperatively. Postoperative patients with increasing abdominal pain, distention, or fever must be seen and evaluated in a facilitated manner. With the use of larger trocars in recent years, the development of incarcerated hernias has become a problem. Patients presenting with postoperative distention and bowel obstruction should be evaluated for an incarcerated hernia within the trocar site. This complication may be prevented by closing the fascia with a single stitch when trocars > 5 mm are used.

Complications of Operative Hysteroscopy

Operative hysteroscopy includes the relatively straightforward procedures of endometrial ablation, myomectomy, and septum division and the management of Asherman syndrome. The overall complication rate for operative hysteroscopy as reported in the AAGL survey was approximately 2% with a major complication rate of < 1%.[16]

Introduction of rigid instruments into a confined space may lead to inadvertent perforation of the uterus or laceration of the cervix. Preexisting cervical stenosis predisposes to these complications. Placement of *Laminaria* tents preoperatively may soften the cervix and allow more gentle dilation. This measure may thus decrease the risk of cervical laceration with the tenaculum and uterine perforation. The presence of uterine anomalies also creates difficulties. Concomitant laparoscopy should be planned when scheduling a procedure to correct an intrauterine septum or for Asherman syndrome.[17]

The use of uterine distention medium for adequate visualization of the intrauterine environment creates unique challenges and hazards during hysteroscopy. Carbon dioxide gas is frequently used for diagnostic procedures, as it provides excellent visualization in a nonbloody field. With the use of low flow, low pressure insufflators specifically designed for hysteroscopic surgery, the risk of embolism is low. Despite the large venous sinuses present within the uterus, which are capable of absorbing large volumes of gas, few problems have arisen. Corson and Hoffman have demonstrated that direct intravenous injection of carbon dioxide gas produces minimal cardiovascular consequences with gas volumes of < 400 cc/min.[18] Current low flow insufflators are designed to deliver less than 100 cc of gas per minute. Several deaths have been reported from carbon dioxide embolism as a result of gas-cooled Nd:YAG fiber tips used for intrauterine surgery. Flow rates for these gas cooled systems are > 1 L/min. The FDA has issued a safety alert warning never to use gas-cooled laser fibers or tips for intrauterine surgery.[10]

Liquid media provide better visualization during operative hysteroscopic procedures. High-molecular-weight dextran has been associated with a rare anaphylactic reaction.[19] Less commonly, intravascular fluid overload has occurred, with development of pulmonary edema. High-molecular-weight dextran is a highly hyperosmolar solution. When large volumes are absorbed intravenously, water is pulled into the intravascular space, and pulmonary edema can develop. This complication can be managed with judicious use of diuretics along with administration of the appropriate electrolyte solutions to provide adequate total body water replacement. This problem can be minimized by limiting the total volume of Hyskon to < 350 cc per procedure.

Low viscosity fluids—sorbitol, glycine, and 5% dextrose in water (D_5W) are popular because they allow excellent visualization while permitting conduction of electrical current. They are used predominantly with the resectoscope for endometrial ablation and myoma resection. Much higher volumes of these solutions can be used because they are miscible with blood. Continuous-flow systems are required to allow adequate visibility. The low viscosity fluid contains no sodium, and therefore rapid intravascular absorption of large volumes may lead to hyponatremia, fluid overload, and pulmonary and cerebral edema. Constant monitoring of intake and outflow volumes during resectoscope procedures and limitation of the total duration of surgery to 60–90 minutes decrease the probability of this serious complication.[20,21] When 1000 ml or more of distention fluid is unaccounted for, serum electrolytes should be assayed and diuretics administered as necessary. For patients with significant underlying cardiovascular disease, it may be prudent to consider central venous pressure monitoring during the procedure for more accurate assessment of volume status.

The major metabolite of glycine is ammonia. There are a few reports of central nervous system (CNS) compromise, with encephalopathy and transient blindness thought to be secondary to high blood glycine level and hyperammonemia.[22]

Infection

Many authors recommend the use of prophylactic antibiotics for all patients undergoing operative hysteroscopic procedures.[23] Serious pelvic infections after hysteroscopic surgery have been reported, especially in patients with a history of pelvic inflammatory disease or hydrosalpinges.[24] These patients are candidates for prophylactic antibiotics and close monitoring postoperatively. Hysteroscopic surgery is contraindicated in patients with active pelvic infection.

Hemorrhagic Complications

Excessive bleeding during hysteroscopic surgery is uncommon, but bleeding problems may be encountered when myomas are resected deep into the uterine wall or during endomyometrial resection for ablation. False passages created during dilation through a stenotic cervix may also bleed profusely. The use of vasoconstrictors, specifically dilute vasopressin (e.g., 10–20 U in 100 ml of irrigation solution) in small volumes, has been recommended.[25] Cardiac arrhythmias have been reported with the use of vasoconstrictors in this capacity. A dilute vasopressin solution injected directly into the cervix can provide adequate hemostasis for most procedures. If it is insufficient, a large Foley catheter may be placed transcervically into the endometrial cavity, inflated with 15–30 ml of fluid, and left in place for several hours. Slow deflation of the Foley bulb and observation ensure that adequate hemostasis has been achieved.[26] This foreign body in the endometrial cavity does create significant postoperative cramping, and it may be useful to place a long-acting local anesthetic in the cervix for patient comfort.

Damage to Adjacent Organs

Injury to the bowel or bladder is an uncommon but serious complication of hysteroscopic procedures. In general, injuries have occurred subsequent to perforation of the uterus with an active electrode or engaged laser fiber. Extreme caution must be exercised, therefore, when resecting or ablating near the cornua because of the thin myometrial wall. Extra care is also required in patients with surgical scars from prior cesarean sections or myomectomy. One case of total necrosis of the myometrium subsequent to high energy YAG ablation has been reported.[27] There are anecdotal reports of resection into the bladder, into adjacent bowel, and even into the iliac arteries during resectoscope surgery (unpublished legal cases). If visualization is lost during a resectoscopic procedure, perforation probably has occurred, and all surgical manipulation must cease immediately. Laparoscopy or, if deemed necessary, laparotomy should be performed to assess intraabdominal damage.

Cancer

Critics of endometrial ablation have postulated that the procedure could bury functioning endometrial glands underneath a scar layer.[28] Theoretically, these glands could undergo malignant transformation with the usual bleeding signs and symptoms obscured by the overlying scar tissue. Although it remains a hypothetical problem worthy of continued scrutiny, to date only one case of delayed diagnosis of uterine cancer has been reported.[28]

Miscellaneous Complications

Creation of cervical stenosis has occurred when endometrial ablation is carried down to the internal cervical os. Patients should be followed postoperatively for development of cervical stenosis with accompanying hematocolpos. The cervical canal may be gently probed at each follow-up visit to ensure patency.

Pregnancy has occurred subsequent to endometrial ablation (personal communication). The procedure does not ensure sterility, and patients must be counseled to use alternate methods of contraception. Significant complications have occurred in the pregnancies subsequent to endometrial ablation due to implantation of the placenta in the myometrium. These pregnancies have had exceptionally poor outcomes, and patients must be forewarned.

Conclusion

Fortunately, serious complications of operative endoscopic procedures are rare. A major injury rate of 2.73% was reported during the first 8 months of 1993 in the AAGL survey of operative laparoscopic complications.[8] This figure compares favorably with that for laparotomy. Nevertheless, many complications appear to be preventable with good surgical experience and training. These procedures are highly technical and depend on properly functioning equipment. Rigid maintenance of equipment, proper patient selection, well trained operating room personnel, and continuing medical education can help develop and maintain excellence. Prompt diagnosis and management of unavoidable complications can lead to improved patient outcomes, and theoretically the chances of complications are then reduced.

References

1. PENFIELD AJ: Trocar and needle injuries. In Laparoscopy, Phillips JM (Ed). Baltimore, Williams & Wilkins, 1977, pp 236–241.
2. HULKA JF, REICH H: Abdominal entry. In Textbook of Laparoscopy (2nd ed), Hulka JF, Reich H (eds). Philadelphia, W.B. Saunders, 1994, pp 85–102.
3. SODERSTROM RM, LEVINSON C, LEVY B: Complications of operative laparoscopy. In Operative Laparoscopy, The Masters' Techniques, Soderstrom RM (ed). New York, Raven Press, 1993, pp 187–197.
4. LOFFER FD, PENT D: Indications, contraindications, and complications of laparoscopy. Obstet Gynecol Surv 1975;30:407.
5. MCDONALD PT, RICH NM, COLLINS GC, ET AL: Vascular trauma secondary to diagnostic and therapeutic procedures: laparoscopy. Am J Surg 1978; 135:651.
6. CORSON SL: Major vessel injury during laparoscopy [letter]. Am J Obstet Gynecol 1980;138:589.
7. JOHNS DA: Perforation of the inferior epigastric vessels. In Complications of Laparoscopy and Hysteroscopy. Corfman RS, Diamond MP, DeCherney A (eds). Boston, Blackwell Scientific, 1993, pp 38–41.
8. LEVY BS, HULKA JF, PETERSON HB, ET AL: Complications of Operative Laparoscopy: American Association of Gynecologic Laparoscopists 1993 Membership Survey J Am Assoc Gyn Laparos 1994;1:301.
9. YACOUB OF, CARDONA I JR., COVERLET LA, ET AL: Carbon dioxide embolism during laparoscopy. Anesthesiology 1982;57:533.
10. FOOD AND DRUG ADMINISTRATION: Gas/Air Embolism Associated with Intrauterine Laser Surgery. FDA Safety Alert. Rockville, MD, FDA, 1990.
11. CHANTIGIAN RC, CHANTIGIAN DM: Anesthesia for laparoscopy. In Complications of Laparoscopy and Hysteroscopy, Corfman RS, Diamond MP, DeCherney A (eds). Boston: Blackwell Scientific, 1993, pp 11–21.
12. SODERSTROM RM: Bowel injury litigation after laparoscopy. Am Assoc Gynecol Laparosc 1993; 1:74.
13. REICH H, MCGLYNN F: Laparoscopic repair of bladder injury. Obstet Gynecol 1990;76:909.
14. GRAINGER DA, SODERSTROM RM, SCHIFF SF, ET AL: Urethral injuries at laparoscopy: insights into diagnosis, management, and prevention. Obstet Gynecol. 1990;75:839.
15. WOODLAND MB: Ureter injury during laparoscopy-assisted vaginal hysterectomy with the endoscopic linear stapler. Am J Obstet Gynecol 1992;167:756.
16. HULKA JF, PETERSON HB, PHILLIPS JM, ET AL: Operative Hysteroscopy American Association of Gynecologic Laparoscopists 1991 Membership Survey. J Reprod Med 1993;38:572.
17. VALLE RF: Cervical and uterine complications during insertion of the hysteroscope. In Complications of Laparoscopy and Hysteroscopy. Corfman RS, Diamond MP, DeCherney A (eds). Boston, Blackwell Scientific, 1993, pp 167–176.
18. CORSON SL, HOFFMAN JJ: Cardiopulmonary effects of direct venous carbon dioxide insufflation. J Reprod Med 1988;433.

19. AHMED N, FALCONE T, TULANDI T, ET AL: Anaphylactic reaction because of intrauterine 32% dextran-70 installation. Fertil Steril 1991;55:440.
20. ARIEFF AI, AYUS JC: Endometrial ablation complicated by fatal hyponatremic encephalopathy. JAMA 1993;270:1230.
21. WITZ CA, SILVERBERG KM, BURNS WN, ET AL: Complications associated with the absorption of hysteroscopic fluid media. Fertil Steril 1993;60:745.
22. HOEKSTRA PT, KAHNOSKI R, MCCAMISH MA, ET AL: Transurethral prostatic resection syndrome: a new perspective: encephalopathy with associated hyperammonemia. J Urol 1983;130:704.
23. SERDEN SP, BROOKS PG: Treatment of abnormal uterine bleeding with the gynecologic resectoscope. J Reprod Med 1991;36:697.
24. COHEN MR, DMOWSKI WP: Modern hysteroscopy: diagnostic and therapeutic potential. Fertil Steril 1973;24:905.
25. CORSON SL, BROOKS PG: Resectoscopic myomectomy. Fertil Steril 1991;55:1041.
26. BROOKS, PG: Complications of operative hysteroscopy: how safe is it? Clin Obstet Gynecol 1992;35:256.
27. PERRY CP, DANIELL JF, GIMPELSON RJ: Bowel injury from Nd:YAG endometrial ablation. J Gynecol Surg 1990;6:199.
28. COPPERMAN AB, DECHERNEY AH, OLIVE DL: A case of endometrial cancer following endometrial ablation for dysfunctional uterine bleeding. Obstet Gynecol 1993;82:640.

26
Adhesion Prevention and Lysis: Indications for Laparotomy and Laparoscopy

Michael P. Diamond and Esat Orhon

Pelvic organs ideally must be in an adhesion-free environment to function properly. Adhesions may interfere with ovum release, pickup, and transport, resulting in primary or secondary infertility. In fact, pelvic adhesions are a major factor contributing to infertility,[1] as they are present in approximately 25% of infertile women.[2] In the presence of adhesions, pregnancy rates range between 22% and 64%.[1,3] If structures adjacent to pelvic organs are affected by adhesions, malfunction and pain due to peritoneal stretch may result. Adhesions are also a major cause of dyspareunia and partial or complete bowel obstruction. Thus the development and, more importantly, the prevention of postoperative adhesions should be a major consideration of all surgeons.

Major advances in operative techniques and instrument design have played a significant role in attempting to reachieve normal pelvic anatomy. The performance of endoscopic surgical procedures is increasing, in part because of technologic innovations and the increasing experience of surgeons. Although laparoscopic procedures, in contrast to those done by laparotomy, are theorized to be associated with a reduction in hospitalization and more rapid recovery, a major question is whether this technology offers an improved outcome. Unfortunately, most clinical studies are descriptive in nature and do not provide an adequate basis for comparison with laparotomy. One must consider whether DeCherney's prediction that laparotomy for pelvic reconstructive surgery would come to an end[4] has yet been fulfilled or there remains a place for laparotomy in the treatment of tuboperitoneal disease.

Definitions

Adhesions are defined as anatomic connections between surfaces at locations where connections do not normally exist. *Adhesion reformation* refers to the recurrence of adhesions after adhesiolysis. *De novo adhesion* refers to existence of new adhesions that developed at sites that did not previously have adhesions.[5] Adhesions may result with any type of surgical procedure involving laparoscopy or laparotomy, but the degree of adhesion formation and subsequent complication rate differs with each surgical approach.[6-9]

Mechanism of Adhesion Formation

Adhesion formation is an integral process of wound healing.[10,11] Once peritoneal surface injury occurs (Figs. 26.1, 26.2), there is an out-

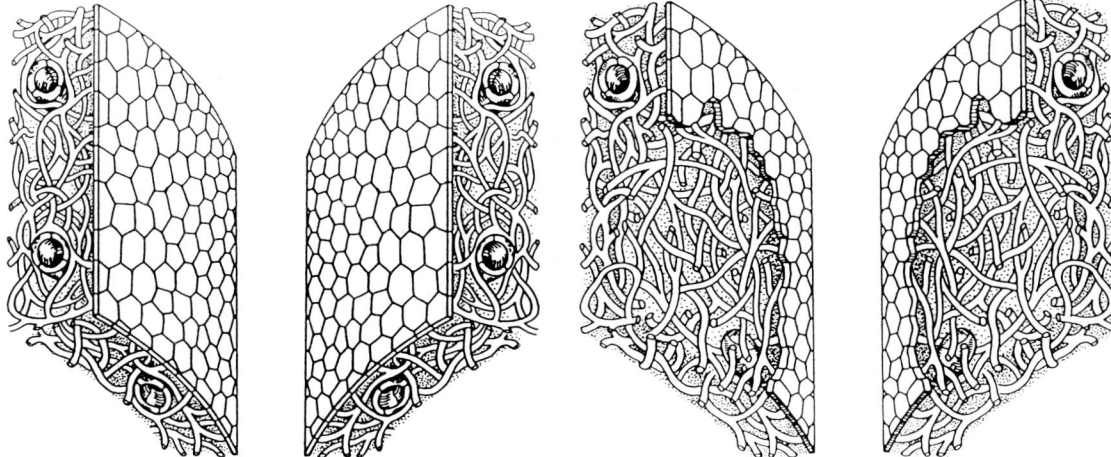

Figure 26.1. Neighboring peritoneal surfaces. (From Diamond.[12] Reprinted with permission.)

Figure 26.2. Peritoneal defect extending into subperitoneal tissues with resultant damage to peritoneum, underlying connective tissue, and vessels. (From Diamond.[12] Reprinted with permission.)

pouring of a serosanguineous exudate that contains histamine and other vasoactive substances. It leads to an increase in capillary permeability that accelerates the flow of serosanguineous fluid(s) and includes inflammatory cells such as monocytes, plasma cells, polymorphonuclear cells, and histiocytes (Fig. 26.3). Within approximately 3 hours, this high protein-containing fluid coagulates, creating fibrinous bands between corresponding surfaces. This process is thought to be initiated and is well advanced within the first 72 hours postoperatively[10,11] (Fig. 26.4). Within this time frame, fibrin accumulation may undergo fibrinolysis, in which case adhesions do not form. If the balance between fibrin deposition and fibrinolysis leads to fibrin accumulation, fibroblast infiltration and proliferation occurs with collagen deposition and subsequent generation of an adhesion[11,12] (Fig. 26.5). The injured peritoneal surface is

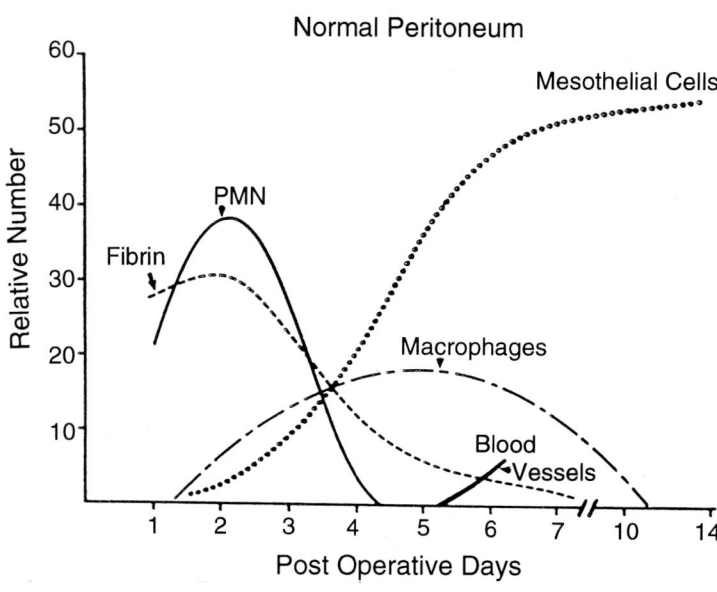

Figure 26.3. Change in the relative number of cellular elements and fibrinolysis (fibrin) at the site of peritoneal injury in mature rats during the course of reepithelialization. (From Gutmann and Diamond.[11] Reprinted with permission.)

26. Adhesion Prevention and Lysis

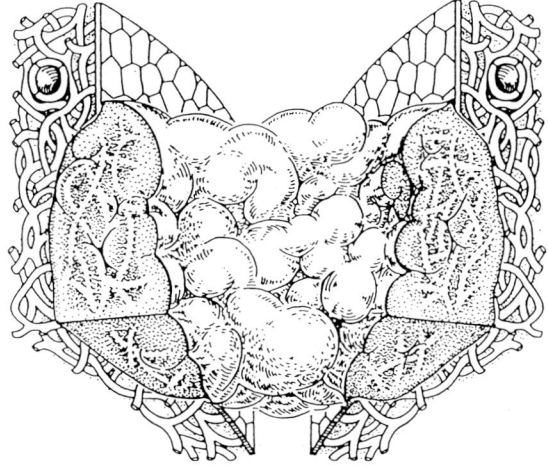

Figure 26.4. Proteinaceous exudate forming over the injured peritoneal surfaces as a consequence of vascular damage and increased vascular permeability. The result is connection of adjoining peritoneal surfaces by the proteinaceous exudate. (From Diamond.[12] Reprinted with permission.)

then repaired within 7 days. The source of the new peritoneal cells is multipotential subperitoneal cells (Figs. 26.6, 26.7, 26.8). The latter stages, which progress over several years, include vascularization and thickening of the adhesive bands.

The question that must be asked, then, is why fibrinolysis occurs? Although answers to this important question are still being sought, one known important factor is that fibrinolysis requires good tissue oxygenation. Whatever interferes with oxygenation and creates tissue ischemia is a nidus for adhesion formation. Ischemia may result from aggressive handling, pressure application, suturing, or stripping of surfaces. Ischemia also induces angiogenesis, which increases the density and thickness of adhesions. Any aggressive procedure or pressure applied to the peritoneum may lead to cell desquamation and resultant fibrin deposition, which elicits adhesion formation mechanisms. The presence of a foreign body may also in-

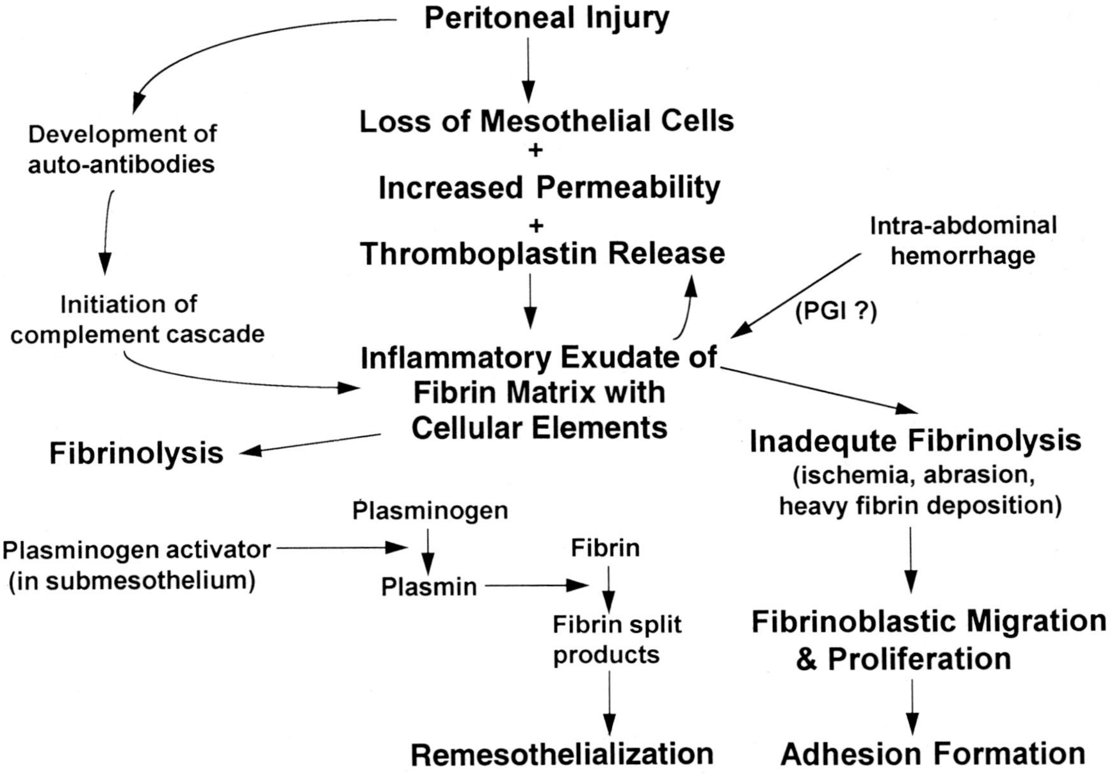

Figure 26.5. Putative mechanism for adhesion formation. (From Gutmann and Diamond.[11] Reprinted with permission.)

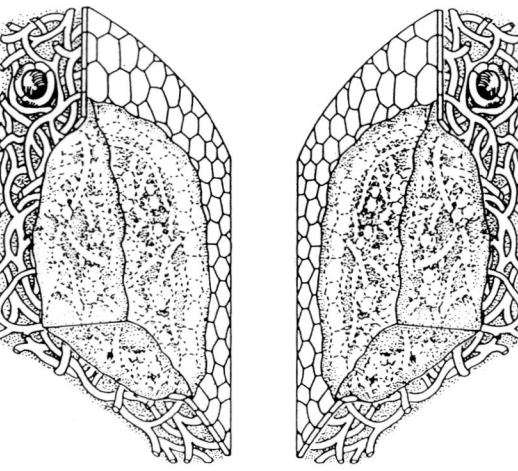

Figure 26.6. As a result of endogenous fibrinolytic activity residing in the peritoneum, the proteinaceous mass has been partially degraded. Note that the mass no longer connects adjoining peritoneal surfaces. Note also the initial generation of new peritoneal cells at the base of the defect. (From Diamond.[12] Reprinted with permission.)

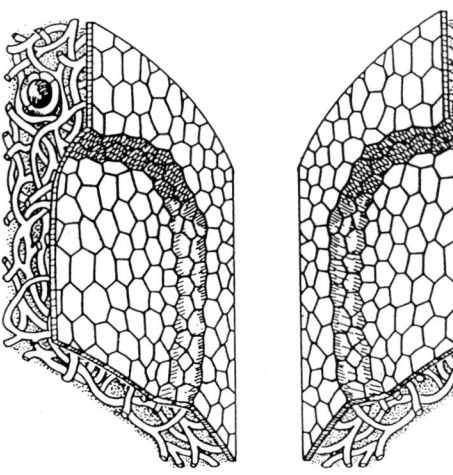

Figure 26.8. Completed healing of the peritoneal surface without adhesion development. (From Diamond.[12] Reprinted with permission.)

crease fibrin deposition, such as during laparotomy when talc or other type of powder is placed inadvertently on the abdominal cavity. This foreign body may be absorbed by mesothelial cells, resulting in an inflammatory process. Any inflammatory process may cause, to a certain extent, cell death or desquamation. Suturing results in fibrin deposition secondary to a foreign body and to tissue ischemia. Lastly, in the past free blood accumulation has been considered to be a major cause for adhesion formation, but this belief has not been supported by any evidence or controlled study. Free blood probably does not cause an adhesion per se without the presence of a foreign body or tissue ischemia.

Significance of Adhesions

Adhesions are widely accepted to be the causative factors of primary or secondary infertility, pelvic pain, dyspareunia, and partial or complete bowel obstruction.[13] The relation of pelvic pain and adhesions is difficult to establish definitively. Pain is not always directly proportional to the amount or density of the adhesions. Pain arising from the uterus or fallopian tubes travels via visceral afferent nerves to the lower thoracic and lumbar sympathetic ganglion and enters the spinal cord at T10–L1. Dysmenorrhea has also been claimed to be secondary to pelvic adhesions.[14] In a study of 100 patients, "pain creating adhesions" was found to be restricting organ motility and expendability. With the exis-

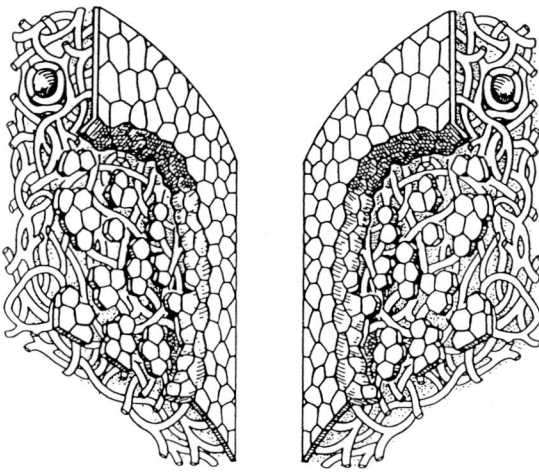

Figure 26.7. Continued fibrinolytic activity has resulted in total resolution of the proteinaceous mass. Peritoneal cells continue to proliferate. (From Diamond.[12] Reprinted with permission.)

Table 26.1. Pregnancy outcome following adhesiolysis

Author	Modality	Surgery	Laser	No. of pts.	Pregnancy No.	%
Wallach et al.	Laparotomy	Macro	—	94	43	46
Jansen	Laparotomy	Macro	—	64	26	40
O'Brien et al.	Laparotomy	Macro	—	41	16	39
Betz et al.	Laparotomy	Macro	—	29	20	69
Grant	Laparotomy	Macro	—	268	94	35
Caspi et al.	Laparotomy	Micro	—	101	38	38
Donnez & Casanas-Roux	Laparotomy	Micro	—	42	27	64
Diamond	Laparotomy	Macro	—	220	55	25
	Laparotomy	Micro	—	140	80	57
Tulandi	Laparotomy	Micro	—	33	17	52
	Laparotomy	Micro	+	30	16	53
Frantzen & Schlosser	Laparotomy	Micro	—	49	20	41
Gomel	Laparoscopy		—	92	54	59
Fayez	Laparoscopy		—	50	23	46
Donnez & Nisolle	Laparoscopy		+	186	108	58
Laparotomy total				1111	452	41
Macrosurgery				716	254	36
Microsurgery				395	198	50
Laparoscopy total				328	185	56

Modified from Diamond.[1] Reprinted with permission.

tence of periuterine adhesions, uterine cramps may cause pain during menstruation due to distortion or "pulling of adjacent" organs or the pelvic side wall.[14] Adhesions are identified in 25% of infertile women[2]; and after adhesiolysis pregnancy is achieved in 35–69%.[1–15] Table 26.1 provides pregnancy outcome following adhesiolysis. Tulandi et al.[16] evaluated the incidence of pregnancy in a controlled study of women with pelvic adhesions with or without laparoscopic adhesiolysis. Of 38 patients, 19 underwent salpingoovariolysis, and 19 were observed expectantly. Pregnancy rates at 12, 24, and 36 months were 27%, 67%, and 67%, respectively, in women undergoing adhesiolysis, compared to 27%, 45%, and 52% in the expectantly managed group. In both groups the presence of severe adhesions significantly reduced pregnancy rates.[16]

There are several studies that correlate relief of pelvic pain, dysmenorrhea, and dyspareunia with adhesiolysis. In one study 43 patients with adhesions were observed for 6 months after adhesiolysis: 28 (65%) noted complete or partial pain relief after 6 months.[17] The rate of pain relief after adhesiolysis was 38–75%.[13]

Reports published to date show great variation in the consistency of adhesion scoring systems.[5] Ideal criteria to achieve consistency in the reporting should include location, extent, severity, and the structures that are adherent.

Prevention

As the clinical importance of adhesions is well understood, prevention has became one of the main concerns in gynecologic surgery, especially in the young or reproductive-age patient. Various modes of therapy are being studied. The following items are known to be the factors that can affect the degree of adhesion development.

1. *Surgical techniques:* With laparotomy the rules of "microsurgery" are well defined.[18,19] Peritoneal injury, foreign bodies (e.g., glove powder), use of dry sponges, tissue dehydration,

and extensive use of suturing and cauterization are but a few of the problems. Appropriate hemostasis with minimal adjacent tissue destruction is essential. Additionally, it has been stated that precise tissue approximation reduces postoperative adhesion formation. However, animal and human studies[20-22] involving second look laparoscopy[11,14,23,24] suggest that leaving the peritoneum without approximation may be associated with fewer adhesions, perhaps because tissue ischemia secondary to suturing is prevented, and may be apparent with both visceral and parietal peritoneum. These studies raise the question of whether leaving the peritoneum or ovary "open" is superior to even microsurgical reapproximation.

2. *Instrumentation:* Many microsurgical fine instruments are available for reproductive open operations as well as endoscopic surgical procedures. Needle cautery, microscissors, atraumatic forceps, and sculptured laser tips are but a few. The effects of various types of cautery and laser are well known,[25] but convincing evidence of distinct advantages of one modality over another is lacking.

3. *Modalities:* When endoscopy was introduced to reproductive surgery, a certain degree of optimism was apparent internationally. After many years of experience authors are now more prudent. There have been no well designed, controlled clinical studies that demonstrate the inferiority of laparotomy compared to laparoscopy.

4. *Adjuvants:* Adjuvants can be classified by the "stage of action" in the adhesion development cascade. Adjuvants target fibrinolysis, coagulation, inflammatory response, and infections; or they serve as barriers. Among the adjuvants are pharmacologic agents administered intravenously or intraperitoneally (e.g., antibiotics, antihistamines, corticosteroids, heparin, and nonsteroidal antiinflammatory drugs, or NSAIDs), hydrotubation (with or without the addition of pharmacologic agents), intraperitoneal dextran, and intraperitoneal (adhesion prevention) barriers. Of the various categories of adjuvants, those that act as a barrier are currently undergoing the most intensive investigation. The mechanism by which such adjuvants appear to be effective is physical separation of the adjoining surfaces of reperitonealization. Barriers can be categorized according to whether they are synthetic products or natural tissues (e.g., amnion, peritoneum, omentum). Among the exogenous types of barrier, some are resorbable whereas others require a second operative procedure for removal.[26] Unfortunately, none is yet "perfect." The use of adjuvants has been reviewed elsewhere[11] and so is only summarized here.

A classification scheme for adhesion-reducing adjuvants is presented in Table 26.2. The ideal adhesion prevention barrier performs a variety of functions. First, its use must be associated with a low risk of complications and side effects. Inherent within this criterion is the property of low tissue reactivity, thereby minimizing establishment of a tissue inflammatory reaction. Second, the barrier should be easy to handle and apply. Third, it should adhere on its own, not requiring sutures or foreign material to secure it in place. Fourth, the barrier should be absorbable so as not to necessitate a subsequent operative procedure for its removal. Finally, the barrier must be efficacious in reducing adhesion formation or reformation.

One barrier used to reduce postoperative adhesions is generic (Interceed, or TC-7). The parent material from which this fabric was derived is oxidized regenerated cellulose. It is relatively simple to apply and conforms to the structure (i.e., adheres in place). The material gelates within hours of placement; and the appearance and postoperative examination (at 2 weeks minimum) usually reveals no gross remnants of it. Thus use of TC-7 does not require a second operative procedure for its removal.[26]

A second barrier that is used is Gore-Tex® surgical membrane (generic). It is a permanent inert microporous implant of expanded polytetrafluoroethylene, which has been shown to decrease adhesion formation in an animal model.[27]

High-molecular-weight substances have also been used as barriers. 32% Dextran 70 (Hyskon) is one example, although it has not been approved for this indication. This material coats surfaces, hydrofloats pelvic organs, and may act as a drug that alters the healing process. Clinical studies have revealed variable results regarding

Table 26.2. Classification of adhesion-reducing adjuvants

Mechanical separation
  Intraabdominal instillates
    Dextran
    Mineral oil
    Silicone
    Povidone
    Vaseline
    Crystalloid solutions
    Carboxymethylcellulose
  Barriers
    Endogenous tissue
      Omental grafts
      Peritoneal grafts
      Bladder strips
      Fetal membranes
    Exogenous material
      Oxidized cellulose
      Oxidized regenerated cellulose
      Polytetrafluoroethylene
      Gelatin
      Rubber sheets
      Metal foils
      Plastic hoods
      Hyaluronic acid
      Photopolymerizable gel
      Reverse thermal gelation gel

Anticoagulants
  Heparin
  Citrates
  Oxalates
Antiinflammatory agents
  Corticosteroids
  Nonsteroidal antiinflammatory drugs
  Antihistamines
  Progesterone
  Calcium channel blockers

Antibiotics
  Tetracyclines
  Cephalosporins

Fibrinolytic agents
  Fibrinolysin
  Papain
  Streptokinase
  Urokinase
  Hyaluronidase
  Chymotrypsin
  Trypsin
  Pepsin
  Plasmin activators

Modified from Gutmann and Diamond.[11] Reprinted with permission.

the ability of 32% dextran 70 to reduce adhesions. Complications such as pleural effusions and rare cases of anaphylactic reactions have been reported.[11]

Fibrinolytic agents and plasminogen activator, which converts plasminogen to plasmin, have also been studied. When used in appropriate doses, plasminogen activator was effective in animal trials and did not cause bleeding complications.[11]

High dose heparin as an anticoagulant can reduce adhesion formation when used intraperitoneally or systemically but is associated with abnormal bleeding.[11] At lower doses, heparin has not been found to be efficacious.

Glucocorticoids act as antiinflammatory agents by decreasing vascular permeability and inhibiting histamines. They have been widely used until recent years, although not all studies demonstrate beneficial effects on preventing adhesions.[11]

The NSAIDs inhibit prostaglandin synthesis and decrease vascular permeability and plasmin inhibitors. However, there have been no clinical studies that demonstrate its effectiveness.[11]

Antihistamines are used to decrease histamine induced vascular permeability.[11] No significant improvement achieved by use of antihistamines has been demonstrated.

Some animal studies have revealed the antiinflammatory and immunosuppressive effects of progesterone, but more clinical studies are needed to judge this agent.[11]

Several new techniques and agents have shown promise in animal trials, including precoating the tissues with hyaluronic acid, films of hyaluronic acid and carboxymethylcellulose,[28,29] a photopolymerizable gel,[30] and a compound that is a liquid at room temperature but forms a barrier at body temperature.[31-34]

Laparoscopy Versus Laparotomy

The choice of laparotomy or laparoscopy as a mode of access into the abdominal cavity should include consideration of the indications, risks versus benefits, and outcome. When comparing these two modes of therapy, one must keep in mind that it is not always possible to compare apples with apples and oranges with oranges because human subjects cannot be easily randomized to laparoscopy versus laparotomy. Surgeons and patients often have preferences perhaps premature concepts of efficacy that result in patients being assigned to one mode of access or another. This point of view often leads the surgeon to decide with a previously laparotomized patient to proceed with laparoscopy for persistent and recurrent infertility or referral to assisted reproductive technologies. Kelly and Diamond[35] reported that more than 40% of patients with endometriosis who underwent laparotomy after prior "surgical failure" subsequently conceive.

Assignment of patients to laparotomy or laparoscopy is often potentially biased. A patient with known extensive tuboperitoneal disease may be more likely to undergo a laparotomy as the first choice. Alternatively, almost all second-look procedures for fertility begin laparoscopically. Lastly, although a number of studies include laparoscopies,[36] we are not aware of any publications that have described performing three laparotomies in the same patient. Thus it is difficult to know the best way to compare these two major modes of access with regard to clinical results, such as intrauterine pregnancy rates, the time required to achieve pregnancy, relief of symptoms, and resolution of presenting complaints.[15]

Gynecologic surgery today may be performed endoscopically in 30–80% of patients currently undergoing laparotomy.[36] Gynecologic operative endoscopy (including laparoscopic and hysteroscopic surgery) includes the techniques of electrosurgery, thermocoagulation, laser (CO_2, KTP, Nd:YAG, argon), sharp dissection, and extra- or intracorporeal suturing. More recently, with an improvement in our ability to establish intraabdominal hemostasis, more complex surgical procedures can be performed laparoscopically.[36] However, these technical innovations are so attractive that the danger of ignoring basic clinical knowledge has been raised. Surgeons should not let themselves be led by personal optimism or expectancy that laparoscopy is "always better" than laparotomy.[10]

One of the main areas of contention has been the superiority of laparoscopy over laparotomy for preventing and treating adhesions. It was widely hoped that laparoscopy would be superior to open surgery in this regard, but many descriptive studies changed this optimism.[5,15,25,37] Thus laparoscopy should be considered a potential "adhesion creator," as is laparotomy.

It is perceived that the potential for postoperative adhesion formation is reduced by using operative laparoscopic procedures rather than laparotomy. Postoperative adhesions may result from intentional injury, unintentional tissue damage, and reformation after adhesiolysis. To study adhesion formation after intentional injury, Filmar et al.[20] made superficial cuts with scissors along the antimesenteric surface of the left uterine horn of 61 female rabbits. They identified no significant differences between the laparoscopy and laparotomy groups. The frequency of de novo adhesion formation can be seen in Table 26.3. De novo adhesions formed despite the use of microsurgical technique and performance by experienced surgeons. It is possible that the use of operative laparoscopy leads to a reduction in de novo adhesion rate.

There are a number of possible mechanisms accounting for the reduction in postoperative adhesions after laparoscopic surgery. Dehydration of the peritoneal surfaces in the presence of bleeding is a major factor in adhesion reformation. Because of the closed environment of endoscopic surgical procedures, peritoneal surfaces are less exposed to dehydration during laparoscopy than with laparotomy. However, nonhumid CO_2 gas is circulating in the abdominal cavity during laparoscopy, which reduces the difference. Another potential advantage of laparoscopy over laparotomy is the lack of need to use bowel packs to expose the operative site, which can abrade or traumatize the peritoneal surface. During laparoscopy, magnifying the image by getting closer is possible, enabling the surgeon to make more precise incisions and coagulate, which is theorized to reduce unintentional tissue damage. Laparoscopy is not totally "foreign body-free"; some sutures or clips can be applied.

26. Adhesion Prevention and Lysis

Table 26.3. De novo adhesion formation

Site of occurrence	Total no. of sites	Adhesions at initial procedure	Structures excised	Sites available for de novo adhesion formation	Sites with occurrence of de novo adhesions	Percentage of available sites with de novo adhesions
Ovaries	164	84	8	72	42	58
Tubes	164	50	10	104	26	25
Omentum	82	4	–	78	13	17
Small bowel	82	8	–	74	19	26
Colon	82	11	–	71	13	18
Cul-de-sac	82	26	56	16	29	
Sidewall	82	27	–	55	30	55
Total	738	210	18	510	159	31

From Diamond.[12] Reprinted with permission.

Gurgan et al.[38] studied the difference between laparoscopic Nd:YAG laser and laparoscopic electrocautery of polycystic ovaries.[7] Among this group, 82% of the patients were noted to have adhesions regardless of the technique used. As seen here, no consistency and confirmation between studies exist, which makes reaching a valid conclusion difficult.

In addition to adhesion development, other criteria may be used to compare laparoscopy and laparotomy. One important criterion should be the rates outcome of intrauterine pregnancies. Several studies failed to show any significant effects of modalities on the rate of intrauterine pregnancies. Success rates vary from 0% to 40% with endoscopic surgery and from 19% to 35% with laparotomy.[10] Moreover, if an adhesion interferes with the tubal mucosa, the results are further impaired. Nezhat et al.[39] reported a pregnancy rate of 48% after laparoscopic neosalpingostomy, but these patients had well preserved cilia and fimbrial folds. If the tubal mucosa is extensively damaged and is a hydrosalpinx, the conception rate is reduced to 6%.[40] The preservation of functional ciliated tubal lumen epithelium increases the success rate regardless of the operative route.[40]

There are no significant differences of pregnancy outcome after ectopic pregnancy treated via laparoscopy or laparotomy. (The rate is 40–50%.) The statistics for ectopic pregnancy after treatment of endometriosis (50–60% in both groups) or adhesiolysis (45–60% in both groups) are similar.

The role of laser therapy in gynecologic surgery continues to be evaluated. As the experience and skills of endoscopic surgeons improve, almost every procedure performed by conventional laparotomy appears efficacious laparoscopically. When the CO_2 laser was first used in gynecologic surgery, many "hopeful expectations" were raised; however, controlled studies comparing laser and conventional electrosurgery revealed that there is no significant difference. Regardless of the tools used, postoperative pelvic adhesions following laparotomy have been reported in 55–95% of cases.[11]

The use of contact lasers has increased in gynecologic reproductive surgery. This technique reduces the potential hazard of unintentional distant injury to intraabdominal organs. Transmission through flexible optic fibers "comforts many surgeons" because it provides tactile sensation similar to that when a scalpel is used. Moreover, various tip shapes are now available that enable the surgeon to make a fine incision and perform dissection, coagulation, or excision of a solid (or cystic) mass.

De Novo Adhesion Formation

De novo adhesion formation is an important issue. To address this point, 68 patients underwent laparoscopic adhesiolysis followed by second-look laparoscopy within 90 days.[5] At the initial surgical procedure the adhesion score was 11.4, and at second-look laparoscopy it was 5.5 ($p < 0.05$), a decrease of 52%; however, adhesion reformation occurred in 97% of patients. This means adhesions that reformed were not as extensive as at the initial procedure, but to a certain extent almost every patient experienced reformation. Despite this fact, de novo adhesion formation was only 12%. As mentioned above, postoperative pelvic adhesions following laparotomy have been reported in 55–95% of cases.[5]

Diamond et al.[37] studied 161 women who underwent laparotomy, followed by second-look laparoscopy 1–12 weeks later. No adhesions were noted at the initial procedure, but at second-look laparoscopy they found that adhesions had developed at 82 sites (51%). Among these 82 women, de novo adhesions occurred at 31% of available sites. Of these 159 sites with de novo adhesions, 130 of 159 (82%) were fine and filmy, whereas only 29 (18%) were dense and vascular.

Second-Look Laparoscopy

There is no consensus as to the best time to perform second-look laparoscopy; the recommendations range from 8 days to 2 years after the primary surgery. Trimbos-Kemper et al. concluded, after a series of third-look laparoscopies, that adhesions that were lysed by second-look laparoscopy did not recur in at least 50% of patients.[41] Unfortunately, they did not have convincing data that it improved the clinical outcome. In the same study, Trimbos-Kemper et al. concluded that neither second- nor third-look laparoscopies improved pregnancy rates; furthermore, they believed that the rate of ectopic pregnancy is significantly reduced by second looks.[41] Second-look laparoscopy allows the surgeon to compare different modalities of treatment and to determine if adjuvants have an effect, information complemented by assessment of outcome. There is no better way for a surgeon to see the surgical results. Table 26.4 conveys rates of pelvic adhesion formation noted at second-look laparoscopy.

The value of second-look laparoscopy was also evaluated by Jansen, who performed a third-look laparoscopy in 38 women.[42] The second-look laparoscopies were done 8–21 days after the initial surgery. The third-look laparoscopies revealed that only 31% of patients were free of adhesions. At the initial operation the mean adhesion score was 12, at the second look laparoscopy it was 9, and at the third-look operation it was 2. Only 8% of the patients

Table 26.4. Rates of pelvic adhesions at the time of second-look laparoscopy

Author	Time of SLL	No. of pts.	No. with adhesions	Predominant type of adhesion	
				Type	%
Diamond et al.	1–12 weeks	106	91 (86%)	Filmy	86
DeCherney & Mezer	4–16 weeks	20	15 (75%)	Filmy	80
	1–3 years	41	31 (76%)	Dense	84
Surrey & Friedman	6–8 weeks	31	22 (71%)	Filmy	100
	> 6 months	6	5 (83%)	Dense	100
Pittaway et al.	4–6 weeks	23	23 (100%)	Thick	26
Trimbos-Kemper et al.	8 days	188	104 (55%)		
Daniell & Pittaway	4–6 weeks	25	24 (96%)	Filmy	7
McLaughlin	6–12 weeks	25	14 (56%)	Filmy	83
Jansen	1–3 weeks	73[a]	42 (58%)	—	—
		183[b]	168 (92%)	Filmy	—
Tulandi et al.	1 year	36	21 (58%)		

From Gutmann and Diamond.[11] Reprinted with permission.
SLL, second-look laparoscopy.
[a]No preoperative adhesions.
[b]Preoperative filmy adhesions present.

were "adhesion reformation-free" despite the second-look laparoscopy.

Pregnancy is generally considered most likely to occur within 1 year of the initial infertility surgery except in women who undergo neosalpingostomy. In a study by Tulandi et al.,[16] 19 of 74 women underwent second-look laparoscopy 1 year after their initial surgery. All patients were followed for up to 3 years. No pregnancy rate difference was noted between those who did versus those who did not undergo second-look laparoscopy. The study of Tulandi et al. revealed one other observation: if a patient did not conceive within 1 year of the primary surgery, she was a strong candidate for an ectopic pregnancy. Ectopic pregnancy was less likely for the women who underwent second-look laparoscopy within the first 8 days of the initial surgery.[16]

When judging laparoscopic adhesiolysis versus adhesiolysis via laparotomy, one cannot easily judge endoscopy by means of complications. There are, of course, a number of reported laparoscopic complications, but many of them are not directly associated with adhesiolysis; they are general complications of endoscopic surgery.[43]

Conclusion

Direct comparison of two modalities of access into the pelvis is not always feasible. Furthermore, the best method may result in a disaster in the hands of an inexperienced surgeon. One must never underestimate the importance of conventional laparotomy. Perhaps it is best to state that a surgeon must never attempt to be a laparoscopist without being cognizant of and experienced in the principles for the surgical procedure at hand using the laparotomy approach. It must also be remembered that laparotomy can be an appropriate alternative and at times a life-saving procedure, as in the presence of laparoscopic complications.

References

1. DIAMOND MP: Surgical aspects of infertility. Mimeo.
2. SEIBEL MM: Working of the infertile couple. In Infertility: A Comprehensive Text, Seibel M (ed). Norwalk, CT, Appleton & Lange, 1990, pp 1–121.
3. JESSEN KL: 45 Operations for sterility. Acta Obstet Gynecol Scand 1971;50:105.
4. DECHERNEY AH: The leader of the band is tired. Fertil Steril 1985;44:299.
5. OPERATIVE LAPAROSCOPY STUDY GROUP: Postoperative adhesion development after operative laparoscopy: evaluation at early second-look procedures. Fertil Steril 1991;55:700.
6. DIZEREGA GS: The cause of prevention of post—surgical adhesions: a contemporary update. In Gynecological Surgery and Adhesion Prevention, Diamond MP, diZerega GS, Linsky CB, Reid RL (eds). New York, Wiley-Liss, 1993, pp 1–18.
7. LA MORTE AL, DIAMOND MP: Adhesion formation after laparoscopy. In Gynecological Surgery and Adhesion Prevention, Diamond MP, diZerega GS, Linsky CB, Reid RL (eds). New York, Wiley-Liss, 1993, pp 51–58.
8. BROSENS I: Prevention of adhesions in ovarian surgery. In Gynecological Surgery and Adhesion Prevention, Diamond MP, diZerega GS, Linsky CB, Reid RL (eds). New York, Wiley-Liss, 1993, pp 121–128.
9. LUNDORFF P: Laparoscopic ovarian drilling in women with 16–21 polycystic ovarian syndrome. In Gynecological Surgery and Adhesion Prevention, Diamond MP, diZerega GS, Linsky CB, Reid RL (eds). New York, Wiley-Liss, 1993, pp 139–147.
10. HESLA JS, ROCK JA: Laparoscopic tubal surgery and adhesiolysis. In Practical Manual of Operative Laparoscopy and Hysteroscopy, Azziz R, Murphy AA (eds). New York, Springer-Verlag, 1992, pp 91–99.
11. GUTMANN JN, DIAMOND MP: Principles of laparoscopic microsurgery and adhesion prevention. In Practical Manual of Operative Laparoscopy and Hysteroscopy, Azziz R, Murphy AA (eds). New York, Springer-Verlag, 1992, pp 55–64.
12. DIAMOND MP: Prevention of adhesions. In Operative Gynecology, Gershenson DM, DeCherney AH, Curry SL (eds). Philadelphia, Saunders, 1993, pp 147–158.
13. PUNCH MR, ROTH RS: Adhesions and chronic pain: an overview of pain and a discussion of adhesions and pelvic pain. In Gynecological Surgery and Adhesion Prevention, Diamond MP, diZerega GS, Linsky CB, Reid RL (eds). New York, Wiley-Liss, 1993, pp 101–120.
14. KRESCH AJ, SEIFER DB, SACHS LB, ET AL: Laparoscopy in 100 women with chronic pelvic pain. Obstet Gynecol 1984;64:672.

15. DIAMOND MP: Review of endoscopic surgical procedures in treatment of the infertile woman. In The Yearbook of Infertility, Mishell DR, Paulson RJ, Lobo RA (eds). Chicago, Mosby-Year Book, 1991, pp 45–64.
16. TULANDI T, FALCONE T, KAFKA I: Second look operative laparoscopy one year following reproductive surgery. Fertil Steril 1989;52:421.
17. STOVALL TG, LING FW: Relieving chronic pelvic pain through surgery. Contemp Obstet Gynecol 1991;36:11.
18. SWOLIN K: Electromicrosurgery. In Gynecological Surgery and Adhesion Prevention, Diamond MP, diZerega GS, Linsky CB, Reid RL (eds). New York, Wiley-Liss, 1993, pp 45–49.
19. GOMEL V: Salpingostomy by microsurgery. Fertil Steril 1978;29:380.
20. FILMAR S, GOMEL V, MCCOMB PF: Operative laparoscopy versus open abdominal surgery: a comparative study on postoperative adhesion formation in the rat model. Fertil Steril 1987;48:486.
21. LUCIANO AA, MAIER DB, KOCH EI, ET AL: A comparative study of postoperative adhesions following laser surgery by laparoscopy versus laparotomy in the rabbit model. Obstet Gynecol 1989; 74:220.
22. TALENT T, MURPHY AA, ROCK JA, ET AL: Effects of Gore-Tex surgical membrane (SM) on post-myomectomy adhesions. Presented at the Annual AFS Meeting, Montreal, 1993.
23. DECHERNEY AH, MEZER HC: The nature of post—tuboplasty pelvic adhesions as determined by early and late laparoscopy. Fertil Steril 1984; 41:643.
24. GRIFFIN A, MALINAK LR: Peritoneal closure. In Gynecological Surgery and Adhesion Prevention, Diamond MP, diZerega GS, Linsky CB, Reid RL (eds). New York, Wiley-Liss, 1993, pp 97–100.
25. DIAMOND MP: Assessment of results of laparoscopic laser surgery. In Lasers in Gynecology, Sutton C (ed). London, Chapman & Hall, 1992 pp 55–72.
26. LINSKY CB, DIAMOND MP, CUNNINGHAM T, ET AL: Adhesion reduction in the rabbit uterine horn model using an absorbable barrier, TC-7. J Reprod Med 1987;32:17.
27. BOYERS SP, DIAMOND MP, DECHERNEY AH: Reduction of postoperative pelvic adhesions in the rabbit with Gore-Tex surgical membrane. Fertil Steril 1988;49:1066.
28. URMAN B, GOMEL V: The effect of hyaluronic acid membrane on prevention of adhesion formation and reformation in the rat model. Fertil Steril 1991;56:568.
29. ZAHRADKA B, YARALI H, GOMEL V: The effect of hyaluronic acid membrane on prevention of adhesion formation and reformation. Presented at the 48th Annual Meeting of the American Fertility Society, New Orleans, 1993.
30. HILL-WEST JL, CHOWDHURY SM, SAWHNEY AS, ET AL: Prevention of postoperative adhesions in the rat by in situ photopolymerization of bioresorbable hydrogel barriers. Obstet Gynecol 1994;83:59.
31. RICE VM, SHANTI A, MOGHISSI KS, LEACH RE: A comparative evaluation of Poloxamer 407 and oxidized regenerated cellulose (Interceed TC7) to reduce postoperative adhesion formation in the rat uterine horn model. Fertil Steril 1993; 59:901.
32. STEINLEITNER A, LOPEZ G, SUREZ M, LAMBERT H: An evaluation of Flowgel as an intraperitoneal barrier for prevention of post—surgical adhesion reformation. Fertil Steril 1992;57:305.
33. LEACH RE, HENRY RL: Reduction of postoperative adhesions in the rat uterine horn model with poloxamer 407. Am J Obstet Gynecol 1990; 162:1317.
34. STEINLEITNER A, LAMBERT H, KAZENSKY C, CANTOR B: Poloxamer 407 as an intraperitoneal barrier material for the prevention of post—surgical adhesion formation and reformation in rodent models for reproductive surgery. Obstet Gynecol 1991;77:48.
35. KELLY RW, DIAMOND MP: Intra—abdominal use of carbon dioxide laser for microsurgery. Laser Surg Obstet Gynecol Clin North Am. 1993; 18:537.
36. AZZIZ R: Advantages and disadvantages of operative endoscopy. In Practical Manual of Operative Laparoscopy and Hysteroscopy, Azziz R, Murphy AA (eds). New York, Springer-Verlag, 1992, pp 1–6.
37. DIAMOND MP, DANIELL JF, FESTE J, ET AL: Adhesion reformation and de novo adhesion formation after reproductive pelvic surgery. Fertil Steril 1987;47:864.
38. GURGAN T, KISNISCI H, YARALI H, ET AL: Evaluation of adhesion formation after laparoscopic treatment of polycystic ovarian disease. Fertil Steril 1991;56:1176.
39. NEZHAT C, WINER WK, COOPER JD, ET AL: Endoscopic infertility surgery. J Reprod Med 1989; 34:127.

40. MAGE G, POULY JL, BOUQUET DE JOLOINIERE J, ET AL: A preoperative classification to predict the intrauterine and ectopic pregnancy rates after distal tubal microsurgery. Fertil Steril 1986;46:807.
41. TRIMBOS-KEMPER TCM, TRIMBOS JB, VAN HALL EV: Adhesion formation after tubal surgery: results of the eighth-day laparoscopy in 188 patients. Fertil Steril 1985;43:395.
42. JANSEN RPS: Early laparoscopy after pelvic operations to prevent adhesions: safety and efficacy. Fertil Steril 1988;49:26.
43. SMITH S: Complications of laparoscopic and hysteroscopic surgery. In Practical Manual of Operative Laparoscopy and Hysteroscopy, Azziz R, Murphy AA (eds). New York, Springer-Verlag, 1992, pp 199–215.

27
Role of Pelvic Ultrasonography and Color Doppler in Laparoscopy

Resad Pasic

Since the 1950s, ultrasonography has gained remarkable acceptance in medicine and surgery for its diagnostic and therapeutic capabilities. With new technologic advances its application in medical practice is widening daily, and there are promising opportunities for further developments in diagnostic and therapeutic use. With improvement in resolution and image display capabilities, three-dimensional scanning, tissue characterization, blood flow measurements, and development of contrast media, there is potential for even wider application of ultrasonography, which has already become an indispensable part of medical evaluation and therapy.

High frequency ultrasonography, providing increased precision and reduced operative trauma, has been used during surgery since the early 1950s. Interventions have ranged from ultrasonic physiotherapy for acute soft tissue injuries,[1] to selective destruction of the vestibule in patients with Meniere's disease,[2] to the destruction of renal calculi with extracorporeally focused shock waves.[3] Ultrasound-guided needle aspiration of cysts and ovarian follicles in a number of circumstances has replaced laparoscopy as a less invasive and just as effective alternative.[4]

A number of those procedures have not withstood the test of time, whereas others have proved useful and have provided the impetus for further research and development of instrumentation and techniques based on the knowledge of ultrasound waves. Examples are the use of ultrasonic surgical aspirators in neurosurgery[5] and recently in laparoscopy[6,7] and the ultrasonic scalpel, which is gaining wide acceptance in operative endoscopy.[8]

The greatest progress has appeared in the area of diagnostics, initially with gray-scale and real-time imaging, M-mode echocardiography, and more recently color flow imaging. With miniaturization of transducers, allowing their placement in a variety of lumens and internal organs, further advances in diagnostic capabilities show promise, including intravascular diagnostics and laparoscopic ultrasonography.

These methods have long been adopted and used by gynecologic surgeons, although for a significant time they have been ignored by most general surgeons and other specialists. The current capabilities of ultrasonography as applied to the field of diagnostic and operative endoscopy are addressed.

Ultrasound Diagnostics

A combination of noninvasive and invasive techniques is used for accurate diagnosis of specific pathologic conditions. Ultrasound imaging provides additional information to the clinical examination, especially with respect to normal anatomy as well as pathologic changes. It is a highly specific and sensitive test. Real-time scanning has made possible the observation of such physiologic phenomena as the fetal cardiac activity and the assessment of other obstetric parameters and intraabdominal abnormalities.

Ultrasonography has proved helpful in the evaluation of trauma. Specifically, it is used for identification and quantitation of intraperitoneal bleeding; it has drastically improved diagnosis of hepatobiliary disease and the evaluation of renal lesions. Abdominal masses, aortic aneurysms, and pancreatic and retroperitoneal tumors are well visualized by ultrasonography and diagnostic accuracy in appendicitis has been reported to be improved.[9] Intraluminal scanning is helpful in the evaluation of prostatic, rectal, and esophageal abnormalities.[10] Endovascular ultrasound scanning is now established as an important tool for the evaluation of vascular and cardiac pathology.[11]

Ultrasonography in Gynecology

Transabdominal ultrasonography of the female pelvis was the conventional method of scanning through the 1970s and 1980s despite its limitation for inadequate depth of penetration. This problem resulted in poor visualization of deep pelvic structures and the prerequisite of a distended bladder, which often led to patient discomfort. Transvaginal ultrasonography has overcome these limitations and has led to widespread application of this noninvasive technique for routine evaluation of the female pelvis. Because a transvaginal probe is placed in greater proximity to pelvic organs, higher frequency ultrasound waves can be utilized, resulting in enhanced resolution and improved imaging of pelvic structures.

Transvaginal sonography plays an important role in the preoperative evaluation of patients with a pelvic mass and provides useful information about the nature of the mass that can influence the clinical decision regarding an operative approach via laparoscopy, versus laparotomy, especially if malignancy is suspected. The accu-

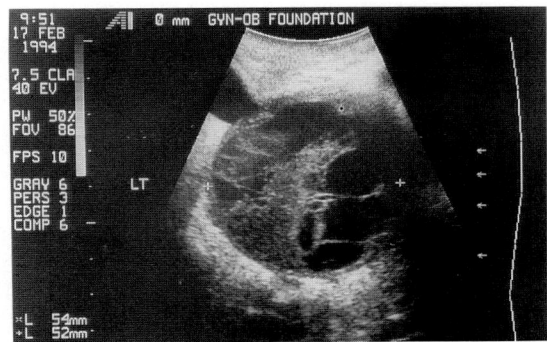

Figure 27.1. Ovarian malignancy demonstrated by vaginal scan.

racy of ultrasonography for detecting the presence, size, location, and texture of a pelvic mass is in the range of 90% according to a number of studies,[12,13] and it is definitely superior to manual examination. Therefore transvaginal sonography provides an excellent means of evaluating ovaries and adnexa-associated structures, and it should be considered prior to pelvic surgery.[14] Most of the ovarian masses in premenopausal women are benign, with the risk of ovarian cancer in premenopausal women with an ovarian mass being 4/1000.[15] The overall risk of malignancy with a persistent mass in postmenopausal women is much higher and is estimated to be 20–30%.[16] Therefore it is important to categorize patients according to their premenopausal and postmenopausal status when planning preoperative management.

A pelvic mass should be suspect for malignancy when it appears solid, fixed, or irregular. Masses of 5 cm diameter are less likely to be malignant than larger masses; when correlating the size of the mass with the likelihood of malignancy, 1% of masses < 5 cm in diameter were noted to be malignant compared to 72% of masses > 10 cm.[17] (Fig. 27.1). If an upper abdominal mass or ascites is present, the diagnosis of ovarian cancer merits strong consideration and laparotomy is given top priority.[18] Parker and Berek have suggested ultrasonic criteria for preoperative evaluation of ovarian masses in postmenopausal women to be managed laparoscopically. According to their findings, cysts

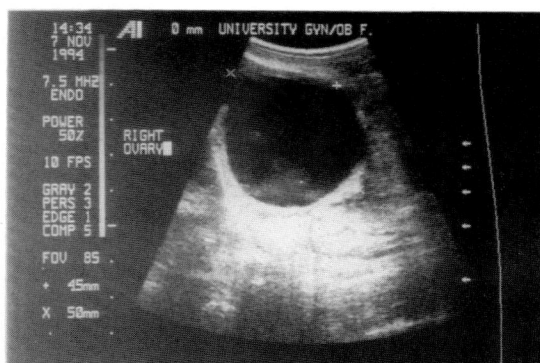

Figure 27.2. Benign ovarian cystic mass is seen on a vaginal scan.

with distinct borders, < 10 cm in diameter, no irregular or solid parts, no thick septa, no ascites, and a normal CA 125 level can be managed laparoscopically.[19]

On the other hand, ultrasonic criteria for low risk of malignancy include small size, unilateral, unilocular cyst with smooth borders, and no peritoneal fluid (Fig. 27.2). Functional cysts often change over time and regress spontaneously. Endometriomas and hemorrhagic cysts also present with regular borders and slightly thicker walls, and sometimes they present with internal echoes. If the cysts that on ultrasonography appear to be functional persist more than 3 months, they should be evaluated for laparoscopic removal. Simple cysts may be good predictors of benign disease, and all masses that meet strict ultrasonic selection criteria should be considered for a laparoscopic approach. Endoscopic removal can be considered for hemorrhagic cysts, dermoids, and endometriomas.[20,21] If during laparoscopy the suspicion of malignancy arises or excrescences are found, the lesion should be biopsied and sent for frozen section. If frozen sections are positive, or large ascites or obvious malignancy is found, a staging laparotomy through a midline incision should be performed without delay.

Sonographic examination has become the most reliable instrument for the diagnosis of abnormal intrauterine pregnancy. It has made a significant contribution to the management of patients suspected of having an ectopic pregnancy. Furthermore, the demonstration of ectopic gestation by transvaginal ultrasonography enables more precise preoperative diagnosis and allows earlier surgical intervention via the laparoscopic approach with the goal of less tubal damage. Ultrasonic signs suggestive of ectopic pregnancy include the presence of a complex or cystic adnexal mass and confirmation of free fluid in the peritoneal cavity. An intrauterine gestational sac should be visible by transabdominal scan if the serum beta human chorionic gonadotropin (β-hCG) is 6000 mIU/ml, and it should be visible by vaginal scan if β-hCG is ≥ 1000 mIU/ml.[22] If the sac is not present in the uterine cavity, an ectopic pregnancy should be suspected and, accordingly, laparoscopy performed.

Transvaginal ultrasonography does not normally delineate the fallopian tubes, which have traditionally been investigated using hysterosalpingography or laparoscopic chromotubation. Hydrosalpinges are readily demonstrated by ultrasonography; and using fluid medium, normal tubes also can be evaluated by ultrasound examination.[23]

Ultrasonography cannot identify small endometriotic implants, and definitive diagnosis of endometriosis requires laparoscopic visualization and tissue confirmation. The sonographic appearance of large endometriotic lesions can be cystic, solid, or both; and the images obtained on ultrasound scans are often highly suggestive of the disease. Recurrent endometriomas are often visible on ultrasound examination, and in women with known pathology transvaginal scanning can be useful for monitoring disease activity.

Transvaginal sonography can be used to evaluate the developmental abnormalities of the reproductive tract. It has an important role in the evaluation of the uterus and endometrium, and it is particularly helpful in patients with leiomyomata. In general, most solid pelvic masses are of uterine, rather than ovarian, origin; and on ultrasound examination leiomyomas present with a hypoechogenic texture within the border of the uterus.[24] Ultrasonography may be superior to hysterosalpingography, hysteroscopy, or laparoscopy[25] for diagnosing uterine leiomyomas (Fig. 27.3). Endometrial thickness can be

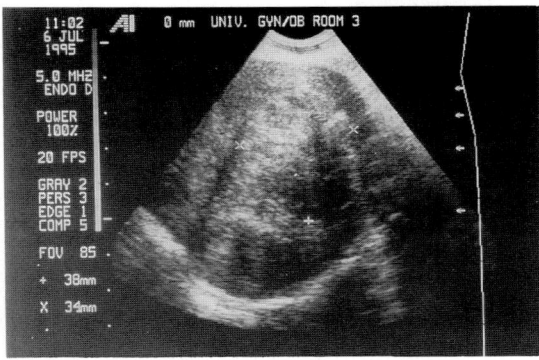

Figure 27.3. Uterine fibroids demonstrated by vaginal scan.

measured throughout the menstrual cycle, and it may prove to be helpful when screening for early changes of endometrial hyperplasia.[26]

Some attempts have been made to detect and map abdominal wall adhesions by ultrasonography in an effort to provide safe abdominal access in patients who are at increased risk for trocar injury of viscera due to previous abdominal surgery,[27] but this procedure has not gained wide acceptance.

Application of the above-mentioned diagnostic possibilities provides accurate diagnosis of most common gastrointestinal and gynecologic disorders. However, laparoscopy is reported to have a higher diagnostic yield with certain conditions, such as carcinoma of the pancreas, peritoneal seeding, appendicitis, endometriosis, ovarian and tubal disease, and the presence of peritoneal adhesions. When routine evaluation has failed to identify the etiology of abdominal or pelvic pain, laparoscopy is accepted as a useful and definitive diagnostic step.

Screening for Pelvic Malignancies

The lifetime risk of ovarian cancer in women is 1/70, with the incidence increasing from 30/100,000 to 70/100,000 as women age from 40 to 60 years. Based on the sonographic findings suggestive of ovarian malignancy (i.e., increased ovarian size, irregular contour of the mass, presence of solid elements, multiple septations, papillary excrescences within the mass, or presence of free peritoneal fluid), Campbell et al. first proposed that ultrasonography could be used as a screening tool for ovarian cancer.[28] The accuracy rates, when using ultrasonic criteria, for prediction of benign ovarian masses range between 92% and 96%.[29-31] Based on the results of the screening studies for early detection of the ovarian cancer and the nature of the disease, there are no data currently available to suggest that routine screening for ovarian cancer can improve survival rates and reduce mortality.[32,33] The screening might prove cost-effective only in women with a family history of ovarian cancer, primarily reflecting the influence of genetic factors in this disease.

Bourne et al.[34] and Kurjak et al.[35] suggested that ovarian cancer could be differentiated from benign ovarian pathology by color flow Doppler studies, which would enhance the specificity of the transvaginal scanning procedure, but further clinical trials must be conducted before the procedure can be properly evaluated.

There is the potential that ultrasonography can be used to monitor postmenopausal women with bleeding to decrease the need for endometrial biopsy. Most women with postmenopausal bleeding present with fragile atrophic endometria. An endometrial thickness of ≤ 4 mm correlates with a relatively low estrogen state and atrophy.[26,36] Those patients could be followed by transvaginal scanning rather than endometrial biopsy, and only patients with evidence of endometrial hyperplasia would be appropriate candidates for endometrial biopsy. Transvaginal ultrasonography with color Doppler imaging has the additional advantage of detecting endometrial[37] tubal and bladder cancers.

Role of Color Doppler Imaging

Saturoma was the first to apply the known scientific phenomenon of Doppler shift in the frequency of back-scattered ultrasound to the detection and measurement of blood flow.[38] This technique was later used to detect and measure blood flow in different organs.[39] The use of pulsed Doppler requires considerable time to select the correct point for observation, especially when small vessels are targeted.

Further advances were made with the introduction of color Doppler imaging,[40] which allows evaluation of blood flow patterns on real-time two-dimensional imaging and provides guidance and accurate placement of the pulsed Doppler to obtain flow velocity measurements, which facilitates the examination. Based on the direction and variance of the detected frequency shift, a color converter assigns color for a specific image. The direction of blood is identified by red and blue colors. The brightness of color is a reflection of the velocity of flow within the vessel. Red indicates flow toward the transducer and blue flow away from the transducer. Various shades of green represent turbulent flow, with a yellow component representing turbulent forward flow, and cyan (greenish blue) representing backward flow of turbulence.

These blood flow color data are superimposed on anatomic tissue data obtained by B-mode scanning for accurate placement of a pulsed Doppler range gate to obtain flow velocity measurements. Thus the color flow Doppler transducer represents a combination of three transducers in a single unit: high-resolution B-mode, color Doppler, and pulsed Doppler. Placing the transducers in a vaginal probe enhances the resolution and image quality and facilitates enhanced presentation of pelvic organs and flow measurements. After visualization of the specific organ by B-mode scanning and focusing it with color Doppler, the blood vessels of interest can be explored with pulsed Doppler to obtain certain spectral waveforms. The peak-systolic and end diastolic frequency shift within the vessel can be recorded and conventional indices of impedance, such as pulsatility index (PI) and resistance index (RI), calculated.

The waveform shape obtained gives a rough indication of the type of flow within the vessels. The tumor vessels typically have continuous high diastolic flow with low pulsatility due to the lack of a muscular layer in the vessel wall and an RI < 0.4. The velocity may also be increased, and there is usually lack of a diastolic notch. The normal arterioles have a muscular layer that helps regulate parenchymal perfusion and is associated with lack of continuous diastolic flow, high pulsatility, RI > 0.4, and the presence of a diastolic notch (Plate 45).

Areas of abnormal vascularity can be used to distinguish benign from malignant masses; and the absence of intratumoral neovascularization and the presence of a high pulsatility index can be used to exclude the existence of invasive primary ovarian cancer. In a patient with a palpable pelvic mass, the optimal therapeutic approach depends on the likelihood that the mass is malignant. By measuring indices of blood flow in an adnexal mass, an effort is made to characterize benign and malignant lesions on the basis of their vascularity, thereby improving the specificity of the ultrasound screening procedures for early detection of ovarian cancer.[41,42] Thus utilizing color Doppler to exclude the presence of malignancy with an ovarian mass allows one to consider a less aggressive surgical approach such as laparoscopy. Data also suggest that by visualizing abnormal blood flow within the endometrium transvaginal color Doppler can depict endometrial carcinoma, determine the depth of the myometrial invasion, and help in tumor staging.[43]

Transvaginal color Doppler can also be used for the diagnosis of early pregnancy and disturbances of blood flow in the trophoblast, embryo, and umbilical cord.[44] Ectopic pregnancy can be evaluated based on the flow measurements within and around the suspected mass.[45] If color flow is not visualized, the assumption is that trophoblast is not active, and expectant management or methotrexate treatment can be instituted. From the opposite perspective, if the flow is present in the adnexal region with an RI < 0.40, strong suspicion for an ectopic pregnancy exists, and appropriate clinical correction must be undertaken.[46]

Laparoscopic Ultrasonography

Ultrasonography has proved to be the important integral part of diagnostic imaging. Miniaturization of transducers has created a new vista for application of laparoscopic ultrasonography that can place scanners in close proximity to the area of interest and obtain better resolution. An ultrasound probe in the 7.5 MHz range that can be introduced through a laparoscopic trocar can provide additional valuable information during endoscopic surgery.

Traditionally, laparoscopic surgery has had certain limitations compared to open surgery, such as lack of three-dimensional presentation and of tactile feedback, which is important for orientation during any surgical procedure. These limitations of endoscopic surgery can potentially be minimized by additional intraoperative ultrasonic scanning, which can determine the nature, consistency, configuration, and size of anatomical structures and provide the surgeon with valuable additional information.

New applications of intraoperative sonography during laparoscopy are currently being evaluated. Laparoscopic ultrasonography has proved valuable for delineating the anatomy of the biliary tree and diagnosing common duct stones during laparoscopic cholecystectomy.[47] Ultrasonic visualization of the cystic duct and biliary tract obviates palpation of the bile duct and portal structures, could lessen the risk of iatrogenic bile duct injury, and may eliminate the need for operative cholangiography during laparoscopic cholecystectomy.[48]

One other potential use of laparoscopic sonography is the evaluation and staging of patients with malignant disorders (e.g., identifying liver metastasis and staging patients with adenocarcinoma of the pancreas).[49] Until now laparoscopic examination could detect only obvious hepatic and peritoneal spread of tumor and prohibit the ability to identify changes in the retroperitoneal area or assessment of a solid organ. These concerns can be eliminated by using laparoscopic ultrasonography. A 7.5 MHz transducer provides high resolution images, facilitating the detection and identification of retroperitoneal lymph nodes. Thus laparoscopic scanning by providing accurate information of the size and extent of an abdominal and retroperitoneal mass can greatly promote laparoscopic techniques for the staging and treatment of intraabdominal malignancies.

Laparoscopic ultrasonography clearly has specific application in gynecologic endoscopic surgery. Potentially it can be used to detect small uterine leiomyomas that are not well delineated by vaginal scan (Plate 46). Moreover, identification of early ectopic pregnancy and evaluation of an ovarian mass are now more feasible (Plate 47). Ovaries and blood vessels in the ovarian fossa can be reliably identified, but the ureters are still difficult to evaluate. Absence of the acoustic "stand off," which enhances visualization of nearby structures, was in part responsible for inadequate visualization of the ureters.[50] It appears that laparoscopic ultrasonography is a valuable adjunct that can enlarge the armamentarium of instruments available for endoscopic surgery.

References

1. LEHMANN JF: Ultrasound therapy. In Therapeutic Heat and Cold, Licht S (ed). Baltimore, Waverly Press, 1965, p 321
2. ARSLAN M: Direct application of ultrasonics on the vestibular apparatus in the treatment of Meniere's disease. Acta Otorhinolaryngol Iber Am 1957;8:358.
3. VALLANCIEN G, AVILES J, MUNOZ R, ET AL: Piezoelectric extracorporeal lithotripsy by ultrasound waves with the EDAP LT01 device. J Urol 1988; 139:689.
4. LENZ S, LAURITSEN JG: Ultrasonically guided percutaneous aspiration of human follicles under local anesthesia: a new method of collecting oocyte for in vitro fertilization. Fertil Steril 1982; 38:673.
5. EPSTEIN FJ, FARMER JP: Trends in surgery: laser surgery, use of the cavitron, and debulking surgery. Neurol Clin 1991;9:307.
6. VASQUEZ JM, EISENBERG E, OSTEEN KG, ET AL: Laparoscopic ablation of endometriosis using the cavitational ultrasonic surgical aspirator. J Am Assoc Gynecol Laparosc 1993;1:36.
7. GROCHMAL SA, WEEKES A, GARRATT D, ET AL: Applications of the laparoscopic ultrasonic aspirator for advanced gynecologic operative endoscopic procedures. J Am Assoc Gynecol Laparosc 1993;1:43.
8. FERLAND R, AMARA J: Harmonic scalpel as a new laparoscopic energy source. Presented at the AALG World Congress, 1992.
9. PUYLAERT JB, RUTEERS PH, LALISANE RI, ET AL: A prospective study of ultrasonography in the diagnosis of appendicitis. N Engl J Med 1987; 317:666.

10. LIU JB, MILLER LS, GOLDBERG BB, ET AL: Transnasal US of the esophagus: preliminary morphology and function studies. Radiology 1992;184:721.
11. PANDIAN NG, KREIS A, BROCKWAY B, ET AL: Ultrasound angioscopy: real-time, two dimensional intraluminal ultrasound imaging of blood vessels. Am J Cardiol 1988;62:493.
12. EL-MINAWI MF, EL-HALAFAWY AA, ABDEL-HADI M, ET AL: Laparoscopic, gynecographic and ultrasonographic vs. clinical evaluation of pelvic mass. J Reprod Med 1984;29:197.
13. LANDE IM, HILL MC, COSCO FE, ET AL: Adnexal and cul-de-sac abnormalities: transvaginal sonography. Radiology 1988;166:325.
14. FREDERIC JL, PAULSON RJ, SAUER MV: Routine use of vaginal ultrasound in the preoperative evaluation of gynecologic patients, an adjunct to resident education. J Reprod Med 1991;36:779.
15. NEZHAT F, NEZHAT C, WELANDER CE, ET AL: Four ovarian cancers diagnosed during laparoscopic management of 1011 women with adnexal mass. Am J Obstet Gynecol 1992;167:790.
16. HULKA JF, HULKA CA: Preoperative sonographic evaluation and laparoscopic management of persistent adnexal masses: a 1994 review. J Am Assoc Gynecol Laparosc 1994;1:197.
17. GRANDBERG S, WIKLAND M, JANSSON I: Macroscopic characterization of ovarian tumors and the relation to the histologic diagnosis: criteria to be used for ultrasound evaluation. Gynecol Oncol 1989;35:139.
18. BEREK J, HACKER N: Practical Gynecologic Oncology. Baltimore, Williams & Wilkins, 1989, p 329.
19. PARKER WH, BEREK JS: Management of selected cystic adnexal masses in postmenopausal women by operative laparoscopy: a pilot study. Am J Obstet Gynecol 1990;163:1574.
20. NEZHAT C, WINER W, NEZHAT F: Laparoscopic removal of dermoid cysts. Obstet Gynecol 1989;73:278.
21. REICH H, MCGLYN F: Treatment of ovarian endometriomas using laparoscopic surgical techniques. J Reprod Med 1987;32:747.
22. CACCIATORE B, TIITNEN A, STENMAN VH, ET AL: Normal early pregnancy: serum hCG levels and vaginal ultrasonography findings. Br J Obstet Gynaecol 1990;97:889.
23. VENEZIA R, ZANGARA C: Echohysterosalpingography: new diagnostic possibilities with S HU 450 Echovist. Acta Eur Fertil 1991;22:279.
24. GROSS B, SILVER T, JAFFE M: Sonographic features of uterine leiomyomas: analysis of 41 proven cases. J Ultrasound Med 1983;2:401
25. FEDELE L, BIANCHI S, DORTA M, ET AL: Transvaginal ultrasonography versus hysteroscopy in the diagnosis of uterine submucous myomas. Obstet Gynecol 1991;77:745.
26. GOLDSTEIN SR, NACHTIGALL M, SNYDER JR, ET AL: Endometrial assessment by vaginal ultrasonography before endometrial sampling in patients with postmenopausal bleeding. Am J Obstet Gynecol 1990;163:119.
27. SIGEL B, GOLUB RM, LOIACONO LA, ET AL: Technique of ultrasonic detection and mapping of abdominal wall adhesions. Surg Endosc 1991;5:161
28. CAMPBELL S, GOSWAMY R, GOESSENS L, ET AL: Real-time ultrasonography for determination of ovarian morphology and volume: a possible early screening test for ovarian cancer? Lancet 1982;1:425.
29. RULIN M, PRESTON A: Adnexal masses in postmenopausal women. Obstet Gynecol 1987;70:578.
30. HERRMANN U, LOCHER G, GOLDHIRSCH A: Sonographic patterns of ovarian tumors: prediction of malignancy. Obstet Gynecol 1987;69:777
31. GRANBERG S, NORSTROM A, WIKLAND M: Tumors in the lower pelvis as imaged by vaginal sonography. Gynecol Oncol 1990;37:224
32. HIGGINS RV, VAN NAGEL JR, DONALDSON ES, ET AL: Transvaginal sonography as a screening method for ovarian cancer. Gynecol Oncol 1989;34:402
33. ANDOLF E, JORGENSEN C, ASTEDT B: Ultrasound examination for detection of ovarian carcinoma in risk groups. Obstet Gynecol 1990;75:106
34. BOURNE T, CAMPBELL S, STEER C, ET AL: Transvaginal color flow imaging: a possible new screening technique for ovarian cancer. BMJ 1989;299:1367
35. KURJAK A, ZALUD I, JURKOVIC D, ET AL: Transvaginal color Doppler for the assessment of pelvic circulation. Acta Obstet Gynecol Scand 1989;68:131.
36. VARNER ED, SPARKS JM, CAMERON CD, ET AL: Transvaginal sonography of the endometrium in postmenopausal women. Obstet Gynecol 1991;78:195
37. BOURNE TH, CAMPBELL S, ROYSTON P, ET AL: Detection of endometrial cancer by transvaginal ultrasonography with color flow imaging and blood flow analysis; preliminary report. Gynecol Oncol 1991;40:253
38. SATUROMA S: Ultrasonic Doppler method for the inspection of cardiac functions. J Acoust Soc Am 1957;29:1181.

39. TRUDINGER BJ, GILES WB, COOK CM: Uteroplacental blood flow velocity-time waveforms in normal and complicated pregnancy Br J Obstet Gynaecol 1985;92:39.
40. KASAI C, NAMEKAWA K, KOYANO A, ET AL: Real time bloodflow imaging system utilizing autocorrelation techniques. Ultrasound Med Biol 1983;(suppl 2):203.
41. KURJAK A, ZALUD I, ALFIREVIC Z: Evaluation of adnexal masses with transvaginal color ultrasound. J Ultrasound Med 1991;10:295.
42. FLEISHER AC, ROGERS WH, RAS BK, ET AL: Assessment of ovarian tumor vascularity with transvaginal color Doppler ultrasound. J Ultrasound Med 1991;10:563.
43. KURJAK A, SHALAN H, SOSIC A, ET AL: Endometrial carcinoma in postmenopausal women: evaluation by transvaginal color Doppler ultrasonography. Am J Obstet Gynecol 1993;169:1597.
44. ALFIREVIC Z, KURJAK A: Transvaginal color and pulsed wave Doppler in the assessment of blood flow in the first trimester of pregnancy. J Perinatal Med 1990;18:173.
45. TAYLOR KJW, RAMOS IM, FEYOCK AL, ET AL: Ectopic pregnancy: duplex Doppler evaluation. Radiology 1989;173:93
46. KURJAK A, ZALUD I: Transvaginal color doppler imaging. In Ultrasound in Obstetrics and Gynecology, Chervenak FA, Isaacson GC, Campbell S (edS). Boston, Little, Brown, 1993, pp 149–55.
47. MOSNIER H, AUDY JC, BOCHE O, GUIVARCH M: Intraoperative sonography during cholecystectomy for gallstones. Surg Gynecol and Obstet 1992;174:469.
48. YAMAMOTO M, STIEGMANN GV, DURHAM J, ET AL: Laparoscopy-guided intracorporeal ultrasound accurately delineates hepatobiliary anatomy. Surg Endosc 1993;7:325.
49. MURUGIAH M, PATERSON-BROWN S, WINDSOR JA, ET AL: Early experience of laparoscopic ultrasonography in the management of pancreatic carcinoma. Surg Endosc 1993;7:177.
50. PASIC R, ROETHLING HP, WOLFE WM: Laparoscopic ultrasound for evaluation of ovarian mass [abstract]. Presented at the International Congress of Gynecologic Endoscopy, 23rd Annual Meeting of the American Association of Gynecologic Laparoscopists, New York, 1994.

28
Operating Room Personnel

Wendy K. Winer

The role of the operating room personnel in gynecologic surgery has changed dramatically.[1] This drastic change has resulted from the development of gynecologic endoscopy and, more importantly, the adaptation of the video camera to the laparoscope and hysteroscope.[1-14] Videoscopic surgery enables everyone present to follow the procedure on the video monitor and appropriately anticipate the surgeon's needs and so has created an entirely new involvement for operating room personnel. This situation has made the contribution by operating room personnel so important that many hospitals have recognized the need for an "endoscopy team" (Fig. 28.1).[1,2,15]

The endoscopy team generally refers to the surgeon, surgical assistant, scrub nurse or technician, nurse circulator, and laser safety officer. For maximum efficiency during endoscopy cases the entire team must be actively involved before, during, and after the procedure. In this chapter we focus on the role of the operating room personnel as part of the endoscopy team in operative gynecologic endoscopy.

Preoperative Preparations

Scrub nurse responsibilities preoperatively include the following.

1. Open the sterile items (i.e., table covers, laparoscopy pack, and instrumentation).
2. Lay out the sterile instrumentation in the most organized way possible.
3. Ensure that all instruments are in proper working order.
4. Verify that all instrumentation required is open.

The *setup* may vary from one institution to another, but in general it includes the following items.

2 Mayo stands (Mayo no. 1: laparoscopic instruments; Mayo no. 2: vaginal instruments)
1 Back table
1 Secondary back table (for additional vaginal instruments to use for more extensive vaginal procedures, e.g., operative hysteroscopy or laparoscopic-assisted vaginal hysterectomy—LAVH)
1 Ring stand with two large basins

The suggested instrumentation to be contained on each of these tables is listed in Table 28.1.

After trocars have been placed, the items from Mayo stand 1 are then transferred to the back table and replaced on the Mayo tray by graspers and routine instruments to be used for laparoscopy, leaving additional laparoscopic instrumentation on the back table easily accessible if required during the procedure. This Mayo

28. Operating Room Personnel

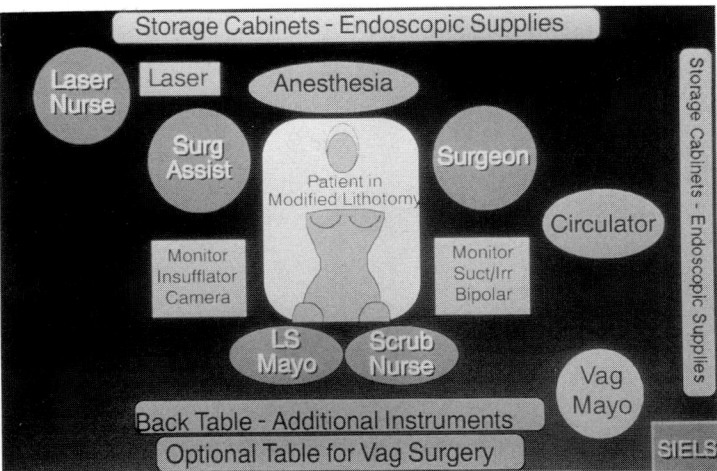

Figure 28.1. Operating room personnel comprise a key part of the endoscopy team.

cart is placed next to the scrub nurse between the patient's legs and close enough to the sterile field that the surgeon and assistant can reach instruments from this stand if needed (Fig. 28.5).

Circulating nurse preoperative responsibilities include the following.

1. Helps scrub nurse open all sterile items prior to setting up the case.
2. Checks surgeon's preference card to verify that all items specific to the procedure and to the individual surgeon's preferences are present.
3. Only open what is planned to be used.
4. Check all video equipment, light cable, light source and bulb, insufflator and gas tank level, irrigation pump and tank level, suction, electrosurgery unit, and laser.
5. Go to the preoperative area. Talk with the preoperative nurse and review the patient's history, laboratory work, consent form, and procedures to be done. Speak with the patient and her family. A warm, caring, reassuring tone is crucial to help ease the patient's anxiety prior to surgery.
6. Accompany the patient to the operating room.

During this time, before the patient is asleep, the number of people in the room should be limited to those who must be there. No visitors may enter until the patient is draped. The noise level should also be kept to a minimum, particularly during the time the patient is being anesthetized. Most often two video carts or ceiling orbiters are used containing the following.

Video cart or orbiter 1 (placed opposite the surgeon)
Surgeon's primary monitor for viewing
Camera box, video recorder, and printer (optional)
Light source
Insufflator
Video cart or orbiter 2 (placed opposite the surgical assistant and adjacent to the surgeon)
Monitor
Electrosurgery unit
Irrigation pump

The suction device is kept on the side where the wall suction is located. The tubing is connected to the canisters with a laser plume filter connected to the tubing or is part of the canister.

Laser nurse responsibilities include the following.

1. Test the laser preoperatively (before the scope is sterilized if using the CO_2).
2. Be responsible for the laser safety guidelines as established by the laser committee of the hospital. These guidelines, which depend on the laser and wavelength being used, must be properly followed.[17-24] The guidelines include information regarding appropriate eye protection for the patient, the endoscopy and anesthesia teams, and anyone else who may be present during the case. In addition

Table 28.1. Suggested instrumentation for Mayo tables, back tables, and ring stand

Mayo cart 1: laparoscopic instrumentation (Fig. 28.2)
  Trocars
  Scalpel
  Surgical sponges
  Veress needle
  Open laparoscopy (optional): Hasson cannula, suture, scissors, hemostats, retractors

Mayo cart 2: vaginal instruments (Fig. 28.3)
  Vaginal speculum
  Uterine sound
  Tenaculum
  Uterine manipulator
  Uterine dilators (optional)
  Uterine curettes (optional)

Back table: laparoscopic instrumentation (Fig. 28.4)
  Graspers with and without teeth
  Endoscopic scissors
  Endoscopic suturing instruments
  2 Bipolar forceps with cords
  Suction/irrigation probe with tubing
  Operative laparoscope
  Claw grasping forceps 10 mm
  Scissors 10 mm
  Endoscopic Kittner or dissector
  Tissue removal instrumentation, e.g., Allis, Kelleys, Lahey clamps
  Curved and straight Mayo scissors
  Endoscopic suture
  Endoloop sleeve (applicator)
  Optional: laser fiber, harmonic scalpel,[16] staples, clips
  Endoscopic organizing pouch
  Light cord
  Camera and cable (camera drape optional)
  Small basins
  Towels, surgical sponges, drapes
  Tray containing extra instruments

Secondary back table: additional vaginal instruments (if operative hysteroscopy is planned)[a]
  Vaginal speculum
  Uterine sound
  Tenaculum
  Uterine manipulator
  Uterine dilators
  Uterine curettes (optional) and telfa (optional)
  D & C set
  Surgical sponges
  Hysteroscope, diagnostic and operative
  Resectoscope if needed (with appropriate tips and electrosurgery cord)
  Y Tubing for fluid
  Light cord
  Camera and cable
  Fluid pouch (attached to the drape and connected to suction for precise measurement of fluid)

Ring stand: two basins for rinsing laparoscope or any instrumentation that has been soaked in disinfecting solutions

[a]If LAVH is to be performed vaginal hysterectomy instrumentation should be included.
Note: Always have a sterile laparotomy set-up readily available in case a laparoscopy needs to be converted to a laparotomy.

to goggles being kept in the room, there should be a sign on the door alerting anyone who may enter during the procedure: "laser in use" and "proper eyewear required" (goggles should be hanging on the door).

3. Check that the fire extinguisher is in place right outside the room.
4. Help connect the laser to the laparoscope—with a laser coupler if using the CO_2 laser or with a laser fiber if using the Nd:YAG laser (or another fiber laser) and any tips if used (Fig. 28.6).
5. Help maintain sterile technique with regard to the laser. It may include draping the arm of the laser or being sure that the fiber is adequately secured to the drape with a clamp.
6. Regulate the laser control board during the procedure. The laser should be placed on "ready" only when the surgeon is ready to activate it. The power setting is determined by the surgeon and the laser then set accordingly.
7. Placing the foot pedal in a convenient location for the physician and one that is separate from any other power source pedal, such as the electrosurgery unit, so the surgeon does not inadvertently press the wrong foot pedal.
8. When the laser is not being activated, the laser safety officer immediately places the laser on "standby." The nurse must follow the procedure attentively to be ready so the surgeon does not have to be delayed when he or she requests that the laser be placed on "ready" (Fig. 28.7).

No one should be operating the laser, or working in a room where the laser is used, without being properly in-serviced trained on that unit. Initial training should come from the manufacturer upon installation and periodically updated. Additional in-service training should be done by the laser safety officer for all other operating room personnel. Anyone who operates the laser must be properly credentialed as determined by the laser committee of the hospital. This credentialing body is generally comprised of physicians and nurses. When appropriate guidelines are not followed as established by the committee, they should be immediately reported verbally and in writing to

28. Operating Room Personnel

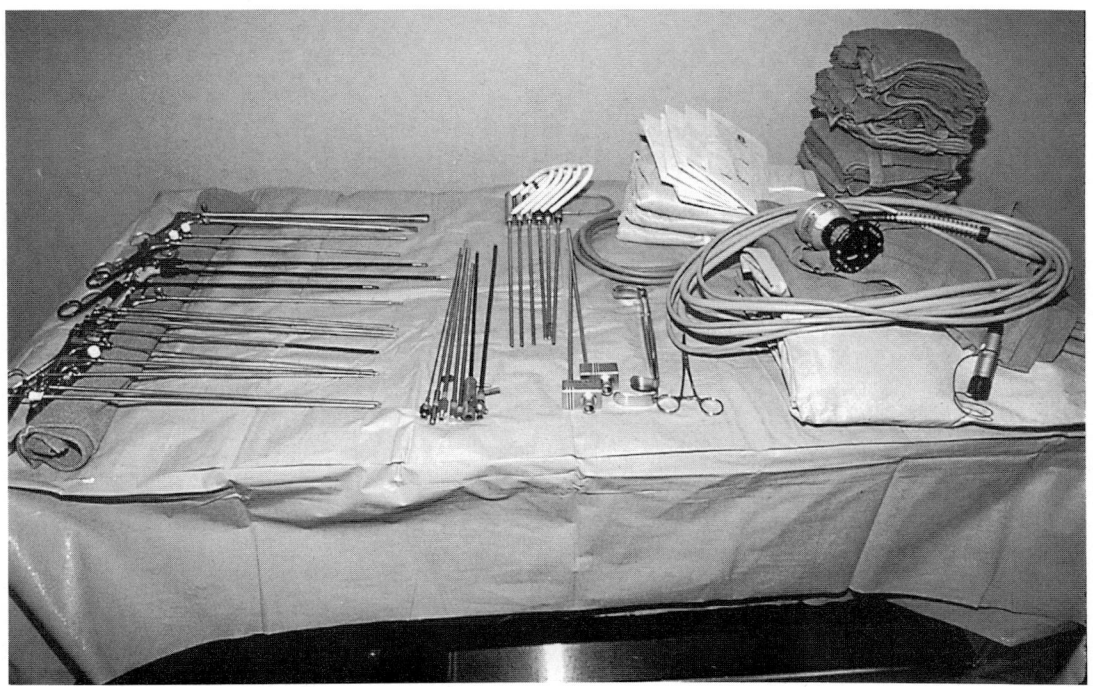

Figure 28.2. Laparoscopic instruments included on back table.

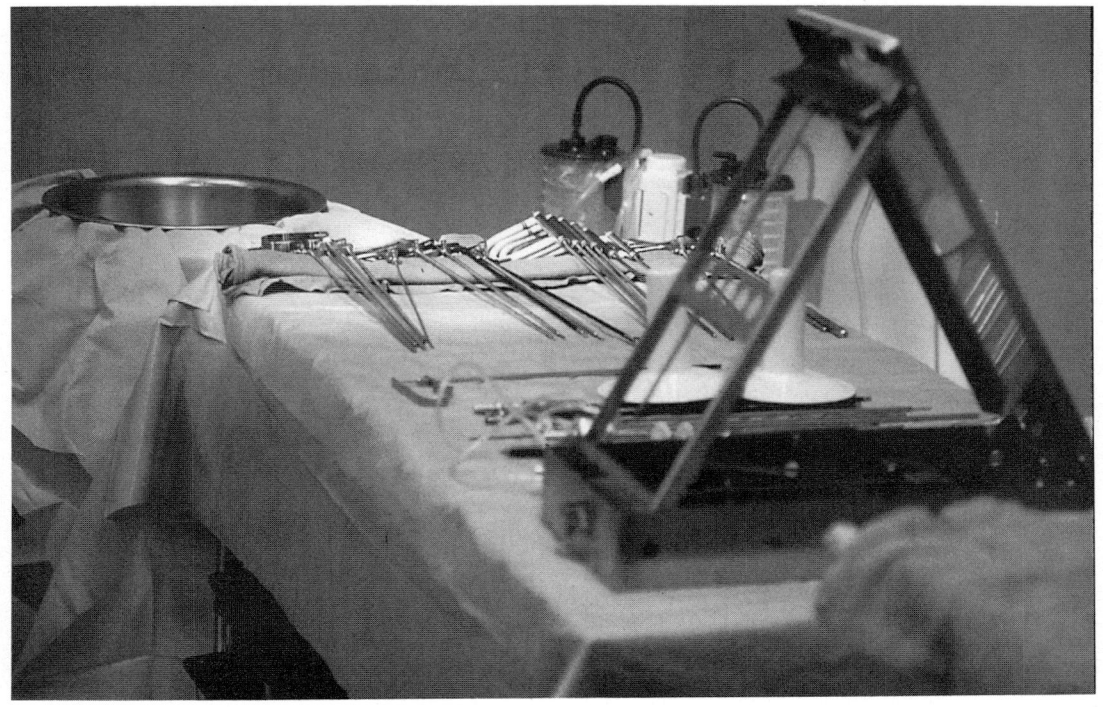

Figure 28.3. Vaginal instruments included on back table.

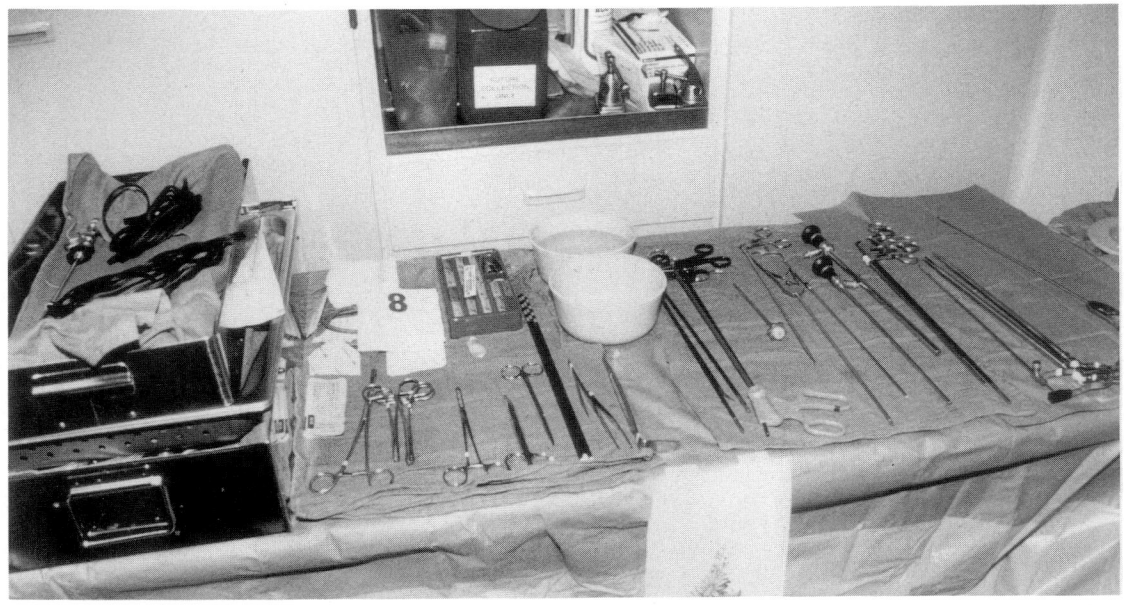

Figure 28.4. Laparoscopic instruments placed on the back table.

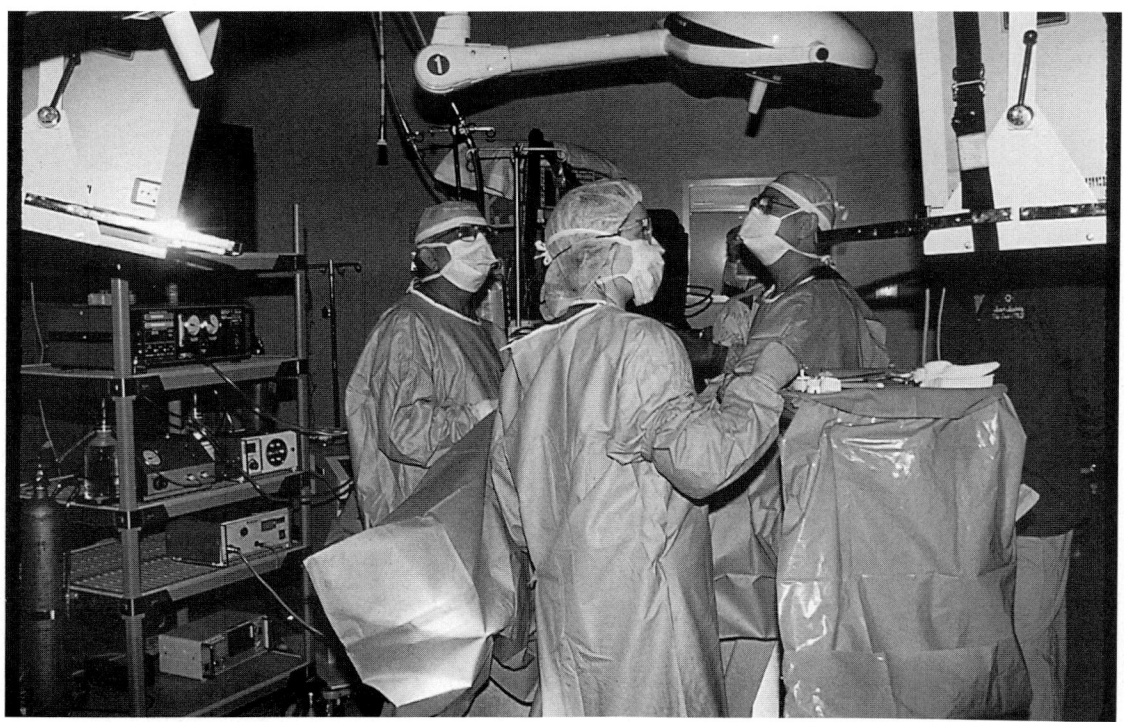

Figure 28.5. Mayo stand should be placed close enough to the sterile field so the surgeon can reach instruments if necessary.

28. Operating Room Personnel

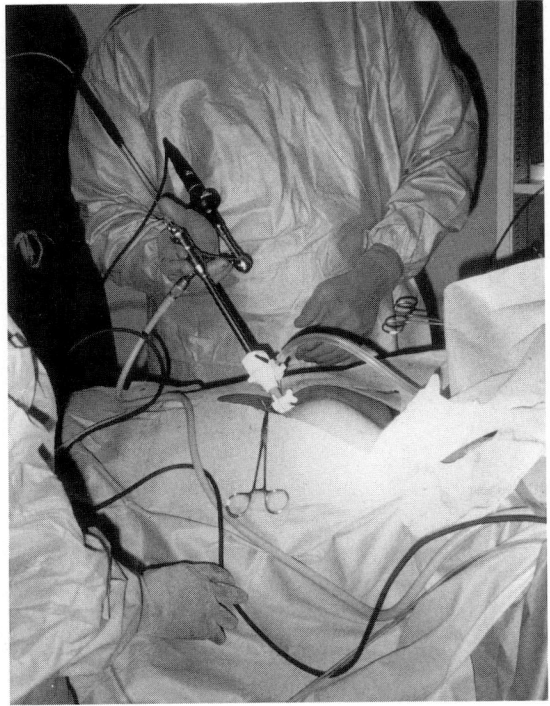

Figure 28.6. Laser is connected at the head of the patient.

the laser committee chairman. It is recommended that members of the endoscopy team attend continuing education programs periodically to remain current on new trends and techniques in operative endoscopy.

Intraoperative Responsibilities

Responsibilities of the endoscopy team as the procedure begins are as follows.

1. Surgical assistant or scrub nurse performs a final review of the instrumentation after it is placed on the Mayo stands and back table, checking that everything is in place and working properly (Fig. 28.8).
2. Circulating nurse positions the patient's legs appropriately in the stirrups (it is suggested that the surgeon check the legs for proper positioning before the patient is prepared and draped (Fig. 28.9).
3. Prepare the patient; catheterize her or place a Foley catheter.
4. After the patient is draped, the instrumentation and equipment are positioned.

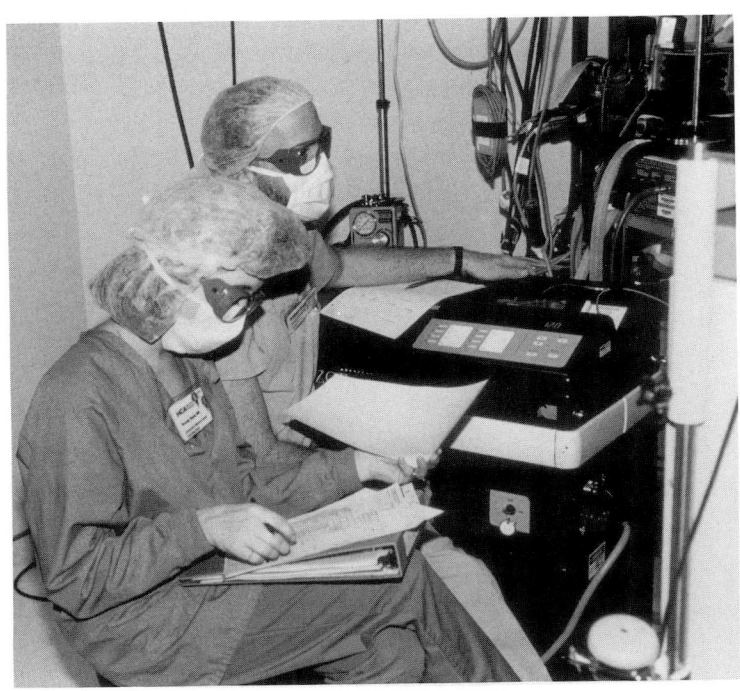

Figure 28.7. Laser safety officer operates the control board during surgery.

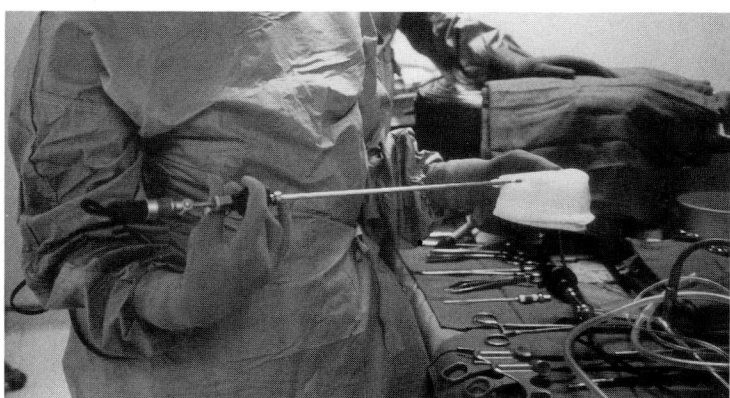

Figure 28.8. Surgical assistant makes a final review of the instruments before the case begins.

The surgeon proceeds with placing the uterine manipulator. During this time the surgical assistant or tech readies the laparoscope (attached to the light cord and camera) on the drape. These cords and the insufflator tubing are secured to the drape and then passed off to the circulator to be connected to the appropriate equipment. On the other side of the table the same thing is done with the suction and irrigation tubes, and the suction and irrigation probe and bipolar forceps are secured. Tubing and cord are passed off and connected to the appropriate equipment by the circulating nurse.

It is helpful to use an endoscopic organizing pouch, which can be secured to the drape over the patient's thigh. Instruments such as the suction/irrigator probe and bipolar forceps may be placed in the organizer while not being used. In this way they can remain connected and on the sterile field, providing quick accessibility throughout the case but not falling off the field or getting in the way when not in use. The bipolar forceps should be tested on a moistened surgical sponge before beginning the case. Because a working bipolar electrode is so crucial, a backup is kept on the back table in case the primary one malfunctions. The suction/irrigator is also tested. A surgical sponge is used to white out the camera after it is connected with the light cord to the laparoscope. A defogging agent is used on the scope. The video carts or orbiters should be in their appropriate positions. At this point everything is ready for the endoscopic procedure to begin, and members of the team

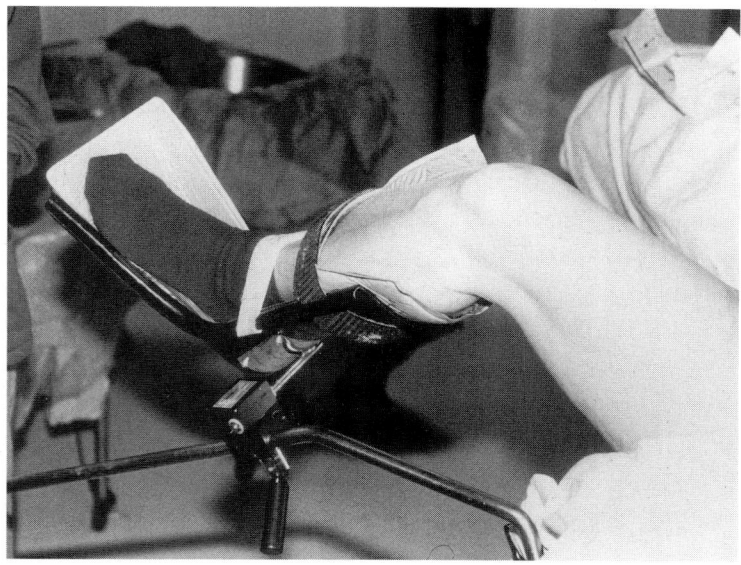

Figure 28.9. Patient's legs are carefully positioned.

Figure 28.10. Registered nurse first assistant handles the scope, freeing the surgeon's hands to operate.

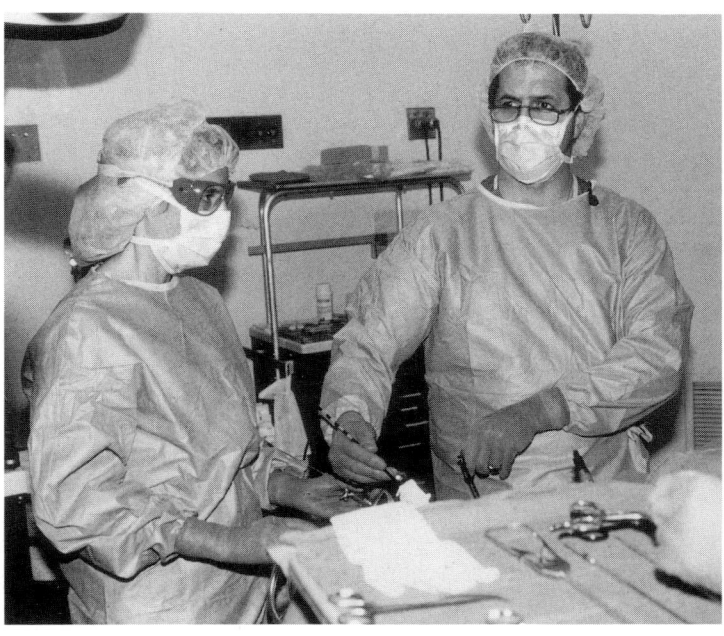

position themselves accordingly. The surgeon is generally on the patient's left side, the surgical assistant directly across from the surgeon on the patient's right side, and the scrub tech between the patient's legs. The laparoscopic Mayo stand is next to the scrub tech. The Mayo cart is elevated over the patient's leg and close enough that the surgeon and assistant can reach instruments on the tray. The insufflator is on video cart 1, where the surgeon can see the insufflation pressure level. Video cart 2, which houses the electrosurgery generator, is adjacent to the surgeon but at an angle so the ammeter (if so equipped) can be seen. The surgical assistant should also be aware of these values during the procedure. For maximum efficiency and safety, everyone should get in the habit of routinely checking the various instrument gauges throughout the surgery.

It is important to keep in mind that advanced operative endoscopy is a "team approach," and the operating room personnel are a key part of the efficiency of the procedure and should continually be watching the monitor to follow the operation. The nurse should be familiar with the anatomy. During the procedure the responsibilities of the circulator include changing irrigation bottles or bags, switching suction canisters when they are full, calculating the intake and output, collecting specimens and labeling them properly, and monitoring the level of CO_2 in the tank for the insufflator and the light intensity of the picture on the video monitor. The surgical assistant often is a "registered nurse first assistant" who handles the scope when the surgeon needs both hands free to suture, manipulate graspers, or coagulate vessels (Fig. 28.10). It is important that this person be aware of the surgeon's routine so as to be able to anticipate the surgeon's moves, particularly when handling the scope. The scope becomes the surgeon's eyes, and moving it automatically generally develops with experience. The assistant's other hand is free to irrigate or suction and to handle graspers, particularly when there are three punctures in addition to the laparoscope. The area where work is being done should be in the center of the monitor if possible. It is important to keep the picture as clear as possible by keeping the scope clean throughout the procedure. During the procedure the scrub nurse passes instruments and often elevates the uterine manipulator as needed. Attentiveness to the monitor enables the nurse to anticipate the instruments to be used. If it is seen that an additional instrument may be necessary, the nurse can then plan accordingly and obtain it from the back table; in some cases the circulator may need to get it, if it is peel-packed or on another set that has not yet been opened. The more a team can work together, the easier it is for the operating room personnel to anticipate and know each surgeon's routine.

Postoperative Considerations

When the case is concluded, great care must be given to careful handling of the delicate instrumentation and to the proper dismantling and cleaning of these items in the work room (Fig. 28.11). Often it is during this process that an instrument is broken, thrown out, or accidentally autoclaved. All scopes, cameras, and light cords should be separated immediately to help avoid accidents. In addition to the scrub nurse, there is generally a technician responsible for the cleaning of all endoscopy instrumentation. It is important to have consistency in this position because this person must be familiar with the many instruments and small parts that attach to them. Small adapters may be costly and could keep a procedure from being performed if they are not in their proper place. It is important that the patient be thoroughly "cleaned up," bandages secured, legs lowered gently together from the stirrups, warm blankets placed, and usual precautions taken as the patient is moved from the operating room table to a bed. The surgical assistant and circulator generally do this task with the aid of other personnel, and the patient is then moved to the recovery room. As the circulator disconnects the cords and gives them to the scrub nurse for cleaning and sterilization, the electrical power should be turned off as carts are moved out of the way. Careful, gentle disconnecting of cords is also crucial. Often additional help comes in for lunch relief or to help in a quick turnover, and these people should not be handling this equipment unless properly in-service trained. As the circulator and anesthesia staff take the patient to the recovery room, they report to the recovery room nurse who will be caring for the patient. The report includes a summary of the procedures, a review of incisional sites and dressings, and a highlighting of anything of which the recovery staff must be aware about the patient or type of procedure done. Once again, it is helpful if there are a group of nurses who usually take care of the gynecologic endoscopy patients, so they are familiar with common postoperative events. For example, patients having this type of surgery often have drainage from their incision sites, particularly in the recovery room, due to frequent irrigation during the procedure. There may also be swelling from the fluid and some fullness in the abdomen. Vaginal bleeding may be present due to uterine manipulation. The Foley catheter is often removed in the operating or recovery room. Depending on the extent of the procedure, these

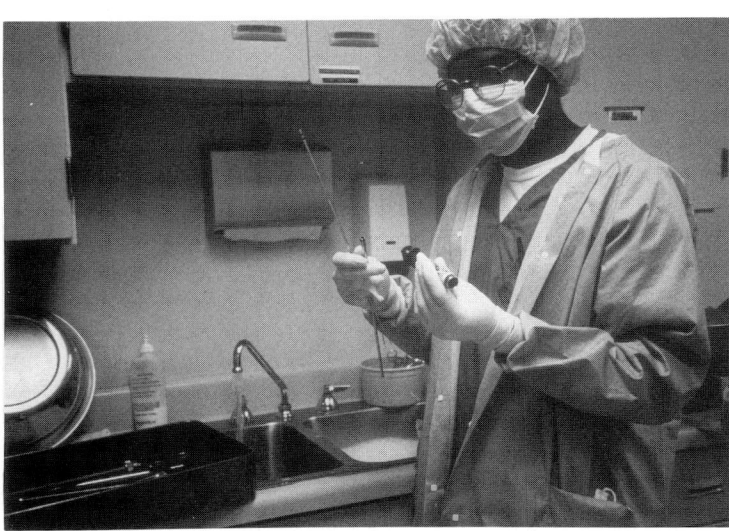

Figure 28.11. Instruments are carefully cleaned after surgery.

patients probably go from the recovery room to a short-stay area. Sometimes they even stay overnight, thus requiring nursing personnel to be familiar with the differences in caring for these patients.

Nursing Responsibilities Specific to Operative Hysteroscopy

When operative hysteroscopy is performed separately or in conjunction with laparoscopy, the nursing roles are similar. The key difference is the paramount importance of an accurate measurement of intake and output with little room for flexibility. Generally, with operative hysteroscopic procedures, glycine or sorbitol solution is used in 3 L bags. These bags are hung on intravenous infusion poles that have been elevated or attached to a hysteroscopic pump. Accurate calculations are crucial. Thus these bags must be closely monitored so the surgeon is kept informed about the amount of intake and outflow. Often a surgeon asks for an update on these figures every 5–15 minutes. The specific guidelines vary, but the important point is that the staff is properly trained along with the physician. These guidelines should be strictly adhered to for the safety of the patient. For accurate calculation of outflow a drainage bag is attached to the sterile drape so all hysteroscopic outflow drains into this bag. This bag is connected to a suction canister on wall suction throughout the procedure. The circulator must constantly check the drainage bag (i.e., Lindeman drape) to be sure it is draining properly and then frequently determine the fluid in the canisters to establish a continual comparison of intake and outflow. If possible during this part of the procedure, it is ideal to have two circulators: one to monitor the intake and outflow and the other to be sure all equipment is operating properly and to keep the inflow solution running, so there are no delays when transferring from one bag to another. During an operative hysteroscopic procedure it is recommended that the staff stay constant to minimize mistakes in intake and outflow calculations.

Conclusion

The 1990s has marked a new era for operating room personnel. The endoscope in conjunction with the video camera has totally refocused the procedure for the operating room staff. Nursing personnel have an enhanced opportunity to play an active role in the procedure and to participate in the team concept. The recommendations in this chapter can serve only as a helpful guide, as each setting varies, and some flexibility may be necessary to provide the most organized, efficient setup for a particular institution. It is important, however, that the entire team be properly trained. Nurses and technicians, should attend training courses perhaps ideally along with the surgeon to receive hands-on practice along with the surgeon. Courses are being taught with hands-on laboratory sessions where nurses and surgeons can work together, each learning their role, to better simulate "real surgery." Learning the procedures, anatomy, and instrumentation, troubleshooting the equipment, and following proper intake and outflow guidelines are key ingredients for a successful endoscopic program. The learning process never ends as techniques are refined, new products are developed, and continued advancement is made in the field of endoscopic surgery. It is the responsibility of the operating room personnel to participate in educational networks through local and national courses and to remain current with the endoscopic literature that is becoming more plentiful as the endoscopic expansion progresses so we may continue to be integral members of the endoscopy team.

References

1. WINER WK: The role of the operating room staff in operative laparoscopy. J Am Assoc Gynecol Laparosc 1993;1:86.
2. WINER WK, LYONS TL: Suggested set-up and layout of instruments and equipment for advanced operative laparoscopy. J Assoc Gynecol Laparos 1995;2:231.
3. GOMEL V: Operative laparoscopy: time for acceptance. Fertil Steril 1989;52:1.
4. NEZHAT C, WINER WK, COOPER JD, ET AL: Endoscopic infertility surgery. J Reprod Med 1989;34:127.

5. GOMEL V: Salpingostomy by laparoscopy. J Reprod Med 1977;18:265.
6. YUZPE AA: Television in laparoscopy. In Laparoscopy, Phillips JM, Corson SL, Keith L, et al (eds). Baltimore, Williams & Wilkins, 1977, pp 306–325.
7. SEMM K: Instruments and equipment for endoscopic abdominal surgery. In Operative Manual for Endoscopic Abdominal Surgery, Semm K (ed). Chicago, Year Book, 1987, pp 46–123.
8. NEZHAT C, WINER WK, NEZHAT F: A comparison of the CO_2, argon and KTP-532 lasers in the videolaseroscopic treatment of endometriosis. Colposc Gynecol Laser Surg 1988;4:41.
9. NEZHAT C, WINER WK, CROWGEY S: Videolaseroscopy for treatment of endometriosis and other diseases of the reproductive organs. Obstet Gynecol Forum 1987;1:2.
10. NEZHAT F, WINER W, NEZHAT C: Salpingectomy via laparoscopy: a new surgical approach. J Laparoendosc Surg 1991;1:91.
11. NEZHAT C, WINER WK, NEZHAT F, NEZHAT C: Videolaparoscopy and videolaseroscopy: alternatives to major surgery? Female Patient 1988;13:46.
12. NEZHAT C, WINER W, NEZHAT F: Laparoscopic removal of dermoid cysts. Obstet Gynecol 1989;73:278.
13. NEZHAT C, WINER WK, NEZHAT F: Is endoscopic treatment of endometriosis and endometrioma associated with better results than laparotomy? Am J Gynecol Health 1988;2(3):10.
14. NEZHAT F, WINER WK, NEZHAT C: Fimbrioscopy and salpingoscopy in patients with minimal to moderate pelvic endometriosis. Obstet Gynecol 1990;75:15.
15. WINER WK: Gynaecology in Minimal Access Surgery for Operating Room Personnel. Radcliffe Medical Press, 1994, pp 149–165.
16. WINER WK: A Comparison of the CO_2 laser and the harmonic scalpel. Minim Invasive Surg Nurs 1993;7:54.
17. DANIELL JF, MILLER W, TOSH R: Initial evaluation of the use of the potassium-titanyl-phosphate (KTP-532) laser in gynecologic laparoscopy. Fertil Steril 1986;46:373.
18. KEYE WR JR, HANSEN LW, ASTIN M, ET AL: Argon laser therapy of endometriosis: a review of 92 consecutive patients. Fertil Steril 1987;47:208.
19. LYONS T: Laparoscopic supracervical hysterectomy, a comparison of morbidity/mortality results with LAVH. J Reprod Med 1993;38:763.
20. LOMANO JM: Laparoscopic ablation of endometriosis with the YAG laser. Lasers Surg Med 1983;3:179.
21. LYONS T: Laparoscopic supracervical hysterectomy. In Laparoscopic Hysterectomy, Garry R, Reich H (eds). Blackwell Scientific, 1993, pp 148–152.
24. LYONS TL, WINER WK: The Nolan-Lyons modification of the Burch procedure. J Assoc Gynecol Laparos 1995;2:95.
22. WINER WK: Nursing aspects of gynecologic endoscopy. In Endoscopic Surgery, B. McLucas (ed). 1995;3:109. Georg Thieme Verlag, Stuttgart, New York.
23. WINER WK: New procedures for women that are being done endoscopically. Minim Invasive Surg Nurs 1995;9:87.

29
Teaching Operative Endoscopy

Michael J. Sammarco

This chapter presents an approach to the development of a teaching program in operative laparoscopy within an obstetrics and gynecology residency program. Unlike more traditional surgical approaches to gynecologic surgery (i.e. abdominal or vaginal routes), the endoscopic approach is much more technical and equipment dependent. Because most of the surgical procedures are performed with the aid of a camera and a video monitor, specific eye–hand coordination skills must be developed. For some these skills are easy to acquire, but for many the initial attempts are often fraught with frustration and anxiety. Operative laparoscopy is a relatively new surgical approach compared to other surgical techiques, and currently most endoscopic surgeons have received their training after completion of a residency. Postgraduate surgical training has not met with the same scrutiny or supervision as the training received during an approved residency program. To ensure that these techniques and skills are properly acquired, incorporation of a structured, comprehensive teaching program dealing specifically with operative endoscopy into residency training is imperative.

The concept of preoperative training of endoscopic procedures is not new. Various programs and techniques for training both residents and surgeons have been described.[1,2] Although many residency programs offer active endoscopic services, it does not ensure that residents are adequately or equally trained. A structured, ongoing, comprehensive resident teaching program was first described in 1993.[3] This program strove to give residents both didactic and hands-on training prior to performing surgical cases. The experience obtained through the development of that program is largely responsible for the information presented in this chapter.

How to Begin

Prior to initiating any formal training program, it is important to identify the learning objectives. Institutional needs vary and are dependent on a variety of factors: the number of residents who require training, the number of laparoscopic procedures performed at that institution, the number of facilities to which the residents are assigned, the number of faculty who are not only available but are able to teach laparoscopy, and the facilities and equipment available for teaching. All of these factors must be considered before developing a successful program. The program must be flexible enough to allow for scheduling conflicts and absenteeism. In addition to the identified objectives, there must be a mechanism to monitor the resident's progress and comprehension. Programs that are offered sporadically, without clearly identified learning objectives or direction, rarely serve as more than a casual, easily forgotten exercise. The program should be challenging enough to hold the participants' attention but not overwhelming or so restrictive as to be unrealistic.

What needs to be learned? The answer to this question serves as the framework for the entire program. All endoscopic training programs should have a didactic and a "hands-on," or practical, component. Regardless of the amount of time spent in the operating room (OR) performing or observing procedures, comprehensive training includes didactic training that explains the reasons for and alternatives to a particular surgical procedure. The primary goal of any endoscopic training program must be to supply both of these components.

The following outline is a suggested list of learning objectives. It can serve as a framework that may be modified by each institution depending on its specific needs. It is helpful to categorize these objectives into two groups: those in which the residents should be skilled and those of which the residents should be knowledgeable (i.e., didactic objectives). To be skilled is to be able to perform a given task or demonstrate a given technique; to be knowledgeable is to demonstrate comprehension. Those objectives requiring the knowledgeability of the residents are to be referred to concepts or to procedures or techniques that are not commonly used but of which the resident should be aware.

I. Preoperative evaluation
   A. Skilled objectives
      1. Demonstrate the ability to obtain an adequate informed consent that includes an indication and diagnosis, the potential benefits, the potential risks, and the medical or surgical alternatives.
      2. Demonstrate the ability to counsel patients regarding the risks and benefits of endoscopic surgery.
   B. Didactic objectives
      1. Be familiar with the necessary diagnostic and clinical examinations pertinent to a diagnosis and procedure.
      2. Be familiar with the need for specific preoperative preparation (i.e., need for bowel preparation, antibiotics, adjunctive medical therapy, or medical clearance).
      3. Be familiar with the medical or surgical alternatives pertinent to a specific procedure.
      4. Know the contraindications, both relative and absolute, to performing an operative endoscopic procedure.

II. Instrumentation and equipment
   A. Skilled objectives
      1. Demonstrate the ability to properly recognize, assemble, and disassemble instruments used for basic operative laparoscopic procedures.
      2. Demonstrate the correct connection of the camera and video system to the laparoscope, including the integration of additional monitors, video printers, and recorders.
      3. Demonstrate the ability to "troubleshoot" the video system and manage the common problems encountered during a surgical procedure.
   B. Didactic objectives
      1. Know the function and application of the commonly used instrumentation not available in their institution.
      2. Know the basic optical physics of the laparoscopic telescope.
      3. Know the appropriate pressure settings used for the insufflating and irrigation devices.

This material is often thought to be mundane and easily obtained during surgery. It is preferable that each resident have a thorough understanding of this material *prior* to performing surgery. This point cannot be overemphasized. The workshops that deal with this basic information are the cornerstones for the remaining workshops. The ability to demonstrate the acquisition of this knowledge gives residents both confidence and security. It greatly improves their operative efficiency. Conversely, it also helps identify those individuals who could benefit from additional instruction lest an adverse event occur.

III. Basic anatomy and insufflation techniques
   A. Skilled objectives
      1. Demonstrate the proper preoperative positioning of the patient for a routine operative laparoscopy.
      2. Demonstrate the proper technique for insertion of an insufflating needle to establish a pneumoperitoneum.
      3. Demonstrate the correct technique for insertion of a reusable and a disposable trocar and cannula.
      4. Demonstrate the ability to identify laparoscopically normal and abnormal anatomy of an abdominal wall and intraabdominal and pelvic organs.
   B. Didactic objectives
      1. Know the acceptable alternative insertion sites for insufflation needles to establish a pneumoperitoneum.
      2. Know the correct technique for open laparoscopy and direct trocar insertion techniques, including the indications and contraindications for each technique.

Many of these objectives are best demonstrated by video review or during a live case with the resident as an observer. Though these objectives appear to be technique oriented, they should be supplemented by the appropriate literature references.

IV. Complications
   Information required to minimize and manage the complications related to operative endoscopic procedures must be understood by the clinician. It is difficult to construct models that accurately demonstrate complications. Therefore these objectives are primarily didactic. The exception is the availability of a live animal model. Such models are beneficial but of limited value when considering the wide range of complications that can occur. Residents should be able to describe how to recognize, minimize the incidence of, and manage the following traumatic (insufflating needle and trocar trauma) and instrumental injuries.

   A. Vascular injuries
      1. Abdominal wall vessels
      2. Intraabdominal vessels (i.e., omental, mesenteric, peritoneal).
      3. Retroperitoneal vessels (i.e., aorta, vena cava, iliac arteries and veins, other major vessels).
   B. Enteric injuries
      1. Stomach, small and large bowels.
      2. Bladder and ureter.
      3. Uterus, ovary, and fallopian tube.

These items refer to all types of injuries: laser, thermal, electrosurgical, crush, laceration, perforation.

   C. Cardiopulmonary
      1. Arrhythmias, hypercapnia, anesthetic complications.
      2. Fluid overload.
      3. Pulmonary edema.
      4. Embolism.
   D. Postoperative
      1. Incisional hernias
      2. Delayed hemorrhage

V. Hemostatic and incisional techniques
   The application of the various energy modalities and of suturing and ligature techniques that are available for laparoscopy is of paramount importance. Because institutions may not have all of these modalities available, the residents should be knowledgeable about all of the technical expertise but must be skilled only in those that are available at their facility. It is recommended that they become skilled in the use of at least one type of laser regardless of whether it is available at their facility. Because the choice of a particular incisional technique is often operator-dependent, the resident should be skilled in more than one technique. This rule also applies to hemostatic techniques. The emphasis should be on both versatility and proficiency. For each technique or energy application, the resident should be able to describe the necessary instrumentation, application technique, tissue effect, patient selection, limitations, complication minimization and management, and relative cost-effectiveness when compared to comparable techniques.

A. Sharp dissection
     1. Instrumentation
     2. Technique and application
  B. Suturing and ligature techniques
     1. Extracorporeal knot-tying
     2. Intracorporeal suturing
     3. Preloaded ligature systems
     4. Hemostatic clips and staplers
  C. Electrosurgery
     1. Basic electrophysics
     2. Tissue effects: fulguration, coagulation, desiccation, cutting
     3. Electrical circuits: bipolar, unipolar
     4. Waveforms: modulated, unmodulated, mixed
     5. Complications: capacitive coupling, direct coupling, faulty grounding
  D. Lasers
     1. Physics: power density, generation of light, wavelength
     2. Tissue effects
     3. Comparison of currently available types of lasers
     4. Safety

The objectives up to this point have pertained to basic information and skills that are needed prior to performing any laparoscopic procedure. The following objectives are more procedure oriented. These are best categorized into those the resident should be skilled in (i.e., able to perform proficiently) and those of which the resident should be knowledgeable (i.e., aware of the technique, indications, contraindications and relative risks and benefits).

VI. Specific procedures
  A. Skilled procedures
     1. Diagnostic laparoscopy and chromopertubation
        a. The resident should be able to discuss the indications and role of diagnostic laparoscopy in the following clinical situations.
           (1) Infertility
           (2) Chronic and acute pelvic pain
           (3) Ectopic pregnancy
           (4) Pelvic mass
     2. Laparoscopic sterilization
        a. The resident should be able to demonstrate at least two techniques and be knowledgeable about the other techniques.
        b. Know the appropriate preoperative evaluation and be able to discuss the risk/benefit ratio (informed consent).
     3. Ectopic pregnancy
        a. Know the risk factors, epidemiology, and necessary evaluation of the suspected ectopic pregnancy.
        b. Choose the appropriate treatment modality, including medical and expectant management, and the laparoscopic and laparotomy techniques.
        c. Perform and select patients appropriately for partial salpingectomy, total salpingectomy, and a linear salpingostomy by laparoscopic and laparotomy techniques.
        d. Be able to adequately manage postoperative elevated human chorionic gonadotropin titers and to diagnose and treat persistent trophoblastic disease.
     4. Lysis of mild to moderate adhesions
        a. Perform adhesiolysis using at least two modalities and be able to discuss the risks and benefits of each.
        b. Know the indications and available techniques for adhesiolysis as it applies to infertility and pain syndromes, including adhesion prevention techniques.
     5. Mild to moderate endometriosis
        a. Select and surgically manage stage I and II endometriosis by resection or ablative techniques.
        b. Discuss the risk factors known to be associated with the development and progression of endometriosis and the role of endometriosis as it relates to infertility and pelvic pain.
        c. Know the signs and symptoms associated with endometriosis,

the revised American Fertility Society scoring system, and the role of medical management and adjunctive therapy.
   6. Pelvic mass
      a. Properly evaluate and select the appropriate patient for a laparoscopic approach.
      b. Be able to perform an oophorectomy by at least two techniques and be knowledgeable about alternative techniques.
      c. Know the available techniques to prevent or reduce intraperitoneal spillage of ovarian contents.
      d. Know the techniques for performing an ovarian cystectomy.
B. Familiar procedures
   The following is a list of procedures of which the resident should be aware, including the correct techniques, indications, risks, and potential benefits. Some of these procedures, have not yet been shown to have proven benefit over more traditional approaches. Because they are generally done with less frequency, the resident may not have the opportunity to perform or even observe them. They are recognized procedures nonetheless, and knowledge of the techniques and indications are useful.
   1. Laparoscopic-assisted vaginal hysterectomy
   2. Appendectomy
   3. Laparoscopic uterosacral nerve ablation
   4. Presacral neurectomy
   5. Ovarian drilling
   6. Ovarian wedge resection
   7. Uterine suspension
   8. Retropubic bladder neck suspension
   9. Myomectomy and myolysis
   10. Fimbrioplasty and neosalpingostomy

The next step is to incorporate both the didactic and the technical exercises into workshop sessions. Workshop sessions that offer only didactic lectures or only technical exercises tend to be less interesting than those in which these two components are offered together. Organizationally, it is easier to design sessions focused on residents at a similar level of training, especially when dealing with the fundamental objectives (I–IV). If this design is not possible and residents with different levels of experience must attend at the same time, workshop sessions should have a variety of exercises that require a range of ability for completion. Alternatively, senior or more advanced residents can serve as assistants or instructors. When structuring the program, all of these factors must be considered. Programs that offer the exercises to all levels tend to be monotonous and ineffective. The pertinent didactic information can be presented in lecture form (which can be time-consuming) or in an interactive format. A syllabus with reading assignments tends to be more time-efficient so long as there is a means to ensure that the material is read. Videotapes and case review supplemented with literature reviews are highly effective teaching tools but can be time consuming for the instructors. Suggestions for workshop sessions are presented later in the chapter. Each institution must critically examine the best way to accomplish the stated objectives. So long as the objectives are met, the program is effective.

Materials and Methods

An integral part of every endoscopic training program is the available instrumentation for the workshops. The instruments used should be similar to those the residents will eventually use for surgery. Endoscopic training programs serve two purposes: to adequately train residents in endoscopic procedures and to familiarize them with instrumentation. It is impractical and ineffective to train residents in specialized procedures on equipment that will not be available to them once they start performing surgery. Optimally, a separate set of instruments should be utilized only in the workshop, as it reduces the risk of damage of those instruments needed for surgery. Occasionally, specialty instruments from the surgical sets must be used to demonstrate their function. It is tempting to reuse discarded disposable instrumentation after it has been properly cleaned and sterilized. Although it is more cost-effective than purchasing a separate set of instruments, it creates an unrealistic situation. The residents must be exposed to a variety of instrumentation if possible. This practice provides more comprehensive education and allows better intraoperative decision-making. The resident will then be able to choose an instrument that relates to its performance rather than that it has been the only instrument to which the resident has been exposed. The following is an example of a typical set of training instruments.

Scissors 5 mm (1)
Graspers 5 mm (2)
Atraumatic graspers 5 mm (2)
Needle holders 5 mm (1 for a straight needle and 1 for a curved needle)
Reducing sleeve 10 mm to 5 mm (1) and 5 mm to 4 mm (1)
0° Laparoscope 10 mm (1)
Trocars and cannulas 10 mm (2) and 5 mm (2)
Unipolar needle electrode 5 mm or 3 mm (1)
Button tip electrode 5 mm or 3 mm (1)
Bipolar forceps (1)
Reducing caps (multiple)

In addition, a videocamera recorder (VCR), camera, monitor, and light source should be available. A Pelvic-Trainer is essential, equipped with an opaque top. Hands-on sessions are best conducted on the Pelvic-Trainer using the video monitor. Groups should be kept small, ideally no larger than three participants per trainer. Residents should wear surgical gloves during the session to better approximate surgical conditions. The instructor should attempt to conduct each session with a "intraoperative attitude," not allowing short cuts or inappropriate techniques because "it is only a workshop." Bad habits developed in the workshop easily find their way into the OR.

Exercises and Models

Ligature Practice Models

There are several models that can be constructed easily and inexpensively. A tying board (Fig. 29.1) is constructed from a block of wood

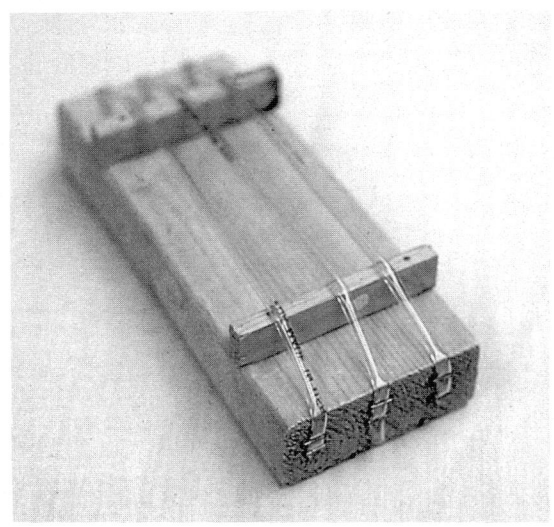

Figure 29.1. Tying board, constructed from a block of wood and tubing, can easily and inexpensively serve as a ligature practice model.

and tubing. An additional model can be constructed from a Penrose drain filled with water. This model performs well because it offers resistance to tie against. These models are used to practice tying extracorporeal knots. The exercises are performed in the Pelvic-Trainer and are uncomplicated. A suture is introduced and passed around either the Penrose drain or the tubing. An extracorporeal knot is then tied and placed. In the case of the Penrose drain, two sutures can be placed and the drain then cut. Knot integrity is confirmed by the absence of leakage. Passing the suture helps develop eye–hand coordination skills, and the placement of extracorporeal knots develops knot-tying skills. It is a practical exercise. Novice residents can use the exercise to familiarize themselves with basic endoscopic instruments and equipment, and the more experienced residents can use the exercise to develop knot-tying skills, practice various tying techniques, and develop better two hand coordination. Because the task is well defined, the resident can concentrate on the technique and not be concerned with the choice of instrument or technique to use.

Figure 29.2. Most easily constructed suture model consists of a piece of decorative fruit mounted to a board. Any material easily penetrated by a needle suffices.

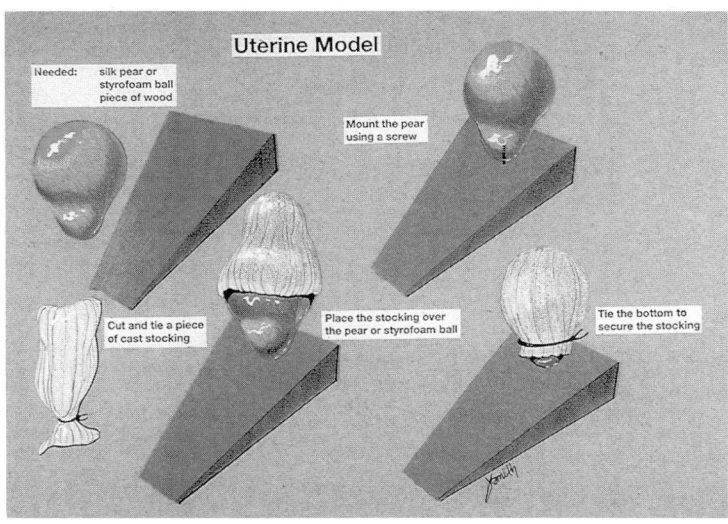

Suturing Models

A variety of models can be used to practice laparoscopic suturing. The easiest to make and use is a piece of decorative fruit mounted to a board (Fig. 29.2). Any material that is easily penetrated by a needle suffices. The important aspect of the model is that it gives the same spatial orientation as would be expected from the uterus in the pelvis. Other useful models are shown in Figs. 29.3 and 29.4. The small bowel model is constructed from enlarged parous pig uterine horns. The bladder model is an extirpated male or female urinary bladder. Each of these models is simply anchored to a towel after being cleaned and rinsed. They offer the advantage of easy assembly; and because they are real tissue they have a feel similar to that encountered during surgery. This point is key to suturing models. The need for suturing arises infrequently, and so it is important that when teaching or learning the technique the model should have some similarity to the clinical application. Suturing is most often used on the uterus, bladder, or bowel. The mounted models offer a similar orientation to the uterus but have a completely different orientation from the bladder or bowel. To teach suturing techniques properly, several models are necessary. The bowel and bladder models can be placed at several locations within the Pelvic-Trainer to require the resident to choose the appropriate

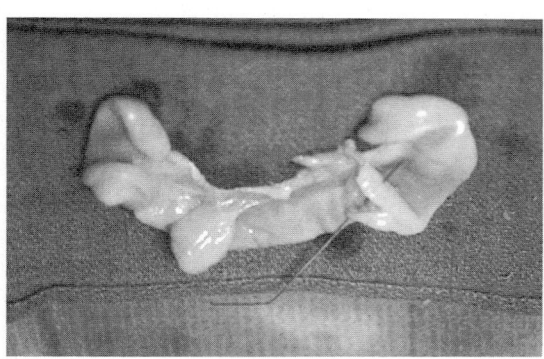

Figure 29.3. Useful model of the small bowel is constructed from enlarged pig uterine horns.

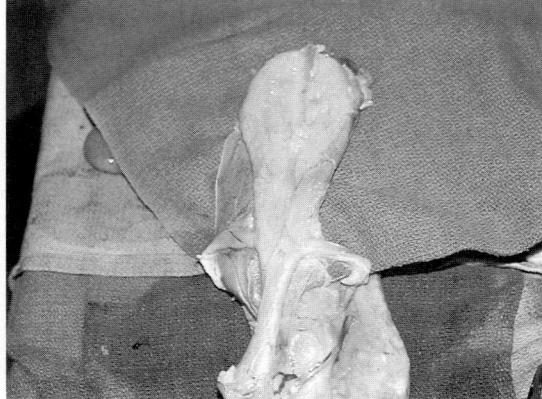

Figure 29.4. Bladder model that is an extirpated male or female urinary bladder.

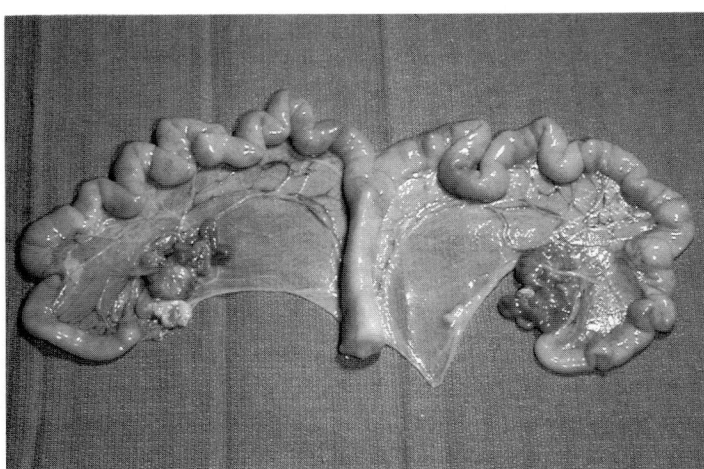

Figure 29.5A. Expirated pig uterus with attached broad ligaments, tubes, and ovaries.

port, type of needle, type of needle driver, and type of knot slider that would perform best in that situation.

Tubal Pregnancy Models

One of the best models for a tubal pregnancy is made from extirpated pig uterine horn (Fig. 29.5A–C). If possible, two "ectopics" should be placed in each uterine horn, so there are four ectopic models for practice on each uterine model. This practice improves the efficiency of the session. This model performs well with all energy modalities. If electrosurgery is to be demonstrated, a grounding wire is simply attached to the tube that is to be used. Once

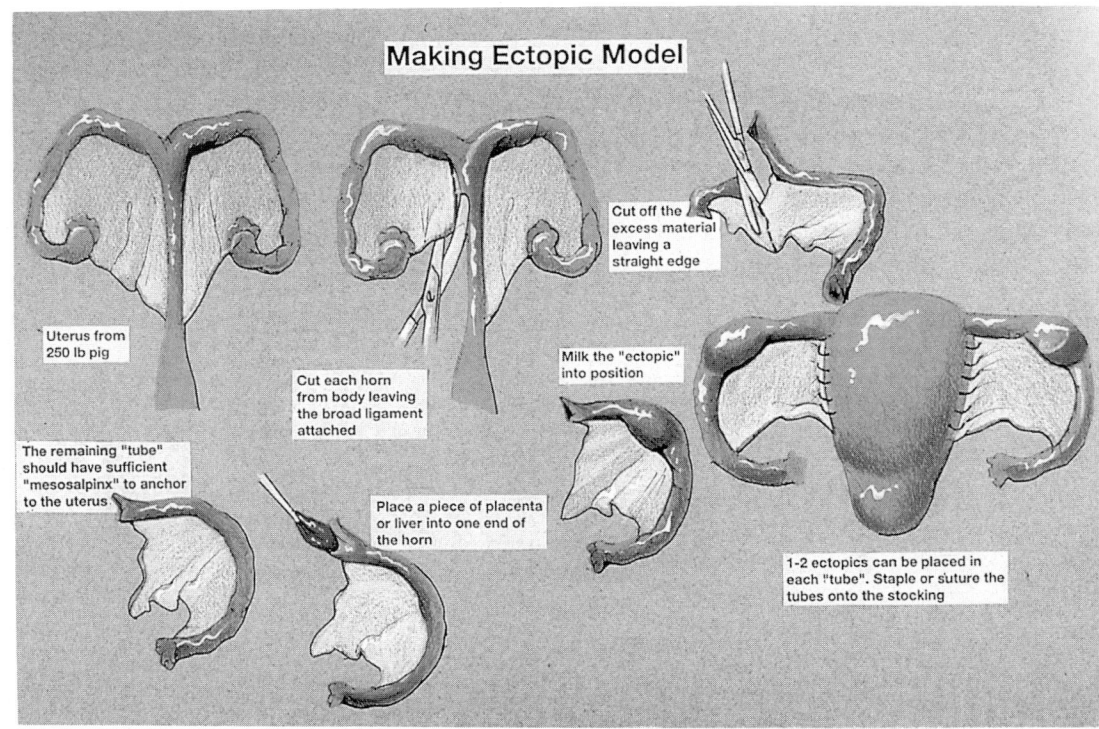

Figure 29.5B. Assembly of an ectopic model.

29. Teaching Operative Endoscopy

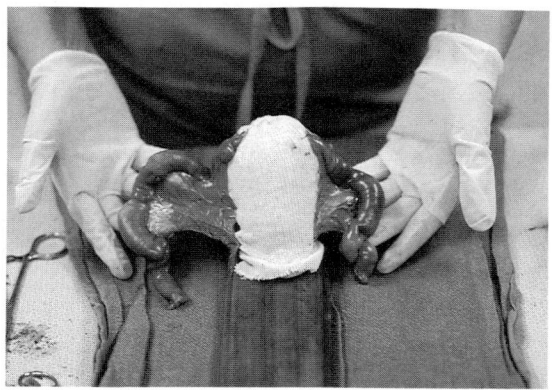

Figure 29.5C. Completed model.

constructed, the model is highly versatile. By adding a large gallbladder (Fig. 29.6A–B), a small gallbladder (Fig. 29.7), ovarian, and hydrosalpinx models are created.

Tissue Effect Models

When comparing the tissue effects of various energy sources, it is important to choose tissue that can readily demonstrate a relative depth of damage. The best model is fresh bovine or porcine liver. Another useful model is a piece of fresh chicken with the skin still attached. This model is best suited for dissection techniques. Models to simulate endometrial implants are made by injecting small amounts of chocolate syrup underneath the chicken skin.

Note

There are many modifications and derivations of these models. The ones described here are useful examples that have been found to be effective.

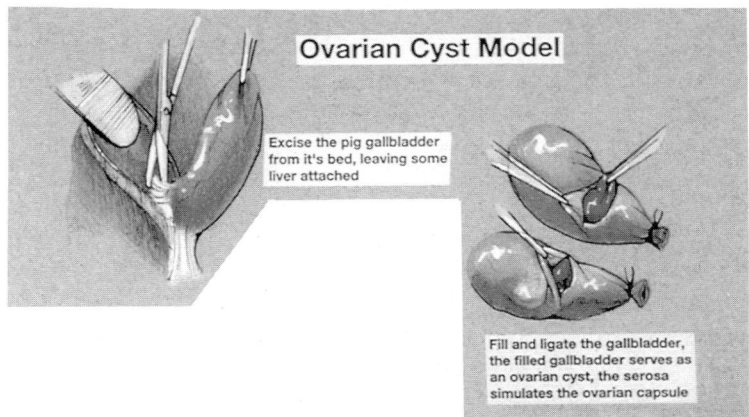

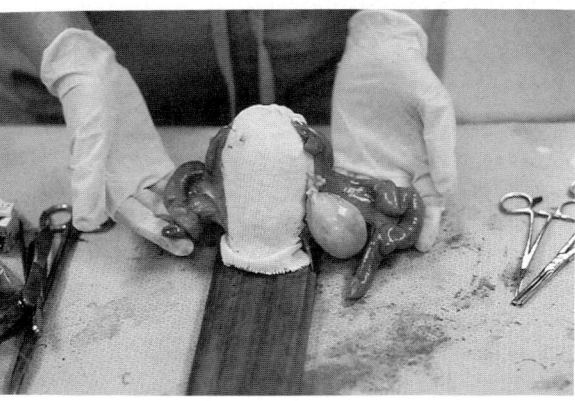

Figure 29.6. After harvesting a pig gallbladder, it can be used as an ovarian cyst model either alone (A) or attached to a uterine model (B).

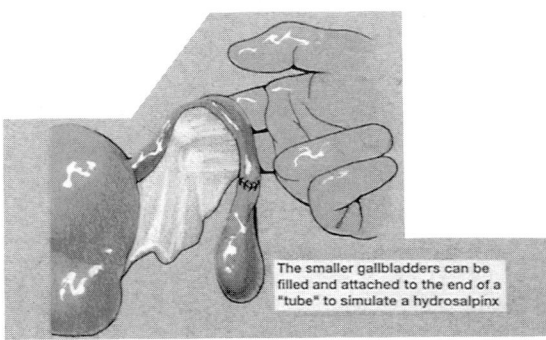

Figure 29.7. With the addition of a small gallbladder, a hydrosalpinx model is created.

Workshop Sessions

Introduction to Operative Laparoscopy

The initial portion of a session on the introduction to operative laparoscopy presents the residents with the general outline of the program and what is expected of them in reference to attendance and participation. The necessary list of reading material or a syllabus is distributed. The session also includes a brief overview of the purpose and direction of operative laparoscopy as it applies to the practice of gynecology at their institution. This session is an excellent time to update the residents on any ongoing protocols or projects that involve endoscopic surgery. The didactic portion of this workshop reviews the institution's available equipment and the instrumentation and additional instruments of which the residents should be aware. It is best done through a slide presentation, followed by a detailed review of general laparoscopic techniques, such as establishing a pneumoperitoneum, trocar insertion, safety of insufflation pressures, and the contraindications to and complications of laparoscopy. Included in this review is a detailed presentation on pelvic and abdominal anatomy and how it applies to operative laparoscopy. These objectives are accomplished with edited video review. When videotapes are used, it is helpful to show only the most pertinent portions and have them well organized. This introductory session tends to be one of the longest workshops and may need to be given in two sessions. If this workshop is a review for more advanced participants, a more interactive approach can be chosen. Videofilms of the equipment or the equipment itself may be shown, with the participants simply answering questions; or the material can be divided between the participants and they can present it to each other. After presenting the didactic information, the hands-on exercises are described. The use of endoscopic suturing has been shown to be an effective introductory exercise, as it can be applied to any level of training.[3]

The hands-on portion presents how to correctly assemble the video setup and various instrumentation, including trocars, irrigation pumps, bipolar forceps, and so on. Appropriate electrical power settings can be reviewed at this time. A list of exercises to be performed on the Pelvic-Trainer follows.

1. Correct technique for introducing an insufflation needle and a trocar (disposable versus reusable)
2. Suture and extracorporeal knot-tying (Fig. 29.1). This exercise should be performed with both an overhand knot and a slip knot with several types of suture material.
3. Correct application of a prepackaged ligature system.
4. Practice laparoscopic suturing (Figs. 29.2, 29.4). Perform this exercise with at least two types of needle driver. This exercise should be done using several types of needle and suture. The various tying techniques should be demonstrated and compared.

Management of the Ectopic Pregnancy

The workshop on managing ectopic pregnancies begins with a review of the current literature pertaining to both the medical and surgical management of ectopic pregnancy. A presentation of the available laparoscopic techniques and their indications and contraindications is appropriate. It should also cover management of a large hemoperitoneum, preoperative considerations, and intraoperative decision-making. Again, videofilm review is helpful but should be concise. This phase is followed by a brief review of the operative laparoscopic setup and knot-tying techniques.

The hands-on portion focuses on the clinical applications of laparoscopic techniques. The following is a list of exercises.

1. Perform a linear salpingostomy (Fig. 29.5).
   With and without injection of the mesosalpinx
   With sharp dissection
   With unipolar instrumentation
2. Perform a segmental resection.
   With suture techniques
   With Hulka clips
3. Perform a total salpingectomy.
   With suture ligatures
   With bipolar techniques

This session can be conducted in a task oriented fashion or in a case-scenario fashion, depending on the level of experience of the participants. Case scenarios add a decision-making component to the exercise and tend to be more interesting. However, they can be overwhelming for the novice who is still learning the basic techniques.

Oophorectomy and Ovarian Cystectomy

The didactic portion of the oophorectomy and ovarian cystectomy session focuses on preoperative and intraoperative decision-making when selecting appropriate candidates for laparoscopic management. It should include an adequate review of the current literature. Videofilm review of the various techniques for oophorectomy and cystectomy is important, as it is difficult to design a comparable exercise. This review includes spill prevention and reduction techniques.

The hands-on session can be used to present the ligature and bipolar electrosurgical techniques used to perform an oophorectomy (Fig. 29.6). This point is also an opportune time to in-service the residents in the use of automatic cutters and staplers. The following is a list of exercises.

1. Perform an adnexectomy using bipolar and ligature techniques.
2. Demonstrate the use of endoscopic stapling devices.
   Linear staplers

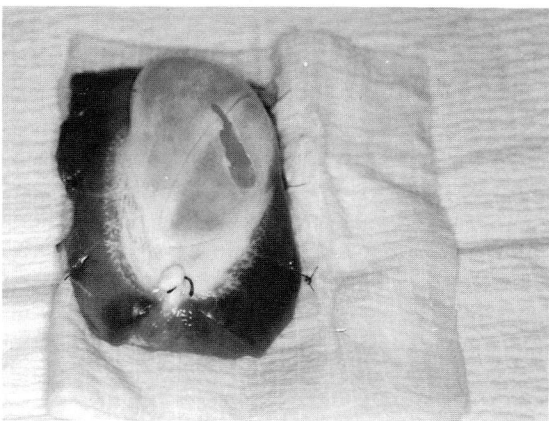

Figure 29.8. Useful exercise for the hands-on session is to simulate an ovarian cystectomy using a pig gallbladder.

   Disposable and reusable clip appliers
3. Perform tissue removal utilizing an endoscopic bag.
4. Perform an ovarian cystectomy on a pig gallbladder (Fig. 29.8).

Comment

Three examples of workshops that can be offered have been outlined. Each workshop can accomplish several objectives, both didactic and practical, efficiently. The key points to remember are to keep the sessions concise and to have the objectives well defined and stick to them. The instructor must adequately prepare for each workshop, prepare the tissue models prior to the workshop, and check on the availability of specific instruments or equipment if appropriate. Exercises must be designed to be challenging for those with different skill levels.

Conclusion

The implementation of a resident training program in operative laparoscopy is a feasible and effective means to properly prepare residents for laparoscopic surgery. Comprehensive and agreed-on objectives should be defined prior to initiating the program. Each session should be comprised of a didactic and a hands-on portion, and it should attempt to cover all of the objectives in an organized, concise fashion.

It is difficult to verify the adequacy of any surgical training. Attendance alone does not guarantee competence. There are useful adjuncts that at least provide some measure of retained information. Written and practical examinations are helpful, especially if a certain level of achievement must be obtained in order to advance to performing surgical procedures. Whatever means is chosen, it should be agreed upon and clearly stated.

References

1. WOLFE WM, LEVINE RL, SANFILIPPO JS, ET AL: A teaching model for endoscopic surgery: hysteroscopy and pelviscopic surgery. Fertil Steril 1988; 50:662.
2. GLOWACKI GA: An in-hospital training program in gynecologic laser therapy. J Reprod Med 1985; 30:93.
3. SAMMARCO MJ, YOUNGBLOOD JP: A resident teaching program in operative endoscopy. Obstet Gynecol 1993;81:463.

30
Learning, Certification, and Credentialing for Endoscopic Surgery

Carl J. Levinson and Raymond H. Kaufman

Most gynecologists learn their basic surgical procedures during residency. Those who pursue a fellowship have more extensive experience with normal and distorted pelvic anatomy. In decades past, further experience was achieved by working with a senior partner or by performing multiple surgical procedures over the years. Unfortunately, to some extent in recent years such common approaches to "learning" have not been permitted. New techniques (laparoscopy, hysteroscopy) and new procedures (e.g., laparoscopic-assisted vaginal hysterectomy, or LAVH) have come upon the scene with great rapidity. The number of surgical cases available to those in training (e.g., hysterectomy) has steadily declined, and the number of practicing gynecologists has increased. As a result of these primary factors (and others), relatively few gynecologists are well trained in the performance of "advanced" gynecologic endoscopy: (1) gynecologists who finished residency before 1988–1990 had no such training (except in specific locations); and (2) practicing physicians generally had limited opportunity to learn and to practice.

The purpose of this chapter is twofold: (1) to direct the physician about the most propitious manner by which to introduce the new endoscopic surgical techniques into his or her practice; and (2) to assist the department chair and the board of directors of a hospital to determine how best to ascertain the competence of a surgeon for the performance of advanced endoscopic and laser surgery.

The recent "surgical revolution" refers to the performance of procedures via endoscopic instrumentation that previously required laparotomy. This shift now seems entrenched, as approximately 50% of previous gynecologic "laparotomies" have been converted to laparoscopic procedures. The underlying reasons for learning the skills of endoscopic surgery are varied: a fundamental desire to learn, to become competent, and to be current; to be the "first on the block"; to keep up with the competition; to enlarge the scope of one's practice; to promote the "new surgery."

The rapidity of change from laparotomy to laparoscopy has been overwhelming, with pressure from all sides: technologic advances, cost containment, new energy sources (e.g., laser), routine use of video (now advancing to three-dimensional pictures), the almost daily development of new instruments, and consumer demand.

The differences between this more recent (1990s) phenomenon of endoscopic surgery and that which occurred during the early 1980s (and even earlier "traditional" surgical training) have been the rapid rate of change, the economic pinch, decreased frequency of traditional gynecologic surgical procedures, lack of endoscopic training in the residency program, proliferation of community-based courses (a plus), impetus from instrument manufacturers, the introduction of laser energy, utilization of video, and problems of credentialing, both standard and economic.

In many respects endoscopic surgery was introduced in the United States much as was all gynecologic surgery. The early U.S. gynecologists were general surgeons, many of whom had come from or had studied abroad, especially in Germany and Austria. This process was repeated during the early endoscopy era, as this surgery was developed in France and Germany. Vaginal hysterectomy may be used as an example, not that all vaginal surgery was embraced by all surgeons. It was slow to gain acceptance in some areas but took hold in others (e.g., Chicago), which subsequently have been strongholds of vaginal surgery. In a classic manner, the procedures were taught by one partner to another, by professor to resident. Where one was located determined how much one saw and did—and how competent one became, much as today. Gradually, however, vaginal surgery was taught to (and practiced by) all.

"The times they are a-changing" and have already changed. New and valid procedures should be learned by all and introduced into their practice modes. Wherein then do the problems lie currently?

1. Residents often do not receive formal instruction in endoscopic surgery.
2. Many resident training programs do not have appropriate teachers for endoscopic surgery.
3. Completion of a 2-day course may not qualify anyone for anything.
4. Performing laparoscopy to cauterize minimal endometriosis, to lyse a few pelvic adhesions, and to ligate fallopian tubes does not prepare a gynecologic surgeon to perform advanced operative laparoscopic procedures, e.g., American Society for Reproductive Medicine (ASRM) class IV endometriosis surgery.
5. The ability to remove an ovarian cyst does not translate directly into being able to perform surgery for ASRM IV endometriosis surgery.
6. Diagnostic hysteroscopy does *not* lead naturally to submucous myomectomy by resectoscope.
7. A laparoscopic salpingostomy in February is not ample preparation for an emergency salpingectomy in August if there has been no intervening experience.

These issues are some of the common and blatant ones that arise on a regular basis. Others are more subtle (e.g., who "proctors, certifies, or credentials"?). Obviously, this responsibility belongs to those who are experienced. The proctor may then be in a "political" bind should the candidate be incompetent or inadequately trained. Usually both physicians are from the same institution, and the inadequate preceptee accuses the preceptor of prejudice. Who would wish to be a preceptor under these circumstances?

The rapidity of change has brought both good and "controversial" results, with of course the inevitable consequences. For the patient, the performance of endoscopic surgery is a boon: there is no inconvenience of a large incision; and there is less disfigurement, a shorter hospital stay, often less expense, and even the possibility of less extensive postoperative adhesions. In addition, the hospital census has diminished, resulting in decreased hospital revenue at a time when more expense is required for highly specialized equipment. More insidious is the fact that most gynecologists perform laparoscopy (almost all physicians perform the simple basic procedures, such as sterilization and adhesion lysis), and in the minds of many the transition to performing advanced laparoscopic surgery requires no specialized training. After all, instruments are available in the operating room, and there is the "need to be current." Furthermore, the results of infertility surgery are not immediately apparent and may be limited regardless of the technique. It is never known what the result might have been in more experienced hands. "Credentialing" is therefore stressed, not in an effort to restrict the number of gynecologic surgeons performing the procedure but to be certain that *all* who perform laparoscopic surgery do so with appropriate training, experience, and competence. (The foregoing remarks are pertinent to advanced operative laparoscopy in general, but they are even more appropriate when these procedures are performed with the use of laser energy.) It is no longer possible for decades to come and go in order to evaluate techniques and therapies; change is so rapid that these evaluations must take place within a matter of years. The groundwork for advanced endoscopic surgery was laid during the 1970s and early 1980s; and the meteoric rise has taken place over the last few years. In all likelihood, it will change the face of gynecologic surgery for years to come. (Consider how the use of vaginal ultrasonography, with markedly improved resolution, has changed the face of in vitro fertilization.) Appropriately rapid accommodations are necessary to remain competent. Proper credentialing *is* in order.

Learning and Preparation

Traditionally, the surgical training sequence follows a certain path: basic medical training (medical school) → laboratory experience and preliminary surgical training as an observer and assistant (medical school and residency) → operative training (residency) → continued surgical experience (practice).

Training for advanced laparoscopic surgery has come to the fore since the mid-1980s while our colleagues in vascular surgery faced and resolved the issue of "specialized training." (As described in an editorial in *Radiology*) Wexler et al.[1] outlined the qualifications for temporary privileges to perform peripheral angioplasty, specifically for those physicians who have *not* had previous formal training in this area.

1. Attend at least one percutaneous transluminal angioplasty (PTA) seminar at which live demonstrations are presented.
2. Learn the nature and anatomy of peripheral vascular disease, indications for angioplasty, risks and benefits of angioplasty, and alternative therapies.
3. Visit a laboratory where peripheral angioplasty is actively performed by experienced personnel and observe at least 10 procedures.
4. Learn the technical aspects and usage of equipment needed for peripheral angioplasty.
5. Learn the theory and practice of thrombolytic techniques as applied in the peripheral circulation.
6. Apprentice with a senior qualified physician who can instruct the candidate in the performance of not fewer than 100 peripheral diagnostic angiography procedures and 50 peripheral angioplasty procedures.
7. Be the primary operator for at least half of all procedures.
8. Apply for temporary PTA privileges to perform 10 procedures under the proctorship of the senior laboratory interventionalist who already has privileges in peripheral vascular disease.
9. Continue under the proctorship until 25 procedures are accomplished (provided no complications occur and the success rate is comparable to the area norm during the 10 procedures).
10. Apply for full privileges if after the 25 cases the success rate has been at least 85% and the complication rate less than 5%.
11. Allow a multidisciplinary panel to review all cases annually and make recommendations to the department chairperson regarding continuance of privileges. (In essence, privileges are not granted until competence is demonstrated.)

Surgery by endoscopy can be substituted for open abdominal procedures in a high percentage of benign cases. It is not difficult to prepare a program as described above, but it is difficult when a large number of surgeons wish to absorb (immediately) a new technique involving new instrumentation and energy sources. As these procedures are performed during the residency program, there is less demand for the training courses that currently exist; instead, the major emphasis is on credentialing and continued evaluation.

Basic Instruction

The previous comments have pointed out an unusual set of circumstances: the need for rapid training of a large number of gynecologists within a short time span during an era of decreasing case load per surgeon. How then can these individuals be prepared properly?

1. *Didactic training* introduces the theoretic issues and the mental knowledge to proceed further.
2. The widespread availability of *video films* allows frequent and minute inspection of techniques. If presented with an explanation and a description, the procedure can be set correctly into the mind of the observer; however, no technical skill can be developed in this manner.
3. The *Pelvi-Trainer* is a simulated situation in which a plastic box (usually covered) contains tissue (real or simulated). The top of the container has holes covered with rubber into which trocars and instruments can be placed. The entire procedure is viewed on a video monitor. Procedures can thus be performed and viewed by many while instruction is given with respect to technical expertise.
4. *Simulators* are now being developed that marry the computer, the video screen (the monitor), and the visual appearance of the pelvis and numerous abnormalities. By manipulating handles the student can perform "mock" procedures on the picture generated by the computer.
5. *Preceptorship* is the modern version of the "apprenticeship," allowing a "student" to train with (and be instructed by) the "master" or teacher. There is no finer method to transmit surgical knowledge and skill. Such training should be pursued because it is the most effective, although not always easy to obtain.

Credentialing/Certification

Certain terms must be defined because they are frequently found in hospital rules and regulations but do not always carry the same meaning.

Credentials are evidence attesting to one's right to credit, confidence, or authority: a written document of specific training and experience (e.g., medical school diploma, Board certification, certificate of attendance at a postgraduate course, statement certifying competence by a preceptor).

Competence is the minimum level of skill acceptable; it can be general or specific in a given technical procedure. Although it is often not written, a program director attests to the cognitive and technical competence of a resident on successful completion of the residency program. Such competence (cognitive and technical), however, may change; and thus periodic reevaluation is required.

Clinical privileges are those functions and procedures bestowed on a physician to allow the physician to perform such activity during the course of caring for patients within a given hospital. It is the hospital governing board that determines the mechanism whereby these clinical privileges are defined. Privileges for separate procedures are necessary for those that are controversial, are risky or have high visibility.

Accreditation does not refer to the physician but, rather, to an academic institution that has met specific requirements of an official review board.

Certification is the most confusing term. This certification (a "certificate") provides a document stating that the individual has completed a course of study and has met specific standards of some official body, which then attests to the individual's ability to practice a certain profession or practice in a specific area of a profession. (As discussed for "competence," all hospitals should require evidence that the cognitive and technical skills remain timely and have embodied new developments in the field.)

Dorsey[2] outlined the goals of credentialing as follows.

Patient protection
Quality assurance
Satisfactory surgical outcome
Evaluation of physicians' skills
Reduction of medical/legal risk

These basic significant goals (required by the hospital governing body) are generally delegated to the chairperson of a department or division. Properly exercised, such decisions are made by a jury of peers. Unfortunately, Dorsey continued, there are few *objective* guidelines for advanced endoscopic surgery at this time by which to determine a physician's competence to perform a specific procedure. These criteria must be rational, justifiable, objective, and fair. The credentialing process must be a cooperative effort between physician and hospital, whereby the surgeon plans the educational experience, fulfills the requirements, and presents appropriate evidence to justify his or her request for certification to perform clinical procedures.

Lessons from the New York Experience

Let us view the experience in New York State pertaining to laparoscopy. In June 1992 it was reported that the State had reviewed 158 major injuries during laparoscopic cholecystectomy over a 19 month period. As a result, the State recommended to hospital trustees that it would be advisable to clarify procedure, process, and evaluation with respect to laparoscopic procedures. It was particularly recommended that the credentialing process be clearly outlined. An accompanying statement was that "the learning curve is no excuse for complications." As a result, all adverse incidents are reportable, and many other changes have been instituted within the State.

Evaluation

In the hospital setting, continued evaluation should be performed by local peers. At least two individuals should provide the peer review: it is necessary to observe numerous procedures, but just how many has never been clear. Occasionally it is necessary to obtain outside evaluation, which is an expensive, time-consuming process. When prepared, the critique should be presented to the physician and a report placed in his or her file. Improvements and further training may be recommended. Reevaluation should be performed at a future time. Most institutions have 2-year cycles, at which point clinical privileges must be reestablished. This area is one of great weakness in our system, as careful scrutiny is rarely performed unless specific problems have developed. The number of operative cases is usually not noted. Perhaps history has indicated that it is not necessary for standard operating procedures, but it is recommended that such standards be provided for *new* operative techniques.

Preliminary Credentials

The physician must be licensed to practice medicine and surgery and be in good standing at the institution. The physician should be Board-certified, with extensive experience in diagnostic laparoscopy and should have privileges for the same surgical procedure by laparotomy as requested for minimally invasive surgery.

In the event that there are physicians at the institution who have been performing endoscopic procedures for 2 years or longer, the applicant may be "grandfathered" for procedures at levels 1 and 2 with required proctoring for three cases.

Levels of Competence: General Requirements

Level 1 privileges (Table 30.1) are extended to all surgeons applying who have met the basic requirements, have sufficient Pelvi-Trainer experience (as attested by an accredited proctor), have attended an appropriate course(s) of at least 20 hours in length including 8 hours of hands-on experience, and have assisted at 5–10 cases. Privileges are continued if good judgment is exercised and consultation sought when appropriate.

Level 2 privileges are extended to those surgeons with level 1 privileges who have completed the required number of proctored cases. (Proctors should not be associated in practice with the surgeon, and it is preferable to have more than one proctor.)

Table 30.1. Levels of competence: specific requirements

Requirements	Required no. of cases
Level 1—basic	
Lysis of adhesions not involving bowel	
Lysis of filmy adhesions involving bowel	
Removal of ectopic pregnancy with conservation of the tube	
Endocoagulation and electrosurgery (fulguration, coagulation)	
Use of Endoloops for	
Hemostasis	
Removal of pedunculated tumors	
Puncture of simple benign cysts	
Level 2—major (procedures)	
Adhesiolysis	
Dense bowel adhesions	2
Mid to upper bowel adhesions	2
Myomectomy	2
Oophorectomy and endometrioma removal	2
Salpingo-oophorectomy	2
Salpingectomy	
Appendectomy	1
Intraabdominal suturing and use of stapling or clips	3
Intra- and extracorporeal knot-tying	
Laser division of uterosacral ligaments	2
Level 3—advanced (procedures)	
Retroperitoneal dissection with ureteral dissection	3
Total hysterectomy (where the uterine artery is occluded laparoscopically) (LAVH)	3
Subtotal hysterectomy	1
Suspension of bladder/urethra	2
Presacral neurectomy and LUNA	2
Level 4—Extra procedures	
Lymphadenectomy	4
Malignancy	3
Pelvic reconstruction	4

LUNA, laser uterosacral nerve ablation.
In view of the fact that many procedures may be performed during the same case, the total number of cases may be fewer than indicated above. In the event that obvious competence is displayed, based on prior documented experience, the department chair may decrease the number of cases required to be credentialed.

Level 3 procedures are advanced, complex procedures that are essentially "new" as performed by endoscopy. Each such procedure is credentialed separately. Requirements include attendance at a course for the special procedure, animal practice, and human work as an assistant surgeon. The procedure itself must be accepted as safe and appropriate with concurrence from the surgeons who performed the procedure by laparotomy. (Complex procedures are best performed by a group of surgeons who perform them on a regular basis. These procedures are generally specialty-specific, and the surgeon must have privileges within that specialty.)

In the event there is a low volume of endoscopic surgical procedures or an inadequate number of proctors, it becomes the responsibility of the chief of service, in accordance with hospital rules, to determine how the surgeons may be credentialed for new procedures. Specialized training, proctoring and careful evaluation are required.

Training

For levels 2 and 3, the surgeon must have been approved for level 1 privileges. (In questionable cases, proctors may be assigned or past performance may be reviewed.)

Training may be in-house if the department has developed a full training program. Outside training may be obtained via a preceptorship or by attending courses. Under a preceptor program the preceptor must attest to the competence of the preceptee. Training courses consist of Basic Laparoscopy Techniques, Laser Physics and Safety, Electrosurgical Principles and Techniques, Approved Faculty Quality, Adequate Didactic Time, and Adequate Time with Tissue or Animals. For level 3 procedures the course(s) must be procedure-specific.

Experience

The surgeon should act as an assistant to experienced surgeon(s) for a variety of cases that increase in complexity (5–10 cases). After having obtained the required training and experience, the surgeon should undergo the proctoring procedure. The proctor should be a surgeon experienced in the area of interest and unbiased, who acts as a reviewer and evaluator of the surgical management. Specifically, the following items must be checked: indication, familiarity with equipment, familiarity with the operative procedure, time involved, knowledge of anatomy, incidence of complications; and general approach. The number of cases required is *suggested* but may be amended by the local institution.

Follow-up Evaluation

Privileges should be reviewed every 2 years, but complications should be reviewed at least annually.

References

1. WEXLER L, LEVIN DC, DORROS G, ET AL: Training standards for physicians performing peripheral angioplasty: new developments. Radiology 1991;178:19.
2. DORSEY JH: Education and credentialling of the gynecologic laser surgeon. Obstet Gynecol Clin North Am 1991;18:661.

31
Legal Issues Regarding Operative Gynecologic Endoscopy

Steven R. Smith

Legal issues related to operative gynecologic endoscopy have grown in importance and complexity as these surgical procedures have become more common and sophisticated. These legal issues include qualifications for practice, informed consent, professional liability (malpractice), hospital practice, equipment failure, treatment of minors, and confidentiality.

Legal issues raised in gynecologic endoscopy generally follow legal principles applicable to other areas of medical practice. In some instances, however, the unusual characteristics of endoscopy require special attention or consideration. For example, the relatively recent development of these techniques and the special skills they require imply that some formal specialty training should be completed before they are undertaken.[1,2]

The major legal principles that influence gynecologic endoscopy and their special application to operative laparoscopy and pelviscopic surgery are addressed here. In most instances, we cannot be completely certain of the application of legal principles to these medical techniques because there are relatively few cases that have specifically involved endoscopy. The basic principles are clear, however; and we can fairly well define the outlines of the law that apply to gynecologic endoscopy. Some caution is called for when applying these principles in any particular state, because as described at the end of the chapter there is variation among states in the application of legal doctrine. This chapter does not include a discussion of topics related to embryoscopy, fetal therapy, ovum donation, and similar reproductive issues.

Formal Training in Gynecologic Endoscopy

The qualifications prerequisite to surgical endoscopy comprise a good example of the potential for legal difficulties that arise from the increasingly sophisticated surgical techniques utilized. In one legal sense, the M.D. or D.O. degree (as part of a license to practice medicine) is the only educational qualification required to engage in the practice of gynecologic endoscopy. A state license permits the holder to practice virtually all kinds of medical or surgical procedures. The broad statement of authority to practice is, however, misleading.

There are substantial ethical and legal limits on physicians practicing in areas in which they are not fully competent, even if the state license permits a full range of practice. For example, a physician "shall . . . obtain consultation . . . when indicated."[3] The practitioner who practices gynecologic endoscopy without formal training risks malpractice liability if that practitioner's quality of care does not conform to that of a well qualified professional. Such a professional is "holding himself or herself out" as an expert and will probably be held to the standard of care of an expert.[4] A physician not well qualified to undertake endoscopic practice must refer the patient to someone who is adequately qualified. The physician who fails to do so is risking malpractice liability.

Emphasis should be placed on *formal* training in endoscopic techniques.[5] Simply reading about new procedures or hearing them described is clearly not sufficient. There should be a period of supervised clinical training in the new techniques. Even a practitioner who has had some formal training in gynecologic endoscopy must engage in additional training when a technique is undertaken that is a material departure from past practice. Given the increasing variety of complex techniques in operative gynecologic endoscopy, it is essential that practitioners have training in the *specific* techniques and equipment they are planning to use. It is also important that institutions ensure that such *specific* training has been completed before a practitioner is permitted to undertake a new procedure in the hospital. Again, the element of adequate supervision by existing experts in the field is of importance.[6]

The specific form of training in terms of its duration, type, location, and intensity depends on the complexity of the procedures to be learned and the experience of the practitioner seeking the training. Ideally, the training leads to a broadly recognized certification by a well respected professional organization or by an accredited institution (hospital or school of medicine).[7] Certification per se, however, does not ensure an adequate education and thus does not ensure legally adequate training. "Box top" or "correspondence" certification would be of little value if the adequacy of training of a physician engaging in gynecologic endoscopy were challenged in a legal proceeding. When obtaining training, the professional should ensure that any formal standards for training in gynecologic endoscopy procedures have been fully met.[8]

In addition to the ethical imperative and liability avoidance value of obtaining good training before gynecologic endoscopy is undertaken, such training is generally necessary before these procedures may be undertaken in hospitals or other institutions. Indeed, to avoid liability and accreditation problems, institutions should have policies and procedures in place to ensure that only those properly trained are permitted to perform gynecologic endoscopy within the institution.[9]

Informed Consent

The primary purpose of the ethical and legal requirement of informed consent is to implement an important personal interest: the right of patients to determine what will be done to their bodies (the right of autonomy privacy).[10] Although informed consent is essentially a legal doctrine, it may have medical benefits as well by preparing the patient for medical or surgical procedures or by increasing trust in physicians.[11] Although we often think of informed consent as of relatively recent origin, legal cases involving liability for failure of consent can be traced back more than 200 years.[12] One of the clearest statements of the requirement of consent is now nearly 75 years old. "Every human being of adult years and sound mind has the right to determine what shall be done with his or her own body and a surgeon who performs an operation without his [or her] patient's consent commits [a tort] for which he [or she] is liable in damages. . . ."[13] In modern times the troublesome part of the informed consent doctrine lies in defining what information must be given for the consent to be "informed" and therefore valid.[14]

Broadly stated, consent is required before any medical treatment or diagnosis is undertaken.[15] Consent for minor, safe, and noninvasive testing or treatment is commonly presumed from the fact that a patient seeks medical attention or does not object to the tests or treatment. As diagnosis or treatment becomes more risky or invasive, however, full consent is no longer presumed; and consent must be preceded by sufficient information for the patient to make an informed decision to accept or refuse the diagnosis or treatment. Gynecologic surgery is within the group of procedures that require specific informed consent.[16] Other treatments, including giving many prescription medications, also require some limited form of informed consent.[17]

Although informed consent need not be in writing in most states, a written document or notation does help prove what information was given and that the patient did consent to treatment. It is not the form that is critical, however; it is the communication of essential information to the patient that is the key.

The doctrine of informed consent sometimes appears to be a mass of ever-changing technical legal rules and regulations, and the law of informed consent is in fact complex.[18] We review various aspects of the legal rules in this section. The physician need not memorize a bundle of legal rules, though, because application of the doctrine of informed consent is relatively simple if the reason for informed consent is kept in mind: *Informed consent is intended to provide the patient sufficient information to permit an intelligent decision on whether to accept the proposed treatment or diagnostic procedures.*[19] The information generally considered to be essential to informed consent includes the following.[20]

1. Description of the procedures or treatments to be undertaken
2. Review of the benefits and the risks or hazards of this treatment or procedure
3. Statement of the alternatives to the proposed treatment or procedure,[21]
4. Consideration of the consequences and risks of rejecting the proposed treatment or procedure

Although the specific information may change depending on the procedure to be performed, the basic question is always the same: What information would a person in this patient's position require in order to make a well informed decision?[22] The decision-making basis for requiring this information is clear. It tells the patient what is recommended and why, the potential problems with that recommendation, and the options available.

Because the consent process is intended to provide information to the patient on which a decision can be made, it is imperative that the information be imparted in a way that is meaningful to the patient.[23] Complexity of language is a good example of an area in which the needs of the patient must be considered. It would do little good to provide a patient with a description of a proposed procedure in complex terms she could not understand.[24]

Specifics of Disclosure

The question of the specific information that must be disclosed is difficult. The question ordinarily arises in relation to the risks that should be identified. On one hand, we want to give the patient as much useful information as necessary. On the other hand, too much information may mislead the patient by needlessly frightening or overloading him or her. Thus it is impossible to answer the question "What information should be disclosed?" with mathematic precision.

As a general matter, a risk should be disclosed as the probability or the magnitude (harm it may cause) increases. A small risk of death should be disclosed, whereas the much larger risk of a transient rash may not require disclosure. The importance of a risk must also be measured in terms of the individual patient to the extent possible. For example, even a small risk of harm to the nerves controlling the hand is likely to be of considerably greater concern if the patient is a surgeon than if she is an attorney.

A physician is generally not required to redisclose information of which the patient is already aware or that is common knowledge. It has been said, for example, that the remote risk of death from anesthesia is such a risk.[25] For several reasons, however, caution is warranted when determining not to disclose information to a patient because the patient probably already knows it.[26] First, physicians may overestimate the knowledge of patients. Second, "common" knowledge is often only partially right at best, and the process of informed consent is a chance to correct mistaken beliefs. Third, some patients emotionally deny some information. This situation can be a problem particularly when patients refuse or delay diagnostic or treatment procedures and such a delay can be dangerous. The consent process may be a way of confronting this denial mechanism.

The obligation to provide information about the consequences of refusing the proposed procedure should not be neglected. This obligation is of significant importance when a patient is rejecting or delaying treatment (or a diagnostic process), and the delay may significantly harm the patient. An example of the importance of this obligation is the case in which a patient refused a Papanicolaou smear, developed cancer that went undetected until a cure was impossible, and sued the physician who had recommended the tests for failure to warn her of the potential fatal consequences of her refusal.[27,28] Although this case goes farther than most in suggesting liability (after all, it is reasonable to assume that the patient should have been aware of the risks she was taking), it does underline the importance of disclosing the risks of refusal of a proposed treatment or diagnostic procedure.

Exceptions to the Requirement

There are a few widely accepted exceptions to the informed consent requirement.[29] The two major exceptions are commonly referred to as the "emergency exception" and the "therapeutic privilege." Both of these labels are somewhat misleading if taken literally.

The *emergency exception* is the common sense rule that when someone is incapable of providing consent and immediate treatment is necessary to avoid death or serious injury, the treatment may be undertaken without informed consent.[30] This exception does not apply each time emergency medical treatment is necessary—only when there is a real emergency and there is no way to obtain informed consent (or refusal). It is important to emphasize that there are *two* requirements for depending on the emergency exception: the absence of any way of obtaining informed consent *and* the existence of a health emergency. Ordinarily, when a patient is incompetent to give (or refuse) consent, the next of kin or guardian gives (or refuses) consent. The emergency exception generally does not apply when it is possible to contact the next of kin or guardian for consent. Also, the emergency exception does *not* apply when a competent patient refuses consent to important treatment. In such cases, the physician or hospital may seek a court order to provide treatment.[31]

The *therapeutic privilege* permits information to be withheld from patients when providing that information would significantly and adversely affect their health. For example, if a patient is likely to become agitated as a result of hearing about certain risks associated with surgery, the information about those risks might be withheld. The decision to withhold information in many circumstances is made in consultation with the patient's family. Great caution should be exercised when claiming the therapeutic privilege. The physician invoking it should be prepared to demonstrate clearly the need to withhold the information and be able to state that serious harm was likely to ensue from giving the information to the patient. The fact that the patient would have refused treatment if given the information is decidedly *not* an adequate reason to invoke the privilege.[25]

Other Values of Informed Consent

In addition to the formal legal aspects involved, the informed consent process may be used to accomplish several other important goals. It can be used, for example, to place in perspective the unrealistic expectations of patients that a procedure is foolproof or guaranteed, to increase patients' feelings of participation in their own health and health care, and to encourage patients to discuss expectations and concerns about treatment.[32] In short, it is an opportunity to improve communication with patients.[33] As such, the process of obtaining informed consent should not be merely a dry, legalistic exercise but, rather, an important part of the total treatment of the patient.[34]

Informed Consent from Minors and Other "Incompetent" Patients

The concept of informed consent assumes that the patient is legally competent to make medical care decisions. In some circumstances, of course, patients are not competent to make their own decisions because of their age (minors) or mental condition.[35,36] When someone is incompetent, the law provides for a substitute decision-maker in the form of a guardian or next of kin.[37]

Traditional common law principles held that minors were not legally able to consent to treatment for themselves. Minors were generally those under the age of 18 or 21 (or somewhere between in some states).[38] A minor is considered "emancipated" from parents because of marriage or a permanent separation from the parental home. They are treated as adults for the purpose of consenting to medical care.[39] Despite considerable evidence that adolescents are able to be effective decision makers well before the age of 21 (or 18),[40,41] as a general proposition the decision to consent is still vested in the parents or guardians of minors.[42–44] There are, however, exceptions to this general rule. A number of states have adopted statutes that give minors the right to consent to treatment in some medical areas, commonly contraception and pregnancy counseling except abortion, obstetric care, and substance abuse treatment.[45] The U.S. Supreme Court has also recognized minors' rights to consent to the use of contraceptives and obtain an abortion in some circumstances.[46,47] The issue of informing parents of an abortion and contraceptive use remains at issue, however, although the consequences of such "squeal laws" may not have yet been fully realized.[46,48] Furthermore, the Supreme Court has upheld state laws that require parental notification of abortion or that require consent prior to abortion if the state statute provides for some legal mechanism to "bypass" the parental consent requirement in appropriate circumstances (i.e., where a minor may go to court to obtain consent to the abortion).[49,50] The issues related to treating minors are considered later in the chapter.

The Process of Obtaining Informed Consent

Ideally, the informed consent process for significant treatment or diagnostic procedures includes a written document that sets out the basic information needed by the patient to make a decision to undergo the proposed procedure plus at least two oral conversations with the patient (and in most cases the patient's family). One conversation should be used to present the information concerning the proposed procedure and to invite questions; the second is used to answer questions and secure consent. It is also desirable for the physician to document these steps as soon as possible after the discussion, summarizing the conversation(s) with the patient.

Obviously it is not always possible, or necessary, to undertake this formal "two conversations plus written consent" process. When there is a need for immediate action or the procedure proposed is not risky or invasive, a much more informal consent process is in order. Even in these circumstances, where consent is obtained more quickly or informally, however, the information necessary to make a decision should be imparted to the patient. Again, it is desirable to keep notes of the conversation with the patient.

Physicians should also remember that it is *their* duty to ensure that adequate informed consent is obtained from the patient. Although in some hospitals it is common for hospital personnel (*e.g.*, nurses) to supervise the signing of the consent form, the physician is ultimately responsible for the consent process, including providing the patient with the information necessary to make the consent decision.

A number of states have adopted informed consent statutes, often as part of malpractice reform efforts. Physicians and hospitals should seek legal advice about the requirements of individual states. For the most part, however, if the suggestions in this chapter are followed, the statutory requirement for informed consent will in all probability be met.

Application of Informed Consent Principles to Gynecologic Endoscopy

The above principles, applied to gynecologic endoscopy, suggest several informed consent guidelines for the practitioner,[51] including the following.

1. Except in the most extraordinary circumstances (e.g., an emergency situation in which the patient is not competent and delay would be harmful), written informed consent should be obtained from the patient. Copies of the written consent should be retained with the patient's hospital records, the medical records, and the physician's records.[52] A copy of the consent could also be given to the patient.

2. The written consent should be supported by oral discussion regarding the procedure. The physician should ensure that all of the patient's questions have been answered.

3. Ideally (except in emergencies), at least two discussions are involved in the consent process. A consent form should be left with the patient at the first meeting and signed at the second. If possible, a member of the patient's family (at the option of the patient) should be present during one of the conversations. Consent is ultimately the responsibility of the physician, not the hospital or nursing staff.

4. Special caution should be exercised when a patient is a minor or is not clearly competent. *State law regarding the "power" to consent to the medical procedure in question must be reviewed.*

5. At a minimum, the patient should be told (1) the nature of the procedure proposed, (2) the risks and benefits of that procedure, (3) alternative procedures or approaches, and (4) the consequences of not undergoing the procedure.

6. Consent should be obtained for diagnostic procedures and treatment and for anything that is significantly invasive, including many prescription drugs.[53] (The consent process for most drugs can be fairly informal.)

7. The informed consent process should be used to reduce unrealistic expectations of the patient. It should be clear that endoscopic treatment or diagnosis involves significant procedures that should not be undertaken lightly, that favorable results cannot be guaranteed, that there are risks associated with them, and that there will be some pain and a period of convalescence.[16]

8. In many instances patients should be informed that it is possible that a much more invasive procedure may be necessary. For example, for laparoscopy the patient should be told that open abdominal surgery may be indicated depending on the circumstances. It should be clear that the patient consents to the more invasive procedure. It is interesting that failure to obtain consent has been a feature of some of the relatively few officially reported laparoscopy liability cases.[54,55]

9. If sterility may result from the endoscopic procedure (or a more extensive procedure as described above), that issue should be raised expressly with the patient.[56] At one time it was thought necessary to obtain the consent to sterilization of a patient's husband, but that is no longer necessary so long as the woman is capable of giving consent.

10. Special consent must be obtained if the patient is a research subject or not receiving generally accepted ("standard") medical care. Special consent should be obtained if the patient is to be used for teaching. (The issue of teaching and research subjects is described later in this chapter.)

Liability and Informed Consent

Failure to obtain informed consent may result in civil liability (malpractice). Negligence is usually the tort resulting from the absence of informed consent, although battery is a remote possibility.

Although informed consent liability occurs, the problems it causes have been overstated because it is not as common as one might expect.[57] A number of states have applied technical legal doctrines in a way that reduces the potential for informed consent liability.[58] For example, by requiring that a patient demonstrate a causal relation between the absence of informed consent and the injury, the patient may have to demonstrate both that she (or, in some states, a reasonable patient) would have refused the diagnosis or treatment if given informed consent and that she was not informed of the risk of harm that in fact occurred.

Informed consent liability tends to be found in cases in which there are factors that aggravate the absence of informed consent, such as when there appears to be malpractice or grossly inadequate information was given to the patient. The absence of informed consent is often raised in malpractice suits as an alternative theory of recovery (i.e., in addition to a claim of bad medical care), but it is not often successful when the overall quality of care has been good, standard treatment has been provided, and the physician has been open and honest with the patient and her family.[59]

Example of an Informed Consent Document

A consent document that might be used for endoscopic surgery is presented below. No single document can be universally relied on as an informed consent document for all occasions, and consent must be undertaken keeping in mind the law of the state in which the procedure is to be performed. This document, therefore is not a "model" consent form.[60] Although there are differing views on this issue, I believe it is wise to develop informed consent documents tailored to specific procedures. Note that this form provides only basic information, and it would have to be accompanied by additional verbally communicated information. In a few instances this informed consent document contains blanks that the physician must complete.

Consent to Endoscopic Surgery

I understand that Dr. _____ is recommending that I undergo endoscopic surgery in order to *[description of the purposes of the endoscopy]*.

Description of the procedure: I understand that during this procedure the surgeons will first perform a diagnostic examination using the laparoscope. This will require creating one or more incisions (cuts) through the abdomen ("belly") near the umbilical area ("belly button"). This incision (or incisions) will probably be one or two inches long (each if there are more than one), although the length of the cut cannot be determined with certainty. Other small incisions may be required to insert additional instruments. I understand that the process that will occur next will depend on the findings during the first part of the operation. If in their judgment, treatment can be undertaken using the same laparoscope, the doctors will use the scope to try to correct identified problems. It is possible, however, that the doctors may decide that it is best to perform additional, more major surgery (laparotomy), which will require a large incision in my abdomen. A hospital stay will be required, which is usually short with laparoscopy, but is likely to be longer if open abdominal surgery is required.

Risks. I understand that laparoscopic surgery is a relatively safe procedure, but it does carry with it risks. There is a small possibility of cutting or puncturing my intestines or other organs (including the ureter or reproductive organs), which might result in serious bleeding or interference with specific function. Allergy to any of the medications used is also a remote possibility. Infection may occur with any form of surgery, although infrequently serious infections are seen with laparoscopy. I further understand that it will be necessary to give me a general anesthetic during the operative procedure, and that anesthesia also carries a risk of adverse reactions.

I have been informed that if it becomes necessary to do additional (major) abdominal surgery there are increased risks, including additional pain after surgery and a period of hospitalization and rest. The risk of infection is increased. Other risks include damage to the stomach, intestines, or other organs, infection or rupture in the surgical wound, burns on the skin, damage to the kidney and urinary system, blood clots in the pelvis and lungs, and allergic reactions.

The significant risks are not great, but there is a small risk of serious complications causing permanent disability or death. *[Insert statement in appropriate cases regarding sterility or the risk of sterility.]*

Alternatives. An alternative to pelviscopic surgery is major abdominal surgery, but that is not recommended because it may be unnecessarily risky and painful until after the endoscopic examination has been performed.

[If there are other diagnostic procedures or treatment alternatives, discuss those possibilities here.]

I also understand that if it is determined that open abdominal surgery is necessary it might be possible for the doctors to not perform it immediately but to wait a short time until I have discussed this matter further with them. Because of the additional difficulties and risks associated with this delay, I have decided that they should proceed immediately if in their medical judgment it is best to do so.

I understand that refusing this procedure might be risky to my health or life. Because the doctors cannot know what, if anything, is wrong with me without this procedure, it would be risky not to undergo this surgery the doctors are recommending. *[If the patient refuses the procedure, it is important to describe the risks in some detail.]*

[See note below concerning research and teaching.]

Consent. Having been informed of the above details and having discussed this operation with my doctor, I consent to Dr. _____ and such assistants as [he/she] may designate to perform the endoscopic surgical procedures, if necessary the abdominal surgery (laparotomy), and removing and disposing of any tissue or organs that may be necessary or medically desirable. This consent extends to the administration of such anesthetics and medicines as may be desirable. I also authorize the doctors to perform such other procedures as they may determine are medically desirable or necessary during the course of this operation. I understand that the doctors cannot guarantee the success of this treatment.

I understand that I may ask any questions about the surgery, and all of these questions have been answered to my satisfaction.

[Signed by the patient (and when appropriate a guardian or member of the family), the physician, and at least one witness (a witness who actually saw it signed).]

A note concerning research and teaching is appropraite here: If anything other than standard, commonly accepted practice is undertaken (including research), additional information must be given and special consent must be obtained. If the patient is to be used as a significant part of a teaching exercise, special consent should be obtained. These possibilities are discussed below.

Malpractice

Malpractice Liability

Civil liability, or malpractice, may arise out of the improper application of gynecologic endoscopic procedures.[61] Most commonly these cases are associated with the tort of negligence (a civil action based on the absence of reasonable care), although in rare instances liability is based on an intentional tort (e.g., battery or intentional infliction of emotional distress) or on a contract (a physician guaranteeing a cure or good result).

Purpose of Negligence

With any undertaking there is a potential for injury. Automobiles are involved in accidents, and some patients are harmed by medical care. When these unfortunate events occur there is harm to someone in terms of damage to property or person (e.g., lost wages, pain, medical bills). Society must determine who is to pay for these losses. It is not a question of *whether* someone should bear these losses. The losses have occurred, and someone *will* bear them. Rather, the question is *who* should bear them. One possibility is that losses should be borne by those who are injured, but this solution may place an extraordinarily difficult burden on those who are unfortunate enough to be injured. This burden, of course, may be reduced if the person injured has paid for insurance to avoid the devastation of injury or if the government provides some form of reimbursement. For the most part, this approach is the one taken by our society; those who experience such events or injuries are expected to bear the burden of the loss. Exceptions to this rule occur when injuries are caused by someone else's carelessness (negligence) or someone intentionally harms someone else. (As we see below special liability may also be imposed for harm resulting from defective products.) Thus negligence shifts the economic burden of someone's carelessness from the person who was harmed to the person whose carelessness caused the harm.

The primary purposes of negligence liability are to compensate someone harmed through someone else's negligence and to provide an economic deterrent to carelessness.[62] The theory is that our concern for having to pay for the injury of others makes us more careful to avoid injuring them. There are, of course, some problems with this system. It is somewhat inefficient in that it requires that two often difficult questions be answered: Did someone's negligence cause an injury? What were the damages caused by the injury? In addition, it is not an effective system of compensation in that many injured parties never recover anything, whereas others recover large amounts.

Principles of Negligence

Negligence liability requires four elements: (1) existence of a duty; (2) breach of that duty; (3) injury to someone; and (4) a causal link between the negligence and the injury. The absence of any one of these elements prevents liability. It is generally said that there is a broad duty of care—a responsibility to act reasonably under the circumstances to avoid injuries. Negligence is simply the failure to act reasonably under the circumstances. Defining "acting reasonably" (reasonable care) under a specific set of circumstances can be difficult. It requires that we set a standard of care against which the conduct of the actor may be judged.

Defining Standard of Care

Put most simply, a person is required to act as a reasonably prudent person would under the circumstances. This general obligation is refined for professionals. A physician is expected to act as a reasonably prudent physician would act under the circumstances. The failure of a practitioner to exercise the degree of care that a reasonably careful professional with similar training and expertise would exercise is negligence. This principle is carried one step further for specialists, who are expected to provide a level of care consistent with that provided by a reasonably careful specialist.

The level of care required is not one of perfection. Not every mistake is negligence. A mistake is negligence only if it is an error that a reasonably careful practitioner (or specialist) would not have made under the same circumstances.[63] Negligence focuses on a single incident rather than on the general competence or reputation of a practitioner. Just as an outstanding driver may infrequently be negligent by missing a stop sign, an outstanding physician may be negligent in providing a particular medical service. Finally, note that the level of care that is expected is defined to include the circumstances under which it is given. The law takes into account circumstances such as emergency conditions when determining what a reasonable person would do. In short, malpractice is based on actions that would be considered by the profession itself to be bad practice.[64]

In any circumstance there may be more than a single reasonable form of care. The law of negligence recognizes this fact. It also provides that the reasonableness of care should be judged in terms of the "school of thought" to which the practitioner subscribes. Where there are reasonable alternative methods of treating a condition, the physician may choose from among those approaches or schools of thought when providing care. At some point a whole school of thought may become negligent (e.g., a school of thought that favored treating appendicitis with aspirin), but that usually occurs when a school of thought has been discredited by a profession.[65]

The level of care expected of someone increases as he or she becomes more expert through special training or experience, or in any way claims to be more expert. Thus a specialist is expected to have a greater expertise in the area of specialty and is expected to maintain a bit higher level of practice in the area of specialty.[66] Those representing themselves ("holding themselves out") as specialists or as being particularly competent in an area are held to the high standard that they imply they have or claim to have. Therefore those claiming special expertise in gynecologic care are held to a higher standard of care, regardless of whether they have the training to justify the higher standard of care.

In some instances, a practitioner performing certain procedures is treated as though he or she were specially trained in that area of practice because (1) it is negligent to undertake this procedure without specialty training, (2) it was negligent not to refer the patient to another physician, or (3) the physician has in effect held himself or herself out as being proficient in the procedure. This principle has special relevance for endoscopic procedures because it is likely that any practitioner performing those procedures would be held to a standard of care of someone adequately trained and proficient in them. By definition, it is negligent to undertake such procedures without adequate training.

Establishing the Standard of Care

Determining whether a practitioner's care was within the standard required is most often determined on the basis of "custom," or the common practice of the profession. (At one time this care was defined in terms of the community in which the physician practiced. This "locality rule" has now been rejected in most areas and is virtually uniformly rejected for specialists.) In addition to custom, courts may rely on formal standards when determining a standard of care. For example, standards of good practice adopted by a specialty board or by a hospital may be used to help define good practice. In rare cases courts have decided that customary practice or adopted standards are themselves negligent. In the most notable case of this sort, a court determined that it was negligent for ophthalmologists not to perform glaucoma tests on those under 40 years of age.[67] Another example is in the area of informed consent. If the custom were to inadequately inform patients of alternatives to treatment, that custom would not define an acceptable standard of care regarding informed consent.[68]

Because determining if care was negligent often requires knowledge of the custom of practice, expert witnesses are called to give opinions about the quality of care and the custom of practice. The question for these physicians is not if they would have given the same care and not if it was the best care possible. Rather, it is what the custom or practice was at the time of treatment and if what the physician did was within the range of what a reasonably prudent practitioner (specialist) would have done under the circumstances.[69]

It is important for the practitioner and the expert witness to remember that not all medical mistakes result in liability. Liability requires the coincidence of (1) a mistake sufficiently outside good practice to be unreasonable, (2) an injury to the patient, and (3) a causal link between the injury and the negligence.[70] Liability is, of course, determined *post hoc*, that is, after everyone knows that an injury resulted from the provision of treatment.[71] There is a natural tendency to see an action (or decision) as unreasonable when it has resulted in an injury.

Expectations play an important role here too. When the expectation is that a procedure is completely safe, anything that goes wrong looks like it was caused by someone's carelessness.

This fact may be part of the reason for the number of obstetric malpractice claims: people have come to expect perfect babies. The principle also applies to gynecologic endoscopy. Patients should not be reassured to the point that they believe there are no risks involved with the procedure. Because of popular reference to the insignificance of endoscopic procedure ("Band-Aid surgery"), unrealistic expectations about the risks of endoscopy may be a problem.

Common Areas of Negligence

Negligence may arise from a number of acts or failures to act. Major sources of negligence include the following.

1. Failure to conduct adequate examination(s) and tests
2. Careless execution of medical and surgical procedures
3. Performing procedures for which the physician is not adequately trained
4. Inappropriate prescription or administration of drugs
5. Carelessness when selecting and supervising of staff
6. Inadequate monitoring of the patient
7. Failure to refer patients to other specialists as needed
8. Unethical conduct that harms a patient

Avoiding Malpractice

Although there are no guarantees that any practitioner can avoid malpractice claims, there are several ways to reduce the risk of malpractice.[61]

1. The most important factor, of course, is to engage in good quality, careful medical practice. You should adhere to the highest professional standards. High quality practice infrequently results in malpractice claims. Most malpractice recovery results from practice that the profession itself would not be willing to label as good, solid care. Most of the following suggestions for avoiding malpractice are other ways of saying "engaged in good medical practice."

2. Be sure that you are adequately trained before undertaking a diagnostic procedure or treatment. In the areas of endoscopic practice it

requires formal training. Be careful not to claim (directly or indirectly) training or qualifications that you do not have; do not "hold yourself out" as being an expert in an area in which you do not have adequate training or experience.

3. Refer a patient to other physicians for care or consultation if the care the patient requires is not within your area of expertise. The desire of the treating physician to develop experience with the kind of case presented by the patient or to "keep" the patient for financial reasons must not be the basis for a legitimate failure to refer.[72,73]

4. Maintain the currency of knowledge in your areas of practice. This point is especially important in areas of gynecologic endoscopy, where knowledge is advancing rapidly. Establish mechanisms to ensure that you stay current of the changes in practice.[74]

5. Be sure that the facility in which care is given is adequately equipped to (1) provide all of the instruments necessary for the procedures undertaken, and (2) provide good emergency care if an unanticipated bad event occurs during treatment. Feel confident in the level of training of the staff at the facility. If you select personnel for your office, do so with care because you will probably be held responsible for their negligence.

6. Use caution when undertaking "nonstandard" treatments, that is, treatments not generally accepted or used by the rest of the medical community.[75] These treatments should be undertaken only after a particularly fully informed consent and only with a clear protocol (preferably written) justifying the deviation from standard practice.[76] It is desirable that the protocol be reviewed by others, such as an Institutional Review Board (IRB).[77]

7. Obtain adequate informed consent as described earlier. Informed consent should be obtained for procedures that are physically invasive. Moreover, at least in an informal way, it should also be obtained for use of prescription drugs.[78]

8. If you treat minors or legally "incompetent" patients, you should have treatment protocols carefully designed to meet the special informed consent requirements of the state in which the treatment is provided.

9. You should be familiar with any special consent or notification requirements in your state regarding sterilization or abortion. These laws have changed with some frequency in recent years.[79]

The above suggestions for avoiding malpractice are directed toward providing good quality medical services. They help avoid engaging in professional negligence. The following are intended to reduce the odds that a liability claim will be made if negligence occurs. Only a small proportion of negligent treatment results in legal claims.[80] It is appropriate therefore to consider ways of avoiding malpractice *claims* (or for dealing with them if filed).[81]

10. Avoid unrealistic expectations by the patient and her family. The unrealistic expectations may not arise from anything you have told the patient but may come from friends, television, or *The Reader's Digest*. Unrealistic expectations suggest that someone is at fault if anything goes wrong. The informed consent process can be used profitably as a way of developing realistic expectations about the diagnostic procedure or treatment.[32]

11. Maintain good communications with patients.[82] Keep them informed. Let them know what to expect in terms of their conditions and their treatments. Except for good medical reasons, do not avoid delivering news, even if it is bad. If something does not go as expected, explain the problem and describe what can be done next.[71] There is considerable debate about whether a physician should tell a patient when the physician has made an error. There is much to be said for being open with patients about error without saying that the error was careless. Others, especially some insurance companies, oppose this form of openness that admits mistakes. In any case, communicate to patients the fact that you care about them.

12. Maintain good records. The records should be as complete an account as possible, explaining *why* you did something (or did not do it) as well as *what you* did. Be aware that others may read these files and do not put con-

fessions of negligence in them. Under no circumstances try to alter records to erase or avoid embarrassing information. This alteration is likely to be discovered and makes you look dishonest.[83]

13. When something goes wrong, contact your malpractice insurance company carrier immediately. Your insurance contract probably requires that you notify the company of possible claims.

14. When something goes wrong, discuss the course of action with your insurance company and others involved (such as the hospital) to determine what should be done regarding the patient. Issues include what to tell the patient and whether to charge the patient for the treatment and, later, whether to offer a settlement. My opinion is that it is often best to be relatively straightforward and not to charge the patient. Although it is true that in some cases this approach gives the patient information that could be used against you, it also is likely to reduce the chance that a claim will be filed.

Hospital Practice

Hospitals have taken on new roles in ensuring the quality of health care in recent years. ("Hospitals" is used here broadly to refer to the wide range of facilities in which health care may be provided.) Hospital accreditation rules, state regulations, and legal liability principles have imposed greater obligations on hospitals.[70,84] It is important that hospitals take seriously these obligations in gynecologic endoscopy in terms of the qualifications of those practicing, staff qualifications and training, and equipment acquisition and maintenance.

Qualifications of Staff

Hospitals have an obligation to ensure that practitioners who undertake complicated diagnosis and treatment within the institution are qualified to do so.[85] The process of granting hospital privileges to practitioners is an important part of this limitation on practice.

Only those who can demonstrate adequate, formal training should be permitted to schedule and undertake gynecologic endoscopy. It is important that hospitals use generally recognized formal standards for determining what training is adequate. They should also determine that their granting of privileges to practitioners is sufficiently specific to limit practice to those areas in which the physicians are adequately trained. Carelessness in the process of granting privileges to a practitioner who turns out to be negligent may result in liability for the hospital.

Hospitals also have a responsibility to review continuously the work of practitioners to ensure that they are staying competent with new technology and knowledge. The usual range of hospital committees and peer review mechanisms should be adequate for this process if those reviews are meaningful in terms of quality and if they are used to make changes in staff privileges when it appears that a member of the staff is no longer at a reasonably high level of competence in some areas. In fact, privilege adjustment (removing authority to undertake some procedures) is probably the "weak link" in hospital privilege qualification reviews. The competition for patients, the economic pressures caused by Diagnosis Related Groups (DRGs) and the like, and the closer ties between physicians and hospitals occasioned by delivery systems such as Preferred Provider Organizations (PPOs) may make it more difficult for hospitals to impose these practice limits on otherwise good practitioners.[86] Nevertheless, the hospital that does not undertake these privilege adjustments is inviting liability for this failure.

In addition, hospitals should determine that practitioners are practicing only within the limits of their privileges and competence. Those who are not privileged to do endoscopy (and the *specific* endoscopic procedures proposed) must not be permitted to perform these procedures. Hospitals should not permit physicians without appropriate staff privilege to schedule those procedures. In addition, nurses and other professionals who see unauthorized practices occurring should report them to supervisors or otherwise try to stop them.[87]

Hospital Support Staff

Hospitals have an obligation to use reasonable care when selecting nursing and support staff. It includes ensuring that those working in sophisticated areas of gynecologic endoscopy are adequately trained. The legal responsibility for employee (whether of the hospital or of the physician) extends beyond care in selection. The concept of "respondent superior," or vicarious liability, means that an employer (principal) is responsible for the negligence of his or her employees (agents). Therefore a hospital may be liable for the negligence of nurses and other employees.[61]

Principal–agent relationships are complicated in medicine, involving as they do the concepts of *shifting agency* (a division of responsibility between hospitals and physicians for the negligence of nurses and others) and *ostensible* or *apparent agency* (treating someone as an agent for liability purposes). This subject is well beyond the scope of this chapter. It should, however, be clear that great care is called for when supervising professional staff assistants.

Equipment

Hospitals have considerable responsibility for the equipment they purchase and maintain for endoscopic procedures.[88] We review the issue of equipment failure below. Briefly a hospital should be aware that it has a particularly strong obligation to provide medical equipment that is not defective and thereby harmful or unnecessarily dangerous.

Records

Like physicians, institutions should be careful that complete and accurate records are kept. Most accredited hospitals now have reasonably good mechanisms for record-keeping. The confidentiality of records must be maintained.[90] All institutions should continue efforts to complete patient records without significant delay. In addition, they should have mechanisms to ensure that records are not altered. There should be some process for protecting a record's integrity, particularly when it may become the subject of litigation or dispute.[83]

Equipment

Equipment is obviously critical to all endoscopic procedures. The U.S. Food and Drug Administration (FDA) regulation of medical equipment[91] and the liability associated with the equipment are complicated matters that could (and do) fill volumes. In this section we only briefly touch on some of the liability issues associated with equipment failure. It is an area in which there is rather considerable disagreement about what the law is and what it should be.[78,92] Liability (in contrast to FDA regulations) is an area that state law generally controls. Hence there is diversity in the way states handle it.

The principles discussed in this chapter suggest that the careless design, manufacture, or maintenance of equipment could give rise to negligence liability—and so they do. A high degree of care is expected of those who provide medical equipment because defects are likely to do serious harm to patients. It requires care not only by the manufacturer of the equipment but also by those who maintain and use it. For example, a hospital is expected to be concerned about the way it sterilizes and cares for its equipment.[88] Both the hospital and the physician using the hospital may be expected to perform reasonable inspections of equipment to determine that it is in good working order.[89]

The potential for liability due to defective equipment may extend beyond negligence. After World War II courts started expanding liability for harm caused by defective products. They now impose "strict liability" for products that are defective and cause injury.[93] The difference between negligence liability and strict liability is that with negligence a plaintiff must prove that a defect in the product resulted from someone's carelessness, whereas with strict liability the patient must prove only that a defect existed and caused injury. As you can imagine, "defective" in this context takes on a somewhat special and technical meaning. Among the reasons for imposing this strict liability are to spread the costs of injuries among those who benefit from using the product, to make product manufacturers and distributors as careful as possible, and to have the prices of products reflect their true costs (including the costs of injuries). Strict liability is generally *not* applied to services such as medical care, but it may be applied to *products* used for medical care.[94]

A product defect may result from an error in manufacturing or packaging (or perhaps maintenance), an error in the design of the product, or defective labeling (notably a failure to give adequate warnings or instructions concerning the product). Determining what is a "defect" has caused some difficulty, and defining a "design defect" has been particularly troublesome.[62] Of course, the fact that someone was injured by a product is not sufficient to prove that the product was defective in a legal sense.

In the area of medical equipment, there is also debate about when the use of the equipment is a "product" and when it is a "service" (services are not subject to strict liability), and if strict liability should be applied at all to medical equipment and devices. In addition, when equipment is produced by the manufacturer, purchased and maintained by a hospital, and used by a variety of physicians, it may be exceedingly difficult to determine who is responsible for the defect or for the injury.[95]

Some generalizations can be made from the current law. When strict liability is imposed for medical devices or equipment, as a practical matter the manufacturer is usually responsible for any defect in design or manufacture or for failure to label or warn. The hospital is responsible for failing to pass on to the physician any warning and for defects caused by its mistreatment of the product. Physicians are usually not part of the chain of distribution through which strict liability is passed. However, they may be deemed negligent for not selecting the proper instrument or equipment, misusing it, or failing to inspect it; this liability usually results in negligence rather than strict liability.[96]

Other Legal Issues

Physicians undertaking endoscopic procedures may face several other important legal issues. This section contains examples of the range of legal concerns that may be encountered.

Confidentiality

Both physicians and patients probably overestimate the degree to which the confidentiality of information from treatment can be maintained.[97] A close study of the law of one state indicated that the exceptions to confidentiality (and to the related concept of testimonial privilege) essentially consumed the rule.[98] What protection of confidentiality the law has given with one hand, it has often removed with the other.[99] This point suggests that gynecologists should be cautious when promising absolute confidentiality to information learned during treatment.[98]

Treating Minors

The traditional rule has been that parents must consent to treatment for their minor children.[100] This rule has now been modified somewhat by statute or court decision in many states.[101] These modifications may permit a minor to consent to gynecologic or obstetric care for herself. These statutes commonly exclude permanent sterilization and abortion from the procedures to which the minor may consent.[102] The U.S. Supreme Court has recognized a constitutional right to privacy that includes the right of a "mature" minor to decide to have an abortion[47] or to use contraceptives even over the objections of her parents.[103] (A mature minor is one capable of understanding the nature and consequences of a decision to have an abortion.[104])

The statutes allowing minors to consent to treatment may permit or require that their parents be notified of the treatment. A number of states have imposed parental notification obligations for minors seeking abortions or contraceptives.[105,106] The Supreme Court has upheld as constitutional state laws that require parental consent to abortions so long as there are "judicial bypass" provisions by which the minor can demonstrate to a court that she is sufficiently mature to make the decision regarding an abortion herself or that the abortion would be in her best interest.[49,50] When such notification is required by the law, the practitioner should inform the minor patient at the beginning of treatment of this reporting requirement.[107]

This area obviously is one in which the practitioner treating minor patients should watch closely for changes in the law. The law concerning abortion and sterilization for minors has been unstable. It is also an area in which those practicing may make a contribution to the public debate. The practical consequences of such laws are sometimes not recognized by courts and legislatures, and obstetricians and gynecologists may help provide this information.[48]

Patients as Research and Teaching Subjects

When patients are used as research subjects (e.g., in clinical trials of new drugs), special care must be exercised to ensure that they are protected from harm. The disclosure of Nazi atrocities committed in the name of research, has focused attention on the risks of experimentation.[108] Much human experimentation now is controlled by federal law, institutional regulations, or ethical principles.[109] Almost any experimentation undertaken should be first examined by some review body, such as an ethics committee or an IRB. IRB approval is required by the federal government for government-funded studies and human trials of new drugs and devices.[110]

The IRBs and other reviewers should ensure that the potential benefits of the study outweigh the potential risks, that there is adequate informed consent, and that the risks are as limited as possible. This review is intended to protect the patient, but indirectly it also helps protect the physician by avoiding unnecessary experimental risks.[111]

No experimental study should be undertaken by a physician without carefully checking to determine if any regulation is applicable and what review is legally required or desirable.[112] IRB review generally takes several weeks and should be completed before a grant application is submitted. Physicians should therefore provide considerable "lead time" when asking for IRB review.

Patients who are used as "teaching subjects," unlike research subjects, are not commonly protected by federal and institutional regulations.[113] Nevertheless, practitioners should consider using the same principles that justify ethical experimentation: The benefits should outweigh the risks, there should be fully informed consent (including the right to refuse to be a teaching or research subject); and the risks should be as low as possible. Too often these principles are not carefully followed.[114]

Note of Caution

A note of caution is in order about the legal principles discussed here. They may not fully describe the law in any given state for two reasons. First, most of the issues discussed are matters of state law, and the law varies from state to state. Although most states follow the same general principles of law, there are some important differences adopted by a few states. For example, several states have modified malpractice principles by statute, and states also vary in their approaches to minors' consent to treatment.[45] Thus in any state there are exceptions or nuances to generally stated legal principles. A second reason for caution is the speed with which the law is changing. In general, the law related to medicine is in flux, particularly in areas affecting reproduction and new technology. This situation affects gynecologic endoscopy in that those practicing in this area of medicine should pay particular attention to the variations and changes affecting their own state(s). Institutions should certainly have their policies and practices related to endoscopy reviewed by an attorney competent in the area of health law. It is an area of the law where early "preventive" activity can avoid some later legal ramifications.

References

1. HULKA JF: Textbook of Laparoscoy (2d ed). Philadelphia, W.B. Saunders, 1994.
2. AZZIZ R, MURPHY AA (EDS): Practical Manual of Operative Laparoscopy and Hysteroscopy. New York, Springer-Verlag, 1992.
3. AMERICAN MEDICAL ASSOCIATION: Revised Principles of Medical Ethics. Chicago, AMA, 1980.
4. BORTEN M, FRIEDMAN EA: Legal Principles and Practice in Obstetrics and Gynecology (Vol 2). Chicago, Year Book, 1990.
5. VITALE G: Credentialing. In Atlas of Operative Laparoscopy for the General Surgeon, Vitale G, Sanfilippo J, Perissat J (eds): Philadelphia, Lippincott 1995.
6. DENT TL: Training, credentialling, and granting of clinical privileges for laparoscopic general surgery. Am J Surg 1991;161:399.

7. SATAVA RM: Establishing an endoscopy unit for surgical training. Surg Clin North Am 1989; 69:1129.
8. CULLADO MJ, PORTER JA, SLEZAK FA: The evolution of surgical endoscopy training: meeting the American Board of Surgery requirements. Am Surg 1991;57:250.
9. MURPHY EK: Liability for noncompliance with hospital policies: national standards. AORN J 1990;52:1060.
10. STUDER M: The doctrine of informed consent: protecting the patient's right to make informed health care decisions. Montana Law Rev 1987;48:85.
11. ROSE RM: Informed consent: history, theory and practice. Am J Otol 1986;7:82.
12. SLATER VS BAKER AND STAPLETON, 95 Eng Rep 860 (KB 1767).
13. SCHLOENDORFF VS SOCIETY OF NEW YORK HOSPITAL, 105 NE 92 (NY 1914).
14. WHITEFIELD A: The meaning of informed consent. Med Leg J 1986;54:11.
15. MORTON WJ: The doctrine of informed consent. Med Law 1987;6:117.
16. SHUGRUE RE, LINSTROMBERG K: The practitioner's guide to informed consent. Creighton Law Rev 1991;24:881.
17. GILHOOLEY M: Learned intermediaries, prescription drugs and patient informed consent. St Louis Univ Law J 1986;30:633.
18. SCHUCK PH: Rethinking informed consent. Yale Law J 1994:103:899.
19. MERZ JF: On a decision-making paradigm of medical informed consent. J Leg Med 1993; 14:231.
20. APPELBAUM P, LIDZ C, MEISEL A: Informed Consent: Legal Theory and Clinical Practice. New York, Oxford University Press, 1987.
21. TERRION HF: Informed choice: physicians' duty to disclose nonreadily available alternatives. Case Western Reserve Law Rev 1993;43:491.
22. SCHULTZ MM: From informed consent to patient choice: a new protected interest. Yale Law J 1985;95:219.
23. WEISBARD AJ: Informed consent: the law's uneasy compromise with ethical theory. Nebr Law Rev 1986;65:749.
24. KAUFER DS, STEINBERG ER, TONEY SD: A model for making medical consent forms more comprehensible. Leg Med 1985; 1985:271.
25. CANTERBURY VS SPENCE, 464 F2d 772 (DC Cir), cert. denied, 409 US 1064 (1972).
26. WADE TC: Patients may not recall disclosure of risk of death: implications for informed consent. Med Sci Law 1990;30:259.
27. TRUMAN VS THOMAS, 611 P 2d 902 (Cal. 1980).
28. WAINESS R: Physician's duty to inform patients who refuse "treatment": Truman v. Thomas in perspective. Med Trial Tech Q 1986;32:444.
29. MEISEL A: The "exceptions" to informed consent. Conn Med 1981;45:27.
30. SMITH SR: Legal issues in trauma care. In Trauma: Clinical Care and Pathophysiology, Richardson JD, Polk HC, Flint LM (eds). Chicago, Year Book, 1987, pp 569–580.
31. KOLDER V, GALLAGHER J, PARSON MT: Court-ordered obstetrical interventions. N Engl J Med 1987;316:1192.
32. DOBSON T: Medical malpractice in the birthplace: resolving the physician-patient conflict through informed consent, standard of care, and assumption of risk. Nebr Law Rev 1986; 65:655.
33. BAKER CH: Comment: informed consent, obligation or opportunity? J Health Hosp Law 1993; 26:214.
34. KATZ J: Informed consent: are miracle, mystery and authority better medicine? J Conn Med 1986;50:457.
35. MARSH FH: Informed consent and the elderly patient. Clin Geriatr Med 1986;2:501.
36. MARGOLIS WM: The doctor knows best? Patient capacity for health care decision making. Oregon Law Rev 1992;71:909.
37. BUCHANAN AE: The limits of proxy decision-making for incompetents. UCLA Law Rev 1981;29:386.
38. HOLDER AR: Legal Issues in Pediatrics and Adolescent Medicine. New Haven, Yale University Press, 1985.
39. WORKING GROUP OF THE NORTHERN REGION IN CURRENT MEDICAL/ETHICAL PROBLEMS: Consent to treatment by parents and children. Child Care Health Dev 1986;12:5.
40. MELTON G, KOOCHER G, SAKS M (EDS): Children's Competence to Consent. New York, Plenum Press, 1983.
41. MELTON G: Children's participation in treatment planning: psychological and legal issues. Prof Psychol 1981;12:246.
42. AMERICAN ACADEMY OF PEDIATRICS: A model act providing for consent to minor's to health services. Pediatrics 1973;51:293.
43. WRIGHT TE: A minor's right to consent to medical care. Howard Law J 1982;25:525.
44. RESTAINO JM JR: Informed consent: should it be extended to 12-year-olds? A surgeon's view. Med Law 1987;6:91.

45. SMITH SR: Legal rights of minors. In Lavery JP, Sanfilippo J (eds): Pediatric and Adolescent Obstetrics and Gynecology. New York, Springer-Verlag, 1985, pp 338–352.
46. CAREY VS POPULATION SERVICES, 431 US 678 (1977).
47. THORNBURGH VS AMERICAN COLLEGE OF OBSTETRICIANS AND GYNECOLOGISTS, 476 US 747 (1986); Bellotti vs Baird, 443 US 4622 (1979).
48. TORRES A, FORREST JD, EISMAN S: Telling parents: clinical policies and adolescent's use of family planning and abortion services. Fam Plann Perspect 1980;12:284.
49. OHIO VS AKRON CENTER FOR REPRODUCTIVE HEALTH, 497 US 502 (1990).
50. HODGSON VS MINNESOTA, 497 US 417 (1990).
51. ROZOVSKY F: Consent to Treatment: A Practical Guide. Boston, Little, Brown, 1984 [with pocket part updates].
52. CONLIN SR: Hospital corporate negligence based on a lack of informed consent. Suffolk Univ Law Rev 1985;19:835.
53. TIETZ G: Informed consent in the prescription drug context: the special case. Wash Law Rev 1986;61:367.
54. COLE VS JORDAN, 288 SE2d 260 (Ga App 1982).
55. HILL VS GILMORE, 326 SE2d 271 (NC App 1985).
56. PIZZALOTTO VS WILSON, 411 So2d 1150 (La App 1982).
57. CARNERIE F: Crisis and informed consent: analysis of a law-medicine malocclusion. Am J Law Med 1987;12:55.
58. SEIDELSON D: Lack of informed consent in medical malpractice and product liability cases: the burden of presenting evidence. Hofstra Law Rev 1986;14:621.
59. RICHARDS BC, THOMASSON G: Closed liability claims analysis and the medical record. Obstet Gynecol 1992;80:313.
60. APPELBAUM P, LIDZ C, MEISEL A: Informed Consent: Legal Theory and Clinical Practice. New York, Oxford University Press, 1987.
61. WARD CJ: Analysis of 500 obstetric and gynecologic malpractice claims: causes and prevention. Am J Obstet Gynecol 1991;165:298.
62. KEETON WP, DOBBS D, KEETON R, ET AL: Prosser and Keeton on the Law of Torts. St. Paul, MN, West Publishing, 1984.
63. FICARRA BJ, CORSO FM: Iatrogenic surgical liability. Leg Med 1985;1985:236.
64. PERDUE J: Medical malpractice 1987: new faces, new facts, new fundamentals. St. Marys Law J 1987;18:955.
65. PENHALLEGON JR: Medical malpractice (update). Defense Counsel J 1993;60:365.
66. MICHAND GL, HUTTON MB: The emergence of a specialty standard of care. Tulsa Law J 1979;16:720.
67. HELLING VS CAREY, 519 P2d 981 (Wash. 1974).
68. NORRIE KM: Medical negligence: who sets the standard? J Med Ethics 1985;11:135.
69. WIENER RL: A psychological and empirical approach to the medical standard of care. Nebr Law Rev 1990;69:112.
70. GERBER P: Medical negligence and legal causation: where the twain do not meet. Med J Aust 1986;144:582.
71. WEXLER DB, SCHOPP RF: How and when to correct for jury hindsight bias is mental health malpractice litigation. Behav Sci Law 1989;7:485.
72. FISCINA SF: Duty to consult: why, whether, how, who, when. Leg Aspects Med Pract 1983;11:5.
73. FRANKEL JJ: Medical malpractice law health care cost containment: lessons for reformers from the clash of cultures. Yale Law J 1994;103:1297.
74. PRILLAMAN HL: A physician's duty to inform of newly developed therapy. J Contemp Health Law Policy 1990;6:43.
75. EPSTEIN RA: Legal liability for medical innovation. Cardozo Law Rev 1987;8:1139.
76. COWAN D: Innovative therapy versus experimentation. Tort Ins Law J 1986;21:619.
77. SMITH SR, MEYER RG: Law, Behavior and Mental Health: Policy and Practice. New York, New York University Press, 1987, pp 192–196.
78. BREST AN: Malpractice liability and drug therapy. Clin Ther 1987;9:138.
79. DUGAN JC: The conflict between 'disabling' and 'enabling' paradigms in law: sterilization, the developmentally disabled and the Americans With Disabilities Act of 1990. Cornell Law Rev 1993;78:507.
80. WEILER PC: Medical Malpractice on Trial. Cambridge MA, Harvard University Press, 1991.
81. TARAGIN MI, WILCZEK AP, KARNS ME, ET AL: Physician demographics and the risk of medical malpractice. Am J Med 1992;93:537.
82. ADAMSON TE, GULLION DS, TSCHANN JM: Educational implications of the relationship between patient satisfaction and medical malpractice claims. Proc Annu Conf Res Med Educ 1985;24:38.
83. MILLER PJ: Documentation as a defense to legal claims. J Am Optom Assoc 1986;57:144.

84. MILLER RD: Problems in Hospital Law. Rockville, MD, Aspen Publications, 1986.
85. MULHOLLAND D III: The evolving relationship between physicians and hospitals. Tort Ins Law J 1987;22:295.
86. FURROW B: Medical malpractice and cost containment: tightening the screws. Case Western Reserve Law Rev 1986;36:985.
87. DARLING VS CHARLESTON COMMUNITY MEMORIAL HOSPITAL, 211 NE2d 253 (Ill. 1965), cert. denied, 383 US 946 (1966).
88. KILLIAN WH: Equipment mishaps may result in lawsuits. Am Nurse 1990;22:34.
89. GOERTH CR: Failure to comply with industry standards can spell negligence. Occup Health Saf 1986;55:50.
90. WEISMAN E: Liability for medical record disclosure is real but rare. Hospitals 1990;64:28.
91. KAHAN JS: Medical devices reclassification: the evolution of FDA policy. Food Drug Cosm Law J 1987;42:288.
92. AGAR J: Labeling of prescription devices for the Food and Drug Administration and product liability: a primer. Food Drug Cosmetic Law J 1990;45:447.
93. AMERICAN LAW INSTITUTE, Restatement of Torts 2d 402A.
94. GRANT LJ: Product liability aspects of bioengineering. J Biomed Eng 1990;12:262.
95. ANDERSON VS SOMBERG, 338 A2d 1 (NJ 1975).
96. MAEDGEN B, MCCALL S: A survey of law regarding the liability of manufacturers and sellers of drug products and medical devices. St Marys Law J 1986;18:395.
97. SMITH SR: Constitutional privacy in psychotherapy. George Washington Law Rev 1980;49:1.
98. SMITH SR: Medical and psychotherapy privileges and confidentiality: on giving with one hand and removing with the other. Ky Law Rev 1987;75:473.
99. KNAPP S, VANDECREEK L: Privileged Communications in the Mental Health Professions. New York, Van Nostrand Reinhold, 1987.
100. EADDY JA, GRABER GC: Confidentiality and the family physician. Am Fam Physician 1982; 25:141.
101. ANDERSON JD: Abortion: state regulations. Marquette Law Rev 1992;76:317.
102. EWALD LS: Medical decision making for children: an analysis of competing interests. St Louis Univ Law J 1982;25:689.
103. CAREY VS POPULATION SERVICES, 431 US 678 (1977).
104. COUNCIL ON ETHICAL AND JUDICIAL AFFAIRS (AMA): Mandatory parental consent to abortion. JAMA 1993;269:82.
105. CROSBY MC, ENGLISH A: Mandatory parental involvement and judicial bypass laws: do they promote adolescents' health? J Adolesc Health 1991;12:143.
106. SCHMIDT CG: Where privacy fails: equal protection and the abortion rights of minors. New York Univ Law Rev 1993;68:597.
107. MORRISSEY J, HOFMANN A, THORPE J: Consent and Confidentiality in the Health Care of Children and Adolescents: A Legal Guide. New York, Free Press, 1986.
108. NUREMBERG MILITARY TRIBUNAL, The Nuremberg Code, 2 The Medical Cases 181–182 (GPO 1947), used in United States vs Karl Brandt et al, Trials of War Criminals Before Military Tribunals Under Control Law No 10 (Oct 1946–Apr 1949).
109. KATZ J: Experimentation with Human Beings. New York, Russell Sage Foundation, 1972.
110. 21 CFR 50 (1992) [contains FDA regulations regarding research under the jurisdiction of the FDA]; 45 CFR 46 (1992) [regulations subject to HHS jurisdiction].
111. ROBERTSON J: The law of institutional review boards. UCLA Law Rev 1979;26:484.
112. GLASS KC, FREEDMAN B: Legal liability for injury to research subjects. Clin Invest Med 1991; 14:176.
113. COHEN DL, KESSEL RW, MCCULLOUGH LB, ET AL: The ethical implications of medical student involvement in the care and assessment of patients in teaching hospitals—informed consent from patients for student involvement: a description of the origin and implementation of policies governing medical student interaction with patients and compliance with federal and JCAH guidelines. Proc Annu Conf Res Med Educ 1985;24:138. [Part I] and 24:163 [Part II].
114. HELMS LB, HELMS CM: Forty years of litigation involving residents and their training: malpractice issues. Acad Med 1991;66:718.
115. MCNOBLE DJ: Expanded liability of hospitals for the negligence of fatigued residents. J Leg Med 1990;11:427.

Section VI
General Surgery and New Horizons

32
Laparoscopic Overview: General Surgical Perspective

Gary C. Vitale

Minimally invasive surgical procedures have revolutionized the general surgeon's approach to surgical intervention over a 5-year period, so it is difficult to imagine that the technique is almost 100 years old. Two slightly different approaches to peritoneoscopy were reported at the turn of the twentieth century in Sweden and Germany. Kelling described creation of a pneumoperitoneum in dogs using a rigid scope designed for cystoscopy.[1] Jakobaeus, working in humans, inserted the cystoscope directly into the peritoneal cavity without creation of a pneumoperitoneum.[2] Their work was essentially diagnostic laparoscopy. These techniques are the ones we use today, although fiberoptics has allowed wider and safer visualization of the tissues.

Modern laparoscopic surgery has its roots in the work of Professor Kurt Semm, who pioneered the development of basic operative laparoscopic skills. Laparoscopic appendectomy was developed by Semm with laparoscopic extraction of the appendix not requiring minilaparotomy.[3] This work and the subsequent increase in gynecologic surgery set the stage for the general surgical revolution, but it was the first performance of a cholecystectomy in a human using standard laparoscopic instruments by Mouret in Lyon, France that served as the true catalyst. After this event in 1987, Dubois in Paris and Perissat in Bordeaux began performing the technique. Dubois and Perissat helped popularize the technique through publications and presentations at international conferences, and it spread rapidly to centers in the United States and Europe.[4,5]

No one could have predicted the explosion of laparoscopic surgery that followed. Innovative surgeons began using a laparoscopic approach for every procedure imaginable. Although issues of safety and adequacy of training have been a source of focus and concern, the field has continued to progress steadily. This chapter outlines recent developments in various surgical disciplines. Gynecologic surgeons should, at least, be aware of the surgical procedures currently being performed within the realm of general surgery and its subspecialties.

Thoracic Surgery

The thoracic cavity is well suited for a thoracoscopic approach, as the ribs prevent collapse of the chest wall. Carbon dioxide is used for insufflation to help collapse the lung, with pressure maintained at 5 mm Hg and a flow rate of < 1.0 L/min to prevent compression of the mediastinum. Thoracoscopy has proved useful for the diagnosis and treatment of pulmonary nodules, pleural disease, and mediastinal tumors. Mesotheliomas can be biopsied via a thoracoscopic approach with less risk of wound seeding than with a thoracotomy.[6] Biopsies may be directed toward areas of pleural abnormality, which increases the diagnostic yield compared to that using a percutaneous approach. Empyemas may be drained thoracoscopically along with decortication and debridement. This approach is more successful with early empyema; the more established cases with a thick inflammatory peel may be better approached with an open procedure.

Ligation and oversewing of bullae is well suited to a thoracoscopic approach. An Endoloop can be passed around the base of the bulla if it can be held up by a forceps. Alternatively, for large bullae inversion and oversewing is possible, or an endoscopic stapler may be used to staple or wedge out the bullae. Pulmonary wedge resections are performed in the same fashion.

Although there are several possible approaches for truncal vagotomy, a thoracoscopic approach is attractive. It is technically simple, requires little dissection, and avoids the need for establishing a pneumoperitoneum. Traditionally, truncal vagotomy is accompanied by a gastric drainage procedure, such as pyloroplasty or gastrojejunostomy. Dubois has advocated endoscopic pyloric balloon dilatation to accompany thoracoscopic vagotomy (F. Dubois, personal communication). If long-term studies confirm the adequacy of balloon dilatation for gastric drainage after vagotomy, this option may become the treatment of choice given its simplicity. Laparoscopic highly selective vagotomy may physiologically be the best operation to perform for peptic ulcer disease, but it is technically complicated.[7]

Esophageal myotomy is performed for achalasia in which there is hypertrophy and hypertension of the lower esophageal sphincter and distal esophageal musculature. A longitudinal myotomy is well suited to a thoracoscopic approach because the functional result depends on the adequacy of exposure and dissection. Exposure of the esophagus is excellent using the thoracoscopic approach. The myotomy can be

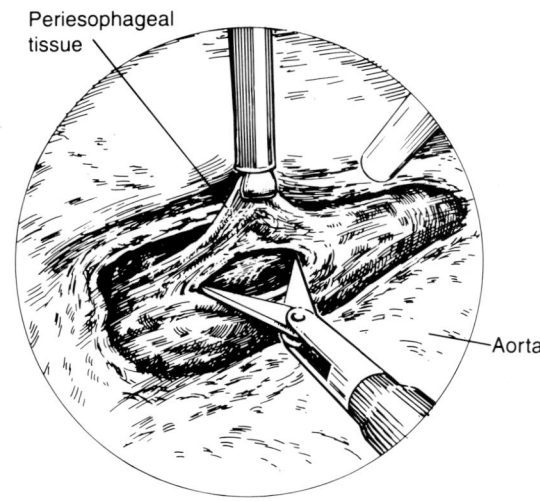

Figure 32.1. Esophageal myotomy, use of cautery scissors.

performed in a precise millimeter by millimeter dissection using a simple grasper, hook dissector, and cautery scissors (Figs. 32.1, 32.2). The precise limits of the dissection are important. If one dissects more than a few millimeters beyond the esophagogastric junction, the patient may have a problem with acid reflux after myotomy. A long myotomy for nutcracker esophagus or diffuse esophageal spasm may be particularly

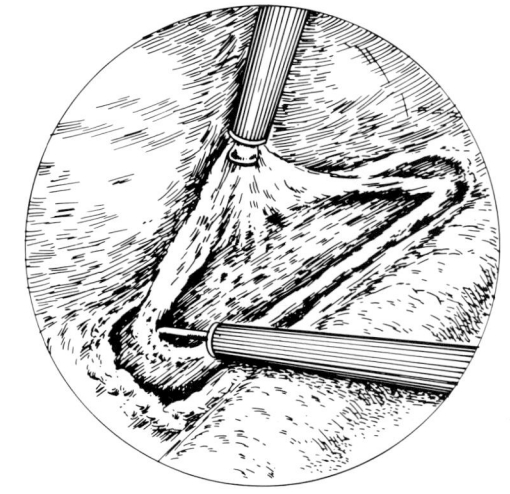

Figure 32.2. Esophageal myotomy, use of hook dissector.

suited to a thoracoscopic approach. The thoracoscopic view of the esophageal hiatus is excellent and may indeed be better than the view with a traditional open surgical approach.[8]

Similar arguments can be made for the thoracoscopic approach to sympathectomy. A thoracoscopic approach allows precise dissection and visualization of the sympathetic chain. The procedure is used most commonly to treat hyperhidrosis and Raynaud's phenomenon. Dissection and excision of the sympathetic chain is performed from below the inferior stellate ganglion to above the T4 ganglion.

Combined laparoscopic/thoracoscopic esophagectomy has been done with cervical anastomosis of the remnant esophagus to the translocated stomach. A laparoscopic approach is used for mobilization of the stomach and a thoracoscopic approach for dissection of the esophagus. The operative time required for such extensive dissection argues against using this approach at present. Advances in instrumentation may improve operative time so as to make it more appropriate for a laparoscopic/thoracoscopic approach or even a mediastinoscopic approach as advocated by Buess et al.[9]

Hernia Surgery

There are several techniques for the performance of laparoscopic hernia repair. Bogojavalensky demonstrated a technique for laparoscopic hernia repair in 1989.[10] The technique he demonstrated involved placing a plug of polypropylene mesh to fill the hernia defect, with suture closure of the internal ring. An early series of laparoscopic hernia repairs reported by Schultz et al. used polypropylene rolled into a tube and placed in the hernia defect. Mesh was then placed over the opening to the hernia defect and the peritoneum closed over it.[11]

Subsequently, the transabdominal preperitoneal approach was developed and involved a wide dissection of peritoneum over the hernia site with a preperitoneal mesh repair and subsequent closure of the peritoneum (Figs. 32.3, 32.4). This technique became favored when problems with plug migration and recurrence

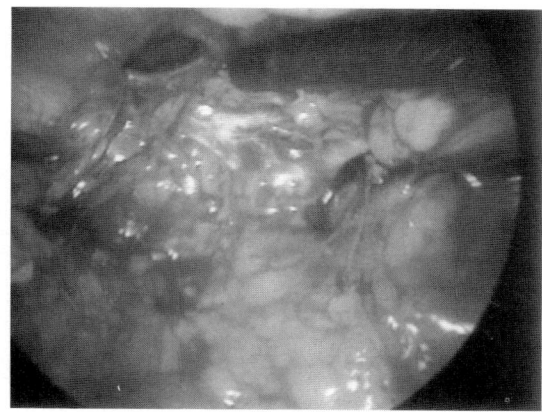

Figure 32.3. Inguinal hernia after dissection of peritoneum from the posterior inguinal triangle. Instrument points to the hernia defect.

were noted with the polypropylene plug method.[12] More recently, a totally extraperitoneal laparoscopic approach has gained popularity. With this variation the laparoscope is inserted through the abdominal wall to the preperitoneal position. The peritoneum is not entered, and the preperitoneal space is dissected with the aid of balloon dilatation. Insufflation of CO_2 then maintains the space adequately for dissection and preperitoneal repair of the hernia with a standard mesh approach. The advantage of this approach is that the peritoneal cavity is

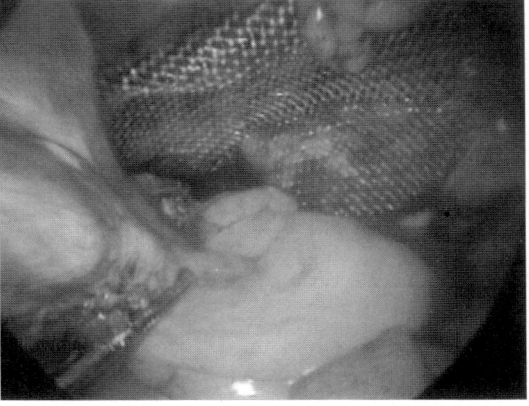

Figure 32.4. Mesh is in place in the preperitoneal space to cover the hernia defect seen in Figure 32.3.

not entered and so there is reduced risk for adhesions and subsequent bowel obstruction.[13]

Laparoscopic hernia repair is appealing given the reduced postoperative pain and early return to work, but long-term results are not yet evaluated. As noted above, the polypropylene plug method has been largely abandoned as a result of a documented high recurrence rate and complications related to the plug. Although recurrence rates are indeed important, complications related to the technique must also be considered when deciding whether to use a laparoscopic approach. Direct bowel or vessel injury from trocar insertion still represents a small but genuine risk. The technique requires general anesthesia with its attendant risks. Additionally, longer-term issues related to infection or erosion of the implanted prosthesis into adjacent structures (e.g., bowel or blood vessels) as well as intraperitoneal adhesions leading to bowel obstruction must be considered, particularly in the young patient who faces a lifetime of having the foreign body in place.

Gastrointestinal Surgery

Antireflux Surgery

Although there have been significant advances in the medical management of gastroesophageal reflux disease, there is still a place for surgical intervention. Histamine receptor antagonists (H_2 blockers such as ranitidine) and proton pump inhibitor (omeprazole) can control acid secretion, but inflammation may be present because of nonacid substances such as bile or trypsin. Progression of ulceration and stricture can occur while on an optimal medical antireflux regimen. Additionally, the volume of refluxed material may cause nocturnal choking and aspiration, which are not improved with acid-reducing agents. Finally, the lifelong cost of intensive medical management with alternating omeprazole and ranitidine courses is significant, and the risk of achlorhydria long term remains unknown. Early reports of experience with laparoscopic antireflux surgery from France and the United Kingdom were encouraging, and subsequent work has indeed shown that antireflux surgery is amenable to a laparoscopic approach.[14,15] It is a functional operation not involving cancer and does not require removal of tissue. Technically, the procedure requires careful dissection around the esophageal hiatus; once this step is accomplished, the fundoplication is relatively easy (Figs. 32.5, 32.6). Recovery is greatly facilitated using this approach, with patients usually taking liquids on the day after the operation and being discharged on the second postoperative day.

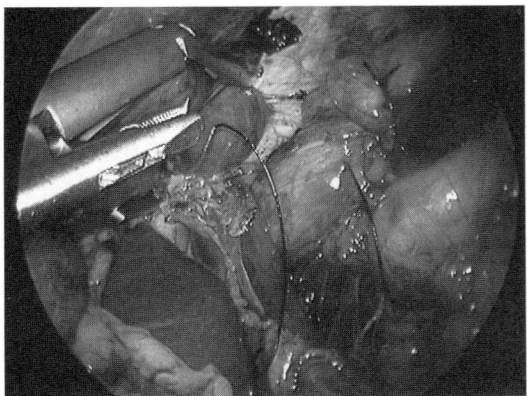

Figure 32.5. Dissection of esophageal hiatus for Nissen fundoplication. Suture in place to close the crura at the esophageal hiatus.

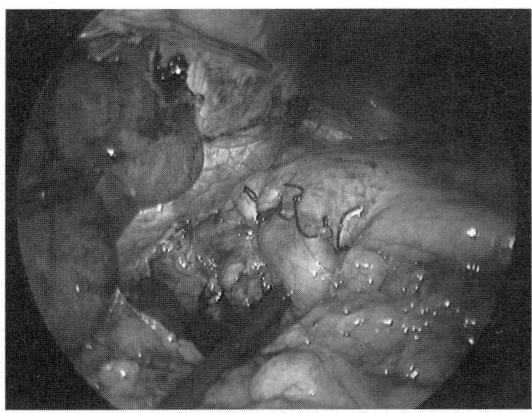

Figure 32.6. Completed Nissen fundoplication; instrument is seen to pass posterior to the gastric fundus behind the fundoplication.

Ulcer Surgery

A laparoscopic approach to peptic ulcer disease is appealing. The choice of operation lies between truncal vagotomy and drainage and highly selective vagotomy. With highly selective vagotomy the innervation of the antrum and fundus is interrupted while sparing the nerves to the pylorus. A drainage procedure is not necessary with this operation because the pylorus still functions. The dissection is a bit tedious laparoscopically, as it involves separating individual nerves in the lesser omentum as they enter the lesser curvature of the stomach. The anterior and posterior leaves of the omentum are best dissected separately, which causes a long dissection time, making the laparoscopic approach difficult.[7,16]

To reduce operative dissection, some surgeons have performed posterior truncal vagotomy, with anterior highly selective vagotomy. This operation is possible because the pylorus functions well with innervation of either the anterior or posterior nerve. That pyloric drainage is not needed makes this operation well suited to laparoscopy. Katkhouda and Mouiel, from Nice, France, first developed a selective vagotomy approach laparoscopically using a posterior truncal vagotomy with an anterior seromyotomy.[17] It involves dividing the seromuscular layer of the gastric wall in order to ablate the lesser curvature innervation. It has the advantage of being complete in that all small vagal fibers coursing through the seromuscular layer are divided before reaching the mucosa, but it has the inconvenience of dividing part of the gastric wall with the risk of inadvertent gastric mucosal perforation. This technique has not become popular in the United States. The use of a stapling device to divide and reanastomose the gastric wall along the lesser curvature represents yet another way to accomplish lesser curvature nerve division. Although this procedure is appealing because of its technical simplicity, it has the disadvantage of entering the gastrointestinal tract and thus obviating one of the attractive features of highly selective vagotomy.

Recurrence rates after open highly selective vagotomy may be higher than after standard vagotomy and pyloroplasty. Thus many surgeons still prefer truncal vagotomy, which may be accomplished endoscopically via either a laparoscopic or a thoracoscopic approach. The laparoscopic approach allows simultaneous pyloroplasty or pyloromyotomy, and the thoracoscopic vagotomy is usually coupled with endoscopic pyloric balloon dilatation. Pyloric balloon dilatation has been used successfully for the treatment of gastric outlet stricture, but its use with ablation of function of the normal pylorus is limited.[18]

Some surgeons have also begun to approach perforated ulcers with an innovative joint laparoscopic/endoscopic approach. An endoscope is first passed through the mouth and into the stomach. The perforation is identified; and under direct vision with the laparoscope in the peritoneal cavity, a snare or grasping forceps is passed through the gastroscope into the perforated ulcer and out into the peritoneal cavity. A segment of previously prepared omentum is then grasped and pulled into the perforated ulcer to seal the hole. Fibrin glue and sutures are used to hold the omentum in place (Figs. 32.7, 32.8).

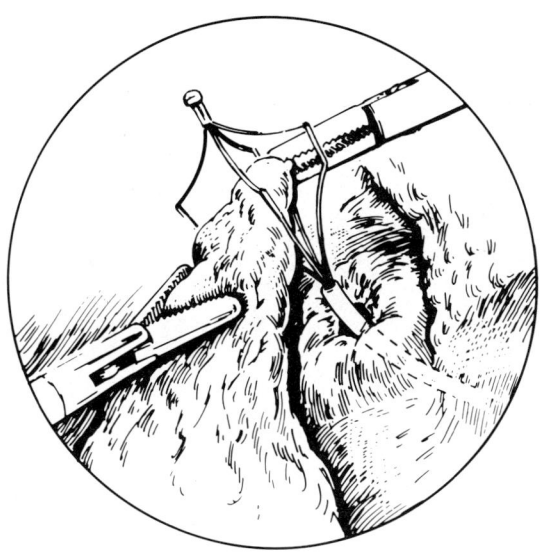

Figure 32.7. Perforated ulcer with the stone basket used to grasp the omentum through the perforation. The stone basket has been passed through a gastroscope, which is passed through the oropharynx.

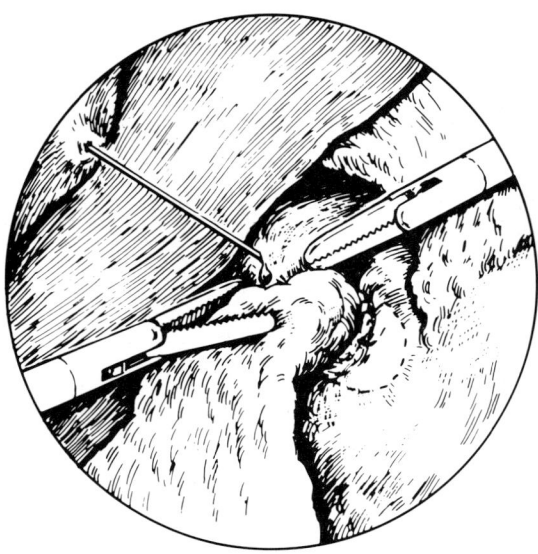

Figure 32.8. Omentum is pulled into place at the site of the perforated ulcer. Fibrin glue is used to secure the omentum. Individual sutures are placed to further secure the omentum.

Biliary Surgery

If there was a single key or, more appropriately, catalyst to the laparoscopic revolution, it was laparoscopic cholecystectomy. There is a report of laparoscopic cholecystectomy by Muhe in West Germany in 1986, although Mouret has generally been credited with performing the first successful laparoscopic cholecystectomy in 1987 in Lyon, France.[19] In either case, laparoscopic cholecystectomy quickly took hold in Europe and then the United States.[20] Dubois et al. in Paris and Perissat et al. in Bordeaux took the lead in Europe.[21,22] Cuschieri, a long time advocate of laparoscopy including laparoscopic cholecytoscopy, led the way in the United Kingdom.[23] Reddick and Olsen,[24] McKernan and Saye,[25] and Berci et al.[26] were among the first to perform and popularize it in the United States. The technique lent itself well to laparoscopy in that the technical aspects of dissection of the cystic duct and cystic artery were straightforward, allowing large numbers of general surgeons to master it. Even so, there were numerous common bile duct injuries during this start-up period and while expertise with the technique was being established. These injuries have now decreased in frequency to a number similar to that seen with open cholecystectomy.[27,28]

Advances in this field include routine use of the laparoscopic approach for acute and chronic cholecystitis (Figs. 32.9–32.14). Intraoperative cholangiography was included early during the development of the operative approach to cholelithiasis by many surgeons (Fig. 32.13). This development has been followed by laparoscopic common duct exploration. The develop-

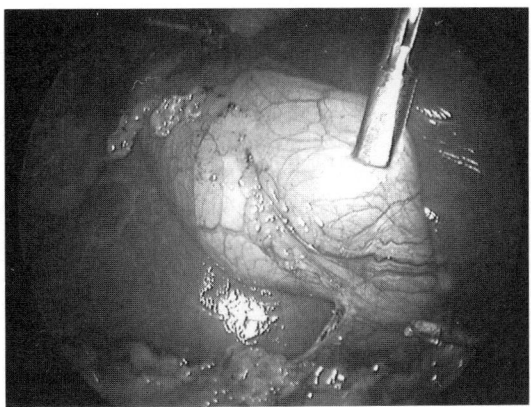

Figure 32.9. Gallbladder is grasped to pull the infundibulum inferiorly and exposes an area of cystic duct and cystic artery.

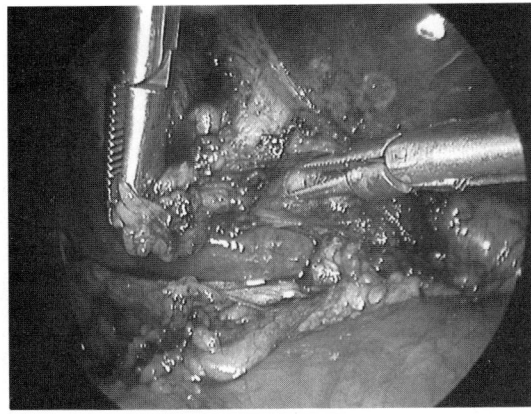

Figure 32.10. Dissection of the cystic duct and cystic artery. Dissecting instrument is used to spread the tissues between these structures.

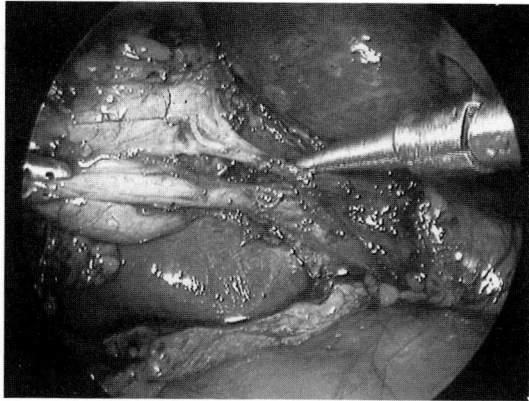

Figure 32.11. Completed dissection of the cystic duct and cystic artery. The instrument points to the cystic artery, and the cystic duct is just below it.

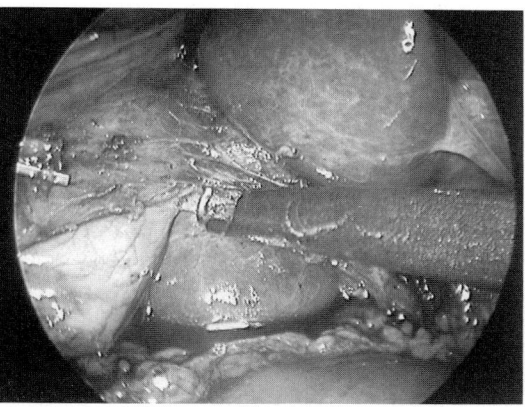

Figure 32.13. Gallbladder is retracted to the left. Hook dissector is used to divide the attachments of the gallbladder to the liver.

ment here has depended heavily on ancillary equipment advances, such as guidewires with dilating catheters and wire/balloon stone extractors. The use of tiny choledochoscopes with thin operating channels has improved the success of locating and extracting stones. The techniques currently utilized include a transcystic route or involve choledochostomy with direct stone extraction. The latter technique should be used only in widely dilated ducts, as suturing techniques are difficult with narrow ducts and could lead to postoperative stricture. Although success is reported in more than 90% of cases, the procedure may take a long time, and stone extraction from the biliary radicles above the cystic duct insertion remains difficult.[29] Uncomplicated intraoperative techniques of sphincterotomy of the ampulla of Vater remain to be developed to treat ampullary stenosis and allow for drainage of stone fragments. Advances in the use of endoscopic retrograde cholangiopancreatography (ERCP) has allowed pre- and postoperative common bile duct stone removal as well, with a success rate in excess of 95%.[30]

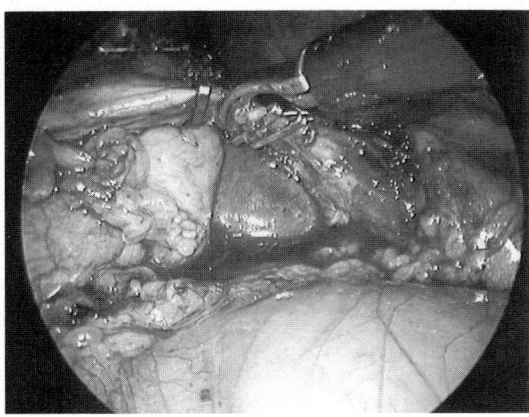

Figure 32.12. Clips are in place on the cystic duct. Scissors are used to divide the cystic duct.

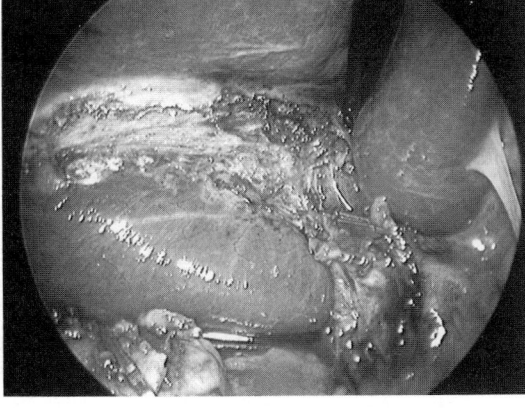

Figure 32.14. Gallbladder bed after removal of the gallbladder. Note the clips on the cystic duct and cystic artery.

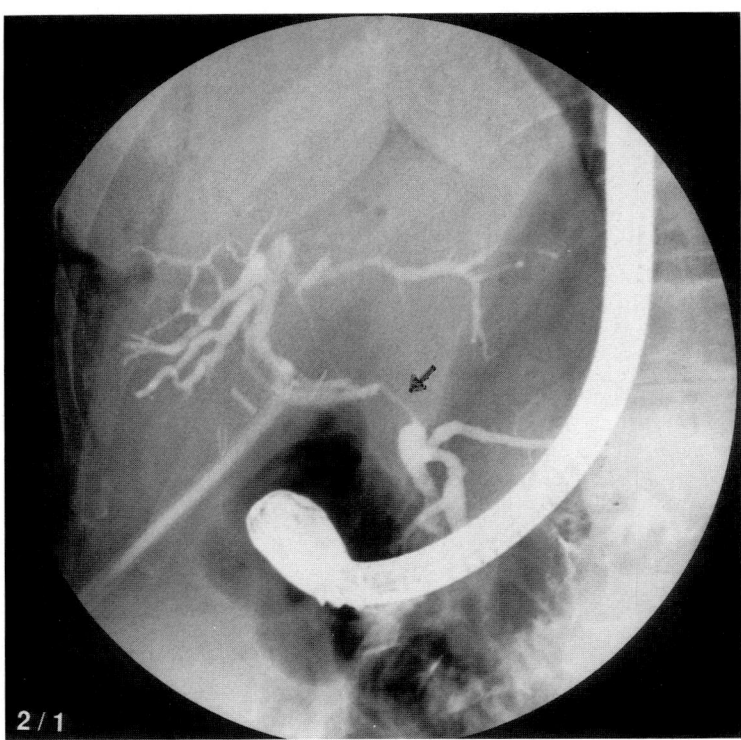

Figure 32.15. ERCP demonstrating a bile duct stricture (arrow) due to a cholangiocarcinoma.

The next level of biliary surgery that has begun to be performed laparoscopically is biliary–enteric bypass for malignant obstruction. A laparoscopic cholecystojejunostomy or choledochojejunostomy can be constructed. These anastomoses must be hand-sewn and are tedious to perform. Advances in suturing devices now being introduced allow simpler passage and capture of needles; these techniques will increase the acceptability of this approach. The wide availability of the endoscopic alternative with ERCP and stent placement under conscious sedation for malignant bile duct obstruction has slowed the development of operative alternatives (Figs. 32.15, 32.16). With economic issues becoming more important in health care management schemes, laparoscopy may become the procedure of choice, as a single procedure results in adequate biliary drainage for a lifetime whereas the endoscopic approach requires stent exchange on a regular basis due to stent obstruction.[31]

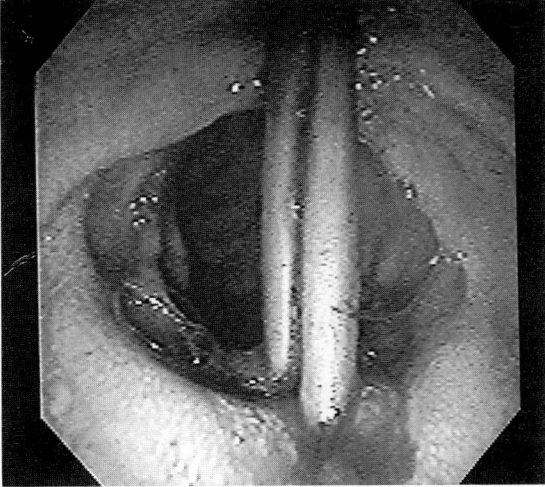

Figure 32.16. Two stents are placed in the biliary system across the bile duct stricture. This endoscopic view shows the end of the stents.

Appendectomy

Professor Kurt Semm, a German gynecologist from Kiel, renowned for his work in advancing operative laparoscopy, performed the first laparoscopic appendectomy in 1983.[32] The patient was a woman with endometriosis involving the cecum and appendix. Semm did not, however, advocate laparoscopic appendectomy for acute inflammation of the appendix and at that time cautioned against it. Gotz further developed the technique and expanded its application.[33] Soon, with advances in laparoscopic instrumentation, surgeons in Europe were removing the appendix for acute inflammation. Schrieber, in 1987 in Dusseldorf, reported results from 70 women undergoing laparoscopic appendectomy, one-fourth of whom had acute appendicitis.[34] By 1991 Pier et al. were able to report a series from Linnich, Germany on 625 patients undergoing laparoscopic appendectomy, 70% of whom had acute appendicitis. The average operating time was 20 minutes. Their conversion rate to open appendectomy was 2%, and abdominal abscess occurred in only two patients, both of whom had perforated appendices.[35]

Our European colleagues continue to have the luxury of keeping patients in the hospital for their recovery, with an average postoperative stay of 7 days reported in the Pier series. Saye et al., however, reported a mean discharge interval of 23 hours for an early series in the United States.[36] Although most general surgeons not performing laparoscopic appendectomy assume that the laparoscopic approach leads to a higher incidence of intraabdominal and wound infections, it has not been borne out in the series reported to date. With proper tissue handling, including placement of the infected appendix in a specimen bag, the incidence of wound-related infections is reduced, which contributes to the shorter average postoperative stay. Laparoscopic appendectomy thus seems to be safe and is a technically approachable operation for the laparoscopic surgeon.

Because open appendectomy can be performed with minimal morbidity and a short hospital stay (1–2 days), with patients going back to work quickly, the cost of the operation is likely to be a focus as well. The use of disposable ports and stapling devices, although appealing and in some cases perhaps contributing to the safety of the operation, must be justified with respect to outcome (Figs. 32.17–32.19). Otherwise, the more economic open procedure may be the procedure of choice, with the laparoscopic approach ending up on the cost-cutting budget director's floor. It is in smaller, simpler operations such as this one that every detail of operating technique and time use under anesthesia must be controlled in order to make the laparoscopic approach competitive.

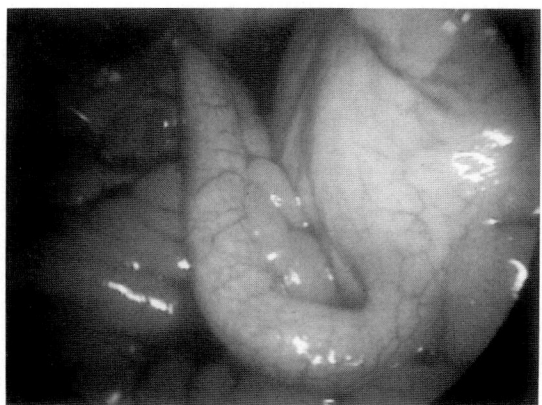

Figure 32.17. Inflamed appendix at the time of laparoscopic appendectomy.

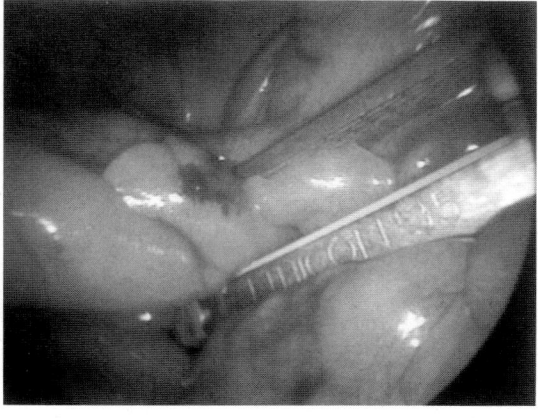

Figure 32.18. Laparoscopic stapling device is placed across the mesentery of the appendix to divide the mesoappendix.

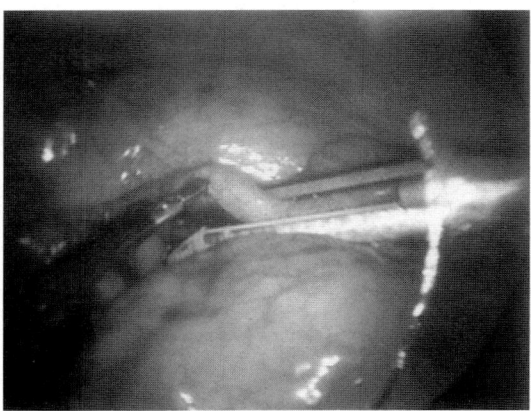

Figure 32.19. Endoscopic stapling device is placed across the base of the appendix to complete the appendectomy. The stump is not inverted.

Colon Surgery

Laparoscopic colon surgery was a natural extension from laparoscopic cholecystectomy. The techniques learned during gallbladder mobilization and resection could easily be applied to colonic mobilization and resection. For lesions on the right side, the anastomosis could be performed by hand-sewing the exteriorized ends of the ileum and transverse colon. The specific skills required for this procedure are mobilization of the right colon and division of colon mesenteric vessels. The exposure of the organ to allow safe dissection and division of vessels is certainly more difficult than exposure of the gallbladder, but with careful rotation and angling of the colon by placement of vessel loops to safely apply traction, exposure is adequate to allow satisfactory colon mobilization. The left colon presents a more difficult problem with splenic flexure mobilization and internal anastomosis. The anastomosis can be handled with a transanal circular stapling device. Splenic flexure mobilization is not difficult if proper countertraction technique is used during the dissection.

Early experiences with laparoscopic colon resection began to appear in the literature shortly after the initial experience with laparoscopic cholecystectomy became widely known.[37] Results were favorable, and surgeons moved quickly from treating small benign lesions of the right colon to treating larger colon cancers. Results are not available at this time from controlled trials regarding the adequacy of colon cancer resection using a laparoscopic technique. Surgeons who are performing the technique regularly are insistent that exposure of the root of the mesentery is adequate, and that complete resection of the mesenteric lymph node-bearing tissue is possible.[38] Time and ongoing clinical trials will answer this question.[39]

Using current technology, the time required to perform a subtotal colectomy, with careful mesenteric dissection, seems excessive. Subtotal colectomy is much easier to perform in thin patients, since vessels are visible through the mesentery. Advancements in the equipment used to expose and ligate mesenteric vessels will certainly reduce the operating time and make larger resections more feasible.

Along with resection, there are several other colonic disease processes amenable to a laparoscopic approach. Repair of injured bowel is easily handled laparoscopically if fecal contamination is limited. The bowel and surrounding peritoneal cavity can be copiously lavaged and direct suture repair of the bowel accomplished. If necessary, a proximal stoma may be created to protect the area of repair. Resection of a full-thickness excision of bowel wall such as is required for treating endometriosis, can be accomplished laparoscopically. Abscesses of diverticular origin can be identified and drained laparoscopically with or without a proximal colostomy. Ileostomy can be performed without a large incision even when laparoscopy is not used. In selected cases, however, it is helpful to assess the bowel more globally at the time of ileostomy formation. In these cases a laparoscopic approach is used, and a small-vessel loop or umbilical tape is passed around the distal ileum and exteriorized through a widened laparoscopic puncture site. Colostomy can be performed laparoscopically for a variety of reasons. The reoperation is made easier because of the reduced adhesions with a laparoscopic approach in an otherwise unoperated abdomen. Cecopexy and rectopexy are possible using a laparoscopic approach. The advisability and success of some of these techniques is question-

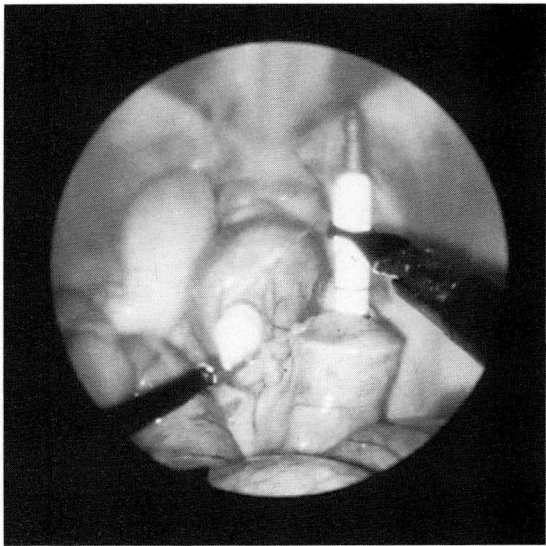

Figure 32.20. Low anterior colon resection. Anvil is in place in the proximal bowel following bowel resection.

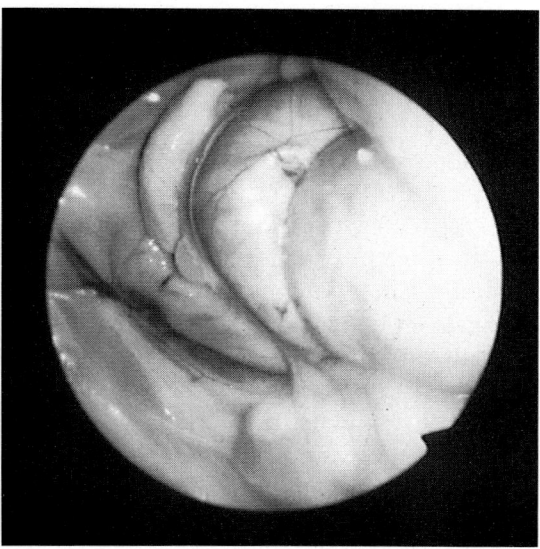

Figure 32.22. Completed colorectal anastomosis.

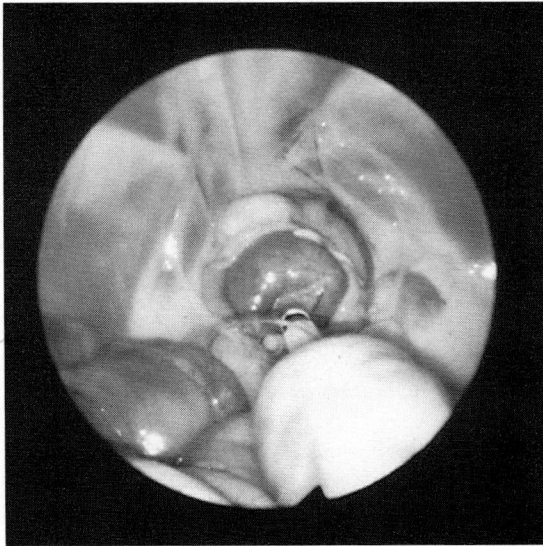

Figure 32.21. Anvil is inserted in the stapling device in the rectum to allow a circular stapled anastomosis.

able even with open surgery, but the ability to perform them laparoscopically is advantageous when indicated. Finally, colostomy closure including dissection and reversal of Hartmann's procedure is possible. An initial approach to the abdomen with an open cannula insertion technique and gentle dissection of adhesions around the colostomy should allow a laparoscopic approach in a significant percentage of these cases. The proximal bowel is mobilized, and attachments to the surrounding peritoneum and fascia at the stoma are divided. The bowel is exteriorized along with the distal bowel and an exterior anastomosis created. In cases of a Hartmann's pouch, the pouch is dissected free from adjacent small bowel, and a transanal stapled anastomosis may be created (Figs. 32.20–32.22). The proximal bowel may be exteriorized to insert the anvil of the end-to-end circular stapler. Dissection of the small bowel is clearly the limiting factor in these cases, particularly if Hartmann's pouch is short.[39–44]

Conclusion

This overview is intended to provide an update on advances in laparoscopy in areas that are no longer considered experimental and that are being implemented regularly into the practice of thoracic and general surgeons. In the hands of a small number of innovators, advances are being made in surgery of the spleen, adrenal glands, pancreas, and liver as well. Vascular surgery, though not yet approachable clinically via laparoscopic or thoracoscopic means, is not lagging far behind. Our vascular surgery colleagues have gone ahead with minimally invasive endoluminal treatments, including balloon dilatation and stenting of strictures, as well as drilling out atheromatous obstruction of small vessels. Clinical trials of endoluminal stenting of abdominal aortic aneurysms are under way. In our own laboratory, thoracic surgeons are developing thoracoscopic techniques of internal mammary artery mobilization and thoracoscopic microvascular anastomosis. Plastic surgeons are proceeding with laparoscopic and thoracoscopic approaches to muscular flaps for use with procedures internally in the abdominal and thoracic cavities. The orthopedists and neurosurgeons are placing scopes in virtually every joint and space in the body. The spine is not exempt, and small scopes can be passed to assist in the treatment of a variety of spinal disorders. Urologists have been heavily involved in endoscopic techniques since the nineteenth century. In fact, modified cystoscopes were the first scopes used for gastrointestinal endoscopy. We, as general surgeons, certainly recognize the contributions made by our gynecologic colleagues in advancing laparoscopy. Gynecologists are now benefiting from all of the attention being given to the development of laparoscopic instrumentation, and it is fair to say that they had developed an extensive repertoire of sophisticated laparoscopic operations, including delicate tubal anastomosis, well before the advent of general surgical laparoscopy. In many centers gynecologists took their general surgical colleagues by the hand through their first laparoscopic procedures. The first cholecystectomy accomplished laparoscopically by Mouret was performed after he completed the gynecologic indication for the operation, namely oophorectomy. The sky is truly the limit with application of these minimally invasive techniques. As we work to advance each of our fields we must remember that the creative ideas of the surgeon next door may have direct and immediate applications in our own field. We must strive to communicate and work together clinically and experimentally to take advantage of special "laparoscopic" opportunities.

References

1. KELLING G: Uber Oesophagoskopie, Gastroskopie und Kolioskopie. Munch Med Wochenschr 1902; 49:21.
2. JAKOBAEUS HC: Uber die Moglichkeit, die Zystoskopie bei Untersuchung seroser Hohlungen anzuwenden. Munch Med Wochenschr 1910; 57:2090.
3. SEMM K: Endoscopic appendicectomy. Endoscopy 1983;15:59.
4. DUBOIS F, BERTHELOT G, LEVARD H: Cholecystectomie par coelioscopie. Presse Med 1989; 18:980.
5. PERISSAT J, COLLET D, BELLIARD R: Gallstones: laparoscopic treatment—cholecystectomy, cholecystostomy and lithotripsy: our own technique. Surg Endosc 1990;4(1):1.
6. KRASNA MJ, FLOWERS JL: Diagnostic thoracoscopy in a patient with a pleural mass. Surg Laparosc Endosc 1991;1:94.
7. LEGRAND M, DETROZ B, HONORE P, JACQUET N: Laparoscopic highly selective vagotomy. Surg Laparosc Endosc 1992;6:90.
8. SHIMI SM, NATHANSON LK, CUSCHIERI A: Thoracoscopic lung myotomy for nutcracker oesophagus: initial experience of a new surgical approach. Br J Surg 1992;79:533.
9. BUESS GF, BECKER HD, NARUHN M, MENTGES B: Endoscopic esophagectomy without thoracotomy. Problems in General Surgery. 1991;8:478.
10. BOGOJAVALENSKY S: Laparoscopic treatment of inguinal and femoral hernia. Presented at the Eighteenth Annual Meeting of the American Association of Gynecologic Laparoscopists, Washington, DC, 1989.
11. SCHULTZ L, GRABER J, PIETRAFITTAS J, HICKOK D: Laser laparoscopic herniorrhaphy: a clinical trial; preliminary results. J Laparoendosc Surg 1991;1:41.
12. SALERNO GM, FITZGIBBONS RJ JR, FILIPI CJ: Laparoscopic inguinal hernia repair. In Surgical Laparoscopy, Zucker KA (ed). St. Louis, Quality Medical Publishing, 1991, pp 281–293.
13. MCKERNAN JB, LAWS HL: Laparoscopic preperitoneal prosthetic repair of inguinal hernias. Surg Rounds 1992;7:597.
14. NATHANSON LK, SHIMI S, CUSCHIERI A: Laparoscopic ligamentum teres (round ligament) cardiopexy. Br J Surg 1991;78:947.

15. DALLEMAGNE B, WEERTS JM, JEHAES C, ET AL: Laparoscopic Nissen fundoplication: preliminary report. Surg Laparosc Endosc 1991;1:138.
16. FRANTZIDES CT, LUDWIG KA, QUEBBEMAN EJ, BURHOP J: Laparoscopic highly selective vagotomy. Surg Laparosc Endosc 1992;2:311.
17. KATKHOUDA N, MOUIEL J: A new surgical technique of treatment of chronic duodenal ulcer without laparotomy by videocoelioscopy. Am J Surg 1991;161:361.
18. GRIFFIN SM, CHUNG SCS, LEUNG JWC, LI AKC: Peptic pyloric stenosis treated by endoscopic balloon dilatation. Br J Surg 1989;76:1147.
19. MUHE E: The first cholecystectomy through the laparoscope. Langenbecks Arch Chir 1986;369:804.
20. PERISSAT J, VITALE GC: Laparoscopic cholecystectomy: gateway to the future. Am J Surg 1991;161:408.
21. DUBOIS F, ICARD P, BERTHELOT G, ET AL: Coelioscopic cholecystectomy: preliminary report of 36 cases. Ann Surg 1989;191:271.
22. PERISSAT J, COLLET D, BELLIARD R: Gallstones: laparoscopic treatment; intracorporeal lithotripsy followed by cholecystostomy or cholecystectomy: a personal technique. Endoscopy 1989;21:373.
23. CUSCHIERI A, BERCI G, SACKIER JM, ET AL: Clinical aspects of laparoscopic cholecystectomy. In Laparoscopic Biliary Surgery. Cuschieri A, Berci G (eds). London, Blackwell, 1990, pp 82–88.
24. REDDICK EJ, OLSEN DO: Laparoscopic laser cholecystectomy. Surg Endosc 1989;3:131.
25. MCKERNAN JB, SAYE WB: Laparoscopic general surgery. J Med Assoc Ga 1990;79:157.
26. BERCI G, SACKIER JM, PAZ-PARTLOW M: Laparoscopic cholecystectomy; mini-access surgery: reality or utopia? Postgrad Gen Surg 1990;2:50.
27. LARSON GM, VITALE GC, CASEY J, ET AL: Multipractice analysis of laparoscopic cholecystectomy in 1,983 patients. Am J Surg 1992;163:221.
28. VITALE GC, STEPHENS G, WIEMAN TJ, LARSON GM: Use of endoscopic retrograde cholangiopancreatography in the management of biliary complications after laparoscopic cholecystectomy. Surgery 1993;114:806.
29. QUATELBAUM JK, DORSEY HD: Laparoscopic treatment of common bile duct stones. Surg Laparosc Endosc 1991;1:26.
30. VITALE GC, LARSON GM, WIEMAN TJ, ET AL: The use of ERCP in the management of common bile duct stones in patients undergoing laparoscopic cholecystectomy. Surg Endosc 1993;7:9.
31. HYOTY MK, NORDBACK IH: Biliary stent or surgical bypass in unresectable pancreatic cancer with obstructive jaundice. Acta Chir Scand 1990;156:301.
32. SEMM K: Die endoskopische Appendektomie. Gynakol Prax 1983;7:26.
33. GOTZ F: Die endoskopische Appendektomie nach Semm bei der akuten und chronischen Appendicitis. Endosk Heute 1988;2:5.
34. SCHREIBER J: Experience with laparoscopic appendectomy in women. Surg Endosc 1987;1:211.
35. PIER A, GOTZ F, BACHER C: Laparoscopic appendectomy in 625 cases: from innovation to routine. Surg Laparosc Endosc 1991;1:8.
36. SAYE WB, RIVES DA, COCHRAN EB: Laparoscopic appendectomy: three years' experience. Laparosc Endosc 1991;1:109.
37. JACOBS M, VERDEJA J-C, GOLDSTEIN HS: Minimally invasive colon resection (laparoscopic colectomy). Surg Laparosc Endosc 1991;1:144.
38. FOWLER DL, WHITE SA: Laparoscopic-assisted sigmoid resection. Surg Laparosc Endosc 1991;1:183.
39. AMERICAN SOCIETY OF COLON AND RECTAL SURGEONS: Policy statement. Dis Colon Rectum 1992;35:5A.
40. BIRNS MT: Inadvertent instrumental perforation of the colon during laparoscopy: nonsurgical repair. Gastrointest Endosc 1989;35:54.
41. REICH H, MCGLYNN F, BUDIN R: Laparoscopic repair of full-thickness bowel injury. J Laparoendosc Surg 1991;1:119.
42. OSTERGAARD E, HALVORSEN JF: Volvulus of the cecum: an evaluation of various surgical procedures. Acta Chir Scand 1990;156:629.
43. BERMAN IR: Sutureless laparoscopic rectopexy for procidentia. Dis Colon Rectum 1992;35:689.
44. LANGE V, MEYER G, SCHARDEY HM, ET AL: Laparoscopic creation of a loop colostomy. J Laparoendosc Surg 1991;1:307.

33
Fetus as an Endoscopic Surgical Patient

Rubén A. Quintero

Prenatal diagnosis of medically and surgically correctable fetal conditions has improved dramatically since the 1970s as a result of the great strides achieved in ultrasound technology, reproductive genetics, pathology, and microbiology. Although most fetal conditions neither require nor are amenable to in utero therapy, others warrant medical or surgical treatment. The decision to offer any form of fetal therapy is based on the balance between the risks and benefits of the therapeutic intervention to the mother and fetus and the concerns about withholding therapy (Table 33.1). The risk/benefit ratio for the fetus depends on the likelihood that the particular condition will disappear, remain stable, or become more ominous during the course of the pregnancy (i.e., knowledge of the natural history of the disease in utero). Transient conditions that do not significantly compromise the health of the fetus, such as transient pleural effusions,[1] may be managed expectantly until they resolve. If the condition is not known to resolve spontaneously, but lack of immediate treatment is also not known to jeopardize the outcome, as in the case of most fetal gastroschisis, definitive treatment may be deferred until after birth.[2,3] On the other hand, if it is known that fetal death or damage may occur unless treatment is undertaken, as with many cases of obstructive uropathy,[4] diaphragmatic hernia,[5] or acardiac twins,[6] prenatal intervention or early delivery is indicated. The risks to the mother depend on the consequences that nonintervention may pose to her health or on the adverse effects that the proposed therapy may entail.

Ideally, the evaluation and treatment of the fetus should have no more limitations than that of the newborn. In reality, the fetus remains a relatively inaccessible patient. The limitations are obviously posed by the intrauterine-intraamniotic location of the fetus and by our relative lack of understanding of the factors responsible for the onset of normal and pathologic labor and for the intact preservation of the fetal membranes.

Despite these limitations, the fetus has increasingly become the subject of various therapeutic approaches. The noninvasive approach, the transplacental route, has been used for the delivery of antiarrhythmic agents to manage complex fetal arrhythmias[7,8] and hyperimmune immunoglobulin for alloimmune thrombocytopenia.[9] Minimally invasive approaches to fetal therapy involve intravascular placement of small-caliber needles under ultrasound guidance for the treatment of fetal anemia.[10] These procedures constitute some of the most successful forms of fetal therapy. The placement of pleuroamniotic[11] and vesicoamniotic[12–14] shunts for

Table 33.1. Conditions and criteria for fetal surgery

Accurate diagnosis
Absence of other major anomalies
Normal karyotype
Knowledge of the natural history of the disease
Previability
Feasibility of the proposed treatment
Fetal benefits outweigh maternal and fetal risks

Table 33.2. Conditions for open fetal surgery in humans

Repair of diaphragmatic hernia
Tracheal ligation for diaphragmatic hernia
Cystostomy or ureterostomy for obstructive uropathy
Banding of sacrococcygeal teratoma
Selective fetectomy for acardiac twin or twin–twin transfusion syndrome

the treatment of pleural effusions and obstructive uropathy, respectively, constitute the second major type of minimally invasive fetal therapy. Major fetal anomalies, such as diaphragmatic hernia, sacrococcygeal teratoma, and cystic adenomatoid malformation of the lung, call for more complicated surgical tasks, which require more direct access to the fetus. The need to perform more complicated surgical procedures led to the development of open fetal surgery.

All forms of fetal therapy have their advantages and limitations. In general, the less invasive the procedure, the less likely it will elicit an untoward response with respect to uterine contractility.[15] In this sense, we have explored the possibility of using minimally invasive endoscopic methods to treat the human fetus. This approach intends to address the limitations of other forms of fetal therapy while offering unique therapeutic options. In this chapter we examine the advantages, disadvantages, and applications of endoscopy to the management of human fetal disease.

Open Fetal Surgery

Attempts to perform open fetal surgery date back to the 1960s.[16,17] Since then, several groups have conducted extensive research to establish the scope and limitations of this approach.[18] During open fetal surgery the mother undergoes laparotomy and hysterotomy. The fetus is partially extracted, undergoes a surgical procedure, and is subsequently returned to the amniotic cavity. The amniotic membranes and uterus are then closed. The fetus is ultimately delivered by cesarean section several weeks later. Table 33.2 shows the conditions for which open fetal surgery has been performed. Although most experience has been gained in the management of fetuses with congenital diaphragmatic hernia,[19] conditions such as obstructive uropathy[20] and sacrococcygeal teratoma[21] have also been addressed using this approach.

A number of concepts have been drawn from the vast experience with these groups: (1) Prenatal intervention is justified under certain conditions and certain circumstances to prevent further organ damage or death, as elegantly shown in animal models of fetal obstructive uropathy.[22] (2) Surgical healing within the amniotic cavity seems to differ from that which occurs in the extrauterine environment, such that scar formation is either absent or significantly reduced.[23] (3) The placenta and the intrauterine environment provide stable and ideal postoperative conditions for the fetus in terms of temperature and nutrient supplies but probably have a limited ability to respond to acute hemodynamic or hydrostatic changes. (4) The incidences of uterine contractions, preterm labor, and rupture of membranes are directly related to the degree of trauma to the uterus and membranes.[15] (5) Most fetal and maternal complications are directly related to preterm labor, which has been difficult or impossible to control.

The complications associated with open fetal surgery (i.e., preterm labor, premature rupture of membranes, abruptio placenta) (Table 33.3) are mostly related to the "unforgiving nature" of the pregnant uterus to the injury inflicted by the incision, and they have limited the array of problems to which this approach can be applied. These limitations and the significantly invasive nature of this type of surgery are responsible for the lack of widespread acceptance

Table 33.3. Maternal and fetal complications of open fetal surgery

Preterm labor
Premature rupture of membranes
Abruptio placenta
Amniotic bands
Fetal intracranial hemorrhage
Maternal pulmonary edema
Need to deliver by cesarean section

of this approach for the management of complex congenital anomalies.

Endoscopic Fetal Surgery: Operative Fetoscopy

Historically, fetal endoscopy preceded ultrasonography and several other diagnostic and therapeutic modalities in fetal medicine. Originally described in 1954 in an isolated report,[24] fetoscopy had its climax during the late 1970s and mid-1980s as a technique to visualize the fetus and to aid in obtaining tissue samples or fetal blood (Fig. 33.1). Despite its initial promise, fetoscopy was performed only in selected centers throughout the world. The invasive nature of the procedure and the limited field and depth of view, particularly if intraamniotic bleeding occurred, limited its use. The development and widespread use of diagnostic ultrasonography and of ultrasound-guided invasive procedures quickly displaced fetoscopy as a diagnostic and therapeutic tool.[25]

Beginning in 1980, an endoscopic revolution began to take place in medicine as a result of the advances made in endoscopic technology and surgical instrumentation. The use of bipolar electrocoagulation, the addition of video technology, and the development of endoscopic surgical instruments changed the outlook of virtually every surgical specialty. These advances have been particularly prominent in gynecologic and general surgery, with the laparoscopic performance of such relatively complex operations as cholecystectomy.[26]

Given that most complications associated with open fetal surgery are related to the degree

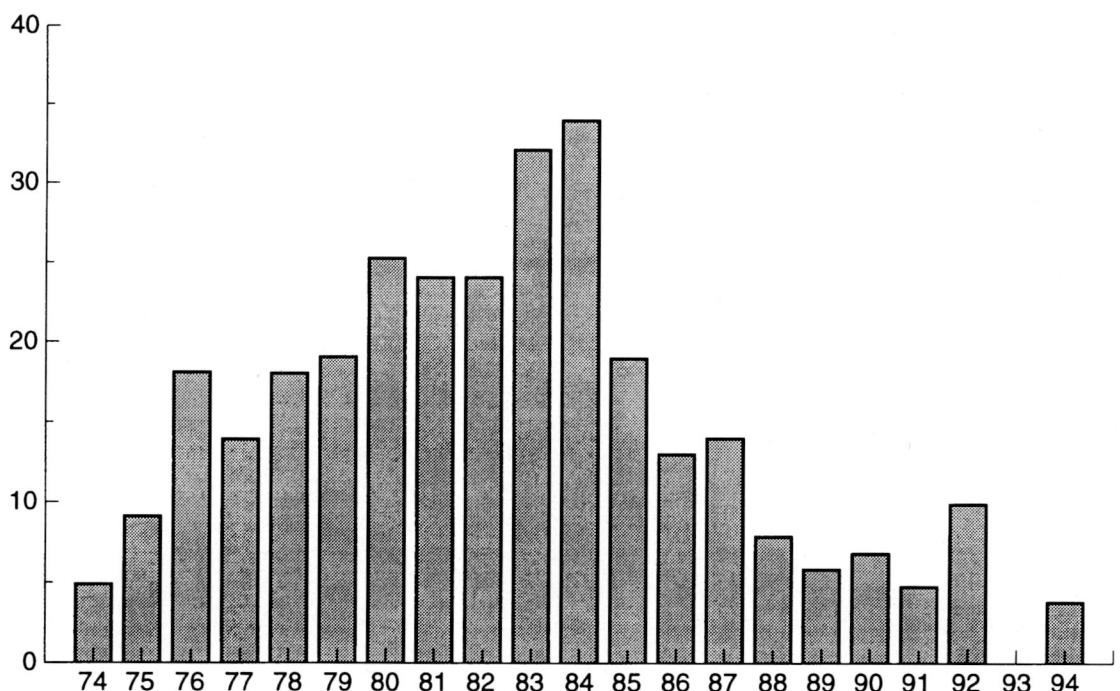

Figure 33.1. Distribution of publications on fetoscopy for two decades.

of trauma to the uterus and membranes, it is only logical to assume that an endoscopic approach to surgically correctable fetal disorders, with its attending lesser degree of trauma to the uterus and fetal membranes, should be associated with better outcomes. The same basic principles that guide endoscopic surgery in other fields (i.e., minimal invasiveness and lower morbidity) take on a different perspective from the savings in cost or length of hospital stay when extrapolated to fetal surgery. Indeed, less morbidity during operative fetoscopy is synonymous with a greater likelihood that the pregnancy will not be lost as a consequence of the intervention. Therefore the efforts in fetal surgery should concentrate on developing endoscopic or minimally invasive techniques to correct birth defects currently managed by open fetal surgery and to address others that may have seemed impossible to address to date.

Developing endoscopic surgical techniques to operate inside the pregnant uterus entails developing practically a whole new surgical field. The unique working environment (the amniotic fluid), access methods, and operating instruments constitute prerequisite areas that require research and development. The following sections address the progress established in these areas by us and other groups and the clinical application(s) of these concepts.

Animal Experimentation

A number of animal experiments have been performed using endoscopic techniques, some specific to the treatment of a particular condition, others addressing the endoscopic techniques per se. We have performed endoscopic procedures in the nonpregnant rabbit under a fluid medium (hydrolaparoscopy) using custom-designed 2 mm instruments.[27] The use of such small instrumentation within a limited space has allowed us to extrapolate our experience more readily to clinical work. With this model, dissection, electrocoagulation, and extracorporeal knots were utilized with excellent results. Estes et al. have used endoscopy and custom-designed 5 mm instruments to repair an experimentally created cleft lip in the fetal lamb. Healing of the lip incision was virtually unnoticeable at birth.[28] De Lia et al. used a YAG laser to photocoagulate placental surface vessels in a pregnant nonhuman primate model.[29] This experience has been extrapolated to humans for the management of pregnancies affected by twin–twin transfusion syndrome[30–34] and acardiac twins (Y. Ville and R. A. Quintero, unpublished results).

Luks et al.[35] have created an endoscopic model of urinary tract obstruction in the lamb by ligating the urachus and the fetal urethra of male fetuses. The urinary tract obstruction was subsequently treated endoscopically via a cystostomy.[35] This group also performed fetal laryngoscopy and bronchoscopy to occlude the trachea.[36] This accomplishment is promising for the management of fetuses with diaphragmatic hernia, as discussed below.

Concepts

A number of concepts and conclusions have been derived from the animal work, although direct application of many of these concepts to humans may not be feasible. For example, most animal endoscopic surgery has been performed with 5 mm instrumentation.[28,36,37] The use of these relatively wide instruments in the human uterus is likely to be associated with greater maternal and fetal morbidity. Second, most animal work has been performed through a laparotomy, without the use of ultrasound, which is essential for clinical work. Therefore additional concepts must be incorporated to make human endoscopic fetal surgery possible.

Access

Entry to the amniotic cavity can be accomplished percutaneously or through a small laparotomy incision. The percutaneous approach is less traumatic, can be performed as an outpatient procedure, and can be used provided the size of the instruments is small (usually < 3 mm). For the technique described at our institution, 2 mm instruments are used, which require a minimal skin incision.[31] If a minilaparotomy is necessary to access the uterus, a 2- to 3-cm

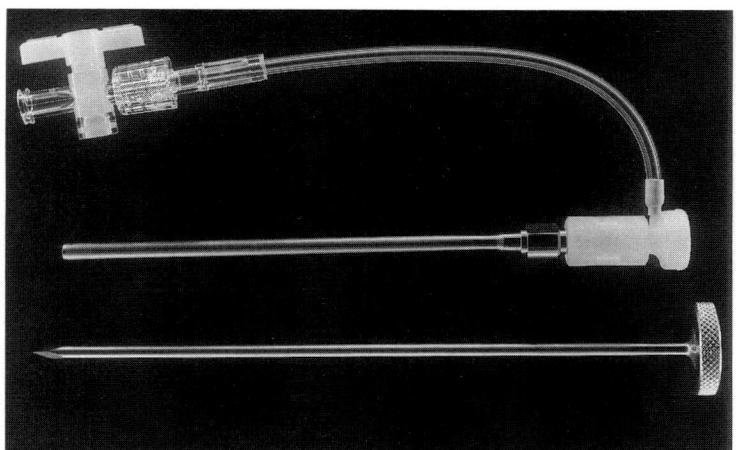

Figure 33.2. Custom-designed 2 mm trocar for use in operative fetoscopy. The checkflow valve prevents amniotic fluid leakage while retaining the endoscope. The side arm plastic tubing allows removal of amniotic fluid or instillation of fluid for better visualization.

incision is made in the maternal abdomen,[30] and the trocar is introduced through the myometrium into the amniotic cavity. A purse-string suture is tied around the entry site to avoid amniotic fluid leakage.

To date there are no trocars specifically designed to enter the amniotic cavity. Most available trocars for adult or pediatric laparoscopy are at least 5 mm in inside diameter (I.D.) and 6–7 mm outside diameter (O.D.). In addition, most rigid endoscopes are equipped with thick protective sheaths that prevent bending. To facilitate work in humans, we have developed special 2- to 3-mm trocars in varying lengths. A check-flow valve at the hub of the trocar prevents amniotic fluid leakage. In addition, a plastic side arm with a valve allows infusion of fluid or removal of amniotic fluid as desired (Fig. 33.2).

Working Environment: Fluid or Gas

Laparoscopy uses gas as a distention medium. Fetoscopic work within a gaseous medium, in contrast to liquid, would have several advantages. First, the techniques used for laparoscopy would be more easily translated into operative fetoscopy. Second, visualization under gas is superior to that under fluid, particularly if the amniotic fluid cavity is turbid or if intraamniotic bleeding has occurred. Unfortunately, fetal acidosis has been reported in fetal lambs when endoscopic work was performed under a CO_2/fluid medium.[28,37] An additional limitation of using gas in the amniotic cavity is that it would not allow concomitant use of ultrasonography. Therefore a fluid environment appears necessary, and unique techniques must be developed to operate within this medium.

Visualization

The exchange of amniotic fluid for lactated Ringer's solution is required for several reasons. We and others have found that light transmission through human amniotic fluid is significantly less than through air or physiologic solution.[38,39] In addition to the baseline limitations, visualization through amniotic fluid may be further hindered by previous blood staining from preoperative cordocentesis, from intraamniotic bleeding during surgery, or from excessive vernix.

The infusion of fluid into the amniotic cavity has been used clinically with protocols designed to decrease the incidence of abnormal fetal heart rate patterns during labor,[40] for the prevention of meconium aspiration syndrome,[41] and for management of certain fetuses with oligohydramnios.[42,43] Extrapolating from this experience, we have developed a technique to exchange the amniotic fluid during endoscopic fetal surgery. With our current technique, a suction/irrigation pump with manual pressure calibration is attached to the side ports of the trocars (Fig. 33.3). This system can rapidly clear the amniotic fluid in case of intraamniotic bleeding without altering the total amniotic

33. Fetus as an Endoscopic Surgical Patient

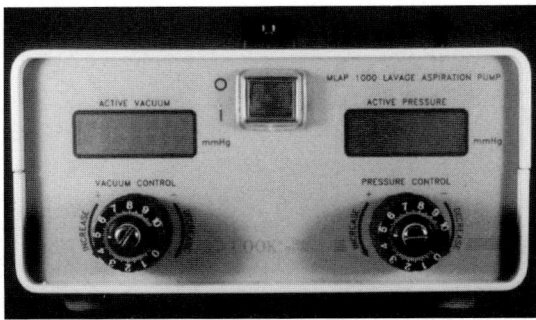

Figure 33.3. Vacuum-pressure pump used for amniotic fluid exchange. The two pressures can be independently regulated. (Cook, Ob/Gyn, Sydney, Australia)

fluid volume. Different ports are preferred for irrigation and suction, although the exchange can also be performed in an alternate fashion through a single port.

Image Display

Given the restrictions in instrument size, the panoramic view provided by large endoscopes (e.g., 10 mm) cannot be enjoyed during operative fetoscopy. Instead, one is limited to the small field of view provided by relatively small endoscopes (1.9 mm). To offset this limitation, ultrasonography is used to guide the insertion of the instruments into the amniotic cavity and for orientation during surgery. To coordinate both images, a video mixer is used (i.e., a device that displays simultaneously or selectively the endoscopic and sonographic images on a single monitor) (Plate 48). By definition, the video mixer reduces by half the number of monitors needed in the room. As with video laparoscopy, we place a monitor on each side of the patient's bed so all members of the surgical team can monitor the procedure simultaneously.

Endoscopes

Endoscopes are a key element when performing endoscopic fetal surgery. A number of endoscopes are currently available for different specialties, but no endoscope is specifically designed for fetoscopic surgery at the present time. Table 33.4 classifies the available endoscopes according to their characteristics. From a practical perspective, different endoscopes are necessary for different procedures.[31] The smallest endoscope is chosen whenever possible. For diagnostic procedures we prefer to use either a 0.7 mm flexible endoscope (Intramed Laboratories, San Diego, CA), or a 1.9 mm rigid scope (Richard Wolf, Vernon Hills, IL), but we have used endoscopes as large as 2.5 and 5.0 mm. Wider fiberoptic endoscopes are not necessarily associated with a better image, as they often retain the same optical resolution but increase the scope diameter with irrigation or working channels.

The length of the endoscope is also important. It must be longer than the trocars, so it can reach the amniotic cavity and preferably be able to span the length of the entire amniotic cavity. This point is particularly important if the fetus changes position intraoperatively. Figure 33.4 displays a number of endoscopes currently in use, including those specifically designed by us.

Surgical Instruments

As with the endoscopes, there is currently no given set of instruments specifically designed for operative fetoscopy. Therefore a significant amount of research time is devoted to either identifying available products that may be adapted to operative fetoscopy or designing them (Table 33.5). Unfortunately, only a small selection of instruments ≤ 3 mm is currently available. If the instruments are ≤ 1 mm in

Table 33.4. Functional characteristics of endoscopes used for operative fetoscopy

Constitution	Consistency	Function	Maneuverability
Fiberoptic	Flexible	Diagnostic	Passive
Solid rod lens	Rigid	Operating	Steerable
Multilens			

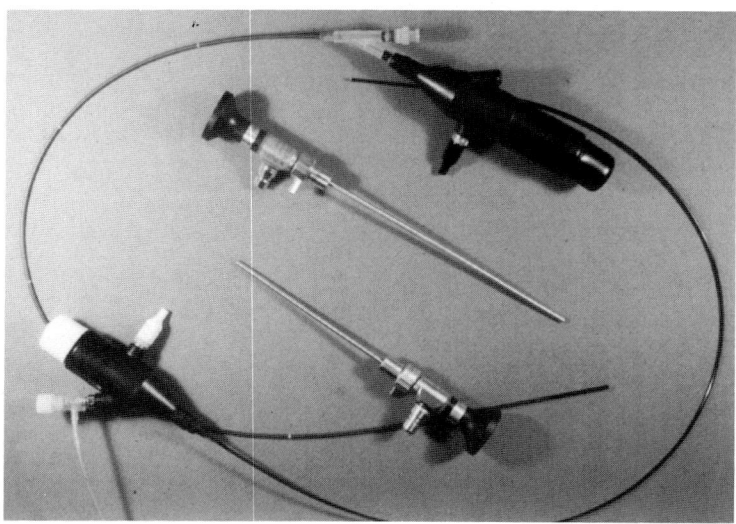

Figure 33.4. Selection of endoscopes currently in use. Modifications of working ports, construction materials, and other technical aspects are often necessary to improve performance.

Table 33.5. Instruments designed and adapted for operative fetoscopy

Designed	Adapted
Trocars	Forceps
Blunt probe	Scissors
Knot pushers	Electrodes
Knot cutters	Wire guides
Bipolar electrocautery scapel	Laser fibers
Bipolar forceps	
Monopolar electrodes	

diameter, they can be introduced through the working channel of several endoscopes (operating endoscopes), obviating the need for a second port (operating endoscopes). If 5 mm instruments can be safely used for intrauterine surgery, a wider variety of instruments are available.

Pressure/Volume Regulation

The amniotic fluid pressure rises linearly by 1 mm Hg/L of physiologic fluid infused.[44] In our procedures, we maintain a baseline level of amniotic fluid, unless it is initially abnormally high or low. In our earliest cases we monitored the intraamniotic pressure several times during surgery. As we did not note significant variations (1–2 mm Hg), we have not continued this practice. However, as many of our cases were performed under general anesthesia, it may have blunted any possible pressure changes. With our current technique, an even exchange of amniotic fluid is performed to diminish the likelihood of significant pressure changes.

Safety

The potential for maternal or fetal injury exists, particularly when wide trocars (e.g., 3.5 mm) are used. As stated, some investigators perform a minilaparotomy when using these relatively large endoscopes to avoid injuring uterine vessels and to place a purse-string stitch around the endoscope to prevent fluid leakage.

Data regarding the pregnancy loss rate associated with fetoscopy is limited to the few series that have been performed in ongoing pregnancies. Hobbins and Mahoney reported two losses among 65 patients (3%) in continuing pregnancies.[45] They used an endoscope 1.7 mm in diameter inserted transabdominally through a 2.2 × 2.7 mm cannula in patients at risk for hemoglobinopathies and other genetic disorders. Rodeck, using a similar endoscope, had a 3.7% pregnancy loss rate among 108 patients who underwent transabdominal fetoscopy for fetal blood sampling, skin biopsy, or evaluation for suspected anomalies.[46] An additional 37 patients underwent pregnancy termination based on the results of the examination. Therefore a 3.0–3.7% figure likely approximates a corrected pregnancy loss rate associated with transabdominal fetoscopy.

Approximately 5–7% of patients in the above-mentioned series experienced amniotic fluid leakage, though most had a successful outcome.[45,46] The corresponding figure of 1.0–1.3% associated with second trimester amniocentesis[47] probably reflects the use of a smaller-bore instrument with the latter technique.

The potential teratogenic effect of light or heat on the developing conceptus has been mentioned since the inception of fetoscopy. However, there is a scarcity of literature evaluating this issue. Hyperthermia is a known human teratogen, primarily affecting the central nervous system (CNS), with the most significant manifestations (neural tube defects) occurring if exposure takes place during days 21–28 postconception. A threshold of approximately 1.5°–2.5°C is required before effects are seen. A considerable amount of heat can be generated at the light cord–endoscope interphase. We have not been able to show any significant temperature elevation at the tip of the endoscope in a waterbath using a 2.7 mm endoscope for more than 30 minutes.[38] In addition, embryoscopy or fetoscopy is performed after the period of neural tube closure. Therefore it is unlikely that the use of endoscopes inside the amniotic cavity is associated with heat teratogenicity.

The potential harmful effect of light on the developing visual pathway has also been a concern for more than 20 years. The human optic vesicle is visible from weeks 6–9 menstrual age. The eyelids are fused beyond 9–10 weeks. Experiments using red laser light focused on the optic vesicles of chick embryos at stages 10–20 have resulted in several anomalies, including microphthalmia and anophthalmia.[48] Other experiments, using white light, have shown alterations in the pineal gland of chick embryos.[49] In our own experiments, we have used a 2.7 mm endoscope and a 300 watt xenon light source for 5 minutes directed at the optic vesicle of chick embryos at stage E10, equivalent to 10–12 weeks' gestation in the human. In this setting, we have been unable to show any histologic alterations in the retina or any alteration in the pattern of neurotransmitter transport from the retina to the optic colliculi.[50] Chick embryos exposed to the above conditions, when allowed to hatch, were able to feed normally when the unexposed eye was covered. Based on these results, white light as provided by an endoscope probably lacks any teratogenic potential on the developing visual organs. Vandenberghe performed light exposure experiments in the fetal lamb and reported no obvious damage to the fetal retina.[39] Despite these negative results, we suggest that fetal endoscopy should probably be performed beyond the time of eyelid fusion, that is, at approximately 9–10 weeks' gestation (menstrual age), as the threshold at which endoscopic white light may cause visual damage has not been established.

Clinical Applications

In the following sections we discuss the specific entities to which endoscopic fetal surgery has been applied and those in which this approach could be potentially used.

Acardiac Twins

Twin reverse arterial perfusion (TRAP) sequence affects 1% of monozygotic twins, or 1 in 35,000 births or 1 in 30 triplets.[51] The proposed pathophysiology for this condition is that in the presence of artery-to-artery and vein-to-vein anastomoses in a monozygotic placenta a hemodynamically advantaged twin (pump twin) perfuses the other twin (perfused twin) via retrograde flow.[52] Inadequate perfusion of the recipient twin is responsible for the development of a characteristic, invariably lethal set of anomalies, including acardia and acephalus. The diagnosis of the acardiac twin is made by pulsed and color Doppler by demonstrating arterial blood flow perfusing the acardiac twin in a retrograde fashion (Plate 49). Typically, the pump twin is structurally normal, but it is at risk for developing in utero cardiac failure and without treatment dies in 50–75% of cases, particularly if the acardiac/pump twin size ratio is > 50%.[6] Subtle signs of hemodynamic decompensation in the pump twin include an enlarged right atrium, increased reverse flow in the infe-

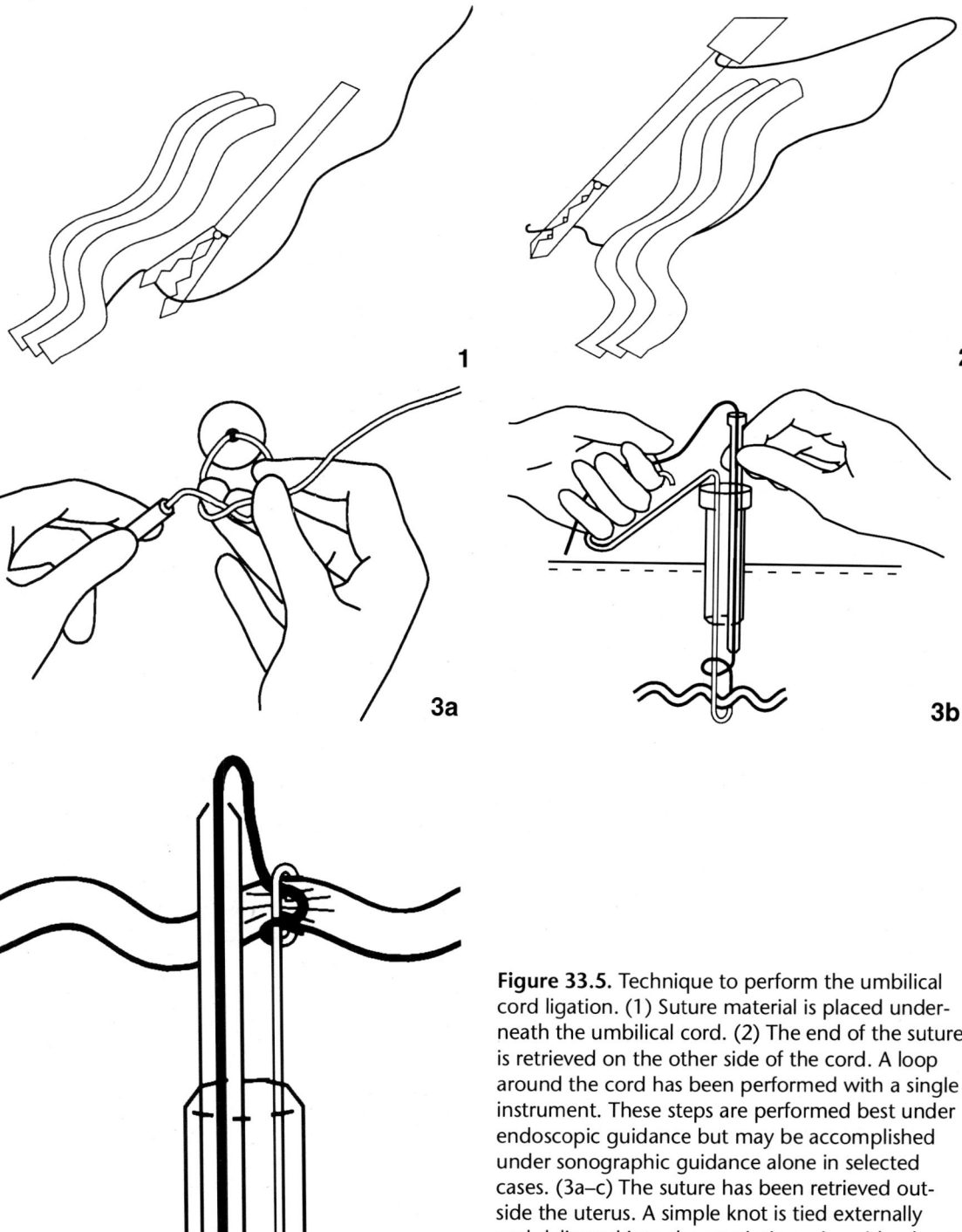

Figure 33.5. Technique to perform the umbilical cord ligation. (1) Suture material is placed underneath the umbilical cord. (2) The end of the suture is retrieved on the other side of the cord. A loop around the cord has been performed with a single instrument. These steps are performed best under endoscopic guidance but may be accomplished under sonographic guidance alone in selected cases. (3a–c) The suture has been retrieved outside the uterus. A simple knot is tied externally and delivered into the amniotic cavity with a knot-pusher.

rior vena cava, reverse flow in the ductus venosus, or pulsatile flow in the umbilical vein, each of which may occur prior to the appearance of ascites and edema.

The therapeutic goal of interrupting the vascular communication between the two twins, although simple in concept,[53] has been difficult to accomplish. Methods previously employed have included removal of the anomalous twin, or sectio parva,[54-46] whereby the abnormal fetus is selectively delivered. Sectio parva requires a hysterotomy and subsequent cesarean section and has been associated with abruptio placenta, preterm labor, preterm birth, and prolonged maternal hospitalization.[53] Another approach consists of ultrasound-directed percutaneous thrombosis of the umbilical cord of the acardiac twin by intraarterial injection of either thrombogenic coils or fibrin superglue in the umbilical cord of the perfused twin circulation.[57-60] Unfortunately, although this method of interrupting the circulation of the acardiac twin may be technically easier, insertion of thrombogenic coils or fibrin glue has been associated with the death of both twins and recanalization of the umbilical arterial flow after the procedure.[58,60]

With the technique proposed by us,[61] one or two 2- to 3-mm ports are introduced into the amniotic cavity under ultrasound guidance. The use of ultrasound guidance is essential for identifying the correct cord to ligate and the placenta-free areas through which the trocars can be introduced. An endoscope is delivered intraamniotically to monitor the surgical procedure. Through the other port, a 3-0 Vicryl suture is passed with a small grasper underneath the umbilical cord (Fig. 33.5). The suture is grasped on the opposite side of the cord and retrieved outside the maternal abdomen. A simple extracorporeal knot is tied and delivered intraamniotically with a knot-pusher to occlude the cord.[62] The procedure is repeated for safety, and the suture is cut with small scissors inside the amniotic cavity (Plate 50). We are now able to perform this procedure by ultrasound guidance alone, which may reduce the number of ports to one.

As the acardiac twin usually lacks any amniotic fluid, access to the umbilical cord may be hindered by the amniotic membrane of this twin. Therefore an amnioinfusion or amniorrhexis of this sac is needed to reach the umbilical cord. This is preferably performed prior to introduction of the 2 mm trocar, so it is done wholly in the sac of the abnormal twin.

Endoscopic umbilical cord ligation is the first surgical procedure to be performed in a human pregnancy using more than one port. It exemplifies many of the concepts needed for operative fetoscopy, including the combined use of ultrasonography, a video mixer, amnioinfusion, suture material, and specialized instruments.

Twin–Twin Transfusion Syndrome

Twin–twin transfusion syndrome appears to result from a net unbalanced flow of blood between two fetuses. In the classic placenta model, an artery from one twin supplies a placental cotyledon, which in turn is drained by a vein to the co-twin.[63] Thus blood is shunted from one twin, the donor, and transfused to the co-twin, the recipient, through placental vascular anastomoses. Monochorionic placentas usually exhibit various degrees of shared fetal circulation.[64] Injection studies of twin placentas[65] have shown that these anastomoses are almost universally present in monochorionic placentas but are rare in dichorionic placentas. In the case of monochorionic placentas the anastomoses commonly take the form of arterioarterial anastomoses, but sometimes venous anastomoses are found.[63] The anastomoses can be superficial, deep, or both superficial and deep. The most common superficial types are artery-to-artery (28%) in conjunction with artery-to-vein (28%) anastomoses,[63] followed by arteriovenous anastomoses (11%). An average of 3.1 anastomoses per placenta are present in each twin pair.

Despite the high frequency of vascular anastomoses in monochorionic placentation, twin–twin transfusion syndrome occurs in only 5.5–17.5%[65-70] of monochorionic gestations. It is important to point out that this variation may be related to the criteria used to diagnose the syndrome.

Standard diagnostic criteria for chronic twin–twin transfusion syndrome at birth are an intertwin hemoglobin difference of > 5 g/dl[71] and a birth weight difference of > 20%.[66] However, these neonatal criteria have been challenged. In a large neonatal series of 178 twin pairs, only four pairs had a hemoglobin difference of > 5 g/dl and a weight difference of > 20%; and none of these pregnancies showed evidence of polyhydramnios or oligohydramnios.[72] Antenatally, an inter-twin hemoglobin concentration difference of > 0.5 g/dl was found by Fisk et al. in only one of three twin pairs sampled.[73] Saunders et al. found a mean difference of only 1.7 g/dl in four twin pairs.[74] Therefore the standard criteria used in clinical obstetrics do not permit a definitive diagnosis of twin–twin transfusion. Sonographic criteria for the syndrome include a discrepancy of more than 10 mm of either the biparietal diameter or the transverse diameter of the trunk between the twins and hydramnios surrounding the larger twin.[75] In addition, the presence of same sex, disparity in the size or number of vessels in the umbilical cords, a single placenta with different echogenicity of the cotyledons supplying the two cords, and evidence of hydrops in either twin or congestive heart failure in the recipient have been suggested.[69] In the extreme presentation, there is polyhydramnios in the sac of one twin and severe oligohydramnios in the sac of the other (stuck twin syndrome). Doppler studies have been equivocal about the prenatal diagnosis of twin–twin transfusion syndrome.[70,76–79] Finally, infusion of pancuronium bromide into one cord to produce paralysis of the other fetus (pancuronium test) to demonstrate transplacental communications has also been suggested as a diagnostic criterion.[80] However, as some form of communication is virtually universally present, this finding per se does not establish the diagnosis.

Expectant or medical management of twin–twin transfusion syndrome has been associated with virtually 100% perinatal mortality.[81] Treatment with digitalis or indomethacin has been attempted with little success.[82,83] Given these poor results, invasive treatment options have been proposed, including serial amniocentesis,[84,85] coagulation of surface placental vessels,[30,32,33] selective feticide,[86] or selective fetectomy.[87] Serial amniocentesis in the sac of the recipient twin (polyhydramnios) frequently results in expansion of the sac of the twin with oligohydramnios, presumably through improved circulation to the stuck twin and increased urine production. This management alternative has been associated with an overall 50–60% survival rate.[88] However, despite initial enthusiasm, support for this approach has dwindled somewhat. Additional risks reported with this technique include infection, rupture of membranes, and abruptio placenta presumably due to rapid removal of large amounts of amniotic fluid. In addition, death of one of the twins has been associated with significant morbidity of the surviving twin, including the appearance of porencephalic cysts and other major neurologic complications.[89–92] Originally, these complications were thought to result from the release of thromboplastic substances from the dead twin into the surviving twin. More recently, however, acute anemia has been documented in the surviving twin, suggesting that perhaps hypotension from acute bleeding into the dead twin may be responsible for the observed complications.[93,94]

Laser photocoagulation of surface placental vessels thought to be implicated in the syndrome has been advocated by several authors.[29,33,34,95] With this technique, an endoscope is inserted in the amniotic cavity and aimed at the surface of the placenta. The purported culprit vessels are photocoagulated using a YAG laser via a fiber passed through the operating channel of the endoscope. As arteries cross over veins on the surface of the placenta, the nature of the vessels can be determined endoscopically.[30] In addition, vessels identified as crossing from one placental territory to the other underneath the dividing membrane may correspond to the abnormal sharing of a cotyledon.[34] Color Doppler identification of a direct communication between the placental insertion of both umbilical cords may offer additional evidence of the involvement of the selected vessels.[32] A 400- to 600- μm fiber and 30–50 watts may be used for this procedure. The larger the fiber, the more reliable is the photocoagulation, as small fibers have a tendency to perforate the vessel and be associated with bleeding. Outcomes using laser photocoagulation for twin–twin transfusion

Table 33.6. Treatment of twin–twin transfusion

Treatment	No.	Both alive	One alive	None alive
Conservative[a]	106	0	5 (4.7%)	101
Amniocentesis[b]	103	39 (37.8%)	22 (21.4%)	42 (40.8%)
Laser[c]	77	27 (35%)	27 (35%)	23 (29.9%)

Comparison between serial amniocentesis and laser treatment shows a trend toward better outcome (survival of at least one fetus) for the latter modality (chi square = 3.0995; df = 1; p = 0.07; 95% confidence limits 0.92–4.64).
[a]Data from Saunders et al.[74]

syndrome have been slightly better than those reported with serial amniocentesis, with an overall success rate of 52–70% of at least one surviving fetus.[34,96] De Lia et al. has reported treatment of 26 twin pairs, with a survival rate of 52.8% for at least one fetus and approximately 35.0% for both twins.[96] Ville et al. treated 45 twin–twin transfusion cases with a YAG laser and reported at least one survivor in 71% of cases (32 of 45) versus 44% (11 of 25) of a previous series treated with amniodrainage, a statistically significant difference.[33,34] We have had experience with photocoagulation in six cases of twin–twin transfusion syndrome, in many of which there was an anterior placenta.[32] Both fetuses survived in two pregnancies, one survived in another two pregnancies, and both fetuses died in the remaining two pregnancies (overall survival rate was 50% of fetuses, or 66% of pregnancies with at least one living fetus). The composite outcome of these series versus that of amniodrainage is shown in Table 33.6. Laser photocoagulation may also be associated with a reduced likelihood of CNS complications in a surviving twin after the demise of its co-twin.[34,96] As hypotension and acute exacerbated anemia are thought to be responsible for these complications, laser photocoagulation may prevent these untoward hemodynamic changes to be reflected in the surviving twin after the death of the affected twin.

Selective feticide has also been proposed for the management of twin–twin transfusion syndrome when one of the fetuses is deemed nonviable. Because of the presence of placental vascular communications, injection of potassium chloride into the cord of this twin may result in the death of both twins.[97] Cardiac tamponade has been reported successful,[98] but this technique may carry risks similar to those of potassium chloride injection. Umbilical cord ligation, under ultrasound guidance or endoscopically, also has been performed successfully.[99,100] It appears that umbilical cord ligation is probably the best option for selective feticide in this context. It should be considered, however, only if there is reasonable evidence that one of the fetuses will die spontaneously.

Amniotic Band Syndrome

The differential diagnosis of the sonographic identification of echoreflective membranes within the amniotic cavity includes amniotic band syndrome, amniotic sheets or shelves, amniochorion separation, and subchorionic hematomas.[101] Useful differential diagnostic criteria have been proposed to distinguish between all of these conditions.[102–104] The sonographic diagnosis of amniotic band syndrome is suggested by the presence of eccentric encephaloceles, cleft lip/palate, abdominal or thoracic wall defects, or amputation of extremities in addition to restriction of fetal movement or evidence of membrane attachment to the fetus.

The etiology of the amniotic band syndrome is not well understood. Streeter[105] suggested that amniotic bands are secondary to an in utero insult, which is also responsible for the fetal anomalies. This theory is supported by the finding of concomitant anomalies of internal organs that cannot be explained by amniotic constrictions.[106–108] On the other hand, Torpin argued that rupture of the amnion early in pregnancy could be associated with limb amputations and other characteristic birth defects; this theory was based on placental pathologic analyses.[109] A third theory suggests that the disorder may be of genetic origin, as occurs with a strain of mice in which the presence of a disorganization gene has been proposed.[110] A familial occurrence of amniotic band syndrome has also been reported.[111]

Some fetuses sonographically diagnosed as having amniotic band syndrome show signs of venous stasis and edema of an extremity without evidence of amputation. It is thought that in such cases endoscopic release of the amniotic bands may be indicated. We have had the opportunity to examine two fetuses thought to have amniotic band syndrome.[31] Endoscopic visualization of the membranes revealed no signs of entrapment or impending fetal danger in one case, but there was significant limitation of movement of the mouth in a second case. Hydrodissection of the membranes in the latter case demonstrated webbing of membranes into the fetal mouth. In addition, a tight membrane could be identified arising from the umbilical cord. The first fetus was born without anomalies. The second fetus showed a constriction ring in one of the extremities. In both cases, the addition of fetoscopy helped establish the correct diagnosis.

It is conceivable that selected fetuses affected by amniotic band syndrome may warrant endoscopic release of the bands. Further experience in this area is needed to evaluate the indications and limitations of operative fetoscopy in these cases.

Lower Obstructive Uropathy

Fetal lower urinary tract obstruction is a sporadic condition that affects 1:5000 to 1:8000 males.[112] Untreated, the obstruction may lead to hydronephrosis, renal dysplasia, and perinatal death.[4,113] Prenatally diagnosed cases of posterior urethral valves have 30–50% mortality. Death is attributable to pulmonary hypoplasia, renal dysplasia, or both.

The sonographic diagnosis of fetal lower urinary tract obstruction is suggested by the presence of a dilated, thickened bladder, hydroureters, hydronephrosis, and oligohydramnios.[114] These findings, in the presence of a male fetus, are highly suggestive of posterior urethral valves. However, other etiologies, such as urethral stricture or atresia, urethral agenesis, ureteral reflux, persistent cloaca, and megalourethra, can present with a similar sonographic image.[114,115] Thus the precise diagnosis can be made only after birth.

The management of patients with sonographic findings of lower urinary tract obstruction is outlined in Figure 33.6. A careful ultrasound examination is performed to rule out associated major congenital anomalies. Sonographic evidence of renal cystic dysplasia and the volume of amniotic fluid are also noted, as they have prognostic value (Table 33.7).[116] Serial vesicocenteses are performed to assess the functional status of the fetal kidneys.[117,118] A single vesicocentesis may not adequately reflect the renal reserve, such that two consecutive samples may be on different sides of the normal cutoff level.[119] Table 33.8 shows the fetal urinary cutoff values used to predict a normal versus an abnormal neonatal outcome.

Ultrasound-guided vesicoamniotic shunts have been suggested for the treatment of fetuses with lower urinary tract obstruction (LUTO) since 1982.[12–14] The diversion of fetal urine into the amniotic cavity serves a dual purpose: it prevents the renal damage that may result from the urinary obstruction, and it allows normal pulmonary development. The rationale for this therapy is based on animal studies in which ligation of the ureters[120] or the urethra and urachus[121] of fetal lambs during midgestation produced renal dysplasia and pulmonary hypoplasia. Decompression of the obstruction resulted in resolution of the urinary obstruction and improved pulmonary status at birth.[122] Experience with percutaneous vesicoamniotic shunting in humans, collected at the International Fetal Surgery Registry, shows a 5% procedure-related loss and a 48% survival rate (40 of 83 treated fetuses). Of the treated fetuses, 74% with posterior urethral valves survived, in contrast to a 45% fetal loss rate reported among untreated fetuses with posterior urethral valves.[4] Survivors with total urethral obstruction, as those with urethral atresia or agenesis, are rare.[123]

Figure 33.6. Algorithm used at our center for the management of fetuses with sonographic evidence of lower obstructive uropathy. The value of fetal cystoscopy for diagnosis and possible treatment of these fetuses is presently being evaluated.

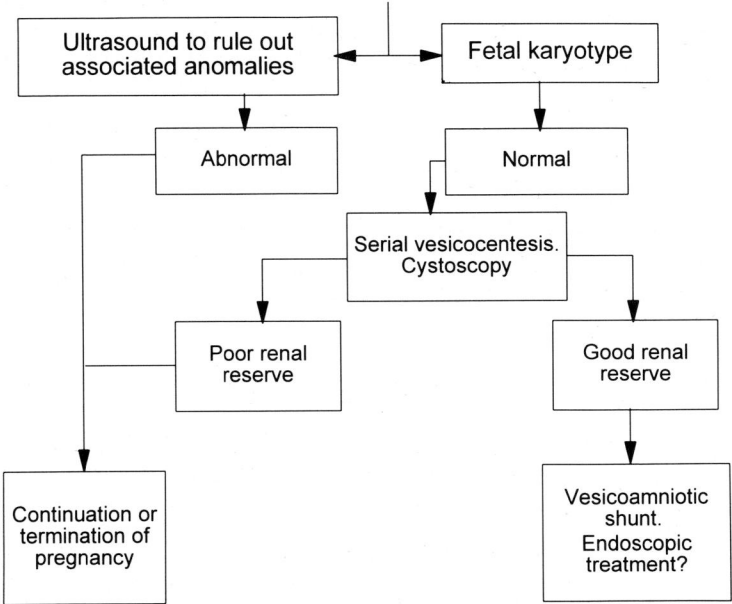

Table 33.7. Prognostic sonographic findings in fetuses with obstructive uropathy

			Predictive value (%)	
Pathology	Sensitivity (%)	Specificity (%)	Positive	Negative
Renal cysts	44	100	100	44
Hyperechogenic renal parenchyma	73	80	89	57
Hydronephrosis	41	73	78	35
Oligohydramnios	35	96	86	69

Modified from ref. 116 and from Muller F, Dommergues M, Mandelbrot L, et al: Fetal urinary biochemistry predicts postnatal renal function in children with bilateral obstructive uropathies. *Obstet Gynecol* 1993;82:813, with permission.

Table 33.8. Biochemical threshold values for predicting the absence of renal dysplasia

			Predictive value (%)	
Biochemical measurement	Sensitivity (%)	Specificity (%)	Positive	Negative
$Na^+ < 100$ mg/dl	56	64	56	88
$Ca^{2+} < 8$ mg/dl	100	27	43	100
Osmolality < 200 mOsm/L	83	82	71	90
β_2-Microglobulin < 4 mg/L	17	36	100	44
Total protein < 20 mg/dl	67	91	80	83

Data from Johnson et al.[119]

Treatment of fetuses with LUTO using urinary diversion procedures has significant limitations. First, they are palliative measures that defer the final treatment of the obstruction until the birth of the child. Second, vesicoamniotic shunts may become obstructed or displaced in up to 25% of cases,[124] requiring additional intervention(s) to replace the shunt, with their attendant complications. Fetal vesicotomy or ureterostomy via open fetal surgery have been proposed[125] to overcome the problems associated with the percutaneous shunts, but they have not gained support.

We have introduced the concept of performing percutaneous fetal cystoscopy to evaluate fetuses with LUTO.[126] This procedure uses the same techniques and skills as fetal vesicocentesis. A thin, flexible endoscope is passed through the lumen of the needle or trocar to observe the fetal bladder at the time of the vesicocentesis (Plate 51). The elements in the trigone can be identified, and the diagnosis of urethral obstruction can be confirmed or ruled out. The endoscope is then removed, and the bladder is drained. Fetal cystoscopy may also be used therapeutically. Indeed, we have performed ablation of posterior urethral valves in a fetus at 24 weeks' gestation.[126] We inserted an operating endoscope toward the posterior urethra and advanced an electrode through the operating channel of the endoscope. The valves were electrocauterized under direct endoscopic visualization (Plates 52–54), and urethral patency was confirmed by instilling physiologic solution into the amniotic cavity transurethrally.

We hypothesize that percutaneous fetal cystoscopy may allow more precise prenatal diagnosis and prognosis in fetuses with LUTO. Because this procedure can be performed at the time of diagnostic vesicocentesis, it should not pose additional risks to the standard assessment of fetal renal function. In addition, those fetuses truly identified as having posterior valves may fare better if the obstruction can be eliminated in utero, avoiding the complications of vesicoamniotic shunts or the morbidity of open fetal surgery. These ideas are currently the subject of intense investigation at our center.

Chorioangioma

Chorioangiomas are the most common placental tumor, occurring in approximately 1% of microscopically examined placentas. The incidence of chorioangioma is higher than previously realized because many small lesions are overlooked on routine examination of the placenta.[127] Chorioangiomas large enough for recognition at delivery occurred approximately once in 13,000 deliveries,[128] and careful sectioning of fixed placentas at 0.5 cm intervals followed by microscopic examinations of all macroscopic lesions detected choriangiomas in 5 of 500 unselected placentas. Chorioangiomas arise from angioblastic tissue. Histologically, they are not considered a true neoplasm but, rather, a hamartoma.

Most tumors are located on the fetal surface of the placenta.[129] A few have been noted at the base of the umbilical cord entirely separated from the placenta, some emerging from the cord.[130,131] The vascular supply to the tumor is established by vessels that come from the umbilical cord vessels[132] or other vessels arising from the placenta. Occasionally a vascular pedicle approaching the tumor has been identified.[128,133–135] The blood supply of these tumors has not been well studied. Chorioangiomas differ in no essential respects from hemangiomas at other bodily sites.[136]

Most of these tumors are asymptomatic,[137] especially if small (< 4 cm in diameter). Larger tumors may be clinically significant and occur in approximately 1:3500 to 1:9000 births.[138,139] The most frequent clinical presentation is the onset of acute polyhydramnios, characterized by a rapid increase of amniotic fluid and marked uterine distention.[140] Common maternal complaints are abdominal pain, nausea, vomiting, and dyspnea in an otherwise normal pregnancy.

Large chorioangiomas have been associated with several fetal complications including polyhydramnios (18–35%), oligohydramnios,[141] nonimmune fetal hydrops,[142] cardiomegaly with or without heart failure, growth retardation, dystocia,[143] premature labor (10%), fetal thrombocytopenia,[144] fetal malformations, microangiopathic hemolytic anemia,[145] and intrauterine fetal death (16%).[146] Maternal complications include thrombocytopenia, coagulopathy,[139] toxemia,[147] abruptio placenta, fetomaternal transfusion, hemolysis, and hemoglobinuria.[148]

Several potential pathophysiologic mechanisms have been proposed to explain the maternal and fetal complications associated with large chorioangiomas. They include excessive transfer of fluid into the amniotic cavity from an increased tumoral vascular area, venous obstruction or functional insufficiency within the placenta, and fetal heart failure. Fetal heart failure may result from poorly oxygenated blood returning to the fetus after circulation through the nonfunctioning placental tissue. Hypoalbuminemia and anemia may also be implicated. Antepartum hemorrhage has been reported in 15–20%[149] of these patients, possibly due to retroplacental bleeding or rupture of the vascular pedicle of the tumor.[150] Intrauterine fetal death may result from congestive heart failure, anemia, or placental bleeding. Neonatal mortality associated with large tumors has been estimated to range between 30% and 40%.[145]

Chorioangiomas can be diagnosed with ultrasonography as uniform and nonuniform echogenic, multicystic masses[150,151] or complex masses.[137] Color Doppler[152] can be used to confirm the vascular nature of the mass. The flow pattern varies with the location of the tumor and the size and number of vascular communications within the tumor. Hirata et al.[153] demonstrated pulsatile blood flow in a placental chorioangioma using color flow imaging and Doppler velocimetry. In addition, pulsed Doppler can help differentiate between maternal and fetal vascular placental abnormalities in utero. α-Fetoprotein has also been used for the early detection of these neoplasms.[154,155]

Management of patients with chorioangiomas should be individualized. Because maternal and fetal complications can lead to premature termination of the pregnancy or to premature birth, serial ultrasound examinations including fetal echocardiography are suggested to determine the optimal time of delivery. Premature labor or acute onset of polyhydramnios may require hospitalization and the use of tocolytic agents.

Most patients diagnosed with chorioangioma have been managed expectantly. A review of the literature shows an overall mortality rate of approximately 30%, half of which deaths are due to intrauterine fetal demise. These figures are undoubtedly biased, as bad outcomes are less likely to be reported. Of the available reports, the most frequent cause of death was prematurity, followed by evidence of fetal heart failure or hydrops. However, since 1986 only 2 of 17 fetuses (11.8%) with chorioangioma have died. Specific risk factors associated with a high risk of fetal or neonatal death have not been identified, particularly as many have been diagnosed retrospectively, and standard parameters of evaluation have not been established. Nonetheless, it is fair to say that fetuses with overt signs of failure diagnosed while still previable constitute the highest risk group and for whom in utero intervention is more clearly indicated.

To date, cordocentesis has been used to manage three patients with chorioangioma. Two fetuses were transfused and delivered within 24 hours for fetal distress.[156] A third case was managed with serial intrauterine transfusions.[153] In this case, a 8.5 cm chorioangioma was diagnosed at 28 weeks. The patient complained of uterine contractions. Ultrasonography showed a fetus with scalp edema and a small pericardial effusion. Color Doppler studies confirmed the vascular nature of the tumor. Serial cordocenteses and intravascular fetal transfusions were performed, increasing the initial hematocrit from 17% to 53%. The scalp edema disappeared. The patient delivered prematurely 25 days later at approximately 32 weeks, and the fetus survived. De Lia et al. suggested that the YAG laser could potentially be used to photocoagulate the vessels that feed such a tumor.[157] We have had a patient with a large chorioangioma (9 cm) and a hydropic fetus at 24 weeks' gestation. Color Doppler disclosed a large artery and vein located subchorionically. Hemodynamic evaluation of the fetus revealed signs of overt heart failure with pulsatile venous blood flow, enlarged right atrium, and tricuspid regurgitation. Cordocentesis revealed moderate fetal anemia and hypoalbuminemia. The vessels feeding the tumor appeared to be too large to be photocoagulated with a Nd:YAG laser. Endoscopically, the artery was dissected from the surface of the placenta, and a suture was placed around this vessel. Remaining vessels were obliterated with bipolar electrocautery. Unfortunately, the fetus did not tolerate the surgery and died 3 days later. Despite the untoward outcome, this case illustrates the possibility of interrupting the blood supply to the chorioangioma and eliminating the shunt through this mass. We speculate that perhaps a combination of intravascular fetal transfusions and endoscopic coagulation or ligation of the feeding vessels may be warranted for severe cases detected prior to fetal viability.

Limitations of Operative Fetoscopy

Table 33.9 provides information on the limitations we have identified while performing operative fetoscopy. The need for better instrumentation cannot be overemphasized. As Semm, a leader in gynecologic laparoscopy, has said: laparoscopic surgery should not be performed with any lesser availability of instruments than open surgery. As no specific instruments are available for operative fetoscopy, this statement is even more relevant and should stress the need to continue to develop the necessary tools for this type of surgery.

Fetal position may be particularly limiting, and techniques to correct it are not available. Occasionally external maneuvers can change the position of the fetus in the uterus, but these measures are neither effective nor reliable. We have attempted to correct fetal position from within the amniotic cavity with limited success. Efforts to address this issue are being pursued.

Table 33.9. Limitations of operative fetoscopy

Placental location
Access
Visualization
Intruments
Fetal position
Premature rupture of membranes

The location of the placenta may also hinder the performance of operative fetoscopy. With open fetal surgery, if the placenta is anterior the uterus is entered posteriorly. Although this technique is significantly more involved, it could be considered for operative fetoscopy as well in selected cases. Although we have been able to avoid entering the placenta in most cases, there has been one instance in which no space free of placenta could be found and in which bleeding from transplacental insertion of the trocars, though not resulting in fetal morbidity, forced us to abandon the procedure.

Some conditions may never become amenable to an endoscopic approach. Such may be the case of cystic adenomatoid malformation of the lung, pulmonary sequestrations, large fetal tumors, or other complex fetal anomalies. These problems should probably continue to be managed by teams with significant expertise in open fetal surgery.

Future of Operative Fetoscopy

A great deal of interest in the management of fetuses with diaphragmatic hernia has been generated. Wilson and others have shown that tracheal ligation in fetal lambs with iatrogenic diaphragmatic hernias reverses the pathophysiologic effects of pulmonary hypoplasia.[158–160] The net accumulation of fluid in the tracheobronchial tree resulted in enhanced lung development. Histologic, molecular, and functional analyses of these lungs demonstrated cell proliferation and lack of arrest of pulmonary development. Using this experience, Harrison et al. have reported three fetuses with diaphragmatic hernias who underwent tracheal obstruction through open fetal surgery (Harrison MR, unpublished data, 1994). One fetus survived and required minimal ventilatory support at birth and intubation for a few weeks after birth due to tracheal instability. The other two fetuses died from postoperative complications. These animal and clinical experiences are encouraging and may completely change our approach to a fetus with a diaphragmatic hernia. If an endoscopic research procedure could be devised to

Table 33.10. Possible future applications of operative fetoscopy

Urinary tract obstruction
Diaphragmatic hernia
Sacrococcygeal teratoma and other fetal tumors
Laryngeal atresia
Aqueductal stenosis
Spina bifida
Gastrointestinal obstruction

obstruct the fetal trachea, it is likely that better results with lesser morbidity would be achieved.

Other conditions for which endoscopic fetal surgery could be potentially used are listed in Table 33.10. Although much research is still needed to understand how these disorders could be addressed endoscopically in utero, it is clear that the list of conditions potentially amenable to in utero surgery is expanding as a result of the lower morbidity associated with this technique. The continued development of operative fetoscopy should make the fetus a true endoscopic surgical patient.

References

1. KERR-WILSON RHJ, DUNCAN A, HUME R, ET AL: Prenatal pleural effusion associated with congenital pulmonary lymphangiectasia. Prenat Diagn 1985;5:73.
2. CARPENTER MW, CURCI MR, DIBBINS AW, ET AL: Perinatal management of ventral wall defects. Obstet Gynecol 1984;64:646.
3. MURAJI T, TWUGAWA C, NISHIJIMA E, ET AL: Gastroschisis: a 17-year experience. J Pediatr Surg 1989;24:343.
4. NAKAYAMA DK, HARRISON MR, DELORIMIER AA: Prognosis of posterior urethral valves present at birth. J Pediatr Surg 1986;21:43.
5. HARRISON MR, ADZICK NS, ESTES JM, ET AL: A prospective study of the outcome for fetuses with diaphragmatic hernia. JAMA 1994;271:382.
6. MOORE TR, GALE S, BENIRSCHKE K: Perinatal outcome of forty-nine pregnancies complicated by acardiac twinning. Am J Obstet Gynecol 1990;163:907.
7. KERENYI TD, MILLER J, STEINFELD L, ET AL: Transplacental cardioversion of intrauterine supraventricular tachycardia with digitalis. Lancet 1980;2:393.
8. DUMESIC DA, SILVERMAN NH, TOBIAS S, ET AL: Transplacental cardioversion of fetal supraventricular tachycardia with procainamide. N Engl J Med 1982;307:1128.
9. BUSSEL JP, BERKOWITZ RL, MCFARLAND JF, ET AL: Antenatal treatment of neonatal alloimmune thrombocytopenia. N Engl J Med 1988;319:1373.
10. GRANNUM PA, COPEL J, PLAXE SC, ET AL: In utero exchange transfusion by direct intravascular injection in severe erythroblastosis fetalis. N Engl J Med 1986;314:1431.
11. RODECK CH, FISK NM, FRASER DI, ET AL: Long-term in utero drainage of fetal hydrothorax. N Engl J Med 1988;319:1135.
12. GOLBUS MS, HARRISON MR, FILLY RA, ET AL: In utero treatment of urinary tract obstruction. Am J Obstet Gynecol 1982;142:383.
13. BERKOWITZ RL, GLICKMANN MG, SMITH GJW, ET AL: Fetal urinary tract obstruction: what is the role of surgical intervention in utero? Am J Obstet Gynecol 1982;144:367.
14. RODECK CH, NICOLAIDES KH: Ultrasound guided invasive procedures in obstetrics. Clin Obstet Gynecol 1983;10:515.
15. NAKAYAMA DK, HARRISON MR, SERON-FERRE M, ET AL: Fetal surgery in the primate. II. Uterine electromyographic response to operative procedures and pharmacologic agents. J Pediatr Surg 1984;19:333.
16. ADAMSON K: Fetal surgery. N Engl J Med 1966;275:204.
17. ASENSIO SH: Surgical treatment of erythroblastosis fetalis. In Diagnosis and Treatment of Fetal Disorders, Adamson K (ed). New York, Springer-Verlag, 1969, p 264.
18. HARRISON MR, GOLBUS MS, FILLY RA, ET AL: Fetal treatment 1982. N Engl J Med 1982;307:1651.
19. HARRISON MR, ADZICK NS, FLAKE AW, ET AL: Correction of congenital diaphragmatic hernia in utero. VI. Hard-earned lessons. J Pediatr Surg 1993;28:1411.
20. HARRISON MR, GOLBUS MS, FILLY RA, ET AL: Fetal hydronephrosis: selection and surgical repair. J Pediatr Surg 1987;22:556.
21. LANGER JC, HARRISON MR, SCHMIDT KG, ET AL: Fetal hydrops and demise from sacrococcygeal teratoma: rationale for fetal surgery. Am J Obstet Gynecol 1989;160:1145.
22. HARRISON MR: Selection for treatment: which defects are correctable. In The Unborn Patient,

Harrison MR, Golbus MS, Filly RA (eds). Philadelphia, W.B. Saunders, 1991, p 159.
23. KRUMMEL TM, LONGAKER MT: Fetal wound healing. In The Unborn Patient, Harrison MR, Golbus MS, Filly RA (eds). Philadelphia, W.B. Saunders, 1991, p 526.
24. WESTIN B: Hysteroscopy in early pregnancy. Lancet 1954;2:872.
25. DAFFOS F, CAPELLA-PAVLOSVKY M, FORESTIER F: Fetal blood sampling during pregnancy with the use of a needle guided by ultrasound: a study of 606 consecutive cases. Am J Obstet Gynecol 1985;153:655.
26. SOUTHERN SURGEONS CLUB: A prospective analysis of 1518 laparoscopic cholecystectomies. N Engl J Med 1991;324:1073.
27. QUINTERO RA, PUDER KS, BARDICEF M, ET AL: Hydrolaparoscopy in the rabbit: a fine model for the development of operative fetoscopy. Am J Obstet Gynecol 1994;171:1139.
28. ESTES JM, SZABO Z, HARRISON MR: Techniques for in utero endoscopic surgery. Surg Endosc 1992;6:215.
29. DE LIA JE, CUKIERSKI MA, LUNDERGAN DK, ET AL: Neodymium:yttrium-aluminum-garnet laser occlusion of rhesus placental vasculature via fetoscopy. Am J Obstet Gynecol 1989;160:485.
30. DE LIA JE, CRUISKSHANK DP, KEYE WR: Fetoscopic neodymium:YAG laser occlusion of placental vessels in severe twin-twin transfusion syndrome. Obstet Gynecol 1990;75:1046.
31. QUINTERO RA, REICH H, PUDER KS, ET AL: Operative fetoscopy: a new frontier in fetal medicine [abstract]. Am J Obstet Gynecol 1994;179:297.
32. QUINTERO RA, GONÇALVES LF, GUEVARA F, ET AL: Color-Doppler guided coagulation of abnormal communicating vessels in twin-twin transfusion [abstract]. Ultrasound Obstet Gynecol 1994;4(suppl 1):93.
33. VILLE Y, HYETT J, HECHER K, ET AL: Management of severe twin-twin transfusion: amniodrainage compared to endoscopic surgery. Ultrasound Obstet Gynecol 1994;4(suppl 1):130.
34. VILLE Y, HYETT J, HECHER K, ET AL: Preliminary experience with endoscopic laser surgery for severe twin-twin transfusion syndrome. N Engl J Med 1995;332:224.
35. LUKS FI, DEPREST JA, VANDENBERGHE K, ET AL: A model for fetal surgery through intrauterine endoscopy. J Pediatr Surg 1994;29:1007.
36. LUKS FI, DEPREST JA, VANDENBERGHE K, ET AL: Fetoscopy-guided fetal endoscopy in a sheep model. J Am Coll Surg 1994;178:609.
37. LUKS FI, DEPREST J, MARCUS M, ET AL: Carbon dioxide pneumoamnios causes acidosis in fetal lamb. Fetal Diagn Ther 1994;9:105.
38. QUINTERO RA, PUDER KS, COTTON DB: Embryoscopy and fetoscopy. Obstet Gynecol Clin North Am 1993;20:563.
39. VANDENBERGHE K: Fetal endoscopic surgery, lessons from animal experiment. Ultrasound Obstet Gynecol 1994;4(suppl 1):129.
40. MIYAZAKI FS, NEVAREZ F: Saline amnioinfusion for relief of repetitive variable decelerations: a prospective randomized study. Am J Obstet Gynecol 1985;153:301.
41. WENSTROM KD, PARSONS MT: The prevention of meconium in labor using amnioinfusion. Obstet Gynecol 1989;73:647.
42. QUETEL TA, MEJIDES AA, SALMAN FA, ET AL: Amnioinfusion: an aid in the ultrasonographic evaluation of severe oligohydramnios in pregnancy. Am J Obstet Gynecol 1992;167:333.
43. SHERER DM, MCANDREW JA, LIBERTO L, ET AL: Recurring bilateral renal agenesis diagnosed by ultrasound with the aid of amnioinfusion at 18 weeks' gestation. Am J Perinatol 1992;9:49.
44. FISK NM, GIUSSANI DA, PARKES MJ, ET AL: Amnioinfusion increases amniotic pressure in pregnant sheep but does not alter fetal acid-base status. Am J Obstet Gynecol 1991;165:1459.
45. HOBBINS JC, MAHONEY MJ: Clinical experience with fetoscopy and fetal blood sampling. In Intrauterine Fetal Visualization, a Multidisciplinary Approach, Kaback MM, Valenti (eds). Amsterdam, Excerpta Medica, 1976, pp 164–170.
46. RODECK CH: Fetoscopy guided by real-time ultrasound for pure fetal blood samples, fetal skin samples, and examination of the fetus in utero. Br J Obstet Gynaecol 1980;87:449.
47. NICHD NATIONAL REGISTRY FOR AMNIOCENTESIS STUDY GROUP: Midtrimester amniocentesis for prenatal diagnosis: safety and accuracy. JAMA 1976;236:1471.
48. SANCHEZ DEL CAMPO F, PUCHADES A, PANCHON A, ET AL: Action of laser light on the ocular development of chick embryos. Anatomisch Anzeiger 1989;169:253.
49. AIGE-GIL V, MURILLO-FERROL N: Effects of white light on the pineal gland of the chick embryo. Histol Histopathol 1992;7:1.
50. QUINTERO RA, CROSSLAND WJ, COTTON DB: Effect of endoscopic white light on the developing visual pathway: a histologic, histochemical, and behavioral study. Am J Obstet Gynecol 1994;171:1142.

51. JAMES WH: A note on the epidemiology of acardiac monsters. Teratology 1977;16:211.
52. VAN ALLEN MI, SMITH DW, SHEPARD TH: Twin reversed arterial perfusion (TRAP) sequence: a study of 14 twin pregnancies with acardius. Semin Perinatol 1983;7:285.
53. PLATT LD, DEVORE GR, BIENIARZ A, ET AL: Antenatal diagnosis of acephalus acardia: a proposed management scheme. Am J Obstet Gynecol 1983;146:857.
54. ROBIE GF, PAYNE GG, MORGAN MA: Selective delivery of an acardiac, acephalic twin. N Engl J Med 1989;320:512.
55. FRIES MH, GOLDBERG JD, GOLBUS MS: Treatment of acardiac-acephalus twin gestations by hysterotomy and selective delivery. Obstet Gynecol 1992;79:601.
56. GINGSBERG NA, APPLEBAUM M, RABIN SA, ET AL: Term birth after midtrimester hysterotomy and selective delivery of an acardiac twin. Am J Obstet Gynecol 1992;167:33.
57. HAMADA H, OKANE M, KORESAWA M, ET AL: Fetal therapy in utero by blockage of the umbilical blood flow of acardiac monster in twin pregnancy. Nippon Sanka Fujinka Gakkai Zasshi 1989;41:1803.
58. ROBERTS RM, SHAH DM, JEANTY P, ET AL: Twin, acardiac, ultrasound-guided embolization. Fetus 1991;1:5.
59. PORRECO RP, BARTON SM, HAVERKAMP AD: Occlusion of umbilical artery in acardiac, acephalic twin. Lancet 1991;337:326.
60. GRAB D, SCHNEIDER V, KECKSTEIN J, ET AL: Twin, acardiac, outcome. Fetus 1992;2:11.
61. QUINTERO RA, REICH H, PUDER KS, ET AL: Brief report: umbilical-cord ligation of an acardiac twin by fetoscopy at 19 weeks of gestation. N Engl J Med 1994;330:469.
62. CLARKE HC: Laparoscopy: new instruments for suturing and ligation. Fertil Steril 1972;23:274.
63. BENIRSCHKE K, DRISCOLL SG: The Pathology of the Human Placenta. New York, Springer-Verlag, 1967.
64. BENIRSCHKE K: Multiple gestation: incidence, etiology and inheritance. In Maternal-Fetal Medicine, Creasy RK, Resnik P (eds): Philadelphia, W.B. Saunders, 1984, p 511.
65. ROBERTSON EG, NEER KJ: Placental injection studies in twin gestation. Am J Obstet Gynecol 1983;147:170.
66. TAN KL, TAN R, TAN AM: The twin transfusion syndrome. Clin Pediatr 1979;18:111.
67. KLEBE J, INGOMAR C: The fetoplacental circulation during parturition illustrated by the interfetal transfusion syndrome. Pediatrics 1972; 49:112.
68. BENIRSCHKE K: Twin placenta in perimortality. NY State J Med 1961;61:1499.
69. BRENNAN JN, DIWAN RV, ROSEN MG, ET AL: Fetofetal transfusion syndrome: prenatal ultrasonographic diagnosis. Radiology 1982;143:535.
70. FARMAKIDES G, SCHULMAN H, SALDANA LR, ET AL: Surveillance of twin pregnancy with umbilical arterial velocimetry. Am J Obstet Gynecol 1985;153:789.
71. RAUSEN AR, SEKI M, STRAUSS L: Twin transfusion syndrome. J Pediatr 1965;66:613.
72. DANSKIN FH, NEILSON JP: Twin-to-twin transfusion syndrome: what are appropriate diagnostic criteria? Am J Obstet Gynecol 1989; 161:365.
73. FISK NM, BORRELL A, HUBINONT C, ET AL: Fetofetal transfusion syndrome: do the neonatal criteria apply in utero? Arch Dis Child 1990; 65:657.
74. SAUNDERS NJ, SNIJDERS RJM, NICOLAIDES KH: Twin-twin transfusion syndrome during the 2nd trimester is associated with small intertwin hemoglobin differences. Fetal Dagn Ther 1991; 6:34.
75. WITTMAN BK, BALDWIN VJ, NICHOL B: Antenatal diagnosis of twin transfusion syndrome by ultrasound. Obstet Gynecol 1981;58:123.
76. PRETORIUS DH, MANCHESTER D, BARKIN S, ET AL: Doppler ultrasound of twin transfusion syndrome at 18 weeks of gestation. J Clin Ultrasound 1983; 11:442.
77. GILES WB, TRUDINGER BJ, COOK CM, ET AL: Doppler umbilical artery studies in the twin-twin transfusion syndrome. Obstet Gynecol 1990; 76:1097.
78. ISHIMATSU J, YOSHIMURA O, MANABE A, ET AL: Ultrasonography and Doppler studies in twin-to-twin transfusion syndrome. Asia Oceania J Obstet Gynaecol 1992;18:325.
79. YAMADA A, KASUGAI M, OHNO Y, ET AL: Antenatal diagnosis of twin-twin transfusion syndrome by Doppler ultrasound. Obstet Gynecol 1991; 78:1058.
80. TANAKA M, NATORI M, ISHIMOTO H, ET AL: Intravascular pancuronium bromide infusion for prenatal diagnosis of twin-twin transfusion syndrome. Fetal Ther 1992;7:36.
81. WEIR PE, RATTEN GJ, BEISCHNER NA: Acute polyhydramnios: a complication of monozygous twin pregnancy. Br J Obstet Gynaecol 1979; 86:849.

82. DE LIA JE, EMERY MG, SHEAFOR SA, ET AL: Twin transfusion syndrome: successful in utero treatment with digoxin. Int J Gynaecol Obstet 1985; 23:197.
83. JONES JM, SBARRA AJ, DILILLO L, ET AL: Indomethacin in severe twin-to-twin transfusion syndrome. Am J Perinatol 1993;10:24.
84. MONTAN S, JORGENSEN C, SJOBERG N: Amniocentesis in treatment of acute polyhydramnios in twin pregnancies. Acta Obstet Gynecol Scand 1985;64:537.
85. ELLIOT JP, URIG MA, CLEWELL WH: Aggressive therapeutic amniocentesis for treatment of twin-twin transfusion syndrome. Obstet Gynecol 1991;77:537.
86. CHITKARA U, BERKOWITZ RL, WILKINS IA, ET AL: Selective second-trimester termination of the anomalous fetus in twin pregnancies. Obstet Gynecol 1989;73:690.
87. URIG MA, SIMPSON GF, ELLIOT JP, CLEWELL WA: Twin-twin transfusion syndrome: the surgical removal of one twin as a treatment option. Fetal Ther 1988;3:185.
88. URIG MA, CLEVELL WH, ELLIOT JP: Twin-twin transfusion syndrome. Am J Obstet Gynecol 1990;163:1522.
89. BEJAR R, VIGLIOCCO G, GRAMAJO H, ET AL: Antenatal origin of neurologic damage in newborn infants. Part II. Multiple gestations. Am J Obstet Gynecol 1990;162:1230.
90. MELNICK M: Brain damage in survivor after in utero death in monozygous co-twin. Lancet 1977;2:128.
91. SCHINZEL AA, SMITH DW, MILLER JR: Monozygotic twinning and structural defects. J Pediatr 1979;95:921.
92. YOSHIOKA H, KADOMOTO Y, MINO M, ET AL: Multicystic encephalomalacia in liveborn twin with a still-born macerated co-twin. J Pediatr 1979; 95:798.
93. DUDLEY DKL, D'ALTON ME: Single fetal death in twin gestation. Semin Perinatol 1986;10:65.
94. OKAMURA K, MUROTSUKI J, TANIGAWARA S, ET AL: Funipuncture for evaluation of hematologic and coagulation indices in the surviving twin following co-twin's death. Obstet Gynecol 1994;83:975.
95. DE LIA JE, KUHLMAN R, HARSTAD T, ET AL: Twin-twin transfusion syndrome treated by fetoscopic neodymium:YAG laser occlusion of chorioangiopagus [abstract]. Am J Obstet Gynecol 1993; 168:308.
96. DE LIA JE, KUHLMANN RS, HARSTAD TW, ET AL: Fetoscopic laser ablation of placental vessels in severe previable twin-twin transfusion syndrome. Am J Obstet Gynecol 1995;72:1202.
97. EVANS MI, GOLDBERG JD, DOMMERGUES M, ET AL: Efficacy of second-trimester selective termination for fetal abnormalities: international collaborative experience among the world's largest centers. Am J Obstet Gynecol 1994;171:90.
98. WITTMAN BK, FARQUHARSON DF, THOMAS WDS, ET AL: The role of feticide in the management of severe twin transfusion syndrome. Am J Obstet Gynecol 1986;155:1023.
99. QUINTERO RA, GONÇALVES L, BERRY S, ET AL: Endoscopic and ultrasound-guided umbilical cord ligation in abnormal monochorionic twin gestations [abstract]. Ultrasound Obstet Gynecol 1994;4(suppl 1):93.
100. LEMERY DJ, VANLIEFERINGHEN P, GASQ M, ET AL.: Fetal umbilical cord ligation under ultrasound guidance. Ultrasound Obstet Gynecol 1994; 4:399.
101. ABUHAMAD A, ROMERO R, SCHAFFER WK: The value of Doppler flow analysis in the prenatal diagnosis of amniotic sheets. J Ultrasound Med 1992;11:623.
102. MAHONY BS, FILLY RA, CALLEN PW, ET AL: The amniotic band syndrome: antenatal sonographic diagnosis and potential pitfalls. Am J Obstet Gynecol 1985;152:63.
103. FINBERG HJ: Uterine synechiae in pregnancy: expanded criteria for recognition and clinical significance in 28 cases. J Ultrasound Med 1991; 10:547.
104. RANDEL SB, FILLY RA, CALLEN PW, ET AL: Amniotic sheets. 1. Radiology 1988;166:633.
105. STREETER GL: Focal deficiencies in fetal tissues and their relation to intrauterine amputation. Contrib Embryol Carnegie Inst 1930;22:1.
106. HIGGINBOTTOM MC, JONES K, HALL BD, ET AL: The amniotic band disruption complex: timing of amniotic rupture and variable spectra of consequent defects. J Pediatr 1979;95:544.
107. DONNAI D, WINTER RM: Disorganization: a model for "early amnion rupture"? J Med Genet 1989;26:421.
108. HUNTER AGW, CARPENTER BF: Implications of malformations not due to amniotic bands in the amniotic band sequence. Am J Med Genet 1986;24:691.
109. TORPIN R: Amniochorionic mesoblastic fibrous strings and amniotic bands. Am J Obstet Gynecol 1965;91:65.
110. HUMMEL KP: Developmental anomalies in mice resulting from action of the gene, disorganiza-

110. tion, a semi-dominant lethal. Pediatrics 1959; 23:212.
111. LUBINSKY M, SUJANSKY E, SANGER W, ET AL: Familial amniotic bands. Am J Med Genet 1983; 14:81.
112. REUSS A, WLADIMIROFF JW, NIERMEYER MF: Antenatal diagnosis of renal tract anomalies by ultrasound. Pediatr Nephrol 1987;1:546.
113. HARRISON MR, FILLY RA, PARER JT, ET AL: Management of the fetus with a urinary tract malformation. JAMA 1981;246:635.
114. GRANNUM PA: The genitourinary tract. In Diagnostic Ultrasound of Fetal Anomalies, Nyberg DA, Mahony BS, Pretorius DH (eds). St. Louis, Mosby, 1990, p 453.
115. NOIA G, MASINI L, CARUSO A, ET AL: Prenatal diagnosis of congenital uropathies. Fetal Ther 1989;4:40.
116. MAHONY BS, FILLY RA, CALLEN PW, ET AL: Fetal renal dysplasia: sonographic evaluation. Radiology 1984;152:143.
117. EVANS MI, SACKS AJ, JOHNSON MP, ET AL: Sequential invasive assessment of fetal renal function and the intrauterine treatment of fetal obstructive uropathies. Obstet Gynecol 1991;77:545.
118. NICOLINI U, TANNIRANDORN Y, VAUGHAN J, ET AL: Further predictors of renal dysplasia in fetal obstructive uropathy: Bladder pressure and biochemistry of "fresh" urine. Prenat Diagn 1991;11:159.
119. JOHNSON M, BUKOWSKI T, REITLEMAN C, ET AL: In utero surgical treatment of fetal obstructive uropathy: a new comprehensive approach to identify appropriate candidates for vesicoamniotic shunt therapy. Am J Obstet Gynecol 1994;170:1770.
120. BECK AD: The effect of intrauterine urinary obstruction upon the development of the fetal kidney. J Urol 1971;105:784.
121. HARRISON MR, NAKAYAMA DK, NOALL R, ET AL: Correction of congenital hydronephrosis in utero. II. Decompression reverses the effects of obstruction of the fetal lung and urinary tract. J Pediatr Surg 1982;17:965.
122. NAKAYAMA DK, GLICK PL, VILLA RL, ET AL: Experimental pulmonary hypoplasia due to oligohydramnios and its reversal by relieving thoracic compression. J Pediatr Surg 1983;18:347.
123. STEINHARDT G, HOGAN W, WOD E, ET AL: Long-term survival in an infant with urethral atresia. J Urol 1990;143:336.
124. ELDER JS, DUCKETT JW, SNYDER HM: Intervention for fetal obstructive uropathy: has it been effective? Lancet 1987;2:1007.
125. CROMBLEHOME TM, HARRISON MR, LANGER JC, ET AL: Early experience with open fetal surgery for congenital hydronephrosis. J Pediatr Surg 1988;23:1114.
126. QUINTERO RA, HUME R, SMITH C, ET AL: Percutaneous fetal cystoscopy and endoscopic fulguration of posterior urethral valves. Am J Obstet Gynecol 1995;172:206.
127. SIDDALL RS: Chorioangiofibroma (chorioangioma). Am J Obstet Gynecol 1924;8:554.
128. FOX H: Haemangiomata of the placenta. J Clin Pathol 1966;19:133.
129. CASH JB, POWELL DE: Placental chorioangioma: presentation of a case with electron-microscopic and immunochemical studies. Am J Surg Pathol 1980;4:87.
130. BARRY FE, MCCOY CP, CALLAHAN WP, ET AL: Hemangioma of the umbilical cord. Am J Obstet Gynecol 1951;62:675.
131. BAYLIS MS, JONES RY, HUGHES M: Angiomyxoma of the umbilical cord detected by ultrasound. J Obstet Gynecol 1984;4:243.
132. DAVIES DV: A benign tumour of the placenta. J Obstet Gynaecol Br Emp 1948;55:44.
133. FISHER JH: Chorioangioma of the placenta. Am J Obstet Gynecol 1940;40:439.
134. ELDAR-GEVA T, HOCHNER-CELNIKIER D, ARIEL I, ET AL: Fetal high output cardiac failure and acute hydramnios caused by large placental chorioangioma: case report. Br J Obstet Gynaecol 1988;95:1200.
135. BURROWS S, GAINES JL, HUGHES FJ: Giant chorioangioma. Am J Obstet Gynecol 1973;15:579.
136. REINER L, FRIES E: Chorangioma associated with arteriovenous aneurysm: a study on hamartoma. Am J Obstet Gynecol 1965;93:58.
137. GRUNDY HO, BYER L, WALTON S, ET AL: Antepartum ultrasonographic evaluation and management of placental chorioangioma: a case report. J Reprod Med 1986;31:520.
138. MARCHETTI AA: A consideration of certain types of benign tumors of the placenta. Surg Gynecol Obstet 1939;68:733.
139. LIMAYE NS, TCHABO JG: Asymptomatic thrombocytopenia associated with chorioangioma of placenta. Am J Obstet Gynecol 1989;161:76.
140. PANACCIONE JL, ESPOSITO WJ, HALLER JO: Acute polyhydramnios associated with chorioangioma: a case report. J Reprod Med 1991; 36:210.
141. RESNICK L: Chorioangioma with a report of a case associated with oligohydramnios. S Afr Med J 1953;27:57.

142. TONKIN IL, SETZER S, ERMOCILLA R: Placental chorioangioma: a rare cause of congestive heart failure and hydrops fetalis in the newborn. Am J Roentgenol 1980;134:181.
143. EMGE LA: Dystocia caused by a hemangioma of the placenta. Am J Obstet Gynecol 1927;14:35.
144. FOX H: Pathology of the placenta. In Major Problems in Pathology, Bennington JL (ed). Philadelphia, Saunders, 1978, p 343.
145. BAUER CR, FOJACO RM, BANCALARI E, ET AL: Microangiopathic hemolytic anemia and thrombocytopenia in a neonate associated with a large placental chorioangioma. Pediatrics 1978;62: 574.
146. ASADOURIAN LA, TAYLOR HB: Clinical significance of placental hemangiomas. Obstet Gynecol 1968;31:551.
147. HEGGTVEIT HA, DE CARVALHO R, NUYENS AJ: Chorioangioma and toxemia of pregnancy. Am J Obstet Gynecol 1965;91:291.
148. STILLER AG, SKAFISH PR: Placental chorioangioma: a rare cause of fetomaternal transfusion with maternal hemolysis and fetal distress. Obstet Gynecol 1986;67:;296.
149. O'MALLEY BO, TOI A, DESA DJ, ET AL: Ultrasound appearances of placental chorioangioma. Radiology 1981;138:159.
150. ASOKAN S, CHADALAVADA K, GARDI R, ET AL: Prenatal diagnosis of placental tumor by ultrasound. J Clin Ultrasound 1978;6:180.
151. CARDWELL MS: Antenatal management of a large placental chorioangioma. J Reprod Med 1988;33:68.
152. CHOU MM, HO ESC, HWANG SF, ET AL: Prenatal diagnosis of placental chorioangioma: contribution of color Doppler ultrasound. Ultrasound Obstet Gynecol 1994;4:332.
153. HIRATA GI, MASAKI DI, O'TOOLE M, ET AL: Color flow mapping and Doppler velocimetry in the diagnosis and management of a placental chorioangioma associated with nonimmune fetal hydrops. Obstet Gynecol 1993; 81:850.
154. MANN L, ALROOMI L, MCNAY M, ET AL: Placental haemangioma: case report. Br J Obstet Gynaecol 1983;90:983.
155. SALAFIA CM, SILBERMAN L, HERRERA NE, ET AL: Placental pathology at term associated with elevated midtrimester maternal serum alpha-fetoprotein concentration. Am J Obstet Gynecol 1988;158:1064.
156. HUBINONT C, BERNARD P, KHALIL N, ET AL: Fetal liver hemangioma and chorioangioma: two unusual cases of severe fetal anemia detected by ultrasonography and its perinatal management. Ultrasound Obstet Gynecol 1994;4:330.
157. DE LIA JE, KUHLMANN RS, CRUIKSHANK DP, ET AL: Current topic: placental surgery; a new frontier. Placenta 1993;14:477.
158. WILSON JM, DIFIORE JW, PETERS CA: Experimental fetal tracheal ligation prevents the pulmonary hypoplasia associated with fetal nephrectomy: possible application for congenital diaphragmatic hernia. J Pediatr Surg 1993;28:1433.
159. DIFIORE JW, FAUZA DO, SLAVIN R, ET AL: Experimental fetal tracheal ligation reverses the structural and physiological effects of pulmonary hypoplasia in congenital diaphragmatic hernia. J Pediatr Surg 1994;29:248.
160. HEDRICK MH, ESTES JM, SULLIVAN KM, ET AL: Plug the lung until it grows (PLUG): a new method to treat congenital diaphragmatic hernia in utero. J Pediatr Surg 1994;29:612.

34

Clinical Perspectives: The Year 2000

Patrick J. Taylor

As the year 2000 rapidly approaches, there is much speculation as to what the future holds for the endoscopic surgeon. Let us remember that Winston Churchill was firmly convinced early in World War II that nuclear power would never replace conventional explosives. With that caveat in mind, three questions concerning the future of operative gynecologic endoscopy should be discussed: What have we accomplished to date? What can we accomplish in the future? What are we capable of accomplishing?

it might be more space-saving to list the surgical procedures that *cannot* be performed endoscopically than to enumerate those that can.

It is clear that the answer to the question, What are we capable of achieving?, encompasses virtually all surgical procedures that until recently were accomplished by laparotomy. Now that the technical feasibility of operative endoscopy has been established, it is perhaps time to reflect and consider in some detail the second question.

What Have We Accomplished?

Had the question of our accomplishments been posed even 10 short years ago the answer would have been laparoscopic sterilization, lysis of adhesions, and destruction of mild to moderate endometriosis (revised American Society for Reproductive Medicine classification stages I and II). Hysteroscopic lysis of adhesions, division of a septum, resection of leiomyomas, and endometrial ablation had been described by a few enthusiasts. None of these procedures, however, with the exception of sterilization, were being performed routinely by obstetricians and gynecologists. Just examine the table of contents of this textbook to appreciate the amazingly rapid development of endoscopic techniques; indeed

What Can We Accomplish?

The breath-taking speed with which new procedures have been introduced has left little time for evaluation of their true place in the surgical repertoire. Before any new technique is adopted universally, it should be subjected to a certain degree of evaluation, including assessment of indications, a cost-benefit analysis, enumeration of complications (not only in the hands of experienced surgeons but in the hands of those with limited experience), confirmation of its efficacy, and consideration of possible alternative treatment options. Given the constraints of space, not every operation can be scrutinized in this manner. Hence illustrative examples are presented.

Laparoscopic Myomectomy and Hysteroscopic Resection of Uterine Septa for Infertility or Habitual Abortion

Indications

Prior to the advent of laparoscopic and hysteroscopic myomectomy, it was unclear whether removal of leiomyomas would enhance an individual's fertility. These lesions occur in 20–25% of women over 30 years of age.[1] In a cohort study, Ross and colleagues demonstrated that 89% of women with leiomyomas had delivered at least one infant at term.[2] The relative risk of spontaneous abortion was slightly, but not statistically, increased. Vercellini et al. summarized 13 series of myomectomy performed in women with a chief complaint of infertility.[3] Of 314 women who wished to become pregnant, 172 (55%) were successful. Unfortunately all of these studies used the patient as her own control, so the outcome, had no surgery been performed, was "unknown." It is reasonable to infer that leiomyomas that distort the uterine cavity or the uterine tube(s) can interfere with conception or early pregnancy. Although many leiomyomas are amenable to hysteroscopic resection, there are indeed lesions for which laparoscopic resection is impractical. At first sight, resection of a uterine septum appears to improve the chances of carrying a pregnancy to term in the face of habitual abortions. DeCherney and coworkers reported a 53% term delivery rate following hysteroscopic resection of uterine septa in a series of 72 patients.[4] Daly et al. achieved a 73% term pregnancy rate.[5] Neither of these studies had a control population. In a small study, 20 women who underwent resection of a septum were compared with 17 matched nonsurgical controls; 70% of the treated and 71% of the nontreated women delivered at viability.[6] This study is too small to state with certainty that a type 2 error is not possible—that a difference does exist but has not been detected; nevertheless, it should at least make us wonder about the efficacy of resection of a uterine septum in managing habitual abortion.

Cost-Benefit Analysis

It is recognized that endoscopic surgery can indeed be cost-effective when compared with similar procedures performed via laparotomy. Daly et al. calculated that hysteroscopic excision of a uterine septum was performed at a net savings of $4000 per case.[5] Certainly the recovery period is shorter and return to work more rapid than for those who have undergone a classic metroplasty. These savings become operant only if the indication for the procedure was correct in the first place. At present, although it is believed that the endoscopic approach is performed for the benefit of the patient, without a properly performed prospective randomized study it remains only a belief, not having been substantiated by solid scientific evidence.

Laparoscopic-assisted vaginal hysterectomy (LAVH) is being performed with increasing frequency. There can be little doubt that—with the elimination of disposable instrumentation—it has the potential to be less expensive than abdominal hysterectomy and, like hysteroscopic metroplasty, causes the patient a great deal less discomfort and time away from normal activities. With this technique, a procedure that would have been performed abdominally can be completed vaginally with the patient recovering more rapidly.

Summitt et al. prospectively randomized 56 patients to either vaginal hysterectomy or LAVH; 29 underwent the former operation and 27 the latter.[7] Outcomes of interest included mean length of operating time, complications, amount of pain medication required, and cost. The incidence of febrile morbidity was similar in the two groups. The mean operating time for vaginal hysterectomy was 64.7 minutes compared with 120.1 minutes for LAVH. Significantly more analgesia was required by the LAVH group. The difference in cost was dramatic. Whereas a vaginal hysterectomy cost $4891, an LAVH cost $7905.

Clearly, similar comparisons must be made between those patients who would have required an abdominal hysterectomy but were able to undergo the procedure vaginally because of the assistance of the laparoscopically performed segment of the procedure. Subtotal laparoscopic hysterectomy may prove to be superior to both LAVH and vaginal hysterectomy.

Complications

No surgical procedure is without risk. Before embracing a new technology it is imperative that an idea of the magnitude of these risks be understood. Because, fortunately, the risks are small, large numbers of patients are required to determine the frequency with which complications occur. Data are available with respect to both hysteroscopic and laparoscopic procedures.

The Royal College of Obstetricians (United Kingdom) has collected data from 147 centers performing hysteroscopic endometrial ablation; information was available from 6850 cases.[8] Major complications occurred in 2.5% and were accounted for as follows: uterine perforation 1.25%, fluid overload 0.4%, infection 0.4%, bleeding 0.2%, and organ injury 0.1%. It seems that purely from the perspective of risk endometrial ablation is a relatively safe procedure. Regrettably, such information simply is not available for other hysteroscopic operations.

Querleu et al. have conducted a multicenter study of operative and diagnostic laparoscopy.[10] In a series of 17,521 cases from seven major centers in France, the following was noted: 8343 were diagnostic and 9178 were operative. There were no deaths in the diagnostic group and one in the operative group (following vascular injury with a trocar). Procedures included in the operative group were lysis of adhesions, conservative surgery for ectopic pregnancy, salpingectomy, distal tuboplasty, ovarian cystectomy, conservative surgery for pelvic inflammatory disease, removal of endometriosis, and uterine suspension. There were 48 major complications, for a rate of 5.23/1000. These data are valuable. Similar information with respect to such procedures as LAVH, myomectomy, and lymphadenectomy is forthcoming.

Efficacy

If a surgical procedure is clearly less effective than the one it is meant to replace, it is difficult to justify its performance. As an example, the satisfactory outcomes following laparoscopic conservative surgery for ectopic pregnancy are well documented. Except under unusual circumstances, it is difficult today—never mind the year 2000—to justify submitting such a patient to a laparotomy.

Endometriosis presents a more puzzling picture. It is clear that a considerable number of women find relief from a primary complaint of pelvic pain after surgical excision of the endometriosis and conservation of their uterus and ovaries. This surgery may be better performed laparoscopically, although from the perspective of efficacy formal comparisons between laparotomy and laparoscopy are required.[11]

It remains controversial as to whether surgical treatment of patients with endometriosis (Revised American Society for Reproductive Medicine[12] stages 1 and 2) can improve their pregnancy rate. A well designed study of treatment-dependent and treatment-independent pregnancies in such patients does suggest a beneficial effect.[13] In terms of efficacy, no differences in outcome were noted when the pregnancy rates after laparotomy or laparoscopy were compared.[14] If laparoscopic surgery is to be justified for the management of endometriosis-related infertility, additional studies are required to demonstrate that the pregnancy rate is improved. If it proves to be the case, the justifications must then become cost savings and alleviation of discomfort.

The same study that evaluated the safety of hysteroscopic endometrial ablation also examined efficacy.[8] Of the 6850 women who had been treated for dysfunctional uterine bleeding, 22% had required further surgery within 1 year. More striking was that 9% had, by the time of study, undergone a subsequent hysterectomy, the very operation that ablation was meant to replace.

Questions remain unanswered and indeed will remain unanswered until after the year 2000. Are women who have undergone endometrial ablation prone to develop carcinoma of the endometrium? Will such cancers, if they develop, be occult because they have been unable to herald their presence by producing vaginal bleeding? Should menopausal women who have had an ablation take estrogen alone, or should a progestin be added if they elect to take hormone replacement therapy?

Letterie et al.[1] have carried out in vitro studies of the histologic appearance of tissues underlying the endometrial coagulum. All specimens contained histologically normal-appearing endometrial glands. If such is the case in vivo, at least on a theoretic basis, there is reason why such women should develop occult carcinoma of the endometrium. Certainly, it seems prudent to prescribe an added progestin.

Options

Just as endoscopic surgery will in many cases replace traditional surgical procedures—if only because patients usually suffer considerably less discomfort and disability—any therapeutic option that is equally or more effective, less invasive, carries a lower rate of complications, or is less expensive will replace endoscopic surgical procedures. An example of this concept is the evolving and complementary roles of laparoscopic tubal corrective surgery and assisted reproductive technology (ART).

For the woman with pathologically damaged uterine tubes, only two viable options exist if she wishes to conceive. Because of the work of several national registries, it is possible to state with reasonable confidence the likelihood of success after one or more in vitro fertilization (IVF) cycles. This information can be used and compared with the probable outcome if laparoscopic tubal surgery were to be attempted. The factors that influence the outcome of tubal surgery are the (1) diameter of the distal ampulla, (2) thickness of the tubal wall, (3) number of tubal mucosa folds, (4) extent of adnexal adhesions, and (5) type of adhesions (vascular or avascular). A simple scoring system exists in which these factors are used to predict probable outcome.[16] Clearly, if a woman's chances would be much poorer with tubal surgery, the ART option merits strong consideration.

These same arguments can be advanced when considering the management of ectopic pregnancy. When 100 patients were treated with methotrexate, 96 were considered to have been treated successfully. Only five experienced significant side effects. The tubal patency rate on the affected side was 84%. Of patients who subsequently conceived, 10% suffered a subsequent ectopic pregnancy.[17]

Whether this option or that of direct injection of methotrexate, prostaglandins, or hypertonic saline into the gestational sac under ultrasonographic guidance[18] will replace laparoscopic surgery remains to be seen. Obviously even as laparoscopic techniques are developed, parallel developments, if proved efficacious, may render them obsolete. Such issues lead logically to a discussion of the final question.

What Are We Capable of Accomplishing?

Surgical practice, as we understand it today, will no longer be carried out in the traditional manner. All of medicine is submitted to intense scrutiny, often partisan and at times perhaps ill-informed. Practice patterns can be as much influenced by public pressure as by scientific data. The question of what we will in fact achieve will therefore be answered by a combination of forces that are both intrinsic and extrinsic to the practice of medicine.

The internal force comprises the countervailing pressures of the "Mallory effect" and the "me too" effect, as well as our willingness (or otherwise) to evaluate what we are achieving. When asked why he wanted to climb Mount Everest, Mallory replied, "Because it is there." Undoubtedly, his was the true pioneer spirit, the same spirit that has led laparoscopists to refuse to believe that a hysterectomy could not be performed endoscopically. To them must go great credit; at the same time we must remember that when Mallory set off on his final assault on the summit he was never seen again.

Although the Mallory effect affects those at the cutting edge of any discipline, its corollary, the "me too" effect influences us all. Have we been just a little too ready to embrace the new approaches before the second part of the internal factor equation has been given an opportunity to exert an influence? There is a remarkable paucity of solid information evaluating the new approaches and comparing them with the old. Some excellent starts have been made with the establishment of national registries and a number of small-scale randomized studies.

A number of pressing questions remain to be answered: How effective is endometrial ablation as a treatment for abnormal uterine bleeding? Does it pose any long-term risks that predispose to the development of uterine cancer? Do uterine septa necessarily need to be resected? Are laparoscopic-assisted vaginal hysterectomy and supracervical hysterectomy better options than vaginal hysterectomy? Which leiomyomas should be excised laparoscopically, and is there a role for myolysis? Might future surgical procedures become commonplace? Which of the various energy sources—electrosurgery, laser, or argon beam coagulator—is the most efficacious and cost-effective? Certainly it is possible to perform laparoscopic lymphadenectomy, but is it a diagnostic or therapeutic maneuver? Querleu et al.[19] have reported their results in a study of 39 patients who were submitted to laparoscopic lymphadenectomy. The procedures required approximately 90 minutes to complete. The mean number of nodes removed was 8.7 with a range of 3 to 22. These data contrast with the mean of 40 nodes removed during abdominal lymphadenectomy.[20] A complete radical hysterectomy performed by laparoscopic methods can take up to 9 hours. It may be that in the future such patients will be treated by a combination of laparoscopic node sampling and Schauta radical vaginal hysterectomy.

The question of applying laparoscopic surgery to the pediatric patient must also be addressed. Given the clearly recognized reduction in postoperative discomfort experienced by most patients who have been managed laparoscopically, there can be little doubt that by the year 2000 there will have been considerable advances in the field of pediatric surgery.

Only with properly conducted observational studies of large numbers of patients and with appropriate methodology can prospective randomized clinical studies gain sufficient statistical power to be credible. Therefore the questions to be answered by the profession for the next millennium are as follows: Do we have the will and resources to begin to collect appropriate answers? Will we modify our practices if the answers are not what we wanted to hear?

The external forces are even more difficult to predict. Undoubtedly, there will be more and more technologic developments. The new world of virtual reality is already being explored as a surgical training mode; undoubtedly, it will soon find clinical application. Robotic scalpels can remove tissue more accurately than the human hand. Telecommunications technology already allows remote performance of manipulative procedures in space. Will the surgeon of the future be assisted in a difficult case by an acknowledged expert who is thousands of miles removed from the operating room?

Present methods of suturing and ligating are cumbersome and inefficient. When the rapidity with which instrument manufacturers have produced a seemingly limitless array of new endoscopic instruments is considered, it seems probable that improved equipment will be appearing forthwith.

Perhaps the single most limiting step to the performance of "truly laparoscopic," in contrast to laparoscopy-assisted, surgery is our inability to remove large pieces of tissue from the abdominal cavity without recourse to colpotomy or a significant increase in the size of an abdominal incision. The search for a new method of tissue removal remains the Holy Grail of laparoscopic surgery. It is to be hoped that by the year 2000 the combined ingenuity of surgeons and the instrument industry will have found this elusive prize. To this end, Steiner et al. have described an "electric cutting device"[21]: a cutting cylinder is introduced through a 14 mm cannula and driven by an externally sited electrical microengine. Fibroids up to 5.5 cm in diameter have been removed successfully with this device.

Patients are no longer passive recipients of our ministrations: They expect to be informed and to play their part in defining their management. Public opinion is remarkably easily swayed by the media. There are probably cases today where we are being asked to perform endometrial ablations in totally inappropriate circumstances because someone has been extolling its virtues on a talk show or in the columns of a magazine. LAVH, for example, may be performed more often to preserve a surgeon's practice than because it is a demonstrably better technique than simple vaginal hysterectomy.

To consumer pressure must be added the effect of fiscal constraint, which is always unpredictable. As an example, bone densitometry is undoubtedly the gold standard for assessment of osteoporosis. The equipment is not available in a number of major Canadian cities because the publicly funded health plan cannot afford to purchase the machines. Extrapolating, it is unlikely that highly technologic adjuncts to the performance of endoscopic surgery will be inexpensive and so also will likely not be readily available.

We live in an era of intense regulatory pressure. Surgical devices and drugs cannot be introduced into practice without approval of the Health Protection Branch in Canada and the Food and Drug Administration in the United States. How much longer will those responsible for public health policy permit the apparently random introduction of new surgical procedures without insisting on a rigorous evaluation process?

The final force external to the purview of the surgeon is the unpredictable advances that can occur at any time in other branches of medicine or the basic sciences. It must not be forgotten that any surgical procedure should rightly be regarded as a failure of medical treatment. Although the early promise that the gonadotropin-releasing hormone agonists would provide a "cure" for leiomyomas has not been fulfilled, who can predict when another medical therapy, perhaps one that interferes with the actions of various growth factors, will appear that renders discussion of the surgical management of leiomyomas "redundant"? By extrapolating from present knowledge and trying to identify at least some of those forces that experience teaches may well exert effects of future surgical procedures, an attempt has been made to forecast where we may find ourselves in the year 2000.

Conclusion

We have indulged in a certain amount of speculation, but we can conclude with some concrete hopes that: (1) Gynecologic endoscopic surgery will continue to evolve. (2) The indications will be refined. (3) Surveys and randomized studies will be performed. (4) The influence of factors external to the practice of medicine theoretically will not exert too damaging an influence. (5) If such is the case, it is probable that invalid procedures will become footnotes to medical history and valid procedures will continue to be refined in order to bring to our patients the undoubted benefits of endoscopy, the next giant step in the evolution of gynecologic surgery.

References

1. VOLLENHOVEN BJ, LAWRENCE AS, HEALY DL: Uterine fibroids: a clinical review. Br J Obstet Gynaecol 1990;97:285.
2. ROSS RK, PIKE MC, VESSEY MP, ET AL: Risk factors for uterine fibroids: reduced risk associated with oral contraceptives. BMJ 1986;293:359.
3. VERCELLINI P, BOCCIOLONE L, ROGNONI MT, BOLIS G: Fibroids and infertility. In Advances in Reproductive Endocrinology—Uterine Fibroids: Time for Review, Shaw RW (ed). Parthenon, 1992, pp 47–56.
4. DECHERNEY AH, RUSSELL JB, GIABE RA, ET AL: Resectoscope management of mullerian fusion defects. Fertil Steril 1986;45:726.
5. DALY DC, WALTERS CA, SOTO-ALBORS CE, ET AL: Hysteroscopic metroplasty: surgical technique and obstetrical outcome. Fertil Steril 1983;39:623.
6. COULAM CB: Unexplained recurrent pregnancy loss. Clin Obstet Gynecol 1986;29:999.
7. SUMMITT RL JR, STOVALL TG, LIPSCOMB GH, LING FW: Randomized comparison of laparoscopy-assisted vaginal hysterectomy with standard vaginal hysterectomy in an outpatient setting. Obstet Gynecol 1992;80:895.
8. Royal College of Obstetricians and Gynaecologists of London, 1993.
9. DICKER RC, GREENSPAN JR, STRAUSS LT: Complications of abdominal and vaginal hysterectomy among women of reproductive age in the United States. Am J Obstet Gynecol 1982;144:841.

10. QUERLEU D, CHEVALLIER L, CHAPRON C, BRUHAT MA: Complications of laparoscopic surgery—a French multicentre collaborative study. Gynaecol Endosc 1993;2:3.
11. The Canadian Consensus Conference on Endometriosis. Taylor PJ (ed) J Soc Obstet Gynaecol Can 1993;15:1.
12. American Fertility Society revised classification of endometriosis 1985. Fertil Steril 1985;43:351.
13. TULANDI T, MOUCHAWAR M: Treatment-dependent and treatment-independent pregnancy in women with minimal and mild endometriosis. Fertil Steril 1991;56:790.
14. GRANT NF: Infertility and endometriosis: comparison of outcomes with laparotomy versus laparoscopic techniques. Am J Obstet Gynecol 1992;166:1072.
15. LETTERIE GS, HIBBERT ML, BRITTON BA: Endometrial histology after coagulation using different power settings. Fertil Steril 1993;60:647.
16. GOMEL V: Distal tubal occlusion. Fertil Steril 1988;49:946.
17. STOVALL TG, LING FW, BUSTER JE: Outpatient chemotherapy of unruptured tubal pregnancy. Fertil Steril 1989;51:435.
18. FEICHTINGER W, KEMETER P: Conservative treatment of ectopic pregnancy by transvaginal aspiration under sonographic control and injection of methotrexate. Lancet 1987;1:381.
19. QUERLEU D, LEBLANC E, CASTELAIN B: Laparoscopic pelvic lymphadenectomy in the staging of early carcinoma of the cervix. Am J Obstet Gynecol 1992;167:296.
20. TROPE C, IVERSEN T: Laparoscopic radical hysterectomy: technical gimmick or surgical advance? Gynecol Endosc 1993;2:83.
21. STEINER RA, WRIGHT E, TADIR Y, HALLER U: Electrical cutting device for laparoscopic removal of tissue from the abdominal cavity. Obstet Gynecol 1993;81:471.

Index

Abdominal entry, complications
  during, 381–383
Abdominal steps, in CISH, 138–139
  abdominopelvic inspection,
    134–135
Abdominoscopy, American
  reinvention of laparoscopy as, 5
Abortion
  minor's consent for, 455
  special consent for, to avoid risk of
    malpractice, 452
  spontaneous, and maternal age, in
    vitro fertilization, 287
Abscesses
  diverticular, laparoscopic treatment
    of, 472
  pelvic, pathophysiology of,
    221–222
  tuboovarian
    infertility following, 279
    laparoscopic treatment of,
      215–226
Acardiac twins, 483–485
  in utero treatment of, 476
  animal model, 479
Accreditation, 438
Acephalus, in acardiac twins,
  483–485
Achalasia, esophageal myotomy for,
  464
Achlorhydria, risk of, in medical
  management of reflux disease,
  466
Acoustic tone, for following
  endocoagulator temperature,
  32

Activated partial thromboplastin
  time (APTT), for regulating
  heparin dosage, 244
Adenocarcinoma, of the urinary
  bladder, 229
Adenomyosis
  appearance of, in surgery for
    leiomyomas, 93–94
  and endometrial ablation, 349, 355
  incidence of, laparoscopic-assisted
    hysterectomy study, 124
Adhesiolysis
  during CISH, 135
  during distal tubal reconstructive
    surgery, 184
  effect of, on fertility, 279, 395
  laparoscopy versus laparotomy for,
    401
  objectives in teaching about, 426
Adhesions
  defined, 391
  diagnosed at oophorectomy, 104
  evaluation and treatment of
    during bladder neck suspension,
      146
    during laparoscopic
      myomectomy, 92
  formation of, 391–394
    de novo, 399–400
    after laparoscopic myolysis, 100
  identification during laparoscopic
    myomectomy, 97
  intraabdominal, first endoscopic
    surgery for, 6
  intrauterine, hysteroscopic
    treatment of, 332–338

  lysis of, 391–401
  microscopic, entrapment of
    oocytes by, 54
  after ovarian drilling, followup to
    evaluate, 112
  after ovarian surgery, study using
    rabbits, 53
  pelvic, treatment of, 279
  due to pelvic inflammatory disease,
    215
  periadnexal
    laparoscopic salpingoovariolysis
      for, 279
    studies of surgical treatment,
      55–56
  peritoneal cavity, lysis of in pelvic
    abscess, 222
  peritubal, and fertility, 279
  postoperative
    in laparoscopic myomectomy,
      97, 99
    in laparotomy, 153
  prevention of, 391–401
  techniques for minimizing
    formation of, 43, 398
Adjuvants, to prevent adhesion
  formation, 396
Adnexal abscess, 215
  defined, 216
Adnexal surgery
  in CISH, 135
  new approaches to, 104
  in ovarian torsion, 113–114
  power density needed for, 50
  torsion requiring, during
    pregnancy, 241

Adnexectomy
    at the time of bladder neck suspension, 146
    workshop for teaching techniques, 433
Age
    and fertility, 284–288
    and fertility treatment, 300
    and incidence of endometriosis, 202
    and reversal of sterilization, 281
    and success of in vitro fertilization, 283–284
Agency, shifting and apparent, legal concepts of, 454
Air embolism, with use of coaxial laser fibers for endometrial ablation, 355
Albukasim (Arab physician, tenth century), 4, 257
Alder's sign, for differentiating appendicitis from uterine pain, 249
Alfentanil (Alfenta)
    premedication with, 368
    for total intravenous anesthesia, 369–370
Allen Stirrups, 23f
    for bladder neck suspension, 146
    for distal tubal reconstructive surgery, 184
    for laparoscopic-assisted hysterectomy, 121
    for oophorectomy, 106
    for rectocele and enterocele repair, 149–150
Alligator jaw forceps, 30
Alloimmune thrombocytopenia, treating in utero, 476
American Association of Gynecologic Laparoscopists (AAGL), 11, 253
    founding of, 8
    survey, 1990, 104
American Fertility Society (AFS)
    award for pelviscopic appendectomy, 12
    classification system
        for endometriosis, 202
        for intrauterine adhesions, 336
        scoring of tubal function, 183–184
    demonstration of laparoscopy at convention of, 8
American Society for Reproductive Medicine, 153, 436
    classification of tubal pregnancies, 155
    See also American Fertility Society
American Society of Anesthesiologists, classification of patients, 375

Aminoglycoside, with laparoscopic treatment for pelvic abscess, 220
Ammeter
    of an electrocoagulator, 31, 65
    of an electrosurgical unit, 108
Amniocentesis
    to monitor in vitro fertilization, 295
    serial, in twin-twin syndrome management, 486
Amniotic band syndrome, 487–488
Amniotic cavity, access to, 479–480
Amniotic fluid, pressure regulation in surgery, 482
Ampicillin
    in fever after endometrial ablation, 353
    prior to endometrial ablation, 355
    in rheumatic heart disease, prior to surgery, 244
Ampullary anastomoses, outcome of, 195
Anaphylactic reaction, to viscous dextran insufflation medium, 387
Anastomoses, twin, in monochorionic placentation, 485
Anatomy
    alterations in pregnancy, 244
    basic, didactic and skilled objectives for teaching, operative endoscopy, 425
Anesthesia, 361–376
    for endometrial ablation, 350
    for pediatric laparoscopy, 258
    during pregnancy, 247–248
Aneuploidy, in embryos of women over age 40, 287
Aneurysms, aortic, 474
Anomalies, in the recipient twin, TRAP, 483–485
Anterior compartment, defects of, 143
Antibiotics
    cefazolin, 334
    cefonocid, 355
    cefoperazone, 220
    cefotaxime, 219, 220
    cephalexin, 334
    cephalosporin, 220
    clindamycin, 223, 244
    in distal tubal reconstructive surgery, 185
    prophylactic
        in pediatric laparoscopy, 258
        for selected patients, 388
        in transvaginal oocyte retrieval, 290
    prophylactic broad spectrum, in pregnancy, 244

for treating pelvic inflammatory disease, 215
        vancomycin, 244
    See also Ampicillin; Cefoxitin; Clindamycin; Doxycycline
Antigens, CA-125, 105
    in endometriosis, 204
Antihistamines, premedication with, 368
Antireflux surgery, 466
Aorta, palpation of, operative laparoscopy, 134
Apparent agency, legal definition of, 454
Appendectomy
    endoscopic, 3, 11–12
    laparoscopic, 242, 308–309, 471–472
        history of, 463
        during pregnancy, 246
    teaching about, 427
Appendicitis
    acute, during pregnancy, 249–250
    differentiating from cholecystitis, 241
    pediatric laparoscopy for managing, 259–261
    retrocecal, 261
Appendix
    ruptured
        differentiating from tuboovarian abscess, 217
        laparoscopic pediatric surgery for, 261
Aquadissection, 207, 218f
Aquadissector, 165
    in laparoscopic surgery for pelvic abscess, 223
    in managing an extraluminal tubal pregnancy, 173
    for mobilizing the tuboovarian complex, 168
Aranzi, Guilio Cesare, 4, 257
Archiving, of videotapes and movies, 82–83
Argenteuil Prize, for invention of the portable endoscope, 4
Argon beam coagulator (ABC), 34, 112
Argon laser, 45, 50
    for dividing the uterine septum, 332
    for managing submucous leiomyomas, 327
Arm rest, Hasson-Levine, 23f
Arrhythmias
    with fluothane use, 369
    and vasovagal reflex stimulation, during laparoscopy, 364
    ventricular, during laparoscopy, 363
    See also Cardiac arrhythmias

Index

Arthroscopy, video visualization in, 78
Asherman syndrome, 387
Aspiration
  of ovarian cysts, 110
  pulmonary, during general anesthesia, mortality due to, 248
  suction, 35–36
Assembly, of laparoscopic instruments, 21
Assisted fertilization, 293–295
Assisted hatching, 295
Assisted reproductive technology (ART)
  as a complement to corrective surgery, 502
  defined, 278
  outcomes of use, 283–288
  techniques of, 288–296
  versus tubal surgery, 278–300
Asystole, during laparoscopy, 363
Atracurium (Tracrium), muscle relaxant for laparoscopy, 370–371
Atraumatic grasping instruments, 29–30
  for ovarian drilling, 113
  for salpingoovariolysis, 184
Atrophy, inducing, before endometrial ablation, 339
Atropine, to block vasovagal reflexes, 364, 372
Audio recording
  care exercised in, 74
  interpretation of, 73

Babcock instrument, 273
Babylonian Talmud
  reference to illumination into the human body, 4
  report of endoscopic surgery in, 257
Bacterial vaginosis, 217
Balanced anesthetic technique, 369–370
Barotrauma, during controlled ventilation, 365
Baseball stitch, to close uterine defect, 94, 94f
Beam guide, helium, for Nd:YAG lasers, 321
Behrman, Jan, 12
Belt stitch, for closing the operative defect, laparoscopic myomectomy, 94, 96f
Benzodiazepines, for preoperative anxiolytic therapy, 367–368, 372
Berkson's fallacy, 202

Bias, in assignment of patients to laparotomy or laparoscopy, 398
Biliary-enteric bypass, 470
Biliary surgery, 468–470
Biopsy
  for diagnosis
    of endometriosis, 204
    of mesotheliomas, 464
    of pelvic inflammatory disease, 217
  hysteroscopic, 325
Birth control pills, for treating endometriosis, 204
Bladder. See Urinary bladder
Bladder neck suspension procedure
  laparoscopic, 144–147
  needle, 144
Blanching technique, for Nd:YAG laser endometrial ablation, 339
Bleeding
  intraperitoneal, evaluation with ultrasonography, 405
  isolated, in endoscopy, 383
  in operative hysteroscopy, 342
  uterine, abnormal, 348–357
  See also Hemorrhage
Blood counts, serial, during recovery, 386–387
Blood flow, in chorioangiomas, 491
Blooming effect
  in carbon dioxide laser radiation, 47–48
  reduction of, by use of CO_2 lasers, 48
Blunt trocar laparoscopy, 28
Bovie, William T., 58
Bowel
  injury to, in hysteroscopic surgery, 388
  resection of, for Meckel's diverticulum, 262
Bradyarrhythmia, during laparoscopy, 363–364
Bridges
  between myomas and the pseudo-capsule, 93
  support, for the surgeon's arm, 22–23f
Bryan's sign, for differentiating appendicitis from uterine pain, 249
Bullae, managing, 464
Bulldog grasper, 30f, 90, 93
Bupivacaine (Marcaine), 373
  in endometrial ablation, 350, 355–356
Burch colposuspension procedure, 144
  compartment deficiency following, 142, 148

Butorphanol (Stadol)
  preoperative medication with, 368
  to reverse respiratory depression from fentanyl, 370
Butyrophenones, premedication with, 368

Calibrated uterine resection tool (CURT), 9–10, 130, 131f
Camera
  for CISH, 132
  manipulation of, by the surgeon, 22–23
  See also Video entries
Camera obscura, medical use of, historic, 4, 257
Cancer
  colon, laparoscopic resection in, 472–473
  risk of, with ovulation induction, 298–299
  See also Carcinomas; Malignancy
Cannula
  for laparoscopic myomectomy, 90
  potential transfer of electrical energy to, 66–67
  Semm vacuum, 23
Capacitance coupling
  ctrosurgical laparoscopy, 66–67
  injury due to, 384–385
Capnography, monitoring patients in laparoscopic procedures, 374–375
Carbon dioxide
  for distention in diagnostic endoscopy, 323–324
  for distention in fetal endoscopy, 480
  See also Lasers, carbon dioxide
Carbon dioxide embolism, due to gas-cooled Nd:Yag laser tips, 387
Carbon dioxide-pneu technique, introduction of, 3, 7
Carcinomas
  adenocarcinoma of the urinary bladder, 229
  cervical, incidence of, 130–131
  endometrial
    evaluating with color Doppler ultrasonography, 408
    risk of delayed diagnosis after endometrial ablation, 355
    risk of delayed diagnosis, after endometrial ablation, 388
  squamous cell, of the urinary bladder, 229
  See also Cancer
Cardiac arrhythmias
  with initial insufflation of the abdomen, 384

Cardiac arrhythmias (*continued*)
  during laparoscopy, 363–364
  from vasoconstrictor administration, 388
Cardiac failure, in utero, 483–484
Cardiac tamponade, in twin-twin transfusion syndrome, 487
Cardiopulmonary complications, in operative endoscopy, 425
Cardiorespiratory disease, as a contraindication to laparoscopy, 364
Cardiovascular complications, in operative endoscopy, 383
Cefazolin, in hysteroscopic treatment of intrauterine adhesions, 334
Cefonocid, prior to endometrial ablation, 355
Cefoperazone, with laparoscopic treatment for pelvic abscess, 220
Cefotaxime
  with laparoscopic treatment for pelvic abscess, 220
  for treating pelvic abscess, outcomes, 219
Cefoxitin
  prophylaxis with, in oocyte retrieval, 299
  for treating pelvic abscess, 223
  postoperative administration, 224
Celioscopy, 5, 7
Central fascial defect versus lateral fascial defect, 143
Central nervous system (CNS)
  damage to, by fetal hyperthermia, 483
  toxicity of glycine to, 323
Cephalexin, in hysteroscopic treatment of intrauterine adhesions, 334
Cephalosporin, in laparoscopic treatment for pelvic abscess, 220
Certification, 438
  value of, 443
Cervical pregnancy, 176
Charge-coupled device (CCD), for digital archiving, 72, 75
Chlamydia trachomatis, 182, 216–217
  culture for, during IVF evaluation, 288
2-Chloroprocaine (Nesacaine CE), for epidural block, 373
  in plasma cholinesterase deficiency, 372
Cholangiography
  intraoperative, 468–470
  in pediatric procedures, 264

Cholecystectomy
  laparoscopic, 242, 468–470
  history of, 463
  during pregnancy, 246–247
  reported injuries, New York State, 439
  ultrasonography use with, 409
  pediatric laparoscopic, 262–264
  stapling used in, 37, 478
Cholecystitis
  differentiating from appendicitis, 241
  during pregnancy, 250–252
Cholecystojejunostomy, 470
Cholecystoscope, introduction of, 3
Choledochojejunostomy, 470
Choledochoscope, 469
Cholelithiasis, in pregnancy, 251
Cholesterol, in gallstones, 251
Cholinesterase, plasma, and chloroprocaine epidural block, 372
Chorioangioma, 490–492
Chorionic villus sampling (CVS), to monitor in vitro fertilization, 295
Chromopertubation, objectives in teaching about, 426
Chromosomal abnormalities, in abortuses of women over forty, 287
Cimetidine (Tagamet), premedication with, 368
Cinematography, 78
  for documentation of operative endoscopy, 74
Circulating nurse
  intraoperative responsibilities of, 417, 419
  monitoring insufflation media, 421
  postoperative responsibilities of, 420
  preoperative responsibilities of, 413
CISH. *See* Classic intrafascial SEMM hysterectomy
Clark, William L., 58
Clarke-Reich knot pusher (ligator), 35, 35f, 112, 146, 273–274
Classic intrafascial SEMM hysterectomy (CISH), 4, 14, 128
  principle of, 130–131, 131f
Classification
  of adhesion-reducing adjuvants, 396
  of endometriosis, RAFS scheme, 202
  of intrauterine adhesions, 334, 336
  of ovarian hyperstimulation syndrome, 298
  of tubal pregnancies, 155

  of vaginal prolapse, 150
Cleft lip, fetal repair of, animal experiment, 479
Clindamycin
  for patients with peritonitis, before surgery, 244
  for treating pelvic abscess, 223
Clinical applications, of endoscopic fetal surgery, 483–492
Clinical privileges, 438
Clips, 36–37
Clomiphene citrate
  challenge with, for assessing ovarian reserve, 285
  treatment for polycystic ovarian disease, 112
Coagulation
  bipolar, in ovarian cystectomy, 112
  in hysteroscopic surgery of uterine septa, 329
  of the operative site, laparoscopic myomectomy, 94
  unipolar, injury to the bowel in, 384–385
  of the vascular pedicle, laparoscopic myomectomy, 93
Coagulopathy, risk of, with high viscosity fluids for distention, 323
Coelioscopy, 3
Cohen, Melvin R., 8
Cohen-Eder cannula, 23
Coherence, of laser beams, 44
Colectomy, subtotal, 472
Collaborative Ovarian Cancer Group, fertility drugs and cancer risk, 299
Collimation, of laser beams, 44
Colon
  endometriosis involving, 208–209, 208f
  surgery on, 472–473
Color, of endometriosis, 204
Color filter, of single-chip cameras, 79
Color imaging, Doppler. *See* Doppler ultrasound, color
Colostomy, laparoscopic, 473
Colposuspension, laparoscopic retropubic, 147–149
Colpotomy drainage, in pelvic abscess, outcomes, 219–220
Communication, through informed consent discussions, 445, 447, 452
Competence
  demonstrating, 438
  levels of, 439–440
Complications
  due to anesthetics, spinal and epidural blockades in pregnancy, 247

Index

of assisted reproductive
technology, 296–299
cardiovascular, in endoscopy, 383
with CISH, 139–140
of endometrial ablation, 353–355
in endoscopy, 380–389
fetal, of large chorioangiomas,
490–491
during gasless insufflation, 26
of gynecologic endoscopy, 362t
of hysteroscopic endometrial
ablation, 501
during insufflation with the Veress
needle, 25
intestinal, in operative laparoscopy,
384–385
of laparoscopic-assisted vaginal
hysterectomy, 117, 124–126
of laparoscopic electrosurgery, 58,
60, 70
potential, 66
of laparoscopic myomectomy, 97
of laparoscopic pelvic lymph node
dissection, 238
after laparoscopic treatment for
pelvic abscess, 225
with local anesthesia, 373
maternal, in chorioangiomas, 491
of multifetal pregnancies, 296
of oocyte retrieval, 299
of open fetal surgery, 478–479
of operative hysteroscopy, 342–343
potential, in laparoscopic pelvic
lymph node dissection,
230–231
rate of
for endoscopy during pregnancy, 253
in laparoscopy, 245
for pediatric laparoscopy in
appendicitis, 259
of retropubic colposuspension, 148
of sacropexy, 151
during secondary trocar placement,
385–386
in surgical treatment of
endometriosis, 210–211
teaching about, operative
endoscopy, 425
of transparietoneal abdominal
incisions, hernia, 309
of vasopressin administration,
169–170
Computer-assisted semen analysis
(CASA), 288
Confidentiality, maintaining, 455
Congenital anomalies, in male factor
infertility and unexplained
fertilization failure, 294
Consumer pressure, effect of, on
surgical decisions, 503–504

Continuous energy delivery, laser, 46
in distal tubal reconstructive
surgery, 184
Continuous flow, of liquid in the
uterine cavity, 322–323
Contraindications
to cholangiography and oral
cholecystography during
pregnancy, 251
to CISH, 131
to distal tubal reconstructive
surgery, 183–184
to endometrial ablation, 349
to endoscopy, 246
to laparoscopic myomectomy, 90
to laparoscopic pelvic lymph node
dissection, 230
to laparoscopic salpingotomy, 161
to laparoscopy, in patients with
cardiorespiratory disease, 364
to methylene blue use, 386
to regional anesthetics, 372
to sacrospinous suspension, 151
to salpingotomy, 159
to spinal and epidural blocks, 372
to tubal conservation in ectopic
pregnancy, 160, 176
to vaginal hysterectomy, 116–117
Controlled Distention Irrigation
System (CDIS), 351
Controlled ovarian hyperstimulation
(COH), 287–288, 289
Cook endoscopic curved needle
driver, 34, 34f
Cook miniretractor set, 37
Cooper's ligament, 309
alternative MMK procedure using,
145
Cordocentesis, for managing
chorioangioma, 491
Cornual ectopic pregnancy, 172–173
Cornual-isthmic anastomoses,
outcome of, 195
Corpus luteum, hemorrhagic cyst of
diagnosing, 217
rupture of, 241
Corticosteroids, to decrease respiratory
distress syndrome in preterm
infants, 243
Cost
of CA-125 antigen for identifying
ovarian malignancy, 105
of fertility treatment, 300
of flexible hysteroscopes, 318
of laparoscopic pelvic lymph node
dissection, 238
of laparoscopy versus laparotomy,
for ectopic pregnancy,
163–164
of laser use, 32

of mesh for hernia stuffing repair,
311
of minilaparotomy for tubal
reanastomosis, 195
of operative laparoscopy, 21,
503–504
vaginal hysterectomy, 117, 126
of semidisposable scissors, 31
and simplification, 306
of stapling
during an LAVH, 36–37
in laparoscopic appendectomy,
308
of transvaginal ultrasonography,
106
of treating ectopic pregnancy,
163–164
Cost-benefit analysis, for hysteroscopic excision of uterine
septa, 500–501
Credentials
preliminary, 439
purpose of, 436–437, 438–439
Cryopreservation, of embryos and
oocytes, 291–292
Cul-de-sac
endometriosis in, 203, 208f
Moschcowitz technique for
obliteration of, 146
removal of an ovarian cystic mass
through, 108f, 112
tenderness of, in endometriosis,
204
Culdocentesis, for verifying ureteral
injury, 386
Culdoscopy, 7
Culdotomy, technique for
in laparoscopic-assisted
hysterectomy, 123
in removing products of an ectopic
pregnancy, 167–168
Cultures, bacterial, in pelvic abscess
laparoscopic surgery, 223
Curettage
intrauterine adhesions caused by,
332
suction, to thin endometrium
before endometrial ablation,
349, 355, 356
Current
division of, risk in electrosurgery,
65
and temperature during
electrosurgery, 59
Curved-needle suturing, 274–277
Cushing, Harvey W., 58
Cutting instruments, 31
automatic, learning to use,
433
electrosurgical, 60–61

Cystadenomas
  benign, oophorectomy for, 104
  serous, cystectomy for, 110
Cystectomy, ovarian, 109–112
  workshop for learning techniques for, 433
Cystic adenomatoid malformation of the lung, in utero treatment of, 477
Cystocele, as an anterior compartment defect, 143
Cysts
  dermoid, managing spill of contents during surgery, 110
  epidermoid pediatric, 265–266
  hemorrhagic, diagnosing, 406
  hepatic pediatric, 265–266
  mucinous, 110
  removal of, 108–109, 109f
  See also Ovary, cysts of
Cytal fluid, for uterine distention, 322–323
Cytoscope, 6f

Dacron mesh, preperitoneal patch repair with, 310
Danazol
  for inducing atrophy prior to endometrial ablation, 339, 349
  for treating endometriosis, 204
Database, for locating documentation, 83
Debridement, radical surgical, for treating bacterial peritonitis, 222
Decibels (dB), measure of signal-to-noise ratio, 80–81
Delay, in recognizing complications, 386–387
Desflurane (Suprane), to maintain anesthesia, 369
Desiccation, with electrosurgery, 63–65
Detrusor instability
  differentiation from stress urinary incontinence, 145
  after retropubic colposuspension, 148
Dexamethasone, treatment for polycystic ovarian disease, 112
Dextrose
  in half-normal saline, for uterine distention, 322
  solution of, for uterine distention with electrosurgery, 322–323
Diagnosis
  of an acardiac twin, 483
  accuracy of endoscopic evaluation of abdominal pain, 242
  of adnexal infection or abscess, 217–218
  of appendicitis during pregnancy, 249
  of chorioangiomas, ultrasonography for, 491
  differential
    of abdominal pain, 309
    of appendicitis during pregnancy, 249
    of distal tubal damage, 182–183
    of ectopic pregnancy, 156–159, 161–162
    of endometriosis, 203–204
    of fetal obstructive uropathy, 488
    of Mayer-von Rokitansky-Kuster-Hauser syndrome, 307
    of pelvic inflammatory disease, error rate in, 225
  postoperative pathologic, CISH, 139
  prior to oophorectomy, 104–106
  of tubo-ovarian abscess, before laparoscopic treatment, 220
  of twin-twin syndrome, 485–486
  ultrasound used for, 404–405
Diagnosis Related Groups (DRGs), 453
Diaphragmatic hernia, in utero treatment of, 476, 477, 492
Diazepam (Valium), premedication with, 368
Dictation, as documentation, limitations of, 74
Didactic training, in new techniques, 438
Diethylstilbestrol, and cholecystitis, 250
Digital signal processing (DSP), 85
Dilatation
  balloon, 474
  pyloric balloon, 467
Dilatation and curettage, for diagnosing ectopic pregnancy, 162
Direct video endoscopy, 79
Direct vision, for removal of accessory trocar sleeves, 382–383
Disposable instruments, relative advantages of, 27
Dissecting hook, coagulation using, 33f
Dissection
  blunt, accompanied by electrosurgery, 207
  noncontact, with electrosurgery, 60–61
  sharp, objectives in teaching about, 426
Distal tube, reconstructive surgery, 182–190

Distention
  medium for, in fetal surgery, 480
  postoperative, indication of delayed damage, 386
  See also Uterine distention
Documentation, 72–85
  defined, 73
Donor insemination, age, and success of, 285
Doppler ultrasound, color, 404–409
  for diagnosing chorioangiomas, 491
  for diagnosing ovarian malignancy, 106
  for evaluating acardiac twins, 483
  for evaluating ovarian cysts, 106
  for identifying communication of placental insertions, 486
  See also Ultrasonography
Doxycycline (Vibramycin)
  for fever after endometrial ablation, 334
  in hysteroscopic treatment of intrauterine adhesions, 353
  for irrigating the peritoneal cavity, 220
  prior to endometrial ablation, 355
  for treating pelvic abscess, 223
  postoperative administration, 224
Dragging procedure, for endometrial ablation with a Nd:YAG laser, 339
Drilling, ovarian, 112–113
Droperidol (Inapsine), premedication with, 368
Duell, Charles H., 39–40
Dura mater transplant, for hernia repair, 310
Dynamic recording, 78–82
Dysmenorrhea, and adhesion formation, 394–395

Ectopic pregnancy, 153–177
  chronic, 176–177
  after distal tubal reconstructive surgery, 186
  evaluating
    with color Doppler sonography, 408
    with sonography, 406
  laparoscopy versus laparotomy for treating, 399
  management of, workshop on, 432–433
  after microsurgical salpingoneostomy, 189
  after neosalpingostomy, 401
  objectives in teaching about, 426
  persistent, 172

Index

radical treatment of, 11
rate of
after fimbrioplasty, 280
in gamete intrafallopian transfer, 292
after laparoscopic salpingoovariolysis, 279
after tubal cannulation, 337
risk of, related to pelvic inflammatory disease, 217
after second-look laparoscopy, 400
in tubal embryo transfer, 292
after tubal reanastomosis, 195
laparoscopic, 197
and tubal reconstructive surgery, 282–283
after tuboovarian abscess, 279
and in vitro fertilization, 297–298
Edema, pulmonary and cerebral, from low viscosity fluids for distention, 387
Effectiveness
of laparoscopic surgery for ectopic pregnancy, 501
of negligence liability, 449
Efficiency, of negligence liability, 449
Electrical devices, placement of, on a support cart, 27
Electric generator for instruments, support cart placement of, 27
Electrocoagulation
in appendectomy, 309
in bladder neck suspension surgery, 146
instrumentation for, 31
for laparoscopic partial salpingectomy, 154, 156
for treating endometriosis, 205–206
Electrodes, for use with unipolar energy, 318f
Electrodesiccation, in oophorectomy, 107, 108–109
Electroexcision, monopolar, for treating endometriosis, 207
Electrolytes
in low viscosity fluids for uterine distention, 322
serum, checking in apparent fluid overload, 355, 387
Electronic imaging, 78–79
illumination needed for, 75
Electronic insufflators, 25–26
Electronic trocar system, 28
Electroshield monitoring system, for protection during laparoscopic electrosurgery, 68–70
Electrosurgery, 58–70
bipolar, in pediatric laparoscopic appendectomy, 260

comparison with CO_2 and Nd-YAG lasers, 54–55
for disengaging leiomyomas, 92
for endometrial ablation, 352–353
outcomes of, 340–341
fluids for uterine distention used with, 322–323
objectives in teaching about, 426
for resectoscopic management of uterine septa, 330–332
for treating endometriosis, 205–206
for treating intrauterine adhesions, 334
Electrosurgical instruments
isolation of, to prevent alternate ground site burns, 65
for laparoscopy in ectopic pregnancy, 164
for ovarian drilling, 113
Electrosurgical unit, for laparoscopic myomectomy, 90
Embryo transfer
cryopreserved, success rate, 283
for in vitro fertilization, 290–291
Emergency exception, to informed consent, 445
Empyemas, thoracoscopic drainage of, 464
Encoding, of a video image, 79–80
Endlurane (Ethrane), to maintain anesthesia, 369
Endocamera, invention of, hysteroscopy, 5
Endocoagulation, 11, 31–32
Endocoagulator
introduction of, 8
for laparoscopic myomectomy, 90
support cart placement of, 27
Endoguide, for laser beam delivery, 50
Endo-Judge needle, for incision closure, 39–40
Endoknots, 272
Endoloop, 464
Endoloop suturing, 270–271
Endometrial ablation, 338
as an alternative to hysterectomy, 348–357
low viscosity fluids, without electrolytes, used in, 387
repeating
choice of instruments for, 353
reasons for, 356
Endometrial hyperplasia, as an indication for hysterectomy, 116
Endometrioma
diagnosing, 217, 406
ovarian, 110

Endometriosis, 199–211
ablation of, laser for, 50
adhesion formation in, 182
bowel resection in treatment of, 472
evaluation and treatment of
during bladder neck suspension, 146
during laparoscopic myomectomy, 92
identification during laparoscopic myomectomy, 97
incidence of, laparoscopic-assisted hysterectomy study, 124
as an indication for hysterectomy, 116
objectives in teaching about, 426–427
outcomes of surgery for, 501
Endometrium versus endometriosis, 199, 200t
Endopath TriStar trocar, device for holding cannula in place, 28, 28f
Endopath Uterine Manipulator, 23–24, 24f
Endopelvic fascia, 142
Endoscopes
for fetal surgery, 481
portable, 5f
Endoscopic bag, learning to use, 433
Endoscopic retrograde cholangio-pancreatography (ERCP), 469–470
in pregnancy, 253
Endoscopy
early history, 3
operative, teaching program, 423–441
team for, 412
Endoscopy, First European Congress for, 15
Endotoxin, in *N. gonorrhoea* infection, 217
Endotracheal intubation, and maternal mortality, 247
Energy, laser, modes of delivery, 46–48
Energy sources
and bowel injury, 384–385
for hysteroscopy and resectoscopy, 321
for laparoscopic myomectomy, 90
for laparoscopy, tissue effect models for teaching about, 431
Enflurane (Ethrane)
for anesthesia during pregnancy, 247–248
to maintain anesthesia, 369

Enteric injuries, in operative endoscopy, objectives in teaching about, 425
Enterocele
  laparoscopic repair of, 149–150
    during vaginal vault suspension, 151–152
  as a posterior compartment defect, 143
  repair of, at the time of bladder neck suspension, 146
Enzyme-linked immunosorbent assay (ELISA), for diagnosing ectopic pregnancy, 158
Epidemiology, of endometriosis, 201–202
Epidermoid cysts, pediatric, 265–266
Epidural anesthesia, 371
  lidocaine for, 373
  lumbar, 372
Epigastrium, laparoscopy of, early work, 7
Epinephrine, administration with lidocaine, 373
Epithelium, glandular, in endometriosis, 200f
Equipment
  hospital, maintenance of, 454
  liability in design, manufacture of, maintenance of, 454
  See also Instrumentation
Eschar, from fulguration, 61
Estrogens
  conjugated, in hysteroscopic treatment of intrauterine adhesions, 334
  effect on cholesterol and bile acids, 250
Etiology
  of amniotic band syndrome, 487–488
  of endometriosis, 199
  of ovarian torsion, 113–114
  of tubal damage, 182
Etomidate (Amidate), for inducing anesthesia, outpatient surgery, 369
Evaluation
  follow-up, for maintaining surgical privileges, 441
  of new techniques, 503
  by peer review, 439, 453
  See also Diagnosis
Eversion technique, distal tubal reconstructive surgery, 188
eXcel-DR puncture closure device, 40f
Excision, of endometriosis, 207–209
Expectant management
  of ectopic pregnancy, 162–163
  of twin-twin syndrome, 486

Expectations
  role in liability claims, 451
  unrealistic, limiting to avoid risk of malpractice, 452
Experience, methods of obtaining, 440–441
Experimentation, animal, for developing endoscopic fetal surgery, 479
Expertise, for performing an appendectomy, 308–309
Extracorporeal endosuturing, 271–274
Extraluminal tubal pregnancy, 173
Extraperitoneal laparoscopic hernia repair, 465–466
Extraperitoneal laparoscopic pelvic lymph node dissection, comparison with the intraperitoneal approach, 237t
Extraperitoneal space, creation of, for laparoscopic pelvic lymph node dissection, 234–235

Facility, reviewing for adequacy, to avoid risk of malpractice, 452
Fallopian tube, abnormalities of, 278–279
Familial disorders
  amniotic band syndrome, 488
  endometriosis, 202
Famotidine (Pepcid), premedication with, 368
Femoral hernia, 309
Fentanyl (Sublimaze)
  premedication with, 368
  for total intravenous anesthesia, 369–370
Fertility
  after fimbrioplasty, 280
  after laparoscopic myomectomy, 99
  after treatment for tubo-ovarian abscess or pelvic abscess, 219
Fertility drugs, and risk of ovarian cancer, 299
Fetal heart rate (FHR), monitoring of, after surgery in pregnancy, 248–249
Fetectomy, in twin-twin syndrome, 486
Feticide, in twin-twin syndrome, 486
Fetoscopy, operative, limitations of, 492
Fetus
  assessing, before surgery during pregnancy, 243
  as an endoscopic surgical patient, 476–493
Fever, postoperative, indication of delayed damage, 386
Fiberoptic cables, introduction of, 3
Fiberoptic endoscopes, 481

Fiberoptic lasers, 43, 49
  contact use of, 399
  for distal tubal reconstructive surgery, 184
  for dividing a uterine septum, 332
  effects on tissues, 45
  for endometrial ablation, 338–339
  Hyskon distending fluid used with, 323
  protective measures used with, 342–343
  sculptured fibers, for treating intrauterine adhesions, 334
Fiberoptic light source, 90–91
Fibrin, deposition of, in *Chlamydia* inflection, 217
Fibrinolysis, and adhesion formation, 392
Fibrin trapping, defense against abscess, 221–222
Fibroid uterus, morcellation of, 124
Fibrosis
  laser surgery versus electrosurgery, 52
  promotion of, by removing retropubic fat, 146
Field of view, in laparoscopic electrosurgery, 66, 81–82
Figure-of-eight sutures
  in laparoscopic-assisted hysterectomy, 124
  in retropubic colposuspension, 149
Fimbrial endosalpinx, examination of, in surgery for pelvic abscess, 224
Fimbrial evacuation, in tubal pregnancy, 170
Fimbriectomy, 193
Fimbrioplasty, 185–187, 280
  teaching about, 427
Fistula formation, complication of laparoscopic-assisted hysterectomy, 126
Fitz-Hugh-Curtis perihepatic adhesions, 223
Fleming, Alexander, 3
Fluid overload
  as a complication in endometrial ablation, 354–355
  as a complication of viscous insufflation medium, 387
  from low viscosity fluids, without electrolytes, 387
  reducing the threat of with electrolytes, 322
Fluids, for uterine distention
  high viscosity, 323
  low viscosity, 322–323, 351, 353, 387
Fluothane (Halothane), to maintain anesthesia, 369

Focus, of laser beams, 44
 and power density, 48–49
Fogging, of laparoscopes and
 cameras, 27
Follicle-stimulating hormone (FSH)
 increase in, with age, 284–285
 inverse correlation of, with success
  of in vitro fertilization, 285
Followup, long term, of laparoscopic
 treatment for pelvic abscess,
 220–221
Food and Drug Administration
 recommendation on trocar composition for single-puncture laparoscopy, 67
 regulation of medical equipment
  by, 454
 warning on use of gas-cooled laser
  tips, 383, 387
Foot pedal, for control of bipolar
 and unipolar electrodes, 31
Forceps
 bipolar, testing and backup supply
  of, 418
 mesoovarian, 29f
 multiprong, 30f
 pronged, 90f
 Seitzinger Tripolar cutting, 31
 Vancaille ovarian, 29f
 See also Kleppinger-type forceps
Frame grabbing, electronic, 77–78
Frame rate, 79
Freeze framing, 72, 76, 77–78
Fulguration, with electrosurgery, 61, 63
Future, advances in laparoscopy, 499–504

Galileon system, for focusing a laser
 beam, 49
Gallbladder, extraction of, pediatric
 cholecystectomy, 263
Gamete intrafallopian transfer
 (GIFT), 278, 292
Gangrene, association with acute
 appendicitis, 249–250
Gas embolism
 choice of medium for
  pneumoperitoneum, 362
 indications of, 364–365, 383
 and intraabdominal pressure,
  pneumoperitoneum, 246
Gastrointestinal surgery, 466–473
General anesthesia, 365–371
Generator, support cart placement of,
 27, 419
Genital prolapse, as an indication for
 hysterectomy, 116
Gentamicin, in rheumatic heart disease
 or peritonitis, prior to surgery,
 244

Glucocorticoids
 for patients with endometriosis, 201
 for preventing adhesions, 397
Glycine
 hyperammonemia from
  metabolism of, 387–388
 for uterine distention, 322–323
Goggles, protective, for using lasers,
 50
Gonadotropin-releasing hormone
 (GnRH)
 for inducing atrophy before
  endometrial ablation, 339
 for treating endometriosis, 204
Gonadotropin-releasing hormone
 agonists (GnRH-a)
 effect of, on leiomyosarcomas,
  99–100
 for preoperative therapy
  laparoscopic myomectomy, 91–92, 132
 in vitro fertilization, 288
Gonadotropins, for treating polycystic
 ovarian disease, 112
Gore-Tex, for barrier adhesion
 prevention, 396
Grasping instruments, 29–30
 bulldog grasper, 90, 93
 forceps for hysteroscopy, 316
 traumatic, 29–30
 See also Atraumatic grasping
  instruments
Greis style needle, 39
Grounding, of the patient, in
 monopolar surgery, 325
Guardian, of an incompetent person,
 informed consent by, 446
Guidelines, for informed consent, in
 gynecologic endoscopy,
 446–447

Half-hitch end knot, for completing a
 continuous suture, 95f
Halothane, for anesthesia during
 pregnancy, 247
Handles, of instruments, suitability
 of, 30
Harmonic Scalpel, 27
 for cutting and coagulation, 32–33
 for laparoscopic myomectomy, 90,
  92
 in ovarian cystectomy, 110, 112
Hartmann's pouch, 473
β-Human chorionic gonadotropin
 (β-hCG), for diagnosing
 ectopic pregnancy, 153, 156
Heart rate patterns, fetal, protocols
 to manage during labor, 480
Heat, for hemostasis, with an
 endocoagulator, 31–32

Hematology, changes during
 pregnancy, 242t, 244
Hematoma, after
 laparoscopic-assisted
 hysterectomy, 124
Hemodynamics
 changes in, during laparoscopy,
  364–365
 decompensation in a pump twin,
  in TRAP, 483–484
Hemoperitoneum, evacuation of, in
 ectopic pregnancy
 management, 165–166
Hemophilus influenzae, 217
Hemorrhage
 as a complication of endoscopy,
  388
 control of, in pediatric
  cholecystectomy, 264
 in endometrial ablation, 355
 intraoperative, managing, 383
 laparoscopically induced, open
  repair of, 236
 See also Bleeding
Hemorrhagic cysts, diagnosing, with
 ultrasonography, 406
Hemostasis
 assuring after oophorectomy, 109
 in bladder neck suspension surgery,
  146
 with carbon dioxide lasers, 47–48,
  49–50
 in distal tubal reconstructive
  surgery, 184–185, 187
 with electrosurgical cutting, 61
 in laparoscopic pelvic lymph node
  dissection, 235
 as protection against postoperative
  adhesions, 97
 with staples, 36–37
 in tubal reanastomosis, 193–194
Hemostatic instruments, 31–35
 endocoagulator, 132
Hemostatic techniques, objectives in
 teaching, operative endoscopy,
 425–426
Heparin
 for obese patients, before surgery,
  244
 for preventing adhesion formation,
  397
Hepatic cysts, pediatric, 265–266
Hepatocystic triangle, 263f
Hernia
 incarcerated, 386–387
 incisional, prevention of, 39–40
 laparoscopic surgery for, 465–466
Herniorrhaphy, 309–311
Hernioscopic stuffing repair, 311
Hernioscopy, 310–311

Hesselback triangle, 309
Heterotopic pregnancy, 297–298
High-risk patients, general anesthesia for, 366–367
Histology, sample for, in pelvic abscess laparoscopic surgery, 223
History, 3–16, 257
   of electrocoagulation as laparoscopic treatment of ectopic pregnancy, 156
   of electrosurgery, 58–59
   of hysterectomy, 128–130
   of laparoscopic treatment for pelvic abscess, 220–221
   of laparoscopic treatment of ectopic pregnancy, 154
   of surgical intervention, in pelvic inflammatory disease, 218–219
History, patient
   for diagnosing malignant ovarian tumors, 105
   for evaluating problems during pregnancy, 242–243
Hoarseness, after intubation, 365
Horizontal resolution, 80
Hospital practice, legal issues in, 453–454
Hulka uterine elevator, 23
Human chorionic gonadotropin (hCG)
   β, relating to intrauterine gestational sac appearance, 406
   verification of pregnancy using, after embryo transfer, 291
   monitoring for, after conservative therapy for ectopic pregnancy, 170–171
   in treatment for polycystic ovarian disease, 112
Human immunodeficiency virus (HIV), test for, in pelvic abscess diagnosis, 218
Hutterites, fertility study as a function of age, 284–285
Hydrodistention, of the fallopian tube, 185
Hydrosalpinx, characteristics of, and success of salpingostomy, 280–281, 399
Hydroxyzine (Vistaril), premedication with, 368
Hyperthermia
   as a human teratogen, 483
   malignant, 375
Hypogastrium, laparoscopy of, risk of early procedures, 7
Hypoglycemia, and hypoxia, 365
Hyponatremia, from low viscosity fluids, 38

for hysteroscopy and resectoscopy, 323
for uterine distention, 354
Hypotension, with regional anesthesia, 372
Hypoxia
   and arrhythmias, during laparoscopy, 364
   and hypotension, during laparoscopy, 365
Hyskon
   for preventing adhesions, 396–397
   for uterine distention, 323
Hysterectomy
   abdominal serrated macromorcellator, 120
   for dysfunctional uterine bleeding, 338, 348
   intrafascial pelviscopic, 128–141
   for leiomyomas, 89
   subtotal, 10, 14
      laparoscopic-assisted, American perspective, 116–126
   at the time of bladder neck suspension, 146
   total, for treating endometriosis, 210
   vaginal, 12, 14, 120f
      adoption of technique, 436
Hysterosalpingography (HSG)
   adjunct to operative hysteroscopy, 342
   to assess distal tubal architecture, 182–183, 193
   of a submucous myoma, 327–328f
Hysteroscopic sheath, 317f
Hysteroscopy
   instruments for, 315–318
      flexible, operative, 338
   observation using a monitor during, 82
   operative, 315–343
      complications of, 387
      nursing responsibilities in, 421
   preoperative
      in pelvic abscess, 223
      for uterine assessment, 349
Hysterotomy
   maternal, for open fetal surgery, 477
   for treating symptomatic uterine septa, 328

Ileostomy, 472
Iliococcygeal muscle, 143
Illumination
   for endoscopy, potential hazards of, 3
   for imaging, variables affecting level needed, 75–76
   See also Light; Light source

Image display, in fetoscopy, 481
Image register, 79
Image transmission, during pelviscopy, 15
Imaging
   for documentation, 72
   in endometriosis, failure of, 204
   of gynecologic endoscopic procedures, 72–85
   illumination for, and image size, 76
   See also Doppler ultrasound
Immune system, role in endometriosis, 200
Implantation, and follicle-stimulating hormone levels, IVF, 285–287
Incidence
   of acute surgical emergencies during pregnancy, 241
   of complications, in laparoscopic surgery for endometriosis, 211
   of hysterectomy, and population of women, 116
Incision
   into ovarian capsules, techniques, 110–112, 111f
   into the pseudocapsule of myomas, 92
   objectives in teaching techniques for, 425–426
   secondary puncture site, in myomectomy, 107
Incompetent patients
   informed consent from, 445–446, 447
   treatment protocols for, to avoid risk of malpractice, 452
Indications
   for endometrial ablation, 348–349
   for hysterectomy, 116
   for laparoscopic myomectomy, 90
   for laparoscopic oophorectomy, 104
   for laparoscopic pelvic lymph node dissection, 229–230
   for laparoscopic surgery during pregnancy, 245
   for McCall-type vaginal vault suspension, 151
Indigo carmine dye
   for evaluating tubal patency, 334
   for hydrodistention of the fallopian tube, 185
   for identifying bladder injury during surgery, 121, 146, 386
   for tubal lavage, in pelvic abscess, 224
Indomethacin, to arrest premature labor, 248
Indwelling catheter, during healing of a perforated bladder, 385–386

Index

Infection, as a complication
  in endometrial ablation, 355
  in endoscopy, 388
  in operative hysteroscopy, 342
Inferior epigastric vessels, potential injury to, in trocar insertion, 382
Infertility
  causes of, 278–279
    adhesions, 391, 395
    male factor, 292–295
  risk of, after pelvic inflammatory disease, 217, 225
  as a symptom of endometriosis, 202–203
Inflammatory bowel disease, and risk during trocar insertion, 383
Informed consent
  to avoid risk of malpractice, 452
  ethical and legal requirement, 443–449
  example of a document for, 448–449
Inguinal hernia, 309
  stuffing repair of, 311
Inguinal herniorrhaphy, pediatric, 264–265
Inguinal ring, internal, herniorrhaphy of, 310
Inhibin, decrease in levels of, with age, 285
Institutional Review Board (IRB), role in approving nonstandard treatment, 452, 456
Instrumentation, 21–41
  and adhesion formation, 396
  development of, 8–9
  didactic objectives in teaching, operative endoscopy, 424
  for ectopic pregnancy management, 164–165
  endoscopes, 5f, 481
  hemostatic instruments, 31–35, 132
  hysteroscopic sheath, 317f
  for hysteroscopy and resectoscopy, 315–321
  intraoperative responsibilities for, 418
  laparoscopes, 26, 27
  for laparoscopic myomectomy, 90–91
  for laparotomy or endoscopic surgery, 132–133
  Lift Retractor System (LRS), 26
  mini-instruments, 37
  for operative fetoscopy, 481–482
  for pediatric laparoscopy, 257–259
  photoendoscope, 5, 6f
  preoperative setup of, 412–413
  scissors, 31, 260

shears, coagulating, 33f
sheaths, 27–28, 107
skilled objectives in teaching, operative endoscopy, 424
for training in operative endoscopy, 427–428
Valtchev uterine mobilizer, 23
See also Ammeter; Argon laser; Bulldog grasper; Endocoagulator; Fiberoptic lasers; Grasping instruments; Harmonic Scalpel; Lasers; Myoma screw/drill; Neodymium-yttrium-aluminum garnet lasers; Optic instruments; Potassium titanyl phosphate (KTP-532) laser; Resectoscope
Insufflation
  didactic objectives for teaching, operative endoscopy, 425
  gasless, 26
  instrumentation for, 24–26
  skilled objectives for teaching, operative endoscopy, 425
Insufflator, 27
  high flow, 25, 132
  for laparoscopic myomectomy, 90
  placement of, during laparoscopy, 419
Insulation, of electrosurgical instruments, breakdown of, 66
Insurance, informing carrier in case of error, 453
Interceed (TC-7), barrier adjuvant to prevent adhesion formation, 396
International Federation of Fertility and Sterility (IFFS), 187
International Fetal Surgery Registry, data on percutaneous vesicoamniotic shunting, 488
International standard, for human chorionic gonadotropin assays, 158
Intestinal complications, in operative laparoscopy, 384–385
Intraabdominal pressure, hemodynamic alterations associated with, 364
Intracorporeal suturing, 274–277
Intracytoplasmic sperm injection (ICSI), 293–294
Intrafascial vaginal hysterectomy (IVH), 14, 15f
Intraoperative responsibilities, of the endoscopy team, 417–420
Intraperitoneal laparoscopic pelvic lymph node dissection, comparison with the extraperitoneal approach, 237t

Intrauterine adhesions
  hysterosalpingography for evaluating, 342
  hysteroscopic lysis of, outcomes in series, 337
Intrauterine devices (IUDs), removal of, using hysteroscopy, 341
Intrauterine embryo transfer, 278
Intrauterine insemination (IUI), 287–288
In vitro fertilization (IVF), 278
  as an alternative to tubal reanastomosis, 193
  as an alternative to tubal reconstruction, 183–184, 189, 281
Irrigation, instruments for, 35–36
Irrigator pump, support cart placement of, 27
Isoflurane (Forane)
  for anesthesia during pregnancy, 247
  to maintain anesthesia, 369
Isthmus-isthmus anastomosis, for reversal of sterilization, 281–282

J-Needle, for incision closure, 39–40
Jones procedure, 328

Ketamine hydrochloride (Ketalar), side effects of, 369
Kleihauer-Bethke test, to evaluate fetomaternal bleeding, 244–245
Kleppinger-type forceps, 31
  for coagulating the tube, in an ectopic pregnancy, 168
  in laparoscopic-assisted hysterectomy, 123
  for oophorectomy, 108
Knot pusher, 270
  Clarke-Reich, 112, 146, 273–274
Knot tying
  half-hitch end knot, 95f
  twist technique, 276
Knowledge, maintaining level of, to avoid risk of malpractice, 452

β-Lactam, treatment for salpingitis, outcomes, 219
Laminaria, use in endometrial ablation, 350
Langmuir-Blodgett thin-film technology, 84
Laparoscopes
  resolution and imaging of, 26
  three-dimensional, 27
Laparoscopic hysterectomy (LH), 118f
  defined, 119
  intrafascial, outcomes of, 139–140
  radical, 120f
  supracervical, 119f

Laparoscopic myomectomy, 89–101, 500–502
Laparoscopic pelvic lymph node dissection (LPLND)
  extended, 233–234
  extraperitoneal, 234–235
  for staging urogenital malignancy, 228–239
Laparoscopic retropubic colpo-suspension, 147–149
Laparoscopic salpingectomy, 166–168
  partial, for ectopic pregnancy, 168
Laparoscopic salpingotomy, 168–170
  versus abdominal salpingotomy, 161
Laparoscopic tubal reanastomosis, 192–197
Laparoscopic ultrasonography, 408–409
Laparoscopic uterosacral nerve ablation, teaching about, 427
Laparoscopy
  adjunct to hysteroscopy, 342
  adjunct to intrauterine surgery, 324
  advantages of, for myomectomy, 89
  diagnostic, 309
    objectives in teaching about, 426
    in pelvic inflammatory disease, 217
  and electrosurgery, issues surrounding, 65–70
  during intrauterine septum correction, 387
  versus laparotomy
    for ectopic pregnancy, cost comparison, 164
    for managing ectopic pregnancy, 153, 397–399
  origination of term, 3, 5
  pediatric, 257–268, 503
  during removal of submucous myomas, 328
  in surgery for uterine septa, 329
  for treating pelvic abscess, 220–225
  for treating tubo-ovarian abscess, 221
  during tubal cannulation, 337
Laparoscopic-assisted vaginal hysterectomy (LAVH), 10, 14f, 118f
  cost-benefit analysis, 500
  defining, 117–120
  indications for, 117
  positioning the patient for, 23
  teaching about, 427
Laparothoracoscopy, 5
Laparotomy
  for assessing damage after uterine perforation, 355
  following blood aspiration into a Veress needle, 381–382

versus laparoscopy
  for managing ectopic pregnancy, 153, 397–399
  for managing endometriosis, 501
  for malignancy staging, 406
  maternal, for open fetal surgery, 477
  for tubal reanastomosis, 193–195
  for tubo-ovarian abscess, outcomes of, 219
Laser fibers or tips, Food and Drug Administration warning on gas-cooled, 387
Laser nurse, preoperative responsibilities of, 413–414
Laser photocoagulation, in twin-twin syndrome, 486
Lasers, 43–56
  carbon dioxide, 43
    for adhesiolysis, 279
    conducting beam to the target site, 26
    for distal tubal reconstructive surgery, 184
    gynecological use of, 49
    for vaporization of endometriosis, 206–207
    for dividing an appendix, 261
    drilling with, in polycystic ovarian disease, 112
  evaluation of, for use in gynecologic surgery, 399
  fiberoptic, 321
  hemostasis using, 32
  for laparoscopic salpingostomy, 164–165
  laparoscopy using, comparison of CO_2 and Nd-YAG lasers, 54–55
  objectives in teaching about, 426
  safety considerations in use of, 375
  surgery with
    laparoscopic myomectomy, 92
    versus electrosurgery, 51–55
  See also Argon laser; Fiberoptic lasers; Neodymium-yttrium-aluminum garnet (Nd-YAG) laser; Potassium titanyl phosphate (KTP-532) laser
Lasing medium, 46
Lateral fascial defect versus central fascial defect, 143
Learning, in endoscopic surgery, barriers to, 435
Legal issues
  in operative gynecologic endoscopy, 442–456
  in video documentation, 83–84

Leiomyomas
  evaluating
    with magnetic resonance imaging, 341–342
    with ultrasonography, 406–407
  incidence of, 89, 500–502
  laparoscopic-assisted hysterectomy study, 124
  as an indication for hysterectomy, 116
  preoperative treatment of patients having, 132
  removal of, endoscopic hysterectomy for, 325–328
  submucous, removing at the time of endometrial ablation, 356
  technique for disengaging, 92–94
Leiomyosarcoma, 99–100
Lesions, in endometriosis, depth of, 205–206
Leukocytosis, in appendicitis, 249–250
Leukoplakia, benign, treatment with the endocoagulator, 8
Leuprolide acetate (Lupron), preoperative treatment with
  in endometrial ablation, 339, 349, 355
  in patients with leiomyomas, 132
Leuprolide screening, for assessing ovarian reserve, 285
Levator ani muscle, 142–143
Levator plate, 150
Levine needle holder, 35, 35f
Liability, and informed consent, 447–448, 451
Lidocaine, for epidural block, 373
Lift Retractor System (LRS), 26
Ligation
  of bullae, thoracoscopic approach, 464
  instruments for, 34–35
  triple-loop technique, 11
Ligature
  loop
    in laparoscopic oophorectomy, 104, 107, 107f
    in laparoscopic partial salpingectomy, 168
  models for practicing, 428
Light
  damage to the fetus by, animal experiments, 483
  for recording images, 74–75
  transmission efficiency of, 75–76
Light source
  illuminating power of, 76
  support cart placement of, 27, 132
Local anesthesia, 373–374
Loop electrode, for endometrial ablation, 348, 353

Index

Loop ligature
  in laparoscopic oophorectomy, 104, 107, 107f
  in laparoscopic partial salpingectomy, 168
Lower urinary tract obstruction (LUTO), treatment of, 488
Luken's trap, to collect culture material, in pediatric appendectomy, 261
Luteal support, exogenous, after embryo transfer, 291
Luteinization, premature, preventing with GnRHa, 288
Luteinizing hormone, monitoring, in transfer of frozen embryos, 291–292
Lymph nodes
  packet of, freeing and removing, 233
  pelvic, operative techniques for dissection of, 231–235
Lymphoceles, after extraperitoneal laparoscopic pelvic lymph node dissection, 235

McBurney's point, pain near, in appendicitis during pregnancy, 249
McCall-type suspension, for vaginal vault prolapse, 150, 151
Magnesium sulfate, to arrest premature labor, 248
Magnetic resonance imaging (MRI), for evaluating uterine leiomyomas, 341–342
Maintenance, of laparoscopic instruments, 21–22
Male factor infertility, 292–295
Malignancy
  bile duct obstruction caused by, 470
  as an indication for hysterectomy, 116
  intraabdominal, color Doppler for staging laparoscopically, 409
  pelvic
    diagnosing, 405–406
    screening for, 407
  potential spillage of ovarian cyst in laparoscopic oophorectomy, 105
  urogenital, LPLND for staging, 228–239
  urologic, laparoscopic pelvic lymph node dissection for, 228–239
  See also Cancer; Carcinoma
Malignant hyperthermia, 375
Mallanpadanti test, need for before surgery during pregnancy, 243
Mallory effect, 502

Malpractice, 449–453
Manual of Endoscopy, 24
Marshall-Marchetti-Krantz procedure, 144
Mattress stitch, for closing the operative defect, laparoscopic myomectomy, 94
Mature minor, defined, 455
Mayer-von Rokitansky-Kuster-Hauser syndrome, 307
Meckel's diverticulum, 261–262
  identifying, 259
Meconium aspiration syndrome, protocols to decrease incidence of, 480
Mediastinal tumor, thoracoscopy for assessing, 464
Medical complications, during pregnancy, 241
Medical therapy
  for endometriosis, 204–205
  for pelvic inflammatory disease, 215
  for tubo-ovarian abscess, historic outcomes, 219
Medica Naturalis (Porta), 4
Medication/anesthesia
  2-chloroprocaine, 372, 373
  cimetidine, 368
  clomiphene citrate, 112, 285
  dexamethasone, 112
  enflurane, 247–248
  fentanyl, 368, 369–370
  fluothane, 369
  glucocorticoids, 201, 397
  halothane, 247
  heparin, 244, 397
  hydroxyzine, 368
  β-lactam, 219
  leuprolide acetate, 132, 355
  lidocaine, 373
  magnesium sulfate, 248
  meperidine, 368
  metoclopramide, 368
  midazolam, 368
  mivacurium, 371
  nalbuphine, 368, 370
  naloxone, 247, 370
  nizatidine, 368
  noxythiolin, 220
  ondansetron, 372
  oxybutynin, 148
  ranitidine, 368, 466
  succinylcholine, 370
  sufentanil, 368
  terbutaline, 248
  tetracaine, 373
  tetracycline, 220, 290
  thiopental, 369
  vecuronium, 371

See also Atropine; Benzodiazepines; Bupivacaine; Butorphanol; Gonadotropin-releasing hormone; Methotrexate; Metronidazole; Nonsteroidal antiinflammatory drugs; Omeprazole; Vasopressin
Memoires Gynécologiques (Arnaud), 4
Menstruation, reflux, and the etiology of endometriosis, 199–201
Meperidine (Demerol), premedication with, 368
Mesenteric cysts, pediatric surgery for, 265
Mesh plug, for hernia repair, 311
Mesoovarian forceps, 29f
Mesotheliomas, thoracoscopy for obtaining a biopsy of, 464
Metal clips, in appendectomy, 309
Metaplasia, of embryologically patterned peritoneum, in endometriosis, 201
Methohexital (Brevital), 368–369
Methotrexate
  for treating cervical pregnancy, 176
  for treating ectopic pregnancy, 161–162, 163–164
    interstitial, 173
  for treating persistent trophoblastic tissue, 172
  for treating uncomplicated trophoblastic disease, 170
Methylene blue, contraindication for, to identify urinary tract trauma, 386
Methylprednisolone, treatment with, after oocyte retrieval for in vitro fertilization, 290
Metoclopramide (Reglan)
  for emesis during pregnancy, 248
  in pediatric laparoscopy, 258
  premedication with, 368
Metronidazole
  with laparoscopic treatment for pelvic abscess, 220
  for patients with peritonitis, before surgery, 244
  for treating pelvic abscess, 223
Metroplasty, hysteroscopic, 330f
  outcomes of, 333t
Metzenbaum endoscopic scissors, 260
Microdiathermy needle versus carbon dioxide laser, for adhesiolysis, 279
Microprocessor chip, for videocameras, 79
Microsurgical tubal reversal, outcomes of, 281–282

Midazolam (Versed), premedication with, 368
β-Mimetics, side effects of, and pregnancy, 248
Mini-instruments, 37
Minilaparotomy
　for access to a maternal uterus, 479–480
　for tubal reanastomosis, 195
Minocycline, for irrigating the peritoneal cavity, 220
Minors
　right of informed consent, 446, 455
　treatment protocols for, to avoid risk of malpractice, 452
Mirroring, historic, tenth century, 4
Mivacurium (Mivacron), muscle relaxant for laparoscopy, 371
Modem, transmission of digitized slides using, 84
Monitoring circuits, to prevent burns at the patient return electrode site, 65, 68–70
Monitoring the patient
　considerations in anesthesia, 374–375
　for fluid balance, 387
Monochromaticity, of laser light, 44–45
Monopolar electrosurgery, use in laparoscopy, 70
Monoshutter, use with lasers in laparoscopy, 50
Morbidity
　postoperative, associated with general anesthesia, 366
　in radiotherapy for bladder cancer, in lymphatic metastasis, 229
　reduction in, with laparoscopy, 21
　in a surviving twin, twin-twin syndrome, 486
Morcellation
　with a calibrated uterine resection tool, 138
　instrumentation for, 38
　motorized instrument, 38
　for removing myomas, 96–97
Morphine, premedication with, 368
Mortality rate
　due to anesthetic complications, in pregnancy, 247
　in endoscopy during pregnancy, 253
　in expectant management of twin-twin syndrome, 486
　in laparoscopy, 245
　in nonperforated appendicitis during pregnancy, 250
Moschcowitz technique, 150
　for cul-de-sac obliteration, 146
Multifetal pregnancy reduction, ultrasound-guided, 297

Multiple gestation, in assisted reproductive technology, 296–297
Multipotential subperitoneal cells, 393
Murphy's sign, in cholecystitis, 251
Mycoplasma, evaluation for, in vitro fertilization, 288
Myolysis, 100–101
　teaching about, 427
Myomas
　instrumentation for enucleation of, 32
　paracervical, removal of, 14
　resection of, use of low viscosity fluids, 387
　submucous
　　corkscrew for fixation of, 318
　　hysteroscopic view of, 327f
　　techniques for enucleation and morcellation, 9, 11
　techniques for removing, 96–97
Myoma screw/drill, 38, 38f, 90, 93
Myomectomy
　and endometrial ablation, 349, 356
　hysteroscopic, for abnormal bleeding, 326t
　laparoscopic, 89–101, 500–502
　teaching about, 427

Nalbuphine (Nubain)
　premedication with, 368
　to reverse respiratory depression from fentanyl, 370
Naloxone (Narcan)
　to reverse respiratory depression from fentanyl, 370
　use in neonates, 247
Narcosis, chloroform, historic introduction of, 3
National Library of Medicine, video applications references, 78
National Television Standards Committee (NTSC), encoding standards of, 80
Natural-cycle ART, 288
Natural killer (NK) cells, in patients with endometriosis, 200
Necrosis, with fulguration, depth of, 63
Needle drivers, 274
　Cook endoscopic curved, 34, 34f
　Szabo-Berci, 35, 35f
Needle holders
　Levine, 35, 35f
　for suturing, 34
　Wisap, 35
Needles
　Endo-Judge, 40
　Greis style, 39
　J-needle, for incision closure, 39–40

　microdiathermy, 279
　Veress, 24–25, 25f, 381
Negligence
　due to lack of informed consent, 447–448
　principles of, 450–451
　purpose of, 449
　responsibility for defective products or maintenance, 454
　sources of, 451
Neisseria gonorrhoea, 216–217
　culture for, infertility assessment, 288
Neodymium-yttrium-aluminum garnet (Nd-YAG) laser, 45
　advantages of, 50
　with air-cooled tips, FDA warning on use of, 387
　for dividing the uterine septum, 332
　for endometrial ablation, 321, 338–339, 348, 352
　for managing submucous leiomyomas, 327
　for ovarian drilling, 112
　for repeating endometrial ablation, 356
　for vaporization of endometriosis, 206–207
Neoplasms, benign, oophorectomy for, 104
Neosalpingostomy
　outcome of, 280, 399, 401
　teaching the procedure, 427
Neovagina, creating, 307
Neural tube defects, association with hyperthermia, 483
Nezhat-Dorsey system, 36
　irrigator pump, 27
Nissen fundoplication, 466f
　pediatric, 266–268
Nitrous oxide
　contraindication for, in laparoscopic pelvic lymph node dissection, 231–235
　discontinuing, in suspected gas embolism, 365
　for general anesthesia during pregnancy, 247
　for peritoneal insufflation hypoxia attributed to, 362–363
　in pregnancy, 248
Nizatidine (Axid), premedication with, 368
Nonstandard treatment, care in using, to avoid risk of malpractice, 452
Nonsteroidal antiinflammatory drugs (NSAIDs), 397
　for pain after endometrial ablation, 353, 356

Index

Noose knot, securing a continuous suture using, 95f
Normal saline, for uterine distention, 322, 332
Noxythiolin, for irrigating the peritoneal cavity, 220

Obesity, and choice of anesthetic, 366
Objective representation, 73
Objectives
   in anti-incontinent surgery, 144
   in formal training for operative endoscopy, 423–427
   in hysterectomy, 116
Observation, components of, 73
Obstruction, atheromatous, drilling, 474
Obturator hernia, 309
Obturator lymph node dissection, 233
Ohm's law, 60
Oligohydramnios
   protocols to manage, 480
   in the sac of one of monochorionic twins, 486
Omentum, sealing a perforated ulcer with, 467–468
Omeprazole, for controlling acid secretions, 466
Ondansetron (Zofran), premedication with, 372
One-loop technique, for appendectomy, 308
Oocytes
   donation of, 295–296
   evaluation of damage to, by method of surgery, 53–54
   quality of, and maternal age, 287
   retrieval of
      complications in, 299
      techniques for, 290
Oophorectomy, laparoscopic, 104–109
   workshop for teaching techniques, 433
Open laparoscopy technique, 28
   with direct placement of a trocar sleeve, 381
Open surgery, fetal, 477–478
Operating instruments, 29–40. *See also* Instrumentation
Operating room setup, for CISH, 133
Operating system, for delivery of laser energy, 46–47
Operative defect, management of, in laparoscopic myomectomy, 94–95
Operative fetoscopy, 478–479
   limitations of, 492
Operative Manual for Endoscopic Abdominal Surgery, 12

Operative techniques
   for adhesion prevention, 395–396
   for appendectomy during pregnancy, 250
   for correcting urinary incontinence, 146–147
   for ectopic pregnancy management, 165–170
   for endometrial ablation, 207–209, 349–352, 355–357
   for endoscopy, objectives in teaching, 425–426
   for hernia repair, 309–311
   for high McCall vaginal vault suspension, 151
   for hysteroscopy, 324
   laparoscopic
      for hysteroscopy, 324
      intestinal complications in, 384–385
      for pelvic abscess surgery, 222, 223–224
      steps in CISH, 134–136
      for laparoscopic-assisted hysterectomy, 121–124
      for laparoscopic cholecystectomy, 252
      for laparoscopic myomectomy, 92–97
      for laparoscopic pelvic lymph node dissection, 231–235
      for laparoscopic sacrospinosus vaginal vault suspension, 151–152
      for oophorectomy, 106–109
      for ovarian drilling, 113
   See also Laparoscopic hysterectomy (LH); Laparoscopic pelvic lymph node dissection (LPLND); Laparoscopic-assisted vaginal hysterectomy (LAVH)
Optical cavity, laser, 46
Optical disk, for archiving documentation, 84–85
Optic instruments, 26–27
   for hysteroscopy, 316
Orange-peel technique, in removing myomas, 96–97, 96f
Organizing pouch, for endoscopy instruments, 418
Osram light sources (mercury vapor), for endoscopy, 76
Outcome
   of excision of endometriosis, 211
   of historic treatments of pelvic abscess, 218–219
   after hysteroscopic treatment of uterine septa, 332

   of laparoscopic pelvic lymph node dissection, 235–239
   of neosalpingostomy, 399, 401
   reproductive
      after persistent ectopic therapy, 172
      with uterine septa, 328
   of treatment of intrauterine adhesions
      hysteroscopic, 334
      resectoscopic, 334
   of tubal surgery, 279–283
   of tubocornual anastomosis, 281–282
   of twin-twin transfusion syndrome, 487
   See also Morbidity; Mortality
Outpatient discharge, information given at the time of, 374
Outpatient surgery, laparoscopy for, 375–376
Ovarian hyperstimulation syndrome (OHSS), 298
Ovarian pregnancy, 176
Ovarian reserve, 285
Ovarian response
   and success rate for in vitro fertilization, 289
   stimulation of, for in vitro fertilization, 288–290
   suppression of, for treating endometriosis, 204–205
Ovarian surgery, 104–114
   drilling, teaching about, 427
   outcomes of, comparison of methods, 52–54
   wedge resection, teaching about, 427
   workshop for teaching techniques, 433
Ovary, cysts of, 109–112
   identification of, during laparoscopic myomectomy, 97
   management of, during laparoscopic myomectomy, 92
Ovary syndrome, palpable, indication for oophorectomy, 104
Ovulation induction, for in vitro fertilization, 289
Oxybutynin (Ditropan), for treating detrusor instability, 148
Oxygenation
   during surgery
      in gas embolism, 365
      special considerations in pregnancy, 243
   of tissues, effect on fibrinolysis, 393

Pain
  abdominal wall, differential diagnosis of, 309
  and adhesion formation, 394–395
  with endometriosis, 202–203
    diagnostic, 203
    outcome of surgery for, 211
  localization of, in appendicitis during pregnancy, 249
  muscle, after intubation, 365
  postoperative, indication of delayed damage, 386
  uterine, alleviation of during pregnancy, 249
Palmer, Raoul, 7
Pancuronium bromide, as a diagnostic tool, twin-twin syndrome, 486
Paracervical block, 356
  protection against bradycardia by, 364
Paravaginal suspension, 144
Partial zona dissection (PZD), 293
Patch repair, of hernia, 310
Pathogenesis, of ovarian hyperstimulation syndrome, 298
Pathology report, for validation of endometriosis surgery, 207
Pathophysiology
  of pelvic abscess, 221–222
  of pelvic inflammatory disease, 216–217
Patient selection
  for general anesthesia, 366–367
  for laparoscopic pelvic lymph node dissection, 228–229
  for in vitro fertilization, 288
Pediatric laparoscopy, 257–268, 503
Pedunculated myomas, disengaging, 92
Peer review
  evaluation for surgical proficiency by, 439
  in hospitals, to maintain competence, 453
Pelvic abscess
  defined, 216
  laparoscopic treatment of, 215–226
Pelvic floor defects
  evaluating prior to surgery for stress incontinence, 145
  managing during retropubic colposuspension surgery, 149
  surgery for, 142
Pelvic inflammatory disease (PID), 182
  chronic, oophorectomy for, 104
  defined, 216
  infertility following, 278–279
  prevalence of, 215
  and risk of infection in oocyte retrieval, 299
Pelvic lymph node dissection, laparoscopic, for staging urogenital malignancy, 228–239
Pelvic mass, objectives in teaching about, 427
Pelviscopic intrafascial hysterectomy, 128–141
Pelviscopy, 3
  development of, 7
Pelviscopy and Hysteroscopy, 12
Pelvi-Trainer, 9, 428
  exercises to be performed on, 432, 438
Penicillin, discovery of, 3
Percutaneous drainage, of pelvic abscesses, 220
Percutaneous fetal cytoscopy, to evaluate lower urinary tract obstruction, 490
Perforation
  of the appendix, 249–250
    fetal morbidity and mortality following, 250
  of the bladder
    during hysteroscopy, 388
    during secondary trocar placement, 385–386
  uterine
    in endometrial ablation, 355
    preventing complications of, 388
Peritoneal cavity
  examination of, at laparoscopic ovarian surgery, 106
  overpressurization of, complications of, 25
Peritoneoscope, for tubal sterilization, 7
Peritoneum, regeneration after excision of endometriosis, 209
Peritonitis
  gentamicin, clindamycin and metronidazole before surgery, 244
  septic complications of, 222
Personnel
  hospital, qualifications of, 453
  operating room, 412–421
  selecting for competence, to avoid risk of malpractice, 452
Pfannenstiel incision, 193–195, 307
pH, arterial, change during carbon dioxide insufflation, 362
Phase alternation by line (PAL), standard for video encoding, 80
Phenothiazines, premedication with, 368
Phillips, Jordan, 8, 12
Phimosis, correction of, 185
Photoendoscope, 5, 6f
Photography
  for documentation of operative endoscopy, 74
  nonsilver, 72
  recording with, 77
Photon emission, 44f
Physical properties, of lasers, 44–45
Physiologic spasm, tubal obstruction caused by, 336–338
Physiology
  changes in, during laparoscopy, 361–363
  maternal, 244–245
Pickwickian syndrome, 366
Pixels, of microprocessor chips, 79
Placenta, monochorionic, of twins, 485
Plasminogen activator, for preventing adhesion formation, 397
Pleural disease, thoracoscopy for assessing, 464
Pleural effusions, in utero treatment of, 477
Pleuroamniotic shunts, 476–477
Pneumoperitoneum, 3
  carbon dioxide, avoiding during pregnancy, 251
  for cholecystectomy, pediatric, 262
  establishing, 134
    in pediatric laparoscopy, 258
  guidelines for, early work, 7–8
  hypotension with, 364
  for pediatric laparoscopic appendectomy, 260
  physiologic effects of, 362–363
Pneumothorax, during controlled ventilation, 365
Polarized glasses, for viewing three-dimensional images, 27
Polycystic ovarian disease (PCOD), 112–113
  laparoscopic laser versus electrocautery for, 399
Polycystic ovary syndrome (PCOS), risk of cycle cancellation in, 290
Polyhydramnios
  association with chorioangioma, 490
  in the sac of one of monochorionic twin, 486
Polyps, endometrial, removal of, 325–328
Polyspermic embryos, in assisted fertilization, 293
Positioning of the patient, 22–24, 121
  for appendectomy, pediatric, 260

for bladder neck suspension, 146–147
for CISH, 133, 134–135
for creation of a neovagina, 307
for diagnostic endoscopy during pregnancy, 245–246
for distal tubal reconstructive surgery, 184
for ectopic pregnancy management, 165
for embryo transfer, 291
at the end of surgery for ruptured appendicitis, 261
and hemodynamic status, 364–365
for inguinal herniorrhaphy, pediatric, 264–265
for laparoscopic surgery, in pelvic abscess, 223
for Nissen fundoplication, 266–267
for oophorectomy, 106
for operative hysteroscopy, 324
physiologic changes due to, 361–362
for rectocele and enterocele repair, 149–150
safety considerations, 374–375
for transperitoneal laparoscopic pelvic lymph node dissection, 232
Posterior compartment defects, 143
Postoperative care
in endometrial ablation, 353
in laparoscopic retropubic colposuspension, 147–148
in laparoscopic surgery for pelvic abscess, 224–225
in laparoscopy, 420–421
Postoperative complications, in operative endoscopy, teaching about, 425
Postoperative hernia, 309
Potassium titanyl phosphate (KTP-532) laser, 45, 50
for dividing uterine septa, 332
for managing submucous leiomyomas, 327
for vaporization of endometriosis, 206–207
Power
accidental transfer of in laparoscopic electrosurgery, 67–70
delivery of, by lasers, 44–45
for electrosurgery, 60
Power density
for desiccation, electrosurgical, 64
of electrosurgical instruments, 60
for excising endometriosis, 207
of lasers, 45
Preceptorship, for learning skills for operative endoscopy, 438

Preeclampsia, prothrombin time in, 244
Preferred Provider Organizations (PPOs), 453
Pregnancy
abnormal, sonographic evaluation of, 406
diagnosis and treatment of ovarian tumors during, 105
ectopic, 153–177
as etiology of ovarian torsion, 113–114
after endometrial ablation, 389
endoscopic surgical procedures, 241–253
loss rate associated with transabdominal fetoscopy, 482–483
ovarian, 176
Pregnancy rate
after adhesiolysis, 395
with tuboovarian reconstruction, 55–56
after cefotaxime treatment for pelvic abscess, 219
after colpotomy drainage of pelvic abscess, 220
comparison of laparoscopy and laparotomy, 399
cumulative, in assisted reproduction, 283–288
from frozen embryos transfer, 291–292
in gamete intrafallopian transfer, 292
after hysteroscopic treatment of uterine septa, 332
after laparoscopic fimbrioplasty, 185–186
after laparoscopic treatment for pelvic abscess, 221
after laparoscopic tubal reanastomosis, 197
after microsurgical salpingoneostomy, 189
after microsurgical tubal reanastomosis, 195
after neosalpingostomy, 401
after oocyte donation, 295–296
after treatment for tubo-ovarian abscess or pelvic abscess, 219
after tubal cannulation, 337
in tubal embryo transfer, 292
after tubocornual anastomosis, 281
after in vitro fertilization, and number of embryos replaced, 290
Premedication, 367–368
dosages for adults undergoing gynecologic endoscopy, 367t
with regional anesthesia, 372–373

See also Medication/anesthesia
Premenstrual syndrome, response to endometrial ablation, 355
Preoperative assessment
for CISH, 133–134
didactic objectives for teaching, operative endoscopy, 424
for laparoscopic myomectomy, 90
for laparoscopic tubal reanastomosis, 192–193
of pelvic floor support, 143–144
skilled objectives for teaching, operative endoscopy, 424
for urinary incontinence correction, 145
See also Patient selection
Preoperative care
laparoscopic pelvic lymph node dissection, 230–231
pelvic abscess, 222–224
Preoperative responsibilities, of the endoscopy team, 412–417
Preparation, of the patient
for CISH, 131–132
for laparoscopic myomectomy, 91–92
Preperitoneal patch repair, with Dacron mesh, 310
Presacral neurectomy, teaching about, 427
Preterm labor, following surgery, management of, 248–249, 477
Prevalence
of endometriosis, 201–202
of infertility, 278–279
Prevention, of adhesions, 395–397
Priming principle, for muscle relaxant administration, 371
Probes, rectal and vaginal, 39
Prochlorperazine, for emesis during pregnancy, 248
Progesterone
effects of, on the gallbladder, 250–251
potential prevention of adhesion formation, 397
serum, for diagnosing ectopic pregnancy, 158, 162
treatment with, in vitro fertilization, 291
Prognosis
in distal tubal damage, 183–184
in ovarian malignancy, factors determining, 105
in surgical treatment of endometriosis, 205
Pronuclear stage tubal transfer (PROST), 292
Properidol, for emesis during pregnancy, 248–249

Prophylactic surgery
　oophorectomy, 104
　removal of the cervix during hysterectomy, 128
　salpingectomy, 283
Propofol (Diprivan), inducing anesthesia with, outpatient surgery, 369
Prostatectomy, radical retropubic, 236
Proximal tubal occlusion, 281
Prying technique, for myoma blunt dissection, 93
Pseudorectocele, identifying, 143
Psychomotor function, return of, after anesthesia, 374
Pubococcygeus muscle, 143
Pulmonary aspiration, during general anesthesia, mortality due to, 248
Pulmonary edema, risk of
　with fluids for distention, 354
　with high viscosity fluids for distention, 323, 387
Pulmonary embolus, 386
Pulmonary nodules, thoracoscopy for assessing, 463–464
Pulse energy delivery, laser, 46–47
Pulse oximetry, for monitoring during surgery, 374
Pumping system, laser, 45–46
Pursestring suture, in appendectomy, 309
Pyloric stenosis, pediatric, 266

Quality of life, hysterectomy to improve, 128–141
Quartz fiber, sculpted conical, for coagulation and cutting, 319f

Radiograph, chest, for preoperative evaluation of cholecystitis, 251
Ranitidine (Zantac)
　for controlling acid secretions, 466
　premedication with, 368
Raynaud's phenomenon, surgery for, 465
Reanastomosis, laparoscopy for, 195–197
Reasonable care, defining, 450
Recommendations, addressing potential malignancy, ovarian cystectomy, 109–110
Reconstructive surgery
　distal tubal, 182–190
　pelvic, use of lasers for, 51
　tubal, outcome of, 281
Recording media, sensitivity to illumination, 75

Record keeping
　to avoid risk of malpractice, 452–453
　institutional, 454
Recovery period, assessment during, 374
Recovery room nurse, postoperative responsibilities of, 420
Rectocele
　laparoscopic repair of, 149–150
　as a posterior compartment defect, 143
　repair of, at the time of bladder neck suspension, 146
Recurrence rate
　for endometriosis, after complete excision, 201, 202, 207
　for myomas, 100–101
Redundant arrays of independent disks (RAID), 85
Referral of patients, to avoid risk of malpractice, 452
Regional anesthesia, 371–373
Repeat pulse energy delivery, laser, 47
Reproductive outcome
　after persistent ectopic therapy, 172
　with uterine septa, 328
Reproductive technology, 278–300
Reproductive tract
　abnormalities of, transvaginal sonography for evaluating, 406
　argon laser for surgery, 50
　diseases of, 348
Research, using patients, special legal obligations, 456
Resecting loop, for removing leiomyomas, 326–327
Resection, of the bowel, following injury, 385
Resectoscope, 318–319
　for endometrial ablation, 339–341, 356
Resectoscopy, 315–343
　indication of perforation during, 388
　non-electrolyte fluids for uterine distention in, 323
　obturator for, 324
　for treating intrauterine adhesions, 334
Resistance, and temperature, in electrosurgery, 59
Resolution of a video system, 80
　chart representing, 81
Resonator cavity, laser, 46
Respiratory depression
　under local anesthesia, in premedicated patients, 363
　as a side effect of fentanyl, 370
Respondent superior concept, 454

Result. See Outcome
Resuscitation equipment, availability of, 375
Retropubic bladder neck suspension, teaching about, 427
Retropubic colposuspension, laparoscopic, 147–149
Retropubic urethropexy, 144
Return electrode, as a potential burn site, in electrosurgery, 65
Rh immune globulin, 244–245
Richter's hernia, 309
　complication of laparoscopic-assisted hysterectomy, 126
Ringer's lactate, for uterine distention, 322
Risk/benefit ratio, of in utero treatment of a fetus, 476
Risk factors
　for ectopic pregnancy, 282–283
　in intubation, 243
　for malignancy, evaluating with ultrasonography, 406
　for malpractice, 451–453
　for pelvic inflammatory disease, 215
Risks
　of cancer, with ovulation induction, 298–299
　of ectopic pregnancy, 156
　of electrosurgery, 65
　of hysterectomy, 338
　of laparoscopic surgery, 117
Roeder loop, 137f
　use in CISH, 133–136, 136f
Roller-ball/roller-bar electrodes, for endometrial ablation, 340, 348, 352–353, 356
Rupture, in an ectopic pregnancy, 173, 176

Sac, for extracting an appendix, 260–261
Sacral colpopexy, for vaginal vault prolapse, 150
Sacrococcygeal teratoma, 477
Sacrospinosus suspension, for vaginal vault prolapse, 150, 151
Safety
　of argon laser use, protective goggle requirement, 50
　considerations in positioning the patient, 374–375
　of electrosurgery, 65
　of fetoscopy, 482–483
　of gas-cooled laser tips, 387
　of hysteroscopic endometrial ablation, 501
　of insufflation, 24
　　pressure maintenance, 25–26

Index

of laser use, guidelines for, 413–414
Salpingectomy
  laparoscopic, 166–168
  outcomes of, 156, 282
  versus salpingotomy, 159–160
Salpingitis, 182
Salpingoneostomy, 187–189
Salpingo-oophorectomy, bilateral, for treating endometriosis, 210
Salpingoovariolysis, and fertility, 279
Salpingoplasty, 11
Salpingostomy, 11
  defined, 154
  hydrosalpinx, 280–281
  workshop on techniques for, 433
Salpingotomy
  defined, 153–154
  laparoscopic, 161, 168–170
  versus salpingectomy, 159–160
  versus segmental resection, in ectopic pregnancy, 160–161
Sampson's theory, of endometriosis, 199–201, 202
Sapphire tips, for Nd:YAG lasers, 321
Scalpel, damage to ovaries, compared with laser or microelectrode incisions, 53
Schiller test, 137, 137f
Scissors, 31
  Metzenbaum endoscopic, 260
Scoring system
  for adhesions, 395
  ultrasonographic, for ovarian malignancy, 106
  See also Classification
Scrub nurse
  intraoperative responsibilities of, 412, 419–420
  postoperative responsibilities of, 420
  preoperative responsibilities of, 417
Second-look laparoscopy
  for adhesiolysis, 99, 215
  for adhesions, 400–401
    formed after surgery, 396
  to evaluate adnexa after ovarian torsion, 114
  to evaluate surgical treatment of endometriosis, 205
  after laparoscopic treatment for pelvic abscess, 224
  at laparoscopy for ovarian suppression, 205
  after reproductive surgery, 189–190
Sectio parva, 485
Segmental resection in ectopic pregnancy, versus salpingotomy, 160–161
Seitzinger tripolar cutting forceps, 31

Semen analysis, before laparoscopic tubal reanastomosis, 192
Semm, Kurt, 463, 471
Semm spoon, 30f
Semm vacuum cannula, 23
Sensitivity, of microprocessor chips in video cameras, 76
Sequential couleur à mémoir (SECAM), encoding standard, 80
Seromyotomy, anterior, 467
Serrated edge macromorcellator (SEMM), 138
  development of, 130
Setup, preoperative, preparation of, 412–413
Sexually transmitted diseases, treating, 215
Sexual partners, of patients with pelvic inflammatory disease, treating with antibiotic, 225
Shears, coagulating, 33f
Sheaths
  disposable versus reusable, 27–28
  trocar, placement in oophorectomy, 107
Shifting agency, 454
Shoulder brace, for patient positioning, 24
Side effects
  of GnRH-a therapy, 91–92
  of midazolam, 368
  of muscle relaxants, 370–371
Signal-to-noise ratio (S/N ratio), and image quality, 80–81
Simplified laparoscopic abdominal morcellation (SLAM), 97
Simpson, James Y., 3
Simulators, computer-generated images for learning, 438
Site, of endometriosis, 203
Slides, color, storing, 82–83
Small intestine, laparoscopic repair of, 11
Society for Assisted Reproductive Technology (SART), reports of, 283–288
Sodium citrate (Bicitra), premedication with, 368
Sonography, for diagnosing twin-twin syndrome, 486, See also Doppler ultrasound; Ultrasonography
Sorbitol, for uterine distention, 322–323
  potential complications, 323
Sounding
  after endometrial ablation, 353, 356
  for identifying free space for a trocar, 134

Space of Retzius, visualization laparoscopically, 149, 234–235
Specimen bags, 38–39
Sphincter, urethral, functioning of, in urinary incontinence, 144
Sphincterotomy
  of the ampulla of Vater, 469
  during pregnancy, 252–253
Spinal anesthesia, 371–372
  agents for, 373
  and infertility treatment, 366
Splanchnoscopy, Italian reinvention of laparoscopy as, 5
Splenic cysts, pediatric, 265–266
Spontaneous abortion, and maternal age, in vitro fertilization, 287
Squamous cell carcinoma, of the urinary bladder, 229
Stable Access Cannula (SAC), 28
Staging
  of intraabdominal malignancy, color Doppler for, 409
  of urologic pelvic malignancy, 239
  See also Classification
Standard of care
  defined, 450
  establishing, 450–451
Staplers, automatic, learning to use, 433
Stapling, 36–37
  in appendectomy, 308
  pediatric laparoscopic, 260
  in laparoscopic-assisted hysterectomy, 123, 125
  for occlusion of an internal hernial ring, 310
  in oophorectomy, 107
Static imaging, 76–78
Step system, for inserting a sheath, 29
Sterility, tubal reconstruction for relieving, 3, 281–282
Sterilization
  laparoscopic
    early application, 6–7
    objectives in teaching about, 426
    minor's consent for, 455
    special consent for, to avoid risk of malpractice, 452
  tubal, 3
    with high frequency current, 11
    history of, 315
    hysteroscopy for, 341
Still photography
  for documentation of operative endoscopy, 74
  lighting for, 76
Storage, of videotapes and movies, 82–83
Storage register, in video imaging, 79
  Y/C output from, 80

Strict liability, for defective products, 454
Studies
  of hCG levels after laparoscopic laser salpingotomy, 170–171
  of laser surgery versus alternative methods, rabbit, 53
  of laser surgery versus electrosurgery, rabbit, 51–52, 54–55
  of myomectomy, 98t
  of total laparoscopic hysterectomy, 124–126
  See also Outcome
Subcutaneous emphysema, complication in laparoscopic myomectomy, 97
Subtotal hysterectomy, debate over, 128
Suburethral sling procedure, 144
Subzonal insertion (SZI) of spermatozoa, 293
Succinylcholine (Anectine), muscle relaxant for laparoscopy, 370
Suction irrigation devices, potential transfer of electrical energy to, 66–67
Suction system, support cart placement of, 132
Sufentanil (Sufenta), premedication with, 368
Superpulse energy delivery, laser, 47
  for distal tubal reconstructive surgery, 184
  versus ultrapulse energy delivery, 48
Support cart, 27
  equipment for CISH, 132
Support staff, hospital, 453–454
Surgery
  minimally invasive
    introduction of, 3
    laparoscopic-assisted vaginal hysterectomy (LAVH), 4
  thoracic, 463–465
  for treating of endometriosis, 205–210
  tubal, versus assisted reproductive technology, 278–300
Surgical assistant
  intraoperative responsibilities of, 417, 419
  postoperative responsibilities of, 420
Surgical techniques. See Operative techniques
Surgiport, device for holding cannula in place, 28
Suturing
  of a damaged bowel, 472
  endoscopic, in herniorrhaphy of the internal hernia ring, 310
  instruments for, 34–35
  laparoscopic
    in laparoscopic-assisted hysterectomy, 123
    techniques for, 270–277
  in oophorectomy, 107
  for reapproximation of the tubal lumen, 194
  teaching techniques
    models for, 429–430
    objectives for, 426
Sympathectomy, thoracoscopic approach to, 465
Symptomatology, of endometriosis, 202–203
Synechiae (intrauterine adhesions), 332–338
Szabo-Berci needle driver set, 35, 35f

Tachycardia, sinus, during laparoscopy, 363–364
Tait's law, 306
Teaching program
  for operative endoscopy, 423–432
  using patients in, 456
^{99m}Technetium iminodiacetic acid, for gallbladder scans during pregnancy, 251
Technician, responsibility for postoperative handling of endoscopy instruments, 420
Techniques
  for administering anesthesia, 368–371
  distal tubal reconstructive surgery, 184–185
  for tubal reanastomosis, 193–195
  See also Operative techniques
Technology, reproductive, 278–300
Telescope, of the hysteroscope, 315
Temperature
  in acute appendicitis, 249
  during electrosurgery, 59–60
  monitoring the patient's, intraoperatively, 375
Temporary privileges, model for training to acquire, peripheral angioplasty, 437
Teratogenic effect, of light or heat, in fetoscopy, 483
Teratomas, benign
  cystectomy for, 110
  oophorectomy for, 104
Terbutaline, brief use of, in pregnancy, 248
Tetracaine (Pontocaine), 373
Tetracycline
  with laparoscopic treatment for pelvic abscess, 220
  treatment with, after oocyte retrieval for in vitro fertilization, 290
Therapeutic privilege, for withholding information from a patient, 445
Thermal injury
  laser surgery versus electrosurgery, 52
  from Nd-YAG lasers, 50, 55
  to the ureter, 386
Thiopental, 369
Third-look laparoscopy, 400–401
Thoracic surgery, 463–465
Thoracoscopy, 463–465
Thrombosis, of the umbilical cord of an acardiac twin, 485
Time, and effects of electrosurgery on tissues, 60
Tissue barriers, for minimizing formation of adhesions, 96
Tissue effects
  of lasers, as a function of power density, 45
  models for teaching about energy sources, 431
Titanium, for stapling clips, 36–37
Tocolysis, consideration in pregnancy at 24 weeks gestation, 243
Tompkins procedure, 328
Torsion, ovarian, 113–114
Total laparoscopic hysterectomy (TLH)
  defined, 119, 119f
  evaluation of, 124–126
Total uterine mucosal ablation (TUMA), 14, 15f
Toxicity, of regional anesthesia, 372
Toxic materials, glycine, to the central nervous system, 323
Training
  formal, in gynecologic endoscopy, 442–443
  in laser use, 414
  preceptorship for, 440
  specialized, 437
  in specific procedures, to avoid malpractice, 451–452
Transabdominal preperitoneal hernia repair, 465–466
Transabdominal ultrasonography, 405
Transfusions, fetal, for chorioangiomas, 491
Transperitoneal laparoscopic pelvic lymph node dissection, 231–233
Transvaginal ultrasonography, 405–408
Trauma, ultrasound evaluation of, 405
Traumatic grasping instruments, 29–30
Treatment
  for ectopic pregnancy

Index

laparoscopic versus nonsurgical, 159–161
selection of, 161–164
of endometriosis, 204–210
of pelvic inflammatory disease, 216t
Trendelenberg position, instrumentation for supporting the patient in, 24
Trendelenburg position, cardiovascular changes associated with, 364
Triangle of Calot, 263f
Trocars
blunt, laparoscopy using, 28
for CISH, 132–133
inserting, 134
disposable versus reusable, 27–28
Endopath TriStar, 28f
for entering the amniotic cavity, 480
umbilical, placing, 381
Trocar sleeves, metal, to reduce capacitance coupling, 385
Tubal architecture, hysterosalpingography for evaluating, 342
Tubal cannulation, hysteroscopic, 336–338
Tubal embryo transfer (TET), 292
Tubal patency, hysterosalpingography for evaluating, 342
Tubal pregnancy
conservative management of, 11
models for teaching about, 430–431
Tubal reanastomosis
comparison of microsurgical techniques, 197t
laparoscopic, 192–197
minilaparotomy for, 195
Tubal rupture, in ectopic pregnancy, 165–166
Tubal surgery versus assisted reproductive technology, 278–300
Tubocornual anastomosis, 281–282
Tuboovarian abscess
infertility following, 279
laparoscopic treatment of, 215–226
Tuboovarian complex, defined, 216
Tumores Praeter Naturam (Aranzi), 4
Tumors
malignant, markers for, 105
vascularity of, color Doppler evaluation of, 408
See also Carcinoma; Cysts; Malignancy
Twin reverse arterial perfusion (TRAP), 483–485
Twin-twin transfusion syndrome, 479, 485–487

Ulcer surgery, 467

Ultrapulse energy delivery versus superpulse energy delivery, laser, 48
Ultrasonography
adjunct to operative hysteroscopy, 341
algorithm for managing fetal lower obstructive uropathy, 489
for confirmation
of leiomyomas, 90
of pelvic inflammatory disease, 218
for diagnosis
of cholelithiasis, 251
of chorioangiomas, 491
of ectopic pregnancy, 153, 157, 158
of obstructive uropathy, 488
fetal
for evaluation before surgery in pregnancy, 243
for guiding surgery, 481
versus fetoscopy, 478
to monitor in vitro fertilization, 295
pelvic, 404–409
transvaginal, 278
for evaluating ovarian cysts, 105–106
vaginal, for diagnosing ectopic pregnancy, 158
See also Doppler ultrasound
Umbilical cord ligation, 484f
Umbilical trocar, placing, 381
Ureteral injuries, 386
Urethra, cancer of, indication for laparoscopic pelvic lymph node dissection, 229–230
Urethral sphincter, functioning of, in urinary incontinence, 144
Urethrocele, as an anterior compartment defect, 143
Urinary bladder
cancer of, indication for laparoscopic pelvic lymph node dissection, 229
perforation of
during hysteroscopy, 388
during secondary trocar placement, 385–386
squamous cell carcinoma of, 229
suspension of, 142–152
Urinary incontinence
restorative surgery to correct, complications following, 142
treatment of, 144–147
Urinary retention, postoperative, 144
Urinary tract obstruction, fetal, animal model for treating, 479
Urogenital diaphragm, 143

Urologic malignancies, laparoscopic pelvic lymph node dissection for, 228–239
Uropathy, obstructive, fetal, 476, 477, 488–490
Uterine dehiscence, after laparoscopic excision of a myoma, 97
Uterine distention
complications associated with, 387
media for, 322–324, 387
as a source of complications, 342
in endometrial ablation, 351
treatment of intrauterine adhesions, 334
Uterine manipulator, 23–24, 90, 134
for distal tubal reconstructive surgery, 185
for ectopic pregnancy surgery, 165
for laparoscopic surgery in pelvic abscess, 223
for oophorectomy, 106
uterine sound as, 121
Uterine septa
hysterosalpingography for evaluating, 342
hysteroscopic treatment of, 328–332, 500–502
Uterosacral ligament
resection of, in treating endometriosis, 208
tenderness of, and diagnosis of endometriosis, 204
Uterosacrocardinal ligament complex, 150

Vaginal manipulator, 149
Vaginal prolapse, 142–152
Vaginal vault suspension, at the time of bladder neck suspension, 146
Vaginosis, bacterial, 217
Vagotomy
selective, 467
truncal, 467
with thoracoscopy, 464
Valtchev uterine mobilizer, 23
Vancaille ovarian forceps, 29f
Vancomycin, prior to surgery in pregnancy, 244
Vascular injuries, in operative endoscopy, objectives in teaching, 425
Vascular surgeon, to repair damage on insertion of instruments, 382
Vasopressin (Pitressin), 135
to control bleeding, 388
in endometrial ablation, 350, 355
injection in CISH, 137
injection in laparoscopic myomectomy, 92

Vasopressin (Pitressin)(*continued*)
   injection in laparoscopic salpingotomy, 169
Vasovagal reflex stimulation, and arrhythmias, during laparoscopy, 364
Vecchietti-Ardillo procedure, 307
Vecuronium (Norcuron), muscle relaxant for laparoscopy, 371
Ventilation, spontaneous versus controlled, during laparoscopy, 363
Ventricular arrhythmias, during laparoscopy, 363
Veress needle
   for pneumoperitoneum, 24–25, 25f
   placing, 381
Vesicoamniotic shunts, 476–477
Vesicocentesis, to evaluate fetal kidney status, 488
Vesicourethral suspension, to correct urinary incontinence, 144–145
Vicarious liability, 454
Videocamera
   for laparoscopic myomectomy, 90
   for pediatric laparoscopy, 258–259
Videocamera recorder (VCR), for training, 428
Video display, laparoscope specifications for, 26
Video films, for training, 438
Videography, for recording salpingoneostomy reconstruction, 189
Video imaging
   for documentation of operative endoscopy, 74, 79–82
   light source for, 75
Video monitoring
   benefits to the operating team, 82, 412
   in laparoscopic pelvic lymph node dissection, 231
   in operative hysteroscopy and resectoscopy, 320–321
Viscus, perforated, 241
Visiport, 29f
Visual documentation, 74–76
Visualization, for fetal surgery, 480
Voltage, and temperature during electrosurgery, 59

Waveform
   in bipolar desiccation, 64
   coagulation, 207
   electrosurgical, 60, 62
Wave guides, laser, 49, 184
Wire loop. *See* Loop electrode
Wisap needle holder, 35
Workshop sessions, for teaching about operative laparoscopy, 432–433
Write-once-and-read-many (WORM) optical disks, 84
Written documentation, 73–74

Xenon lamps, 319
   for endoscopy, 76

YAG laser. *See* Neodymium-yttrium-aluminum garnet (Nd-YAG) laser
Y/C output, 80

Zona drilling, 293
Zygote intrafallopian transfer (ZIFT), 278, 292